RHINOPLASTY
PROBLEMS AND CONTROVERSIES
A Discussion with the Experts

Contributors

Daniel C. Baker, M.D.

Professor, Institute of Reconstructive Plastic Surgery, New York University School of Medicine; Attending Surgeon, Manhattan Eye, Ear and Throat Hospital, New York, New York

Thomas J. Baker, M.D.

Clinical Assistant Professor, Department of Plastic Surgery, University of Miami School of Medicine; Senior Attending Surgeon, Department of Plastic Surgery, Mercy Hospital, Miami, Florida

Walter E. Berman, M.D.

Clinical Professor, Department of Head and Neck Surgery, University of California, Los Angeles, Center for the Health Sciences, Los Angeles, California

Anthony R. Bull, M.D., F.R.C.S

Consultant Surgeon, The Royal National Throat, Nose, and Ear Hospital, Charing Cross Hospital Charing Cross Hospital Senior Lecturer, The Institute of Otolaryngology London University London, England

Harvey Caplan, M.D.

Associate Professor of Medicine, Department of Otolaryngology, McGill University; Chief, Department of Otolaryngology, Reddy Memorial Hospital, Montreal, Quebec, Canada

Eugene H. Courtiss, M.D.

Associate Clinical Professor, Department of Surgery, Harvard Medical School, Boston, Massachusetts; Chief of Plastic Surgery, Department of Plastic Surgery, Newton Wellesley Hospital, Newton Lower Falls, Massachusetts

Mark Gorney, M.D.

Associate Clinical Professor, Department of Plastic Surgery, Stanford University, Stanford, California; Chief of Plastic Surgery and Training Program Director, Division of Plastic and Reconstructive Surgery, St. Francis Memorial Hospital, San Francisco, California

Guy Jost, M.D.

Professeur au Collège de Médecine Des Hôpitaux de Paris; Chief of Plastic Surgery, Hôpital Lariboisière, Paris, France

Frank M. Kamer, M.D.

Associate Clinical Professor, Department of Head and Neck Surgery, University of California, Los Angeles, School of Medicine, Los Angeles, California

Eugene B. Kern, M.S., M.D.

Professor of Otolaryngology, Department of Otorhinolaryngology, Mayo Medical School, Rochester, Minnesota

Rodolphe Meyer, M.D.

Professeur-Adjoint à l'Université de Lausanne; Médicin-Adjoint, Chirurgien-Plasticien à l'Hôpital Cantonal, Lausanne, Switzerland

Wolfgang Mühlbauer, M.D.

Professor of Plastic Surgery, Medical Faculty, Technical University, Munich; Chief, Department of Plastic, Reconstructive and Hand Surgery, Burn Center, München-Bogenhausen, Munich, West Germany

Alvaro Olmedo, M.D.

Chief, Division of Surgery, Department of Surgery, Clinica Londres, Mexico, D.F., Mexico

Fernando Ortiz-Monasterio, M.D.

Professor of Plastic Surgery, Department of Surgery, Universidad Nacional Autonoma de México; Chief of the Division of Plastic Surgery, Plastic and Reconstructive Surgery, Hospital General Manuel Gea González, México City, México

George C. Peck, M.D.

Clifton, New Jersey

Thomas D. Rees, M.D.

Clinical Professor of Plastic Surgery, New York
University School of Medicine; Chairman,
Department of Plastic Surgery, Manhattan Eye, Ear
and Throat Hospital; Attending Surgeon, New York
University-Bellevue Medical Center, New York, New
York

Jack H. Sheen, M.D.

Associate Clinical Professor, Department of Surgery,
Division of Plastic Surgery, University of California,
Los Angeles, Los Angeles, California

Nicolas Tabbal, M.D.

Clinical Instructor, Department of Plastic Surgery,
New York University; Assistant Attending Surgeon,
Department of Plastic Surgery, Manhattan, Eye, Ear
and Throat Hospital, New York, New York

M. Eugene Tardy, M.D.

Associate Professor and Director, Division of Head
and Neck Plastic Surgery, Department of
Otolaryngology, University of Illinois School of
Medicine, Chicago, Illinois

Claus Walter, M.D.

Professor, Department of Hals-Nasen-Ohrenklinik,
Universität Bonn, West Germany; Head, Abteilung
für Plastische Chirurgie und Hals-Nasen-
Ohrenkrankheiten Klinik am Rosenberg, CH-9410
Heiden, Switzerland; Clinical Professor, Department
of Otolaryngology, University of Texas, Health
Science Center, San Antonio, Texas

Preface

For many years, the Department of Plastic Surgery at the Manhattan Eye, Ear and Throat Hospital, in conjunction with the Institute for Reconstructive Plastic Surgery at New York University, has sponsored symposia each fall in New York City. Every other year the subject has been rhinoplasty—a subject whose popularity is reflected by the overflow registration at each meeting. These symposia are also of special note because they bring together otolaryngologists and plastic surgeons and allow the intermingling of these diverse specialties in a fascinatingly complementary manner. The participants have the opportunity to exchange information and, we hope, gain mutual enhancement.

This unique volume represents the results of some especially stimulating discussions at these meetings. The contributors are world-renowned authorities on the art of rhinoplasty from the disciplines of plastic surgery and otolaryngology. The chapters herein reflect an interdisciplinary exchange, particularly the Point & Counterpoint sections, where dialogue is often spirited and controversial issues are highlighted, including the varying points of view regarding technical approach and philosophy of each contributor. It is my hope that the reader will enjoy and learn from the differences that emerge from the controversies presented here.

For those of us who perform rhinoplasty frequently, it is comforting to confirm our suspicion that the rules are not cut and dried, and that there is still plenty of room for individual differences of opinion not only in the philosophical approach to rhinoplasty, but also in the planning and technical execution of the operation as well. There are also alternatives, wherein lies much of the true value of a book such as this, for no one surgeon can have at his command all of the variations or "tricks" that might be useful when confronted by the varying technical problems that can be encountered during the course of rhinoplasty. Reading about these options and how they are exercised in the hands of experts can only add to the armamentarium of the reader.

None of us knows all of the answers to rhinoplasty, and each of us who is deeply interested in the subject welcomes any expansion of our knowledge that widens our surgical horizons. It is our hope that this presentation will be useful in providing the reader with some different points of view that will eventually be useful in problem solving.

There is repetition throughout the book; however, repetition is to some extent inevitable because each chapter represents the viewpoint of an individual surgeon regarding a particular problem as stated in the title of the part. For example, Part I, Tip Projection, comprises five approaches to this area and, necessarily, each surgeon is allowed to fully describe his technique, regardless of overlap. I have tried to limit repetition as much as possible; what remains, I feel, is necessary to give the reader a complete presentation.

Thomas D. Rees

Acknowledgements

We are grateful to the individual faculty members of these rhinoplasty symposia for their patience and forbearance in polishing their spoken words into written ones for this book. The original concept to produce this volume and much of the planning was shared between Ms. Karen Berger and the senior editor. Ms. Berger moved on to other publishing endeavors during production of the manuscripts; however, her tasks were ably taken up by Ms. Elaine Steinborn, Ms. Eugenia Klein, and Ms. Laurel Fuller.

We impart particular thanks to Ms. Karola Noetel for her patience and hard work in coordinating all of these efforts between publisher, authors, and editors, especially in the early months of preparing the manuscripts.

Thanks also to Mrs. Francine Leinhartt, who worked ceaselessly on these symposia as an organizer and general secretary.

Thomas D. Rees
Daniel C. Baker
Nicolas Tabbal

Contents

1

Patient Selection and Medicolegal Responsibility for the Rhinoplasty Patient

Mark Gorney

The desire to appear normal or aesthetically pleasing is older than plastic surgery. The puritan ethic that has, until recently, dominated our culture and disapproved of narcissism is rapidly breaking down. The growing popularity of rhinoplastic surgery has, unfortunately, created in our country a carnival-like atmosphere of which advertising by unqualified practitioners is only one aspect. In this climate it becomes imperative to establish clear criteria for patient selection; without these, there will be an inevitable parallel increase in patient dissatisfaction and litigation.

Who, then, is the "ideal" candidate for rhinoplasty? There is no such thing; however, the surgeon should certainly seek those personality factors that will enhance the physical improvements desired. There are, in most cases, clear indications of who will do well and enjoy the results. A person who is obviously intelligent, preferably educated, and who listens (rather than merely hearing) and clearly understands the pros and cons of what is sought is a good candidate. Individuals who have a clearly discernible physical problem about which they have an understandable but not neurotic concern are good candidates.

Persons whose jobs require them to look attractive or who must compete with younger people are probably good candidates. Someone, with a sense of humor is always a better candidate than a dour, anxious individual. Rinoplasty patients are in a category by themselves and should be evaluated with the utmost care. Generally speaking, men make more

difficult patients than women. They do not tolerate pain as well and are generally more fussy.

There are basically two major categories for rejection of a patient seeking rhinoplasty. One is anatomical unsuitability; the other is emotional inadequacy.[1] Of these, emotional inadequacy is by far the more important. It is reviewed here on a purely pragmatic basis. The inexperienced surgeon must learn early to differentiate between healthy and unhealthy reasons for seeking aesthetic improvement. It becomes absolutely critical to develop a sixth sense regarding motivation because a substantial number of poor results are based on emotional dissatisfaction rather than technical failure.

In our civilization, there is still a certain stigma attached to seeking aesthetic improvement. This may add a significant element of guilt to a preexisting distorted body image. Jacobson and others[2] neatly liken the body image to a gyroscope. When it is functioning well, we do not notice it. It does not decide the course or steer the ship. In a storm, however, the ship becomes difficult to steer if the gyroscope is not functioning.

The concept of body image is a familiar one to most plastic surgeons but not to lay people. It can be easily explained to the patient by using the following analogy: when one thinks of oneself in the third person, in dreams or fantasies, one tends to think of the best period in one's life—age 20 or 30, for example. With advancing age, the image in the mind stands in sharp contrast to the image in the mirror. The greater the disparity between these two

1

images, the more likely it is to disrupt functioning in one's peer group.

Obviously, every patient seeking rhinoplasty cannot be referred for a psychiatric evaluation, nor is it necessary. Patients seeking plastic surgery believe that they are trying to do something positive about their problems. If they are asked to see a psychiatrist, they might consider themselves failures. It is seldom that patients have sufficient self-awareness to realize that their problems lie more in their minds than in the physical parts they wish corrected.

There are no objective criteria in this gray zone. The criteria are not only subjective, but also totally different for patient and physician. The patient has an idea of what he or she wants; the surgeon knows, more or less, what can be done. The problem is for the two to communicate as accurately as possible beforehand. It is much easier to arrive at a prior mutual understanding than to look back with regret in retrospect.

Obviously, there is a significant difference in the psychodynamics of the male versus the female rhinoplasty patient. Jacobson and others[2] have pointed out that both sexes have positive psychological expectations and a conscious wish for attractiveness; women, however, more frequently wish to change themselves to feel more attractive whereas men seem more interested in changing others' attitudes toward them.[2,3] The male patient, according to Jacobson and others[2], more often than the female patient has the following:

1. A family or cultural background conflicting with his present life
2. Difficulties in heterosexual adjustment
3. A self-deprecating attitude and feelings of inadequacy
4. Familial conflict and either conscious or subconscious shame related to ethnic background

The characteristics of the individual least likely to be satisfied with his postoperative result can be formed into a useful acronym—*SIMON:*

> *Single*
> *Immature*
> *Male*
> *Overexpectant*
> *Narcissistic*

There are often identifiable, common traits in certain types of aesthetic surgery candidates. Patients with outstanding or "lop" ears often demonstrate a hostile, aggressive, "chip on the shoulder" attitude. Most often, they have inherited this deformity from a parent who also suffered ridicule in childhood. Patients seeking rhinoplasty, on the other hand, frequently show a guilt-tinged, second-generation rejection of their ethnic background masked by excuses, such as not photographing well. Often it is not so much a desire to abandon the ethnic group as it is to be viewed as individuals and to rid themselves of specific physical attributes associated with their particular ethnic group.[2,4,5,6]

Motivation, rather than specific psychodynamics, should be the plastic surgeon's overriding concern. Is there a pragmatic desire to improve appearance, or is there a pathological projection of subconscious problems onto a physical fault? Contrast these two commonly heard statements:

- I don't like my nose. It's too big for my face and I don't photograph well.
- I've always been terribly self-conscious about my nose. My father's family all have noses like this. I hate it!

Many patients can say anything convincingly, but the second statement should trip a red flag and invite further inquiries into the patient's real motivation.

Strength of motivation is important and has a startlingly close relationship with patient satisfaction. A strongly motivated patient will have less pain, a better postoperative course, and a significantly higher index of satisfaction—regardless of the result.

PATIENT SELECTION AND LIABILITY POTENTIAL

Despite all this, it is possible to establish some nearly objective criteria for patient selection and liability potential in order of descending importance.

Objective deformity versus patient concern

Figure 1-1 shows graphically a plot of the patient's objective deformity as judged by the surgeon versus the patient's degree of concern about the deformity. Two extremes of patient selection are as follows:

1. The patient who has a major deformity but demonstrates minimal concern (lower right-hand corner)
2. The patient who has a minor deformity that causes extreme concern (upper right-hand corner)

The latter represents the poorest candidate. One seldom sees the patient in the lower right-hand corner, but the majority of patients seeking aesthetic surgery fall somewhere on a diagonal band between the contralateral corners. The decision to accept or reject a

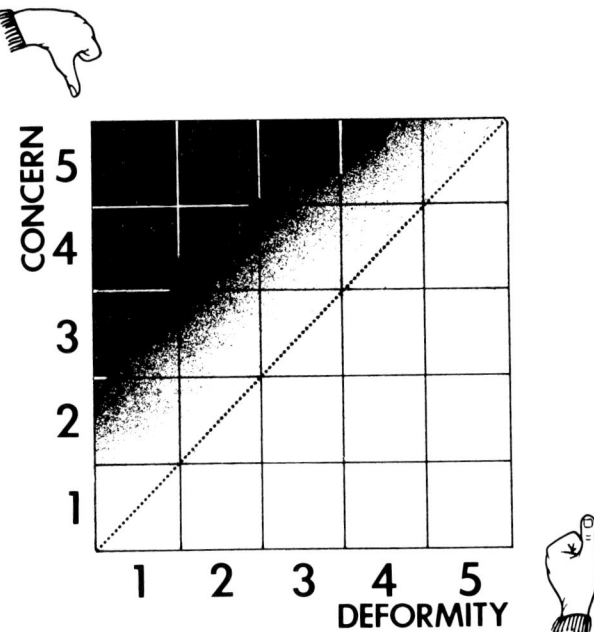

Figure 1-1. "Gorney gram." There is a close relationship between final outcome of any elective procedure and the patient's "concern ratio." The greater the patient's preoccupation with his or her problem, the less satisfactory the final outcome, even if the problem is minimal in the surgeon's objective evaluation. The opposite is also true. Most patients fall in a broad band indicated by the diagonal line.

patient for surgery must be the surgeon's ultimate responsibility. I have found it very useful to note, sometime during the initial visit, on a "tic-tac-toe" type of diagram (see Figure 1-1) my coded impression of where the patient falls. Thus when a patient whom I dimly recall expresses interest in proceeding with the surgery, a glance at the chart with the X in the appropriate square serves as a reminder about this patient's candidacy.

Great expectations. Experience invariably teaches the plastic surgeon to avoid patients who expect surgery to change their whole lives. If the surgeon operates on someone who has a large, crooked nose and significant hang-ups, the result likely to be someone with a smaller, straighter nose and even greater hang-ups—or worse. Certainly, a reasonable degree of positive change is expected and usually occurs; however, aesthetic surgery, regardless of excellence, is dubious therapy for severe personality disturbances.

The demanding patient. The individual who brings pictures, drawings, and exact specifications should be suspect, as a general rule. Such a person

has little insight into the realities of reconstructive surgery and, by definition, forces the surgeon to attempt to fulfill expectations that cannot be realized. More than likely, this type of patient is very explicit, very fussy, and very demanding about tiny imperfections and will not understand the fact that the surgeon is working with human tissue, not clay.

The indecisive patient. We have already discussed the relationship between motivation and result. To the question: "Doctor, do you think I ought to have this done?" The correct answer is, "This is a decision that I cannot make for you. I can neither encourage nor discourage this operation. I can only tell you what I think we can accomplish. If you have thought about it carefully and feel strongly that you would like to have it done, you will probably be satisfied with the results. If you have any doubts at all, I strongly recommend that you think about it further or not have it done at all."

It is very difficult to dissuade a jury or an arbitration panel when one of the patient's principal claims is that he or she was "talked into" the surgery.

The immature patient. For reasons other than growth and development, one should carefully evaluate the degree of maturity in the young candidate. There is, of course, no linear relationship between maturity and age. Immature individuals often have excessively romantic and unrealistic expectations regarding the effects of the change. When confronted with a mirror postoperatively, they sometimes exhibit disconcerting shock reactions and alarming behavior. If they have been talked into the surgery by a relative or friend, this only compounds the problem.

The important patient. Beware of patients who make a conscious effort to impress others by their stature, profession, community standing, peer groups, and the like. Such individuals often suggest that a successful result on them will immediately bring on a flood of referrals and undying fame. They will also turn out to be very difficult patients who have weak egos and need constant shoring up. They are difficult to satisfy and tend to forget their financial obligations.

The secretive patient. Some applicants make a fetish of absolute secrecy about their surgery. Besides the fact that such arrangements are difficult to guarantee, exaggerated concern regarding this aspect of the operation indicates a certain degree of guilt about what they are about to do.

Familial disapproval. I prefer that the immediate family be in agreement with the proposed operation and often refuse to do it if they are not. Too often, failure to communicate or an unsatisfactory result produces an automatic "See, I told you so!" reaction. This only intensifies the patient's feelings of guilt and dissatisfaction, and the associated difficulties.

Failure to establish rapport. An experienced aesthetic surgeon can usually determine within minutes of entering the examining room whether the individual sitting in the chair will become a patient. Within moments of the opening conversation there are often discernible "bad vibes." One of the most significant mistakes in plastic surgery is to take on as a patient someone whom one truly dislikes. A clash of personalities cancels out all other factors, regardless of the "challenge" of the case.

The truly ugly patient. The patient whose deformity borders on the monstrous usually has grave mental or deep psychiatric problems. With the exception of persons who may be helped by the brilliant craniofacial surgery techniques of Tessier, such individuals are rarely candidates for aesthetic surgery in the traditional sense. Once again, the challenge may prove to be too much of a temptation, and, in the end, the surgeon winds up converting the truly grotesque into the simply ridiculous.

The "surgiholic." Beware of the patient who has had multiple or repeated aesthetic procedures. Such a patient obviously has a severe and probably incorrigibly distorted body image. Aside from the technical difficulties involved, you will suffer comparison to the other surgeons. If you are more successful, you may be harrassed by requests for "just one more, please."

AN OUNCE OF PREVENTION

There should be a frank discussion of fees and costs—if not by the surgeon, then by someone in the surgeon's office. Experience has shown that payment in full and in advance for cosmetic surgery tends to diminish subsequent unhappiness with the final results.

One of the most valuable and least expensive investments you can make is a chalkboard in every examining room. All illustrations and diagrams should be on the chalkboard and not on the permanent record. Unless you can exactly duplicate what you have drawn, a permanent record may come back to haunt you.

In counseling the patient, avoid the use of complex medical terminology. Use simple, understandable language and tailor your explanations to your impression of patient's capacity to understand. Do not make any promises—stated or implied. Do not patronize your patient but do encourage questions; an informed patient is a good patient.

I recommend that you not use "painful" language. Do not say "cut" or "chisel"; say "incise" and "remodel."

The "laying on of hands" is never more important than when talking to an anxious patient. Your reassuring touch during the course of the examination will often give the patient a subconscious impression of the kind of surgeon you are.

It is an ironclad rule in our office never to accept patients at the first visit. I ask them to go home, think about what I have told them, and return (at no fee). I ask them to write down any questions, and, at the second visit, I go over the highlights of our original conversation and cover, once again, the most significant complications that may occur. When I am convinced that the patients are well and truly motivated and understand clearly what I have told them, then, and only then, do I allow them to book the surgery.

At surgery, it is axiomatic that all patients under local anesthesia should be adequately sedated. No permit should be signed after sedation is administered, since it may be held to be invalid. All members of the surgical team should understand clearly that the patient, under the influence of narcotics, can misinterpret the most innocent words or jokes and that these can come back to haunt them. Under no circumstances should there be arguments of any kind, even in jest. There should be no swearing for any reason. Assistants and observers should be warned to save voicing their doubts for later. There is no such word as "oops" in the operating room, whether the surgeon drops a hemostat or comminutes the nasal bones. It helps to talk to the patient and be highly visible at the beginning and end of the procedure. It is extremely therapeutic to have music in the operating room if the surgery is being performed while the patient is under local anesthesia; it not only diffuses the unfamiliar and terrifying atmosphere, but also tends to cover up the sounds of the operating room, which of themselves are extremely anxiety producing.

The surgeon should always report to the family immediately after the operation. If they are not present, a telephone call may be the least expensive investment the surgeon could make. A visit on the evening of the operation is immensely reassuring to the patient. The surgeon should be the last person the patient sees before going under the anesthetic and the first face that the patient focuses on in the recovery room. Discharge instructions should be clear, specific, and in writing. Availability during the first few days is essential. If the surgeon signs out, it should be to someone equally competent, and the patient should be notified of this ahead of time.

When dressings come off, there will be innumerable questions, all of which require simple, reassuring answers. There will be fewer questions and the patient will be less anxious if these questions have been addressed preoperatively.

SUMMARY

Litigation and misunderstanding between patient and physician in plastic surgery have as a common denominator not poor results, but poor communication. Underlying all dissatisfaction is a failure to establish or maintain rapport between patient and surgeon. This vital relationship can be shattered by the surgeon's arrogance, hostility, or indifference (real or imagined), but especially by the patient's feeling that "the surgeon didn't care."

There are only two ways to avoid this debacle. One is to make sure the patient has no reason to feel this way. The other is to learn to avoid the patient who is going to feel this way no matter what is done.

REFERENCES

1. Gorney, M.: Psychiatric and medical-legal implications of rhinoplasty, mentoplasty, and otoplasty, Symposium of Aesthetic Surgery of the Nose, Ears, and Chin, vol. 6, 1973.
2. Jacobson, W.E., and others: Psychiatric evaluation of male patients seeking cosmetic surgery, Plast. Reconstr. Surg. **26:**356, 1960.
3. MacGregor, F.C., and Shaffner, B.: Screening patients for nasal plastic operations, Psychosom. Med. **12:**277, 1950.
4. Meyer, E., and others: Motivational patterns in patients seeking elective plastic surgery (women who seek rhinoplasty), Psychosom. Med. **22:**193, 1960.
5. Palmer, A., and Blanton, S.: Mental factors in relation to reconstructive surgery of nose and ears, Arch. Otolaryngol. **56:**148, 1952.
6. Stern, K., Fournier, G., and LaRiviere, A.: Psychiatric aspects of cosmetic surgery of the nose, Can. Med. J. **76:**469, 1957.

Point & Counterpoint

Question: How do you deal with teenagers?

Comment (Tom Rees): Although we all aesthetically agree on the importance of maintaining a high dorsal profile in noses, our practices differ significantly in geography and patient profile. Many of my patients are teenagers, 15- and 16-year-olds, and I find it difficult to talk a teenager into keeping a straight profile. They complain, "You didn't curve it enough." I say, "But aesthetically it looks wonderful and you are going to like it 10 years from now." They reply, "I don't care, doctor. I wanted a bit of a curve, like Mommie has. I don't want that retroussé look; I want a little curve." By following our established standards we sometimes impose our own feelings onto our patients, even if it will be appreciated later. I find this to be a problem.

When I discuss a rhinoplasty with adult patients and plan with them, I always ask the patient what he or she wants. I never start talking to the patient until I hear what he or she has to tell me because sometimes it is completely different from what I am thinking.

I ask all my patients, "What view of your nose bothers you the most? When you look in the mirror what don't you like?" About 90% of the time they complain about the bump on its profile. The tip may look like a cauliflower, yet my patients often say it does not even bother them from the front. I urge all rhinoplastic surgeons to listen to these patients, because even when you do a beautiful job on the tip, if the patient sees a little bump on the profile afterward, he or she will be unhappy, especially if the patient is a teenager. In adults we can leave a little bump and keep the profile high; this is usually well accepted. Teenagers, however, are different. They have their own desires and needs, and for me, sometimes it is a dilemma.

Question: How do you deal with teenagers?

Comment (Jack Sheen): First of all, I can't agree more with the idea of listening to the patient. I always listen and try to understand the patient's perception of his problems and desires regarding his nose. I will ask, "If you could have only one thing changed, what would it be?" I then ask for a detailed account of what the patient does not like about his nose. I write these points on the chart at the time of consultation and on the patient's photograph envelope, which goes with me to the operating room. Only after I have noted the patient's remarks do I begin my analysis and discussion of the problems.

Whether or not to have a retroussé look is a critical point with all patients, not only teenagers. Perhaps teenagers need a little more convincing. When the patients are of Mediterranean or Middle Eastern descent, I try to encourage them to accept a straight dorsum in line with the tip. I usually show comparative photographs: one with an absolutely straight dorsum and another with a straight but lower dorsum and a slightly projecting tip. I ask them to focus just on the relationship of the dorsum to the tip and to state which of the two they like better. If they strongly favor or dislike one or the other, I then have a definite idea of how to proceed. If, after I've offered my best arguments and opinions, a thick-skinned or Middle Eastern type of patient still insists that he prefers the retroussé nose, I will do it because I believe in satisfying the patient. I also know that if the patient has regrets later, I can simply raise the dorsum.

Question: How long do you spend in consultation?

Comment (Jack Sheen): I can spend as little as 10 minutes or as much as 1 hour or more in consultation. I see many secondary rhinoplasty patients who are usually extremely anxious and require much time and patience. I spend three consultative sessions with secondary rhinoplasty patients, but that is my limit. During these consultations, I discuss problems, pitfalls, surgical procedure, and realistic expectations. I think this is time well spent.

Question: If you decide you don't want to do a case, what do you say to the patients? Don't they beg you, and then ask why you are refusing? Don't they say, "You did my cousin or my uncle or my Aunt Sally? Why won't you do me?"

Comment (Jack Sheen): When I decide not to do a case, I tell the patient, in clear terms, that I do not feel that I could satisfy him, or that I could not achieve the kind of result that would justify a surgical procedure. I have learned to trust my instincts about certain patients, especially hostile patients.

For example, on one occasion I refused to operate on a patient referred by a colleague who later called me and all but insisted that I operate on her. Going against my own feelings about this patient, I relented and performed the secondary rhinoplasty. The problems from this case still plague me. First, she employed a team of attorneys to try to pressure me to indict the first surgeon, which I refused to do. Then, she refused to pay my fee and continued to haunt my office, bellowing complaints and accusations.

At times, it can be difficult to refuse a patient, but in the long run saying "No" at the outset is much easier than dealing with a patient's disappointment and hostility following surgery.

Comment (Harvey Caplan): I have had patients say, "Do you really think I should have my nose done?" I feel philosophically that at no point in aesthetic surgery should I get involved and say, "Yes, you need a rhinoplasty. I think you should have your nose done." If patients ask me, I ask them what they think is wrong with their nose. If they can tell me, then my obligation as an aesthetic surgeon is to explain whether it is feasible, in reality, to correct the defect.

A psychiatrist at the hospital where I work is quite interested in cosmetic surgery, and, because we participate in a national health program, it is not expensive for me to refer patients to this psychiatrist.

About 3 or 4 years ago we decided to send everybody to the psychiatrist. In reviewing 300 consecutive cases, he arrived at the following statistics: 76% of the patients he interviewed were frankly neurotic, obsessive, compulsive, and anxious. Yet after we did the surgery, 95.5% were satisfied. He warned me about psychotic patients, who make up 3% of our practice. The conclusion was that we shouldn't be afraid to operate on individuals who are psychoneurotic and have feelings of anxiety or compulsion, or maybe a certain degree of narcissism, but we should beware of the psychotic people, those who are probably a bit out of touch with reality.

I admit that I could not readily recognize psychotic individuals; the psychiatrist could. I think we should develop a system to determine who is frankly psychotic. One clear sign of a psychotic patient is the inability to look you in the face. These people look around the room, everywhere but at you. Another sign of psychosis is the nonblinking, expressionless, staring patient. I always refer patients with these characteristics to the psychiatrist.

PART

I

TIP PROJECTION

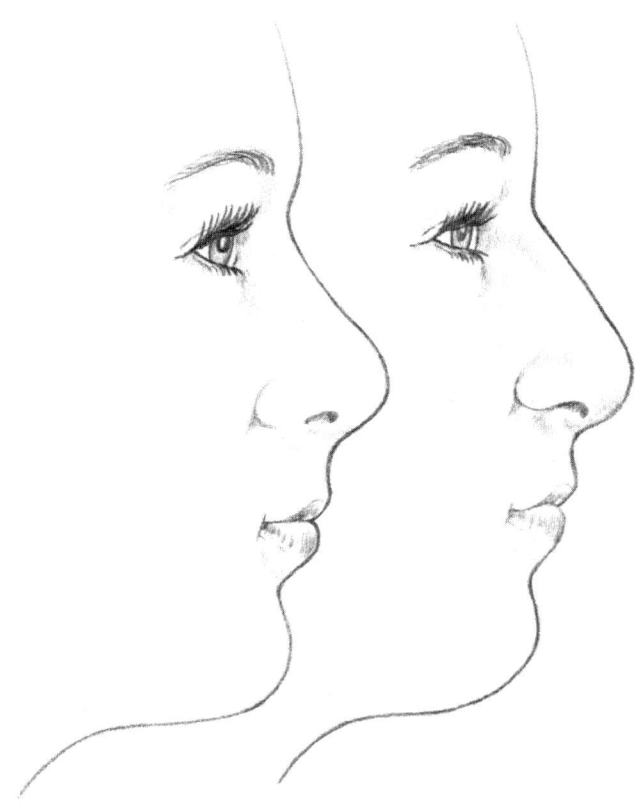

2

Nasal Tip Projection: Goals and Maintenance

George Peck

Nasal tip projection is one of the most important concepts in rhinoplasty. There are two basic components of nasal tip projection. Lobule tip projection is the subtle tip projection we all look for in our rhinoplasties with the nasal tip projecting gracefully from the straight line of the bridge. Septal support is the basic structural support of the nasal tip. When the nose lacks septal support, the entire nasal tip can collapse. This tip deformity can only be recon-structed with a strut type of graft. The following paragraphs address some of the problems with tip projection and suggest methods of solution.

LOBULE TIP PROJECTION

I initially saw the 34-year-old patient in Figure 2-1 in consultation for a primary rhinoplasty. Examination of the preoperative profile revealed a short nasal tip projection. At the time of the con-

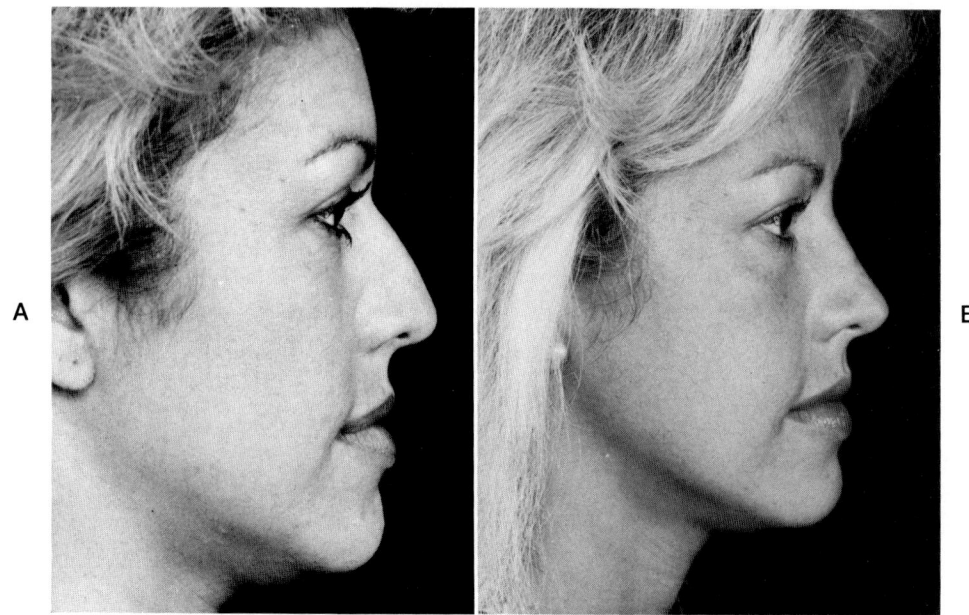

Figure 2-1. A is a preoperative view before secondary rhinoplasty associated with an onlay tip graft to improve tip projection. In this patient a standard correction would have been insufficient. A tip graft was necessary to complete the procedure. **B** shows the result.

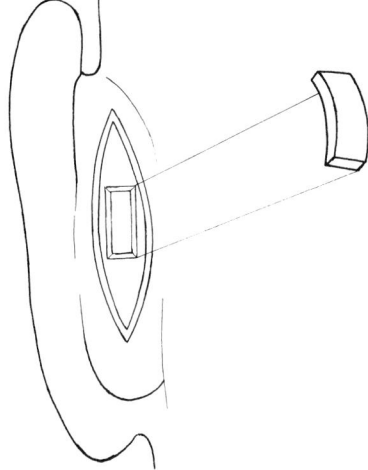

Figure 2-2. The conchal site of a typical cartilage graft from the posterior surface of the ear, useful in nasal tip reconstruction.

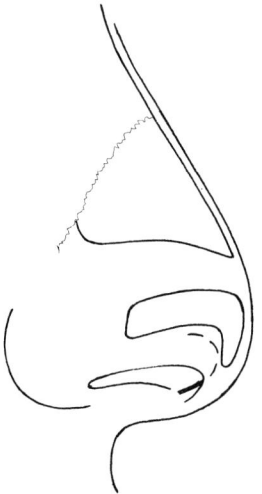

Figure 2-3. The dotted line represents the infracartilaginous incision, which aids in dissecting the tip pocket, especially for insertion of a graft.

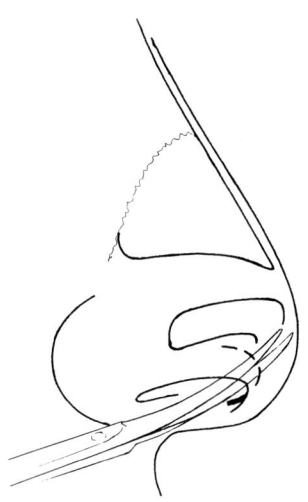

Figure 2-4. The dissection is carried out through the infracartilaginous incision.

sultation we must recognize this deformity and immediately consider augmentation. Conventional rhinoplastic techniques in this nasal tip will not produce the necessary projection.

My technique for solving this tip problem is to begin with an intracartilaginous incision in the lower lateral cartilage areas. This incision creates the sculpturing line in the nasal tip. The bilateral incision creates a gull-wing highlighting to the nasal tip. Then the cephalad portion of the lower lateral cartilage is removed, preserving all vestibular skin lining. In this particular patient the sculpturing of the lower lateral cartilages produced the necessary lines but did nothing to augment the nasal tip. Thus I recognized the need for enhancement of the subtle tip projection.

I prefer to use a cartilage graft taken from the auricular concha, although I have satisfactorily used cartilaginous hump and septum. Figure 2-2 shows the relative size and shape of the cartilage graft, which is usually 4 × 9 mm.

Figure 2-3 shows the infracartilaginous incision made in the dome of the lobule. In Figure 2-4 a pocket is dissected over the domes in a relatively virgin area, since the major portion of the intracartilaginous incision lies more cephalad. A rimming incision would skeletonize the entire nasal tip, making it impossible to create a pocket; therefore, I prefer an intracartilaginous incision.

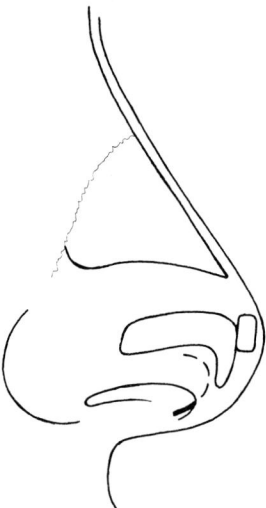

Figure 2-5. The placement of the tip graft is shown anterior to the alar cartilage rim.

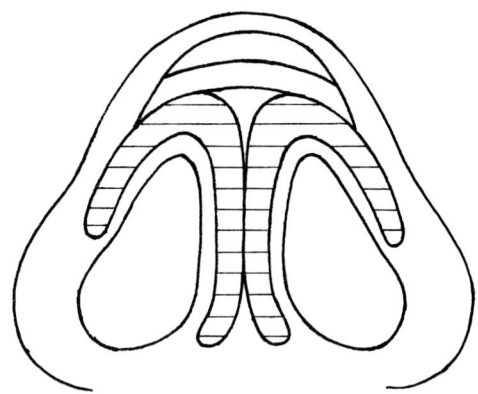

Figure 2-6. A two-layered graft may be required in some patients.

In Figure 2-5 the cartilage graft is placed in the pocket so it lies horizontally across the domes. Figure 2-6 shows a double graft, which may be used if necessary.

The cartilage graft is not under tension but is merely an onlay graft overlying the lower lateral cartilage domes. In essence, the thickness of the lower lateral cartilage is increased at the domes.

The complications I have seen with this type of graft are few. The graft must be placed horizontally to prevent crooked lines. In thin skin, the graft edges may show through.

Figure 2-7 offers preoperative and postoperative photographs that show the shape of the tip in smiling. There is no drooping of the nasal tip. Figure 2-8 shows the natural lines and highlighting achieved with the cartilage graft.

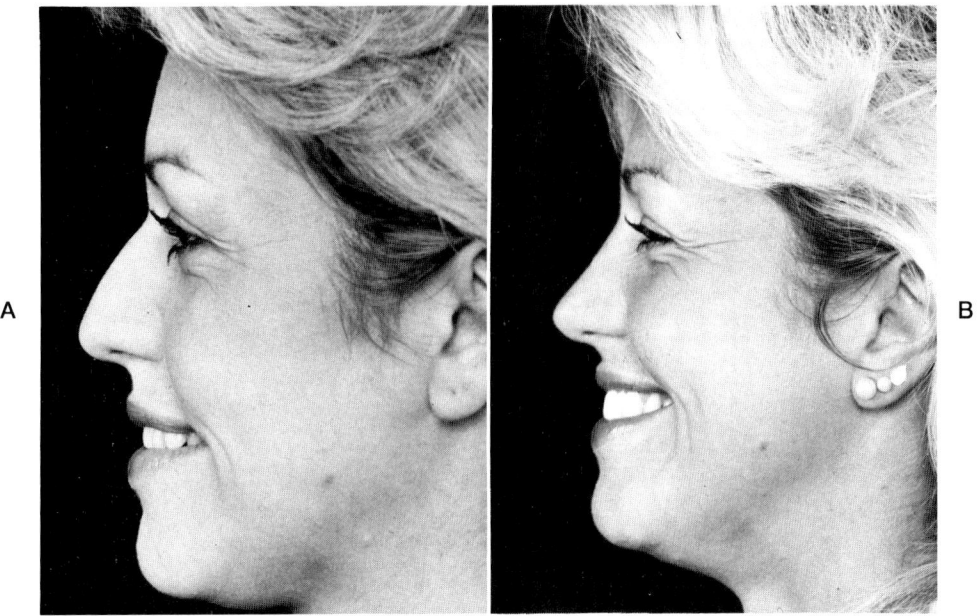

Figure 2-7. **A** is a preoperative photograph with animation. A tip graft was used to prevent downward plunging of the tip following operation. The postoperative result is seen in **B** (same point as in Figure 2-1).

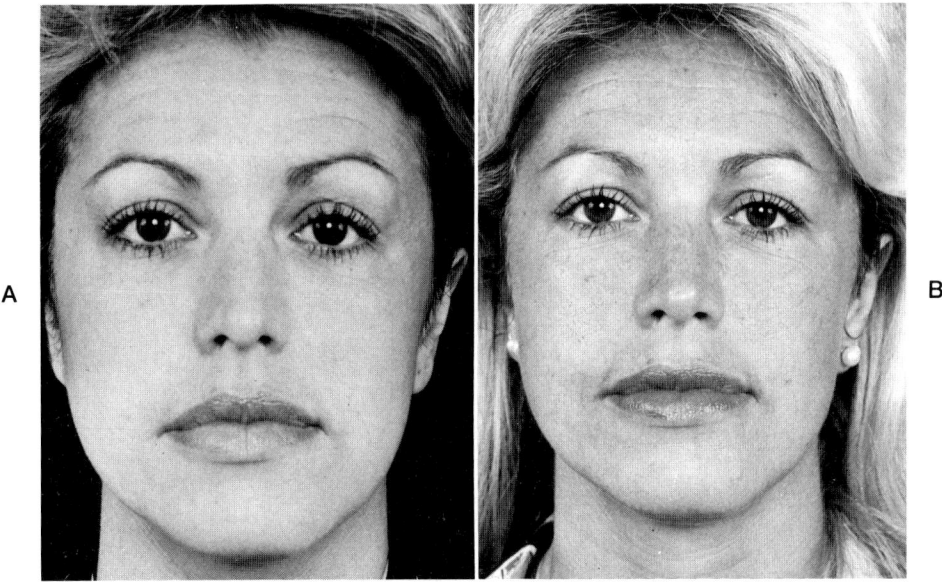

Figure 2-8. **A** and **B,** Preoperative and postoperative (front view) photographs of the patient shown in Figures 2-1 and 2-7.

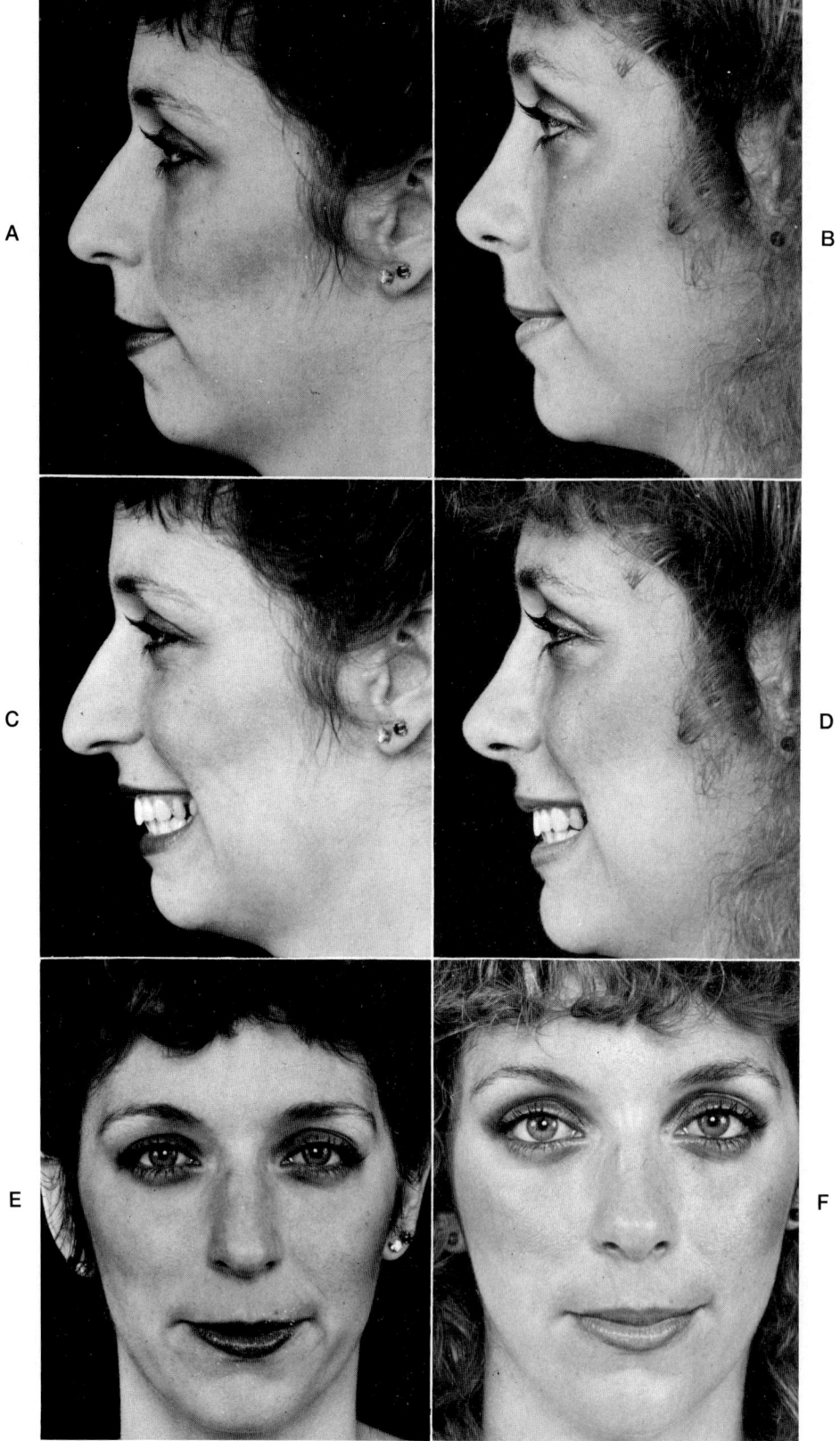

Figure 2-9. Preoperative and postoperative photographs of a patient showing the typical results of tip grafts to improve projection.

In Figure 2-9 we see a 25-year-old patient who had a primary rhinoplasty augmented by an autogenous cartilage onlay graft in the nasal tip. We can readily see the result of the augmentation in the postoperative photograph. A chin augmentation was also necessary. The smiling view (Figure 2-9, C and D) shows the relative stability of the graft. The front views (Figure 2-9, E and F) show the normal architecture and highlighting achieved with this technique.

SEPTAL SUPPORT

Figure 2-10 shows a 59-year-old patient who had a previous rhinoplasty performed. At consultation it was noted that she had a saddle deformity and complete loss of all septal support to the nasal pyramid.

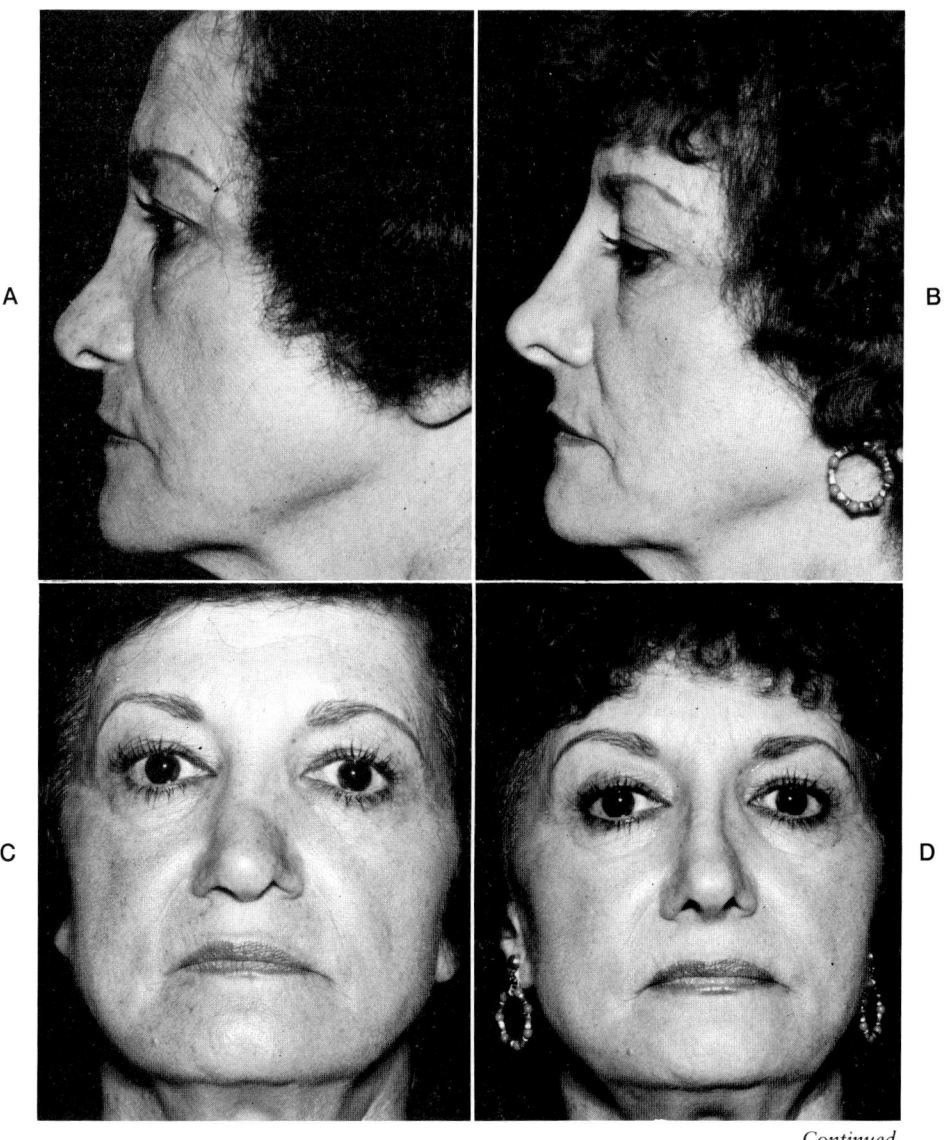

Continued.

Figure 2-10. Preoperative and postoperative views of tip and dorsal reconstruction with two-layered tip graft (Figure 2-11) and dorsal iliac bone graft (Figure 2-12) to correct a saddle-nose deformity.

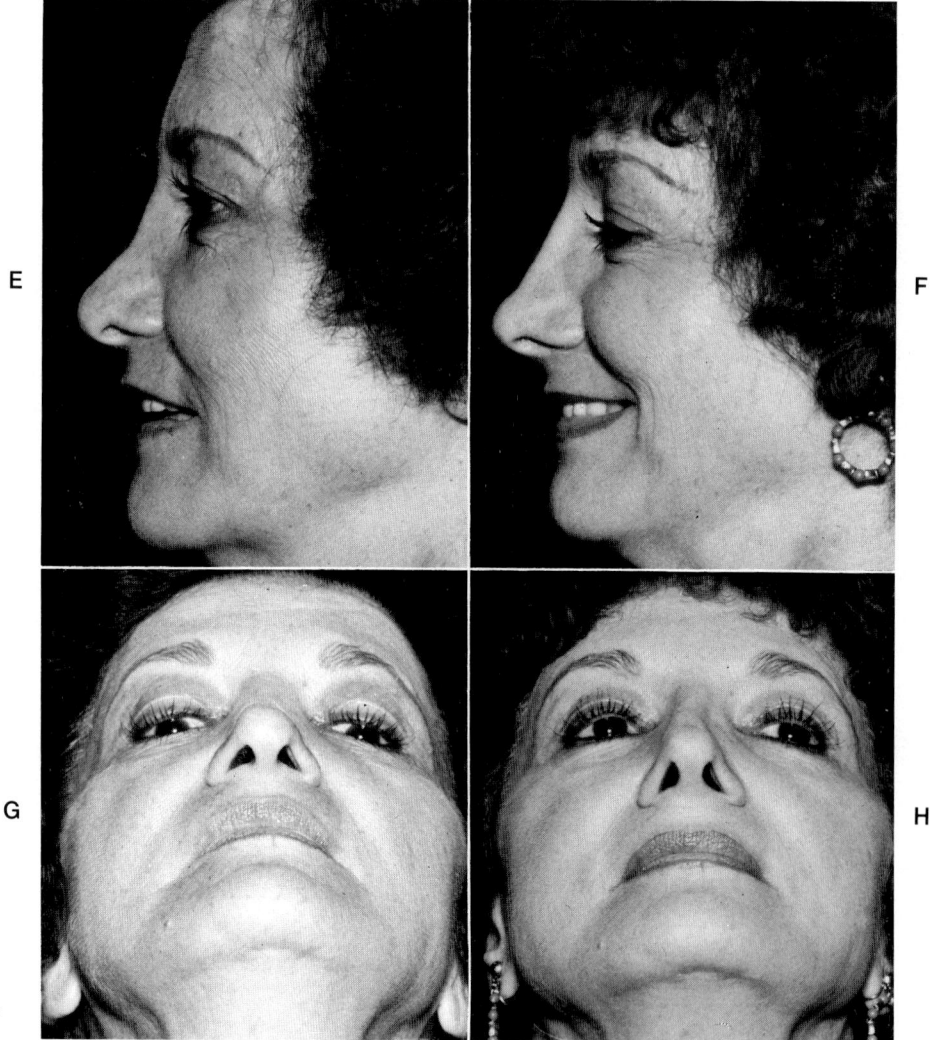

Figure 2-10, cont'd. Preoperative and postoperative views of tip and dorsal reconstruction with two-layered tip graft (Figure 2-11) and dorsal iliac bone graft (Figure 2-12) to correct a saddle-nose deformity.

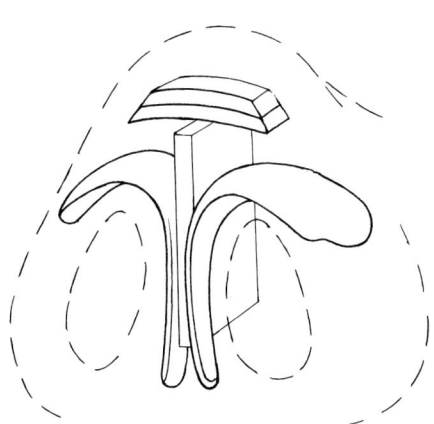

Figure 2-11. Two-layered cartilage onlay graft to the tip.

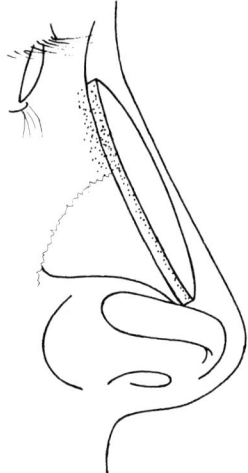

Figure 2-12. Correction of the saddle nose deformity in the patient in Figure 2-10 with an iliac bone graft.

Reconstruction involved use of an "umbrella" graft in the nasal tip pyramid (Figure 2-11). The septum was reconstructed with a strut graft obtained from the patient's auricular conchal cartilage. This graft was placed in a pocket developed between the medial crurae. An infracartilaginous incision was made on the right side at the mid-columella. With the sharp-pointed dissecting scissors, a pocket was developed between the medial crurae from the nasal spine to the nasal tip. The cartilage strut was placed between the crurae, much as the filler in a sandwich, and sutured in place by a transfixion suture. The double onlay graft, which completes the umbrella, was placed through a separate incision at the domes.

The saddle deformity was corrected by use of an iliac bone graft (Figure 2-12). This graft was placed through an incision made at the septal angle. The pocket made was large enough to accommodate the graft but no larger, thus eliminating the need to fix the graft. The nasal bridge was rasped before insertion of the graft to create a raw surface. Although the bone graft leans slightly to the right, an overall acceptable result was obtained (Figure 2-10, C and D).

In the smiling profiles shown in Figure 2-10, E and F the reconstruction of bridge, nasal tip pyramid, and nasolabial angle is evident. Figure 2-10, G and H offers worm's eye views of this patient, making the increased height of the nasal tip together with the change in external nares shape clearly evident.

3

Tip Projection and Contour

Jack Sheen

Although this discussion will focus on the various struts and grafts used to achieve tip projection, it is first necessary to understand the aesthetics of the nasal tip and its relationship to the aesthetics of the face as a whole. In general, the ideal nasal tip is suitably projecting and softly faceted. It is characterized by subtle projections that correspond to the domes of the lower lateral cartilages, by a defined angle at the columellar lobular junction, and by a point of differentiation from the dorsum that emphasizes the tip as the most projecting nasal part. This last point—the tip as the most projecting part (from any point of view)—is crucial to a successful rhinoplasty, so this is what we try to achieve, either by modifying the patient's existing tip structure or by creating a new structure using autogenous cartilage grafts.

CARTILAGE GRAFTS

Grafting cartilage to the tip became an important part of my rhinoplasty technique when I first had a clear concept of the problem of the tip with inadequate projection (TIP). During the years, rhinoplastic surgeons have observed this problem from many points of view and have suggested various causes, the most popular being the short columella. Contrary to this view, I feel that it is not so much the columella as a structural deficiency of the tip. To correct this structural deficiency, a special tip graft was designed. Since 1969 I have placed well over 1,000 tip grafts of various types and combinations. As certain problems became apparent, it became necessary to modify the original single graft technique. For comparison, I will briefly describe the tip graft as originally reported and the modifications in technique that have since evolved.

The original tip graft was designed to expand and project the tip and to recreate the projections of the domes of the lower lateral cartilages. The notch at the base provided lateral stability. Importantly, the design also ensured a favorable mechanical relationship between the widths of the ends of the graft, since a too narrow base would not support the graft if excessive pressures were placed on the projecting end.

With the original design, two major problems became evident: unnatural-appearing contour and shifting of the graft. To correct an unnatural flatness inferiorly, I began placing small crushed cartilage grafts anterior to the primary graft to fill out the tip contour. This produced a less angulated, more natural tip.

The next problem, shifting of the graft, was manifest by postoperative asymmetries of the tip. To correct this problem, I placed a second tip graft to project the flat side, thereby making the tip symmetrical. To avoid the problem of shifting, I now place multiple grafts in the tip during the primary procedure. These grafts consist of one or more main "support" grafts, small cartilage fragments placed posterior to the main grafts to fix them in position, and small cartilage fragments or crushed cartilage placed anteriorly for improved contour.

The decision to use a tip graft is almost always made preoperatively. Patients with a TIP problem are advised of the necessity and possible complications of tip grafts. I explain that I cannot achieve a well-defined, projecting tip without using a graft, but warn that there may be some unnatural angularity; however, since I have modified the original technique, the results have improved. During the last 5 years, shifting of the graft has not been a problem nor has loss of projection. Originally some single grafts (less than 20%) lost a measure of projection.

I do not know if this was caused by absorption of the cartilage, improper placement of the graft, or a shifting of the graft's position.

CASE REPORT

The 38-year-old woman shown in Figure 3-1 had a primary rhinoplasty at age 25. She was seen in consultation for airway obstruction and aesthetic improvement of her nose.

Preoperative evaluation

The soft tissues are of good quality; there are no scars, adhesions, or discolorations. On lateral view, a supratip deformity is evident, with no differentiation of the nasal tip. The tip contour is poorly defined. The nasolabial angle is open, with slight retrusion of the lip. On palpation, the nasal bones are of average length; the bony pyramid is open at the roof. The walls of the middle vault are medially

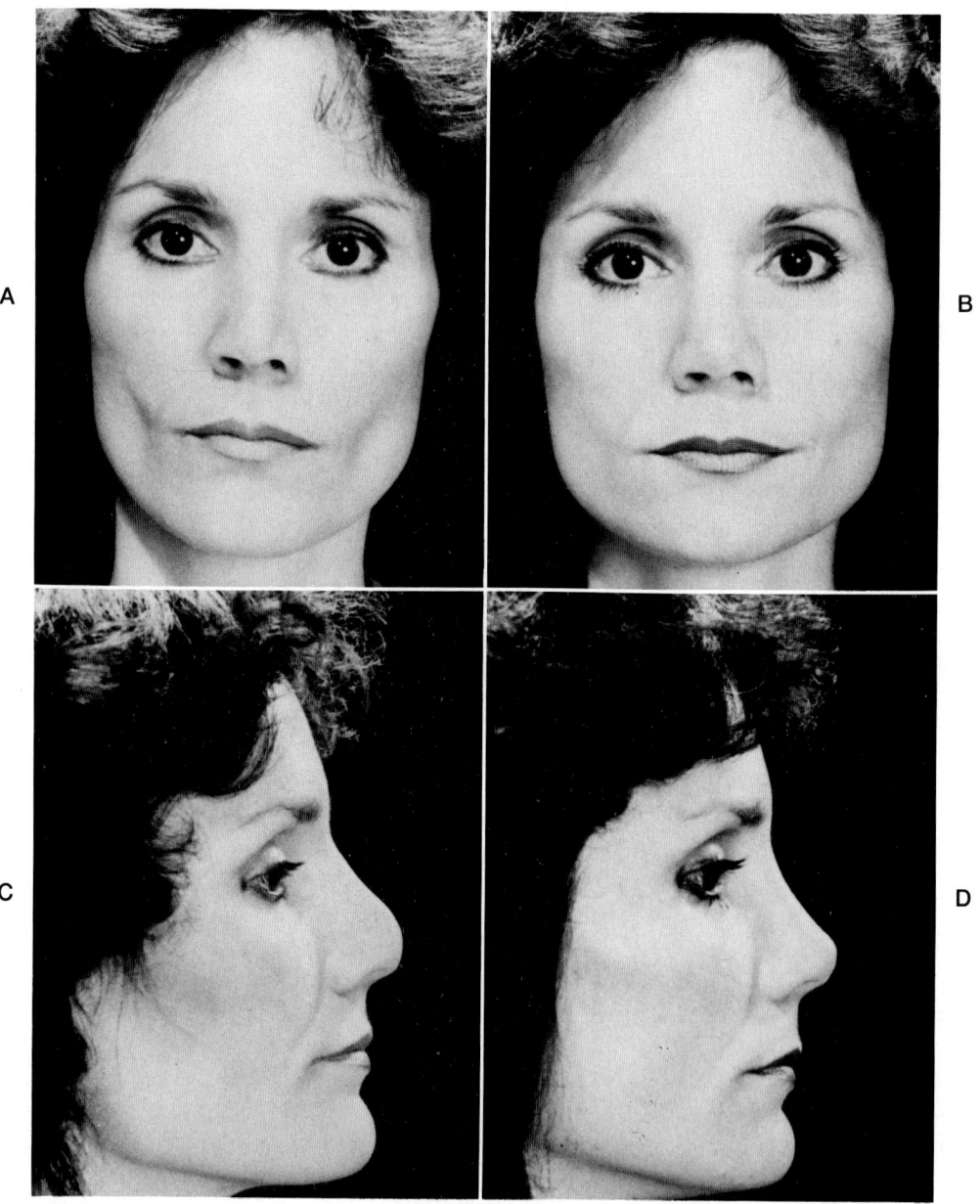

Figure 3-1. A and **C,** Patient with unsatisfactory rhinoplasty. In addition to functional impairment, a primary complaint was lack of tip projection and definition. **B** and **D,** Patient 14 months after secondary rhinoplasty with tip reconstruction.

displaced. Internally, both valves are narrow; the right side is narrower than the left. The septum, which deflects to the right, is intact. There is also a high anterior septal deviation.

Surgical approach

The surgical design incorporates a submucous resection for correction of the airway and use of the resected cartilage for aesthetic reconstruction. In addition to a dorsal graft and bilateral spreader grafts, multiple tip grafts are needed to adequately expand and project the tip.

Surgical procedure

1. Maxillary augmentation
2. Limited skeletonization
3. Anterior edge of the septum lowered slightly
4. Submucous resection
5. Partial bilateral inferior turbinectomy
6. Graft of crushed cartilage placed over open dorsal roof
7. Placement of spreader grafts
8. Placement of grafts at the base of columella
9. Placement of multiple crushed tip grafts
10. Type II alar base resection
11. Routine packing and dressing

Postoperative results

The patient is shown 14 months after secondary rhinoplasty with tip reconstruction (Figures 3-1 and 3-2). She has excellent, functional airways. On front view (Figure 3-1, B), the lateral walls are in good continuity. There is an appropriate light reflex at the nasal tip. On lateral view (Figure 3-1, D), the tip

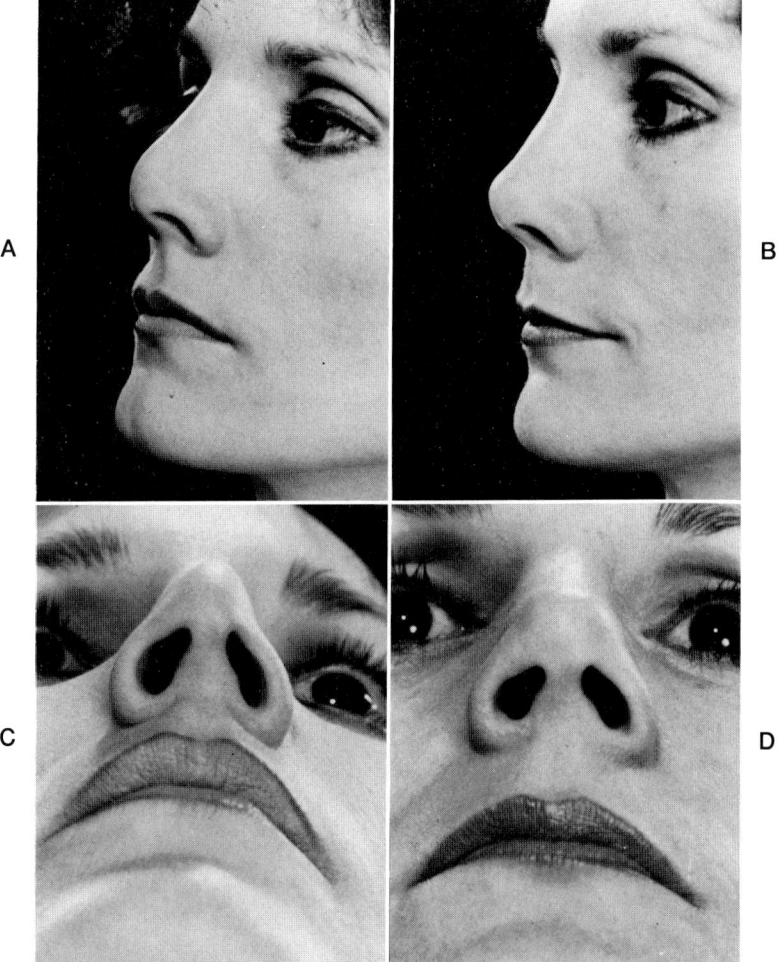

Figure 3-2. **A** and **B,** Comparative photographs before and after tip reconstruction. **C** and **D,** Same patient before and after secondary rhinoplasty from basal view. The apparent projection of the tip in the preoperative photograph results from the projection of the supratip.

reconstruction has improved the profile: a smooth line extends from the root to the tip, which has become the highest point in the profile. The length of the nose is visually increased by moving the most projecting part to a point over 1 cm, caudal to the preoperative point of the supratip projection. The effects of maxillary augmentation and grafts at the base of the columella are subtle. Oblique views verify symmetry of the tip (Figure 3-2, *B*).

SUMMARY

This case represents both functional and aesthetic problems. Functionally, the airways were impaired because of narrowed internal valves and a septal deviation. Aesthetically, the nose had the stigmatic of a postoperative, "surgical" nose, with a characteristic supratip deformity and lack of tip differentiation and definition. A submucous resection and spreader grafts improved the airways. Tip projection and definition were achieved by multiple crushed cartilage grafts placed in the tip.

4

Nasal Tip Sculpturing

Frank Kamer

The nasal tip is one of the most difficult areas to correct in rhinoplasty, presenting a surgeon with the greatest problems as well as offering the most satisfaction. During my residence, a single technique was taught for handling the tip—marginal incision and delivery of the tip cartilage. This provides excellent exposure for analysis of the cartilage anatomy, but because of the great ethnic diversity in noses and faces, variations in technique are necessary to create a natural-appearing tip. Different techniques are indicated, depending on the individual patient and the specific problem.

My personal philosophy in surgery views rhinoplasty as an art, not just a technical, surgical exercise. I feel the preservation of tissue is of utmost importance, for both function and aesthetics. To preserve and yet enhance the natural tip characteristics, grafts are sometimes necessary. My goals in surgery focus on achieving a balance between the preservation of natural and normal features and the correction of the offending characteristics.

I believe aesthetic surgery of the nasal tip can be represented by a gradual continuum of greater difficulty and increasing technical intervention (Figure 4-1). The degree of surgical reconstruction needed depends on the severity of the deformity, the aesthetic goals and philosophy of the surgeon, and

a thorough grasp of the dynamics and vagaries of healing. Natural tip defining points, highlights, facets, and projection, if present, should be preserved whenever possible. If not, then appropriate grafts, battons, or distinct rearrangement of the lower lateral cartilages should be considered.

OPERATIVE TECHNIQUES

There are three ways to approach the nasal tip cartilages (Figure 4-2): (1) Using an intercartilaginous incision in the retrograde fashion, (2) splitting the cartilages in varying ways and removing a specified portion of that cartilage, and (3) delivering and inspecting the anatomy while doing what surgery is necessary to the cartilages.

Preservation of the natural shape and contour of the tip is accomplished by removing appropriate portions of the cephalic margin of the lobular cartilages in a retrograde fashion or via a cartilage-spitting approach. If the tip presents problems of asymmetry or bifidity or if it requires a change of projection, then it can be delivered and the cartilages sutured, vertically or horizontally split, or more completely studied for diagnostic purposes. The tips with more problems can also be augmented with grafts or battons of autogenous material. The open method is best reserved for cleft noses or Binder-

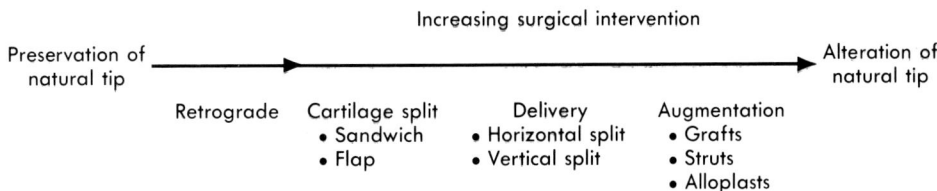

Figure 4-1. Continuum of increasing technical intervention on the tip.

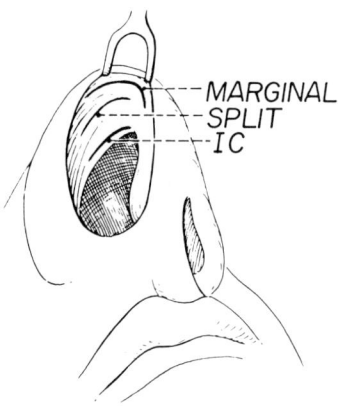

Figure 4-2. Types of incisional approaches to the nasal tip.

type syndromes. I will show how each of these approaches is applied to the simple cases and then proceed to the more difficult ones.

Retrograde technique

I use a retrograde technique for the symmetrical tip that requires minimal refinement. In those cases, the rim cartilages and support of the tip are left intact and minimal rotation is obtained. The disadvantages of this approach stem from difficulty in viewing the dome area upside down and backwards; access is gained to the cartilage via an intercartilaginous incision. The external and vestibular skin layers are separated from the lobular cartilages in a retrograde fashion and a strip, wedge, or ellipse is removed to

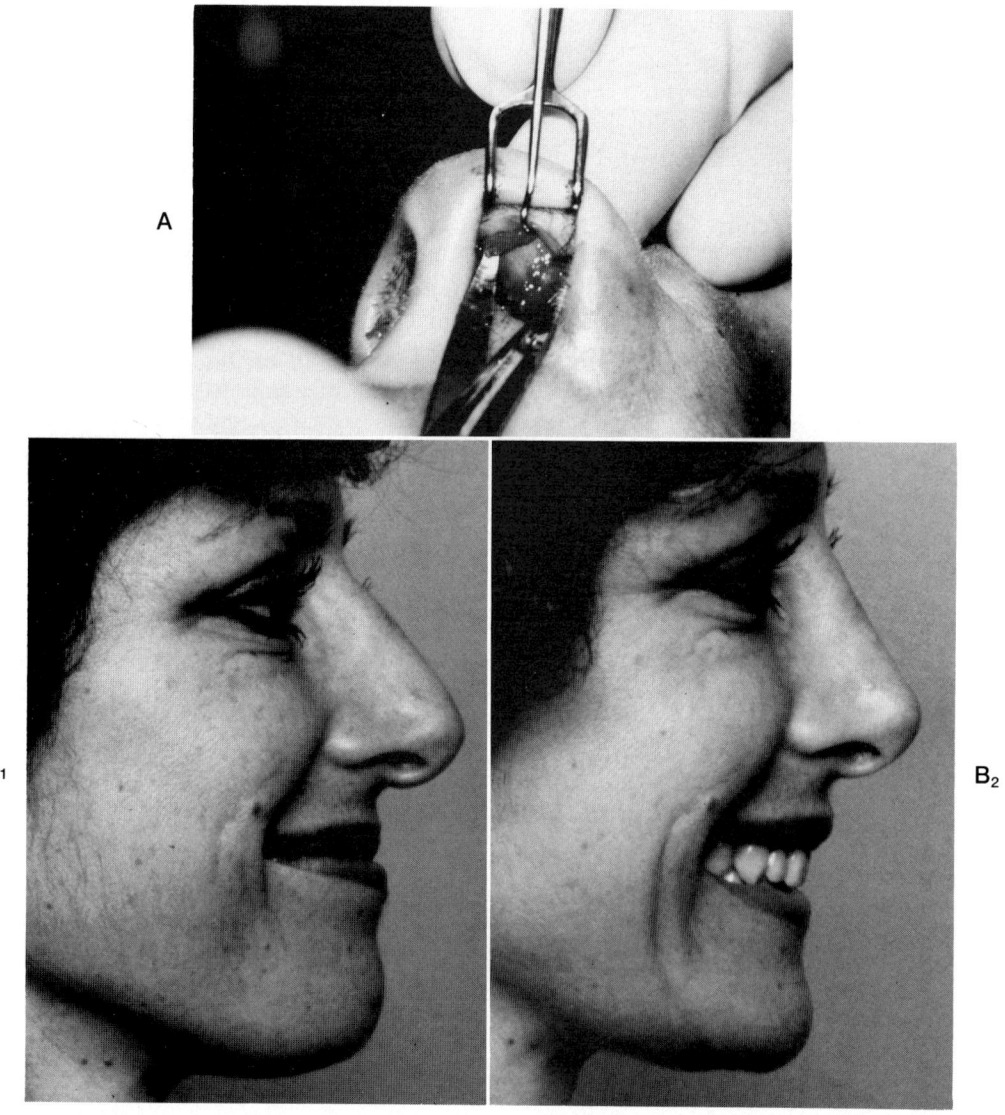

Figure 4-3. Retrograde approach. **A,** Intraoperative view showing scissor dissection. **B₁,** Preoperative view. **B₂,** Postoperative view. Tip rotation is unaffected.

give the necessary definition to the tip without changing projection or rotation (Figures 4-3, *A*). Refinements of the tip can be done in this manner, resulting in minimal alteration (Figures 4-3, *B₁* and *B₂*).

Cartilage-splitting technique

When tips require more refinement and definition or if more rotation is needed, I prefer a cartilage-splitting technique. This can be done by removing cartilage from between the sandwich of the vestibular and external skin layers or by using a bipedicle chondromucosal flap (Figure 4-4, *A₁*). Both techniques leave an intact rim strip. By preserving the rim cartilage, support of the tip is relatively well-maintained and projection is minimally lowered, depending on the amount and size of cartilage removed. An ellipse or strip of cartilage can be removed from the superior margin of the lateral crus to give the tip required definition (Figure 4-4, *A₂*). Variations of the technique can be used to gain access to the dome or to remove a small wedge of cartilage from that area and achieve some narrowing without disturbing the intact rim (Figure 4-4, *B*). A flap technique can also be used that creates a slightly different type of tip definition with a bit more rotation. Tip projection is inherently lowered slightly, depending on the amount of cartilage removed (Figure 4-4, *C₁* to *C₄*).

Delivery and inspection

To gain or lower projection, it is best to do a delivery technique and inspect the cartilages. A complete transfixion through a septocolumella incision, by virtue of linear scar contracture postoperatively, lower projection just a bit, even without cartilage removal. By removing cartilage, even greater lowering of tip projection is accomplished. I reserve the delivery technique for problem cases—asymmetrical, bifid, overly projected, underprojected, or severely drooping tips. For an open rhinoplasty, there is no better way to visualize the anatomy than delivering the tip cartilages. As a learning tool, it is superb.

While performing a rhinoplasty, the surgeon should always be aware of the areas of tip support that Janeke and Wright[3] described some years ago (Figure 4-5). When completely transfixing a nose and delivering the cartilage, we are interrupting most of these supports—the base of the medial crura at the spine, the interdomal ligaments, the attachment of the cartilages of the upper and lower lobules, and, laterally, the attachment at the sesamoid cartilages. Weakening these areas diminishes projection postoperatively. In addition, delivering the cartilage creates a greater potential for tip ptosis postoperatively. Therefore, it must be emphasized that only those tips requiring such a procedure should undergo delivery techniques.

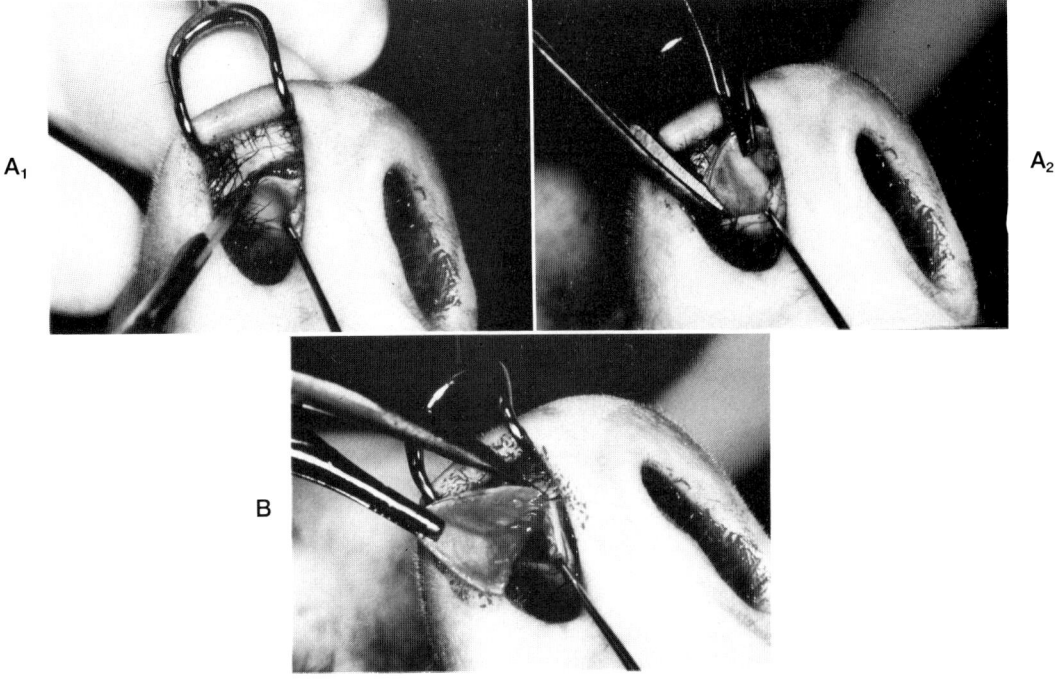

Figure 4-4. Cartilage splitting technique. **A₁,** Incision. **A₂,** Dissection. **B,** Removal of a wedge from dome without sectioning through rim.   *Continued.*

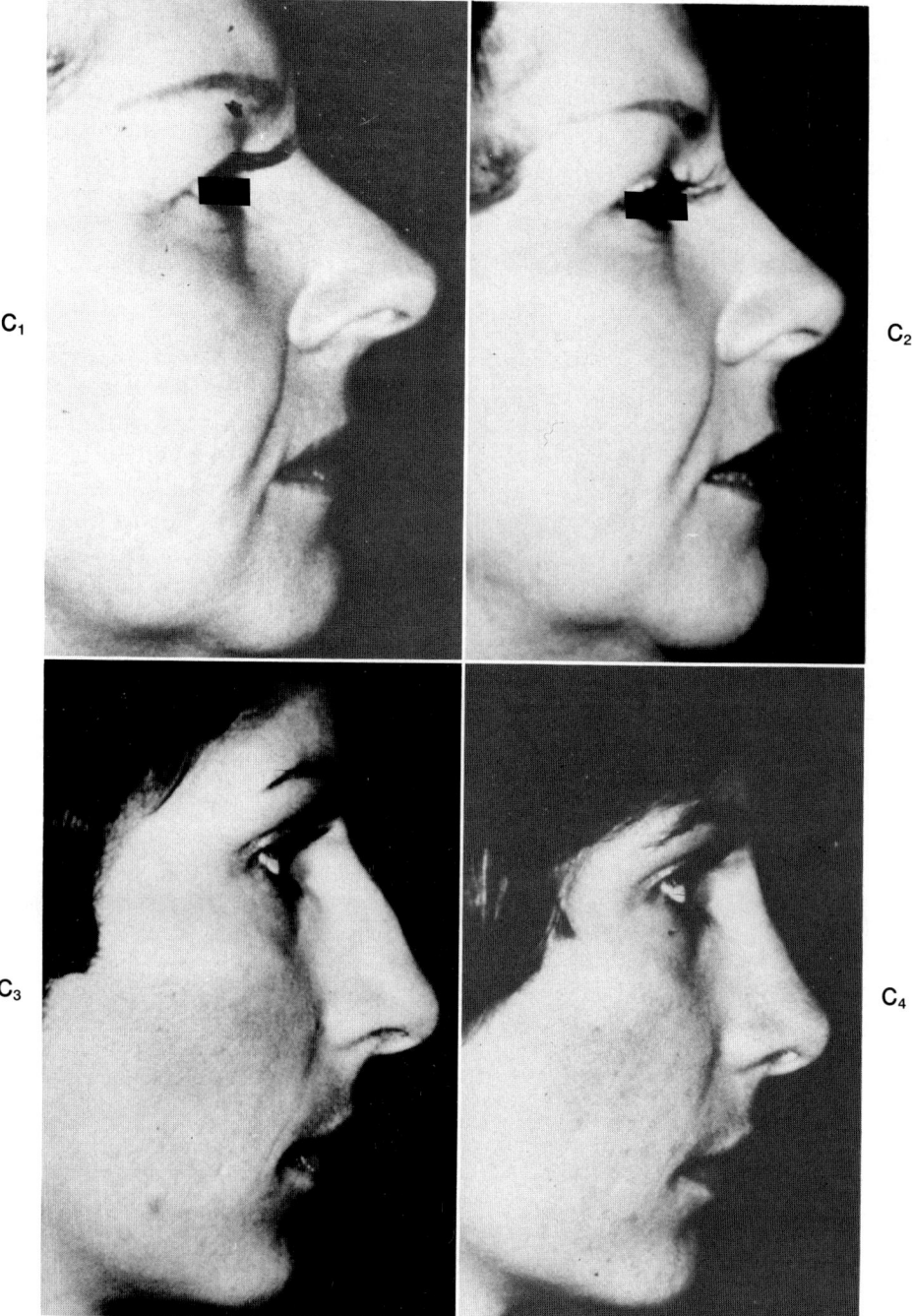

Figure 4-4, cont'd. Cartilage splitting technique. C_1, Preoperative view. C_2, Postoperative view. C_3, Preoperative view of cartilage splitting technique using crural flap. C_4, Postoperative view of the same patient.

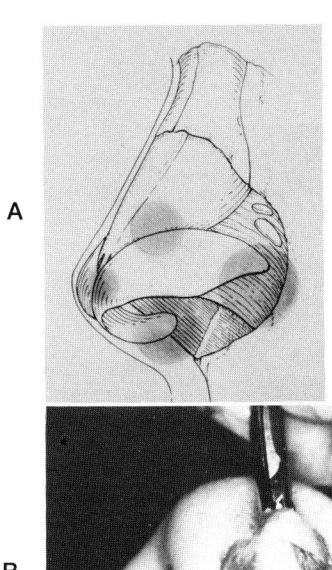

A

Figure 4-5. A, Areas of tip support. B₁, Delivery technique with vertical split. B₂, Cartilage delivery technique with resection of cephalic portion of lateral crura. C₁, Preoperative view showing severe underprojection and bifidity. C₂, Postoperative view. C₃, Preoperative view. C₄, Postoperative view.

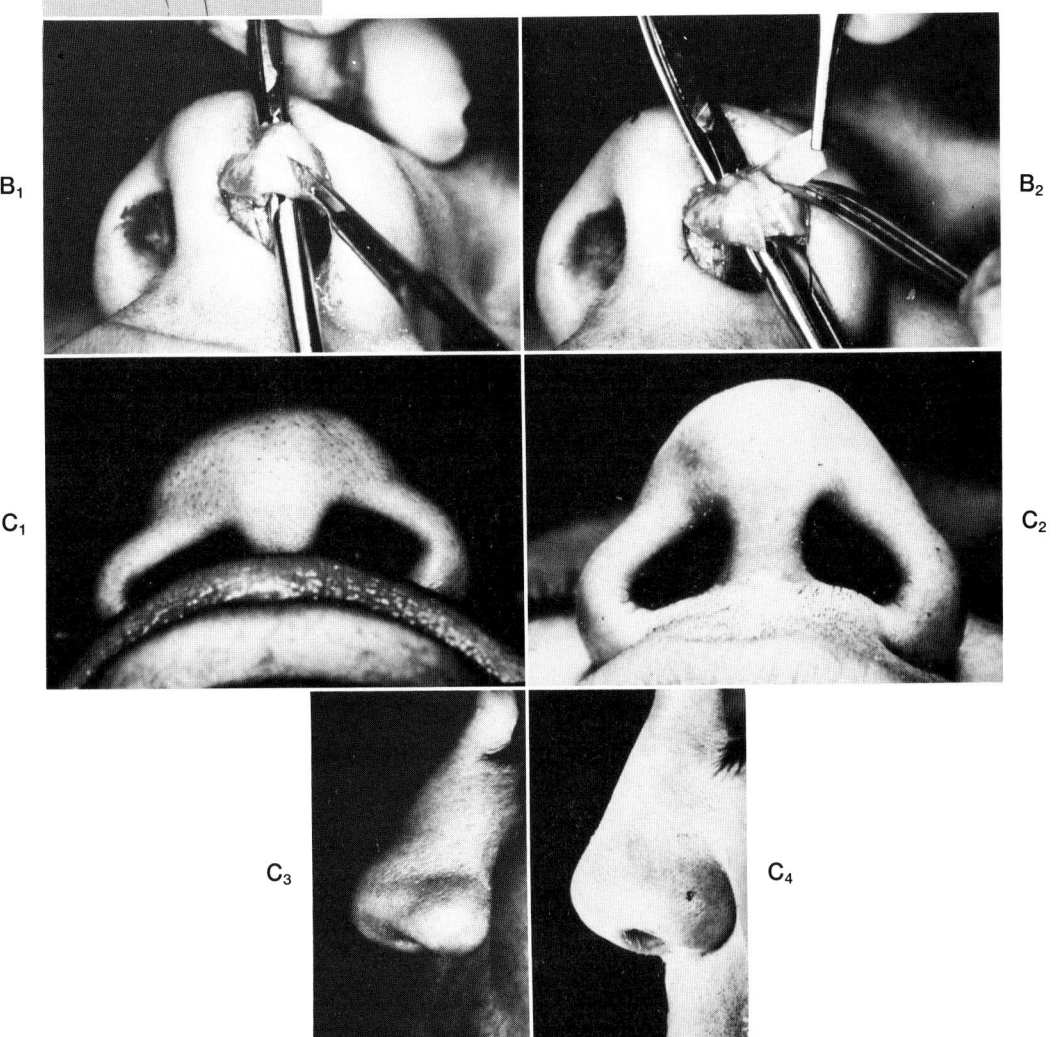

Applications

Severely drooping tips require radical alteration by vertical splits made through the cartilage (Figure 4-5, B_1 and B_2). These were described by Fomon,[1] Goldman,[2] and Lipsett,[4] among others. All of these vertical tip incisions radically alter the tip. Postoperatively, the patient may have difficulty in healing, although the result is often a magnificent and dra-matic alteration of the nasal tip. Problems of asymmetry, pinching, bossa, polly-beak formation, and ptosis are not uncommon. These tip techniques, in my opinion, are best reserved for tips that require more dramatic changes, such as those with severe bifidity or underprojection (Figure 4-5, C_1 to C_4). One of my teachers, Dr. Irving Goldman,[2] de-scribed suturing the medial crura together to gain

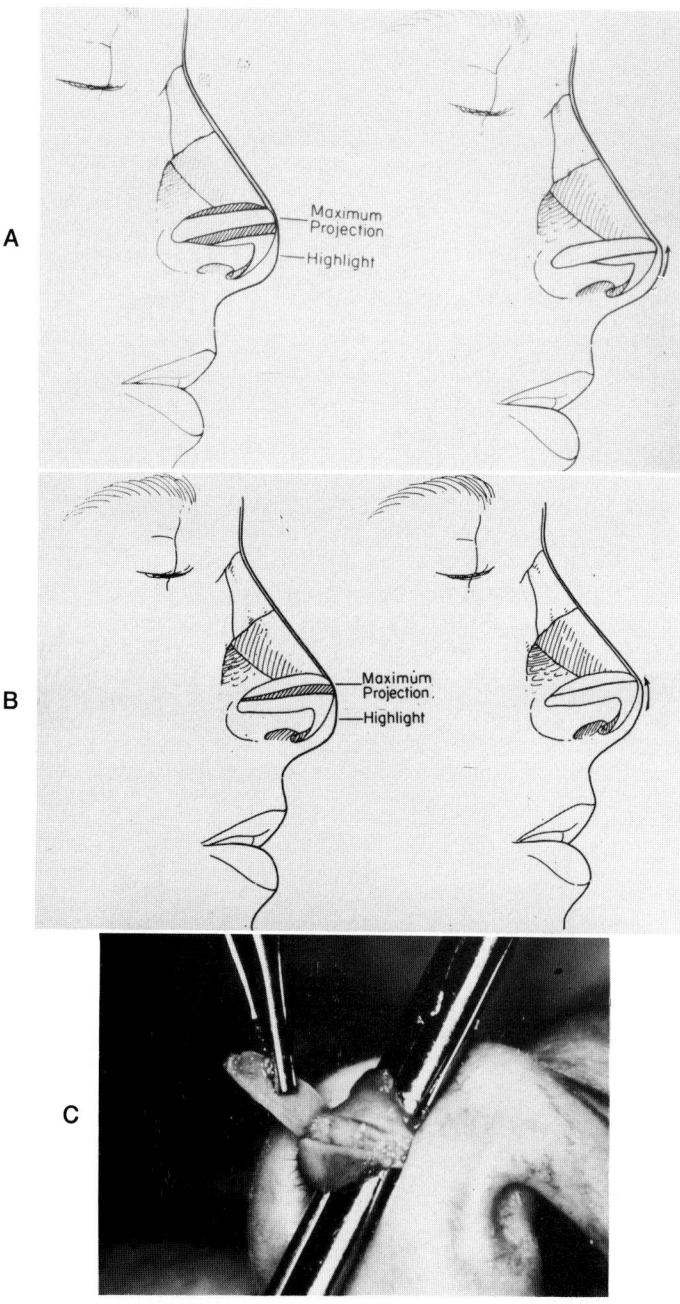

Figure 4-6. Horizontal strip technique. **A,** Maximal rotation. **B,** Minimal ro-tation. **C,** Removal of horizontal strip. *Continued.*

more projection by borrowing from the lateral crura. Suturing a cartilaginous graft to the medial crura as a sandwich can provide even more projection and added bulk to the tip. Dramatic alteration can be gained, but often at the expense of natural aesthetics.

When the nose has normal highlights and projection, it is best to preserve them even if they are a distance apart. To maintain the highlight, facets, and tip-defining points while preserving a projection at a variable distance from the highlight of the caudal margin of the tip cartilages, I elect to remove an intervening horizontal strip of cartilage and preserve both the entire rim and the more cephalic projecting margin of the alar cartilages (Figure 4-6, *A*). This allows preservation of the highlight without endan-

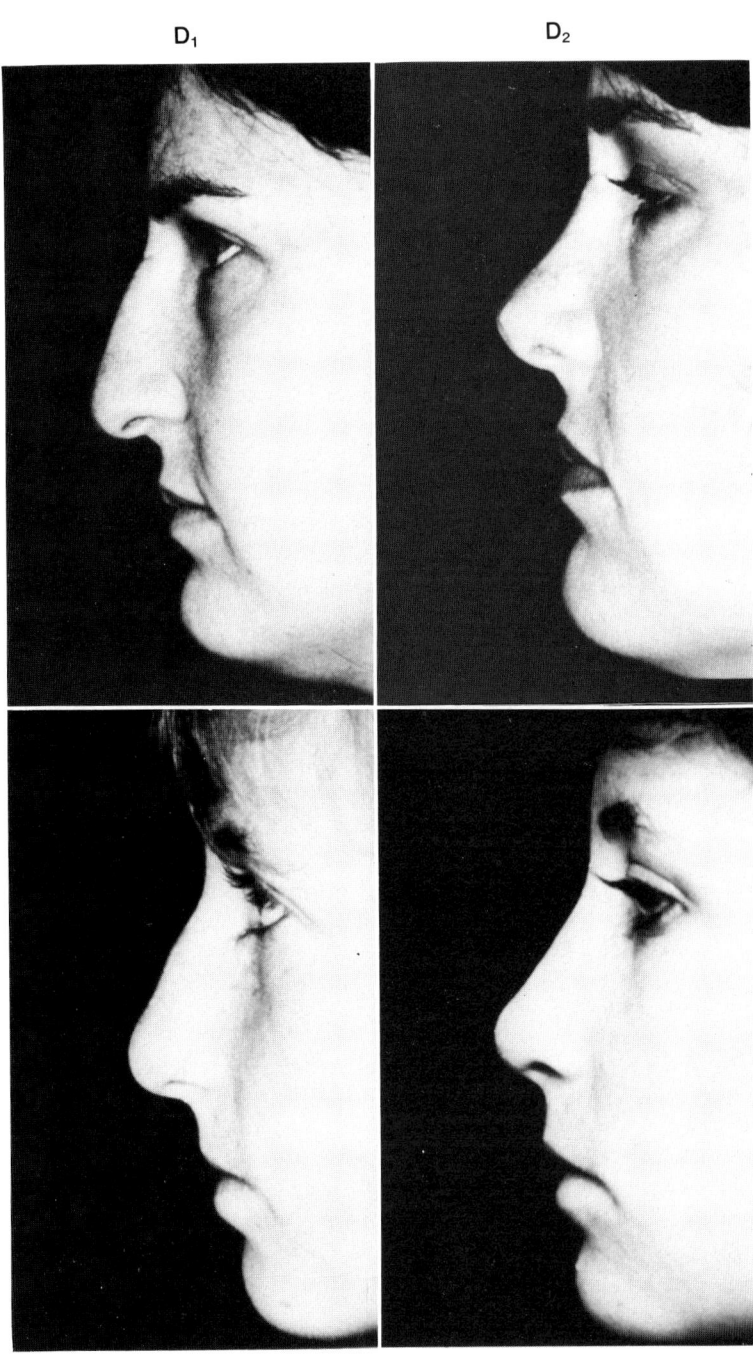

Figure 4-6, cont'd. D_1, Preoperative view of horizontal strip technique, maximal rotation. D_2, Postoperative view. D_3, Preoperative view of horizontal strip technique, minimal rotation. D_4, Postoperative view.

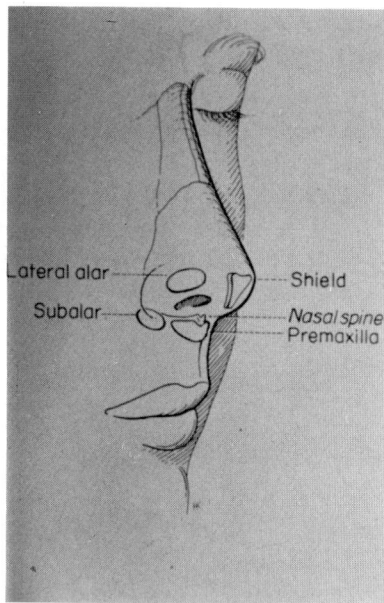

Figure 4-7. Location and types of nasal grafts.

gering the facet. Before injecting local anesthetic, the highlight and most projecting point of the lobular cartilage are marked (Figure 4-6, B_1 and B_2). An intervening horizontal strip of cartilage is removed and the cartilage both superior and inferior to it is preserved. When maximal rotation is required, the incision is carried out laterally to the rim and a strip removed from the midline to the lateral end of the incision (Figure 4-6, C). Bulk can also be removed from the cephalic margin of cartilage. The maximal projection and the highlight can then be brought into apposition.

When less rotation but more definition is required of the tip, the excision is placed within the limits of the cartilage. The projected and highlighted areas are still brought into apposition, but with more limited rotation. Underlying mucosa is preserved, and the cartilages are not sutured. The median horizontal strip technique allows for maintenance of both highlight and projection, but the technique is best reserved for those tips in which one wishes to preserve these features but bring them closer together (Figure 4-6, D_1 to D_4).

In more difficult noses where there is little projection, we can vertically split the cartilages and borrow from the lateral or medial crura. I find columella base struts not very helpful. If they are too long, they present an unnatural tent-pole appearance. If too short, they seem to do little except add support to the tip. Grafts can be very useful to increase projec-

tion and add highlights in the tip. The so-called "shield" graft described by Sheen[5] is a particularly helpful technique for this purpose. Pseudoprojection or lowering of the dorsum to try to match a natural but underprojecting tip is only useful in a patient of short stature with a small face; otherwise the nose can appear unbalanced with the face and body. Rotation is a maneuver that does not add projection, but in the severely ptotic tip, it does help to give an illusion of projection and possibly eliminate the need for a graft.

Grafts are indicated to fill, elevate, or contour (Figure 4-7). Grafting of the premaxilla and nasal spine appears to help with projection and tip support. Subalar grafts can also aid in tip support and, to a lesser degree, projection. In some noses, such as the one illustrated in Figure 4-7, it is not necessary to rotate or excise caudal septum. Augmentation simply by the addition of autogenous cartilage at the nasal spine and premaxilla area could suffice to give the illusion of shortening or rotation (Figure 4-8, A). The graft is placed in its pocket through the transfixion incision and gives additional support and projection to the nasal tip as well as improving the highlight (Figure 4-8, B_1 to B_4).

The hypoplastic underprojecting immature lobule is an excellent indication for a shield graft in primary cases. Added projection and definition in these cases are needed, and it is difficult to use the natural cartilage because of its softness. The surgeon can enhance projection by adding to the tip while maintaining a higher dorsal profile (Figure 4-9, A).

In revision tip surgery, the tip graft is most useful. The graft is best taken from the thicker areas of the cartilaginous septum. It must be fashioned so it is not too wide, making the tip appear bifid, or too narrow, giving an amorphous or pointed appearance (Figure 4-9, B). The cartilage is placed through a small slot incision at the margin of the dome (Figure 4-9, C). Whenever possible, I attempt not to connect the graft pocket with the incision used to alter the tip. The pocket is small, made just large enough to admit the graft. The graft is shaped and placed to sit on the lobular-columella junction. When placed properly, it creates a dramatic and extremely natural improvement, often without doing much else to the nose (Figure 4-9, E_1 and E_2).

Tip grafts are useful in the rather difficult cases that would ordinarily require radical alteration of the cartilage to gain projection and definition of the tip. In problem revision cases where the cantilever effect of the nose is lost by excessive bone removal, and scar tissue provides much of the support of the

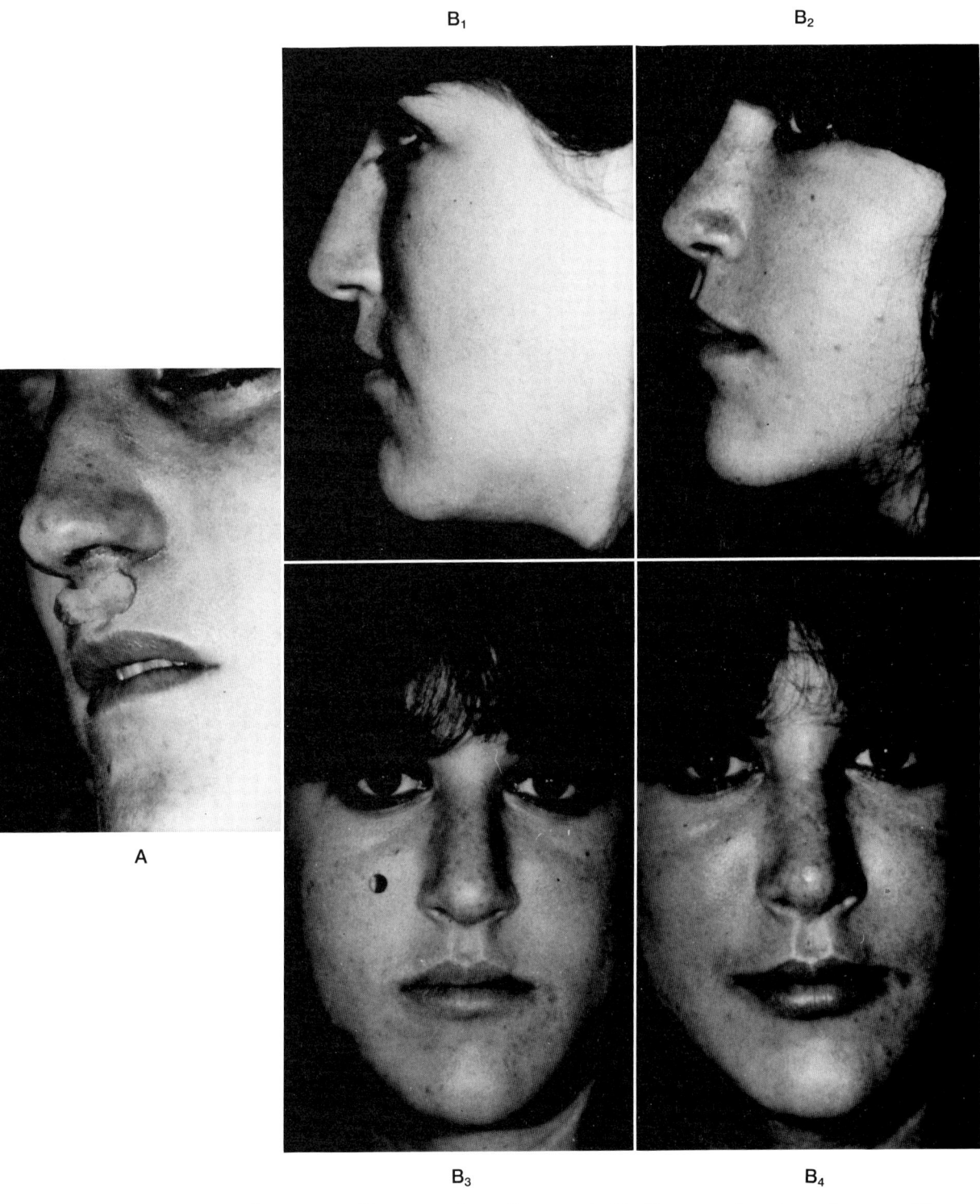

Figure 4-8. A, Location for premaxillary septal cartilage graft. **B₁,** Preoperative view of premaxillary cartilage graft. **B₂,** Postoperative view. **B₃,** Preoperative view of premaxillary cartilage graft. **B₄,** Postoperative view. Preoperative and postoperative views demonstrate the projection of nasal tip achieved by the additional support of such a graft.

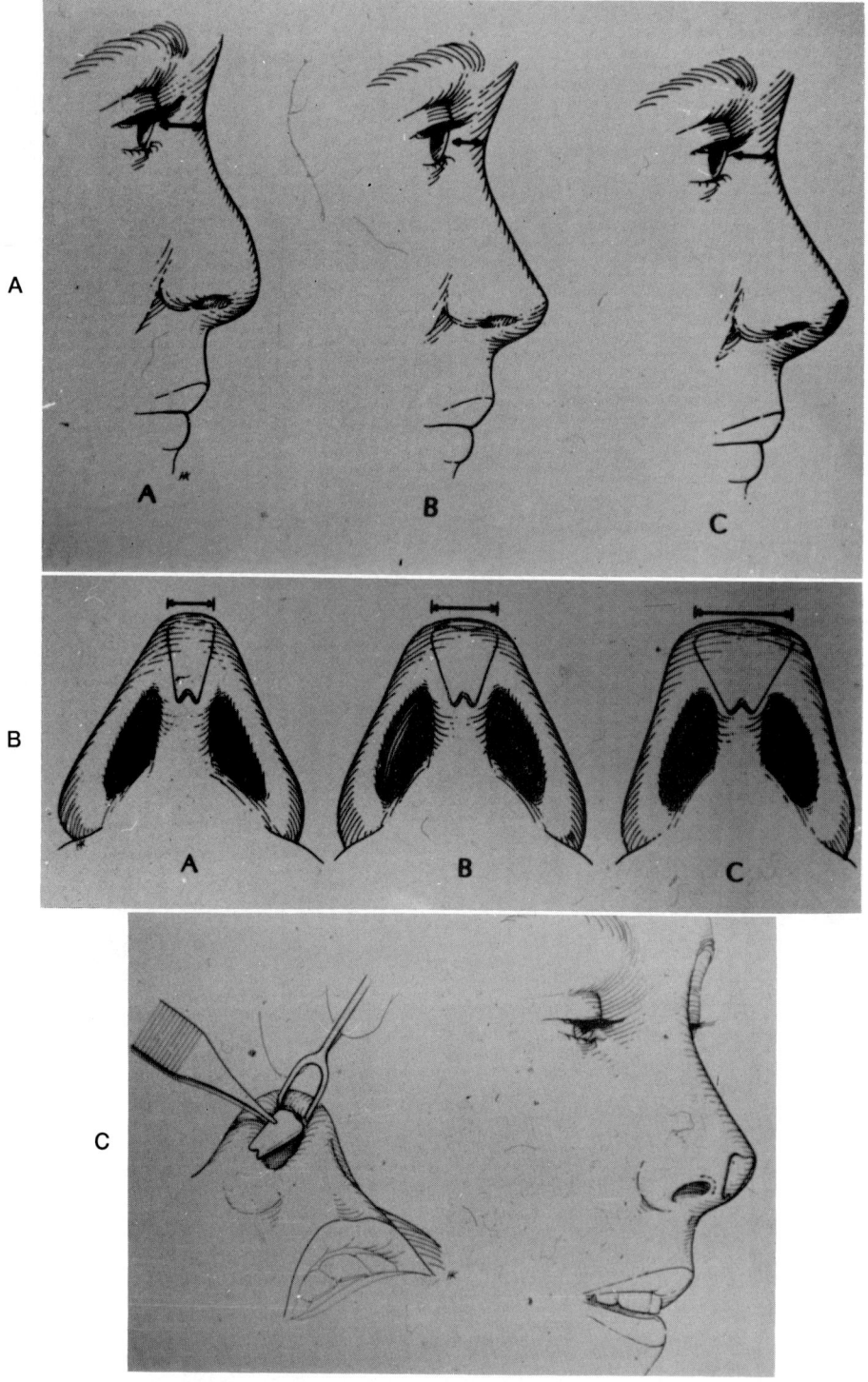

Figure 4-9. A, Indication for shield graft: **A,** High dorsal profile with poor projection. **B,** Pseudoprojection by lowering dorsum. **C,** Maintenance of high dorsal profile with tip projection by shield graft. **B,** Proper sizing of shield graft: **A,** Tip may appear pointed. **B,** Represents appropriate size. **C,** Tip may appear bifid. **C,** Insertion of shield graft through small incision.   *Continued.*

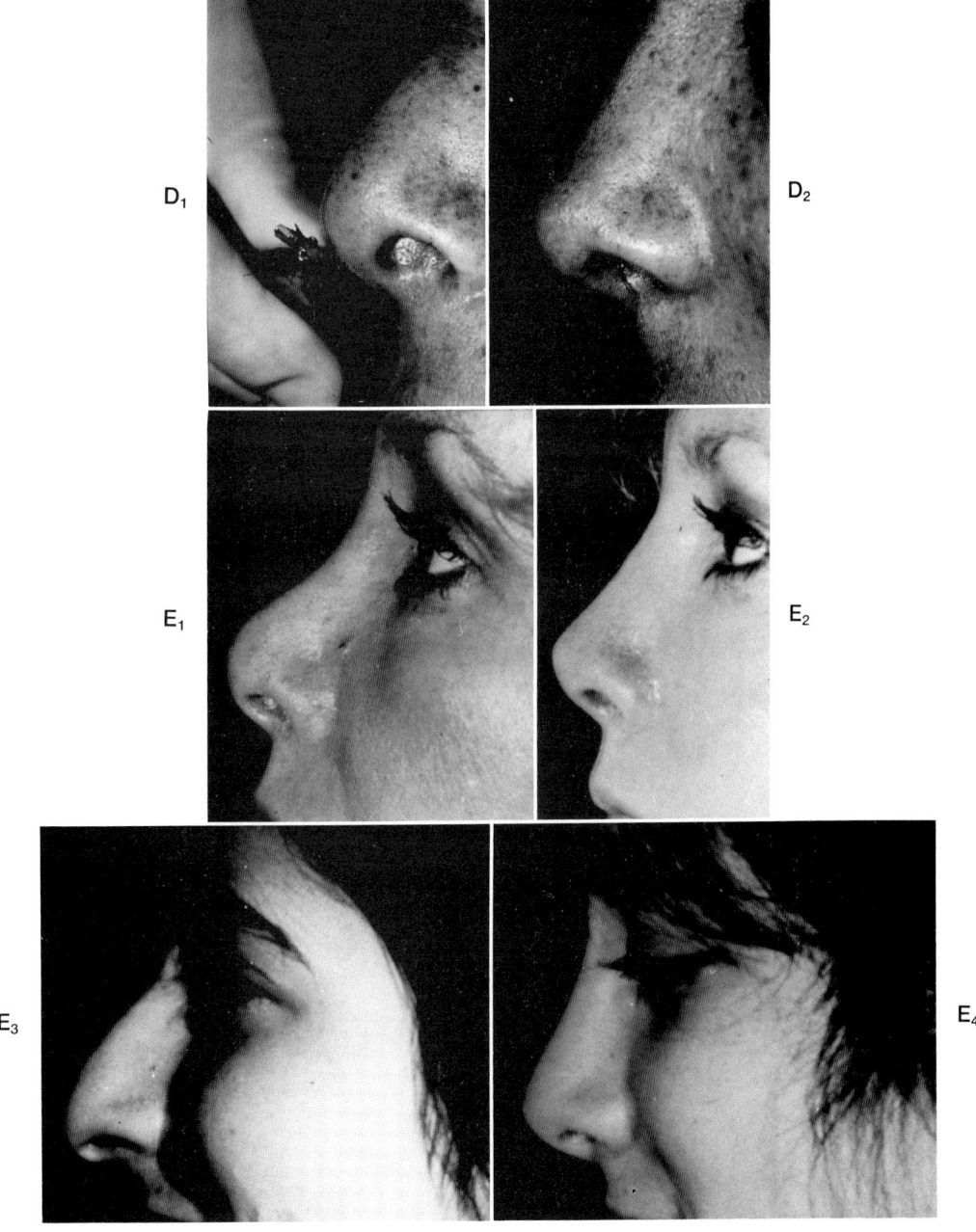

Figure 4-9, cont'd. D_1, Intraoperative view showing proper placement and angle of shield graft. D_2, Postoperative view shield graft in place. E_1, Preoperative view of shield graft, dorsal and lateral alar grafts. E_2, Postoperative view of patient with shield, lateral and dorsal grafts. E_3, Preoperative view of rhinoplasty using shield graft. E_4, Postoperative view of rhinoplasty using shield graft.

tip because of excessive cartilage removal, a tip graft and removal of scar tissue with an added dorsal graft often help a great deal (Figure 4-9, F_1 to F_4). I find this tip graft to be one of the most versatile and useful of all grafts to return the scarified tips to a more normal appearance. Autogenous tip grafts can also be harvested from the concha. Conchal cartilage is especially helpful when most of the septal cartilage has been removed by previous surgery. As it approaches the external canal, the conchal cartilage becomes thicker. It has a helpful curvature that mimics the double break of the nasal tip and, when judiciously used, can create remarkably idealized nasal tips.

Most primary cases do not need grafts. Grafting should be used only when the natural cartilages cannot be rearranged or altered because of their size, shape, or consistency. The grafted nose sometimes presents very unnatural, overprojecting, stiff, stylized tips. It is usually more advantageous, if possible, to reshape the alar cartilages and the tip rather than resort to grafts, especially in primary operation. In recent years I have seen considerably more overuse of these grafts, creating nasal tips that often look nice but amorphous and large, indicating some overgrafting and a dorsum that is too high. The tips may then appear stiff, immobile, and unnatural. In my opinion, grafts should be indicated only in cases that require additional support, projection, contouring, or filling.

The open rhinoplasty is best reserved for extremely difficult nasal presentations, such as the cleft nose or Binder's syndrome. In these extreme cases of asymmetry, underprojection, and lack of tissue, visibility for both diagnosis and treatment is essential. Replacement techniques must be used and adequate frats placed properly. However, I do not believe that a horizontal transcolumella scar is a necessary addition to most noses that can be corrected via a closed technique. It is unfortunate that so many noses today are being violated by this uncommonly indicated technique.

REFERENCES

1. Foman, S.: Management of deformities of the lower cartilaginous vault, Arch. Otolaryngol. 54:467-472, 1951.
2. Goldman, I.B.: New technique for corrective surgery of the nasal tip, Arch. Otolaryngol. 58:183-218, 1953.
3. Jancke, J.B., Wright, W.K.: Studies on the support of the nasal tip, Arch. Otolaryngol. 93:458-465, 1971.
4. Lipsett, E.M.: New approach to surgery of the lower cartilaginous vault, Arch. Otolaryngol. 70:42-47, 1959.
5. Sheen, J.H.: Achieving nasal tip projection by the use of small autogenous vomer or septal cartilage graft, Plast. Reconstr. Surg. 56:35-40, 1975.

5

The Tip

Tony Bull

In the early days of rhinoplasty the tip was relatively ignored compared to the nasal bones and dorsum. Surgical deformities often resulted from excess work on the dorsum. The "ski-slope" nose resulted when excess bone and cartilage was removed from the nasal dorsum and relatively little work was done on the nasal tip, giving a characteristically "scooped out" defect. Also, removal of an overly large bony hump with the standard thick-edged Joseph saw and minimal removal of cartilage was a common cause of polly-beak. Failure to provide an infracture of the nasal bones produced "open-roof" or "plateau" appearance. In the past, tip surgery involved routine excision of a large triangle of caudal septal cartilage, resulting in an excessively upturned nose with a very obtuse and unnatural-looking nasolabial angle, the so-called pug nose deformity. These were the "old" surgical appearances of faulty rhinoplasty (Figure 5-1).

CARTILAGE-SPLITTING INCISION

In the last two decades more thought has been given to, and more elaborate work carried out on, the alar cartilages. Specifically, a cartilage-splitting incision parallel to the rim of the alar cartilage (but clearly not parallel to the margin of the nasal vestibule) allows delivery of the upper two thirds or three fourths of the alar cartilage and permits precise and symmetrical removal of the cephalic portion of this cartilage under direct vision with preservation of the vestibular skin (Figure 5-2). I feel this delivery approach is preferable to the retrograde approach to the cephalic portion of the alar cartilage via the intercartilaginous incision.

In rhinoplasty most nasal tips require removal of the cephalic portion of the alar cartilage. They do not require a rim incision with complete delivery of the cartilage. Removal of the cephalic portion of cartilage gives a consistently subtle but definite change in the nasal tip, allowing narrowing and rotation (Figure 5-3). It also maintains alar rim anatomy and tip facets, which may be made less apparent after a rim incision.

Two relevant factors with removal of the cephalic portion of the alar cartilage are symmetry and amount excised. Related important factors are skin thickness and cartilage texture. Thick seborrheic skin conceals underlying irregularities that may follow asymmetrical or piecemeal removal of alar cartilage. On the other hand, extensive improvement or refinement of these nasal tips is not possible. With thin skin, however, the anatomy of the underlying strong resilient cartilages is obvious. Therefore, great care is needed with nasal tip work to be sure that the excision is symmetrical and precise. A cartilage-splitting incision demonstrates the cartilage anatomy well. The alar margin, which is not always clearly delineated, is made more apparent with pressure from the back of the scalpel. The vestibular hairs also usually mark the alar rim fairly reliably, for they are usually absent or less apparent on the skin overlying the cartilage (see Figure 5-2).

RIM INCISION

The cartilage-splitting incision does not suffice in the square of round nasal tip. The bifid nasal tip also requires a rim incision and full delivery (Figure 5-4), as does a radical tip change. A rim incision is usually necessary in a projecting tip, especially when the projection is marked. Sometimes, however, the nasal spine is so prominent that it lifts and projects the entire tip of the nose. If so, no work is needed on the tip cartilage; the anatomy needs no change other than to be receded.

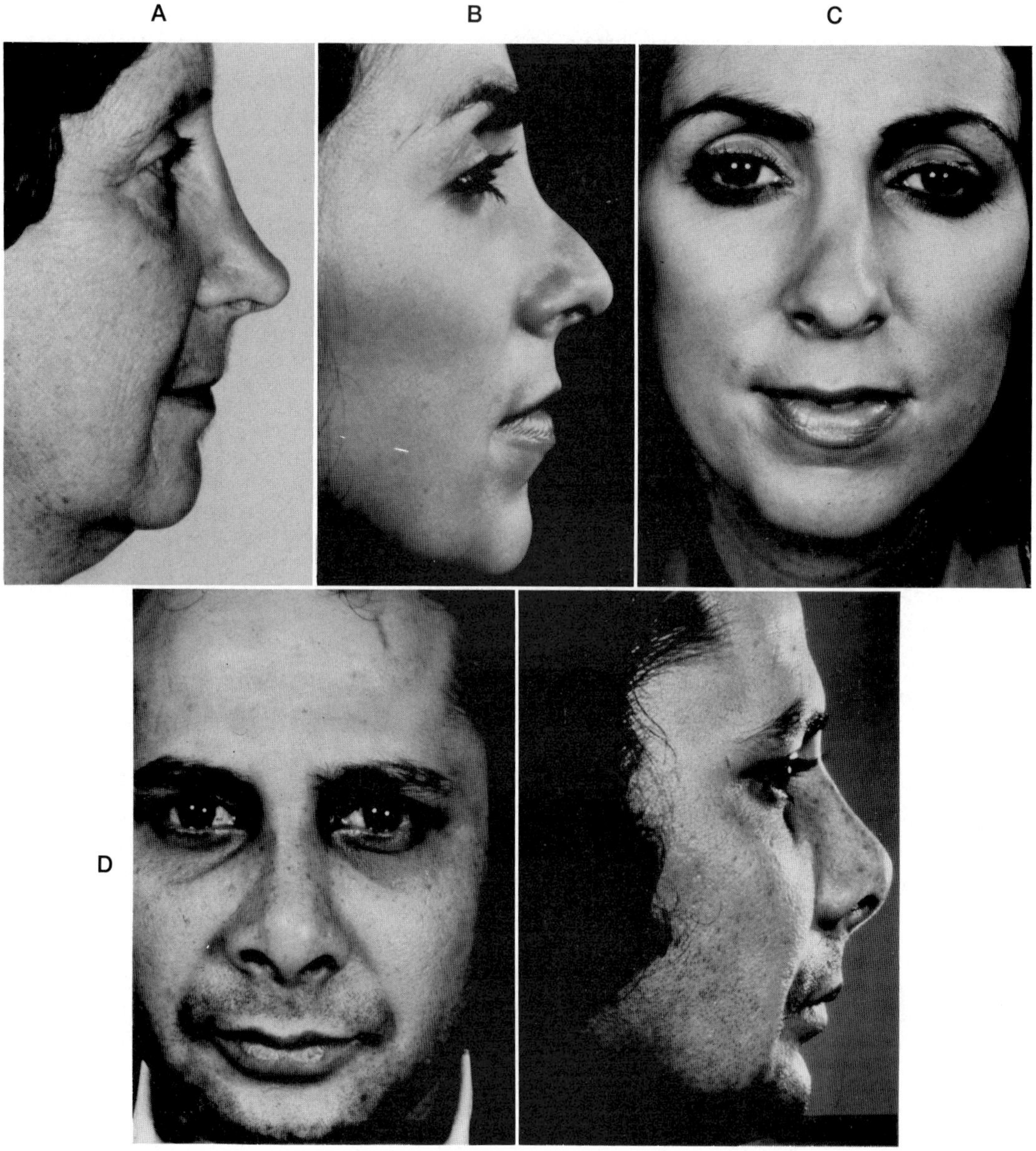

A   B   C

D

Figure 5-1. Old types of rhinoplasty stigmata. **A,** The ski slope, an excessive rhinoplasty carried out in an elderly patient where relatively small changes should be made. **B,** A polly-beak, in this case caused by excessive hump removal rather than failure to remove septal and upper lateral cartilage. **C,** "Open-roof" deformity, failure to infracture the nasal bones. **D,** "Pug nose" caused by excessive removal of caudal septum. The nasolabial angle in a male should be approximately 90 degrees.

Figure 5-2. The cartilage-splitting incision gives an excellent delivery and exposure of the cephalic margin of the alar cartilage, which can be excised accurately under direct vision with preservation of the vestibular skin.

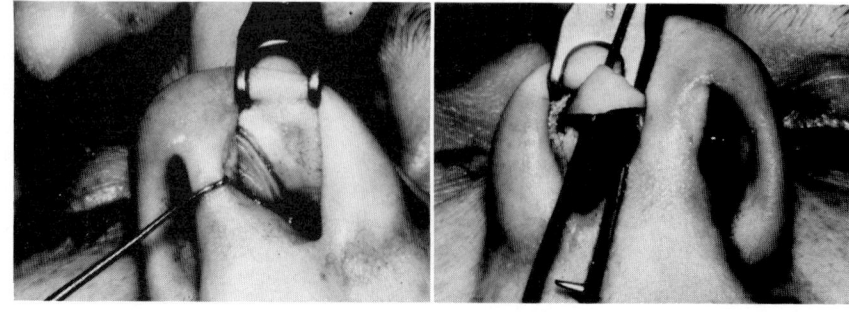

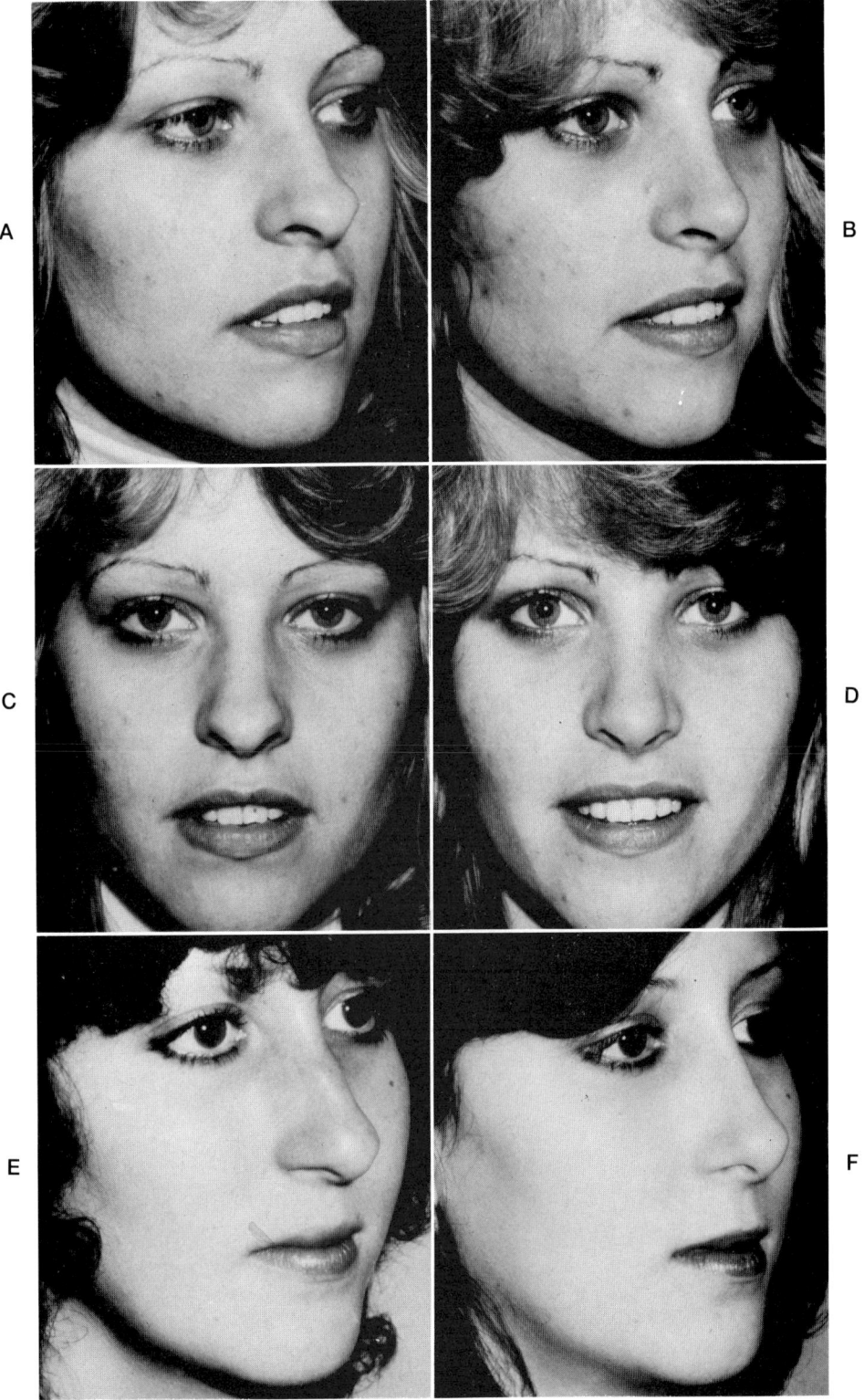

Figure 5-3. A-F, Removal of the cephalic margin of the alar cartilage achieves narrowing and rotation of the tip, which is the most common requirement in tip surgery. A subtle but definite change with narrowing also seen in the postoperative photograph.

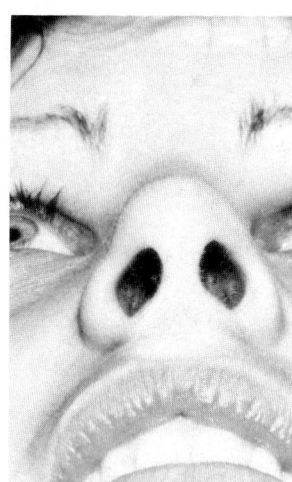

Figure 5-4. Rim-incision and full-delivery technique of the alar cartilages is necessary for gross tip deformities such as this bifid tip.

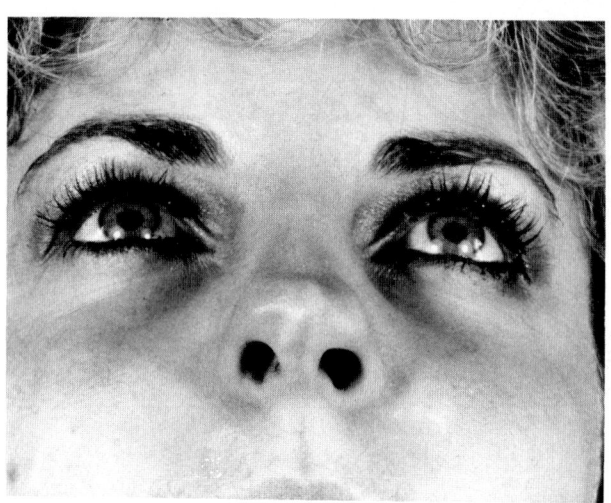

Figure 5-5. Morcellization techniques, particularly on strong cartilages with thin skin, can produce gross tip asymmetries, as in this case.

A difficult nose to manage is one with a projecting pointed tip, strong alar cartilages, and thin, aging, and atrophic skin. Problems can arise with morceling and dicing techniques, which aim to give a minimal change but in fact may cause conspicuous irregularities apparent through thin skin (Figure 5-5). If the dome is divided asymmetrically the cartilage tends to spring apart, producing a conspicuous deformity that may be awkward to revise. With a rim incision tooth forceps may break a brittle cartilage; these types of coarse forceps are better avoided in handling alar cartilage.

SHORT COLUMELLA

The short columella is a trap, certainly in early rhinoplasty experience, particularly when combined with a nasal hump. Not infrequently only the nasal tip needs raising to the level of the nasal hump, which is therefore apparent rather than real (Figure 5-6). One technique popularized by Goldman is to suture the medial crura back to back, after having delivered them and divided them lateral to the domes (Figure 5-6). Lengthening the columella and performing tip projection with this technique achieves long-term maintenance, which may not always be the case with

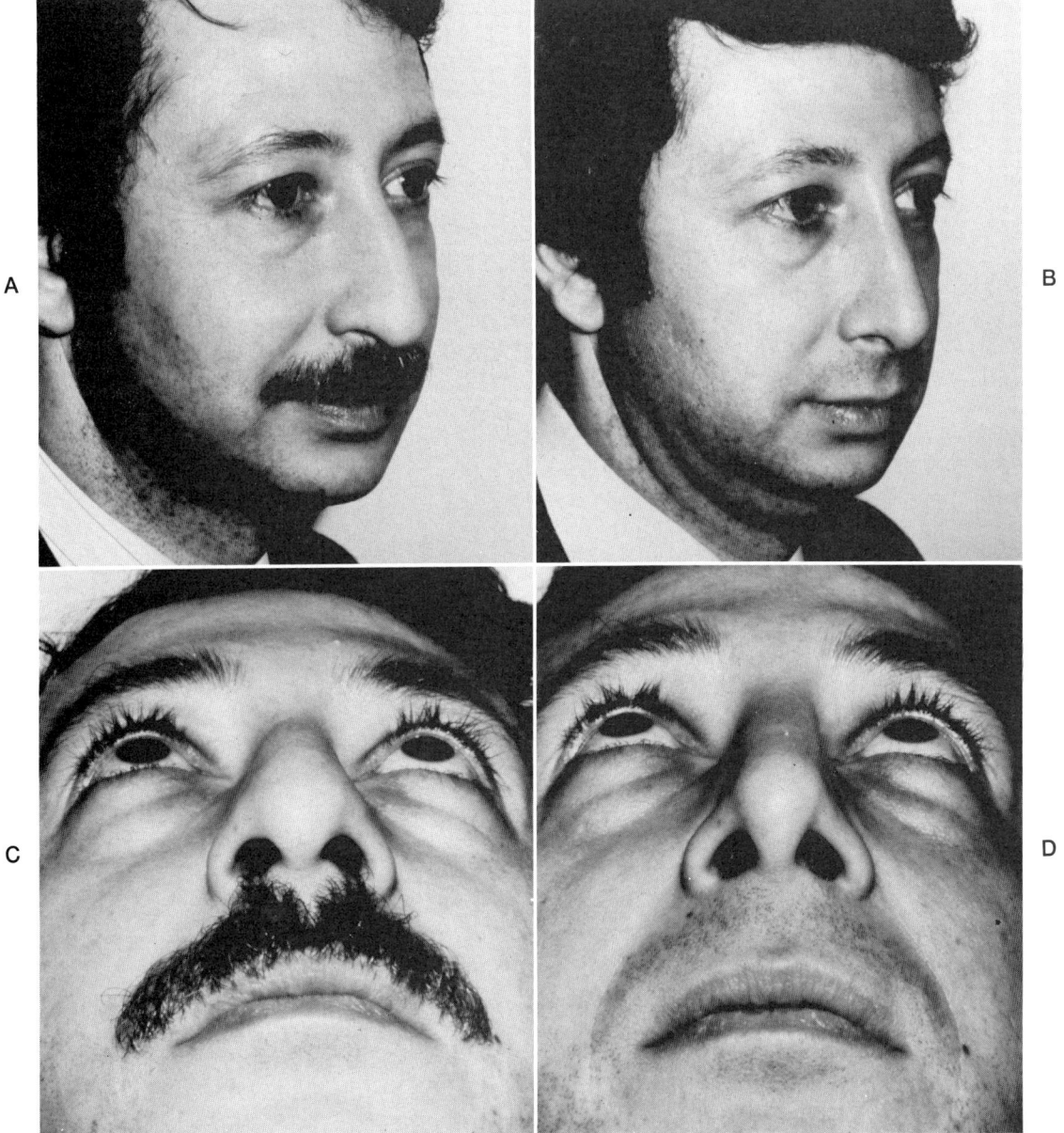

Figure 5-6. A-D, A short columella in which a deformity (of the polly-beak type) can be caused by excessive removal of the nasal hump. In this case, simple elevation of the tip is all that is required to achieve a satisfactory result.   *Continued.*

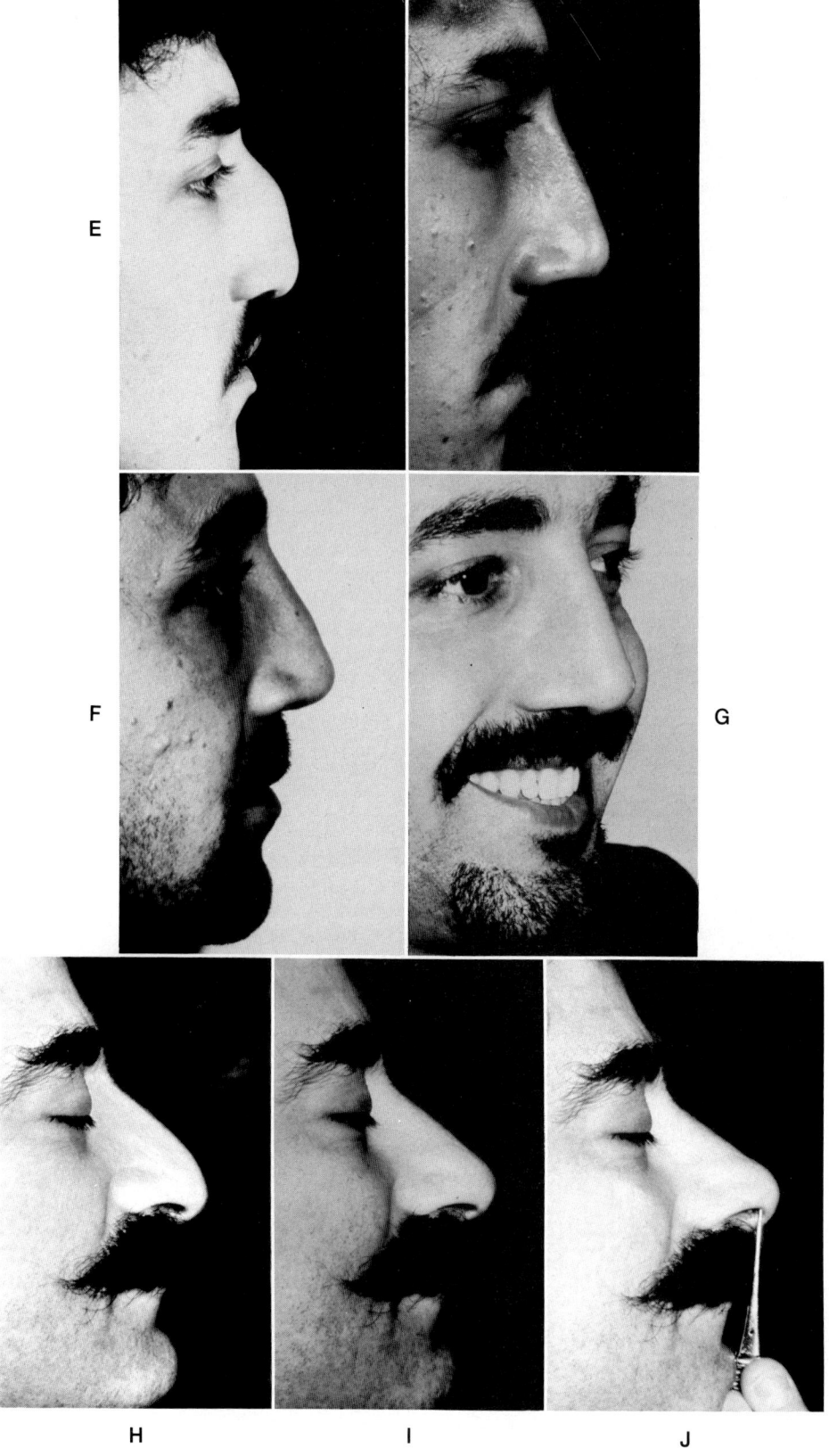

Figure 5-6, cont'd. **E** and **F,** A Goldman-type technique was used to lengthen this extremely short columella. **G,** Fifteen years later the tip remains well projected and exhibits no tendency to pull down when smiling. **H** and **I,** The hump that presents is eliminated by raising the tip. **J,** This is achieved as a preoperative demonstration by elevating the tip of the nose with a probe from the opposite side.

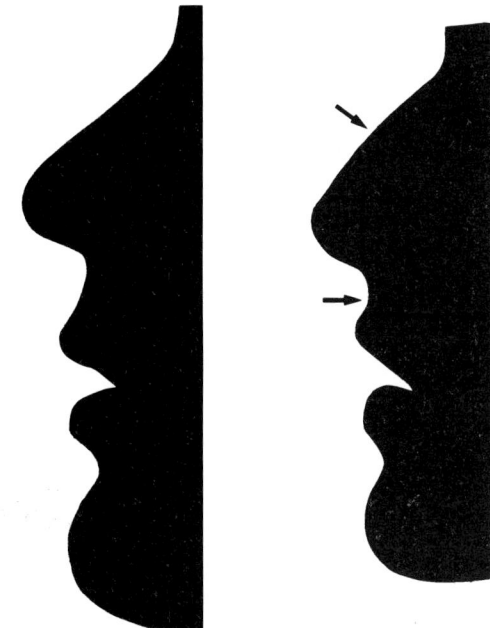

Figure 5-7. The pull of the musculus depressor septi may produce a polly-beak appearance, pulling down the nasal tip, and also curl and "crowd" the upper lip, resulting in excessive gum exposure.

struts and battons. It is a perfectly useful technique for the long, curved nose with a short columella. In a male, reducing the size may emasculate the nose; raising the tip and removing little or no nasal hump avoids this untoward result.

DEPRESSOR MUSCULUS SEPTI

One nasal muscle is surgically relevant in tip rhinoplasty—the depressor musculus septi. With smiling, the nasal tip is often pulled downward by this muscle and the upper lip curls upward, exposing gum (Figure 5-7). This muscle is particularly important in the nose with the short columella because it accentuates the short columella with the pull exerted during talking and smiling at its insertion into the alar cartilage. Surgical division of the muscle releases the lip and reduces the curled, crowded appearance as well as releasing the pull on the nasal tip (Figure 5-8, A and B). The muscle is also important in the hypermobile nasal tip where excessive movement is noticed while talking, as the muscle causes the cartilage domes to move excessively and obviously.

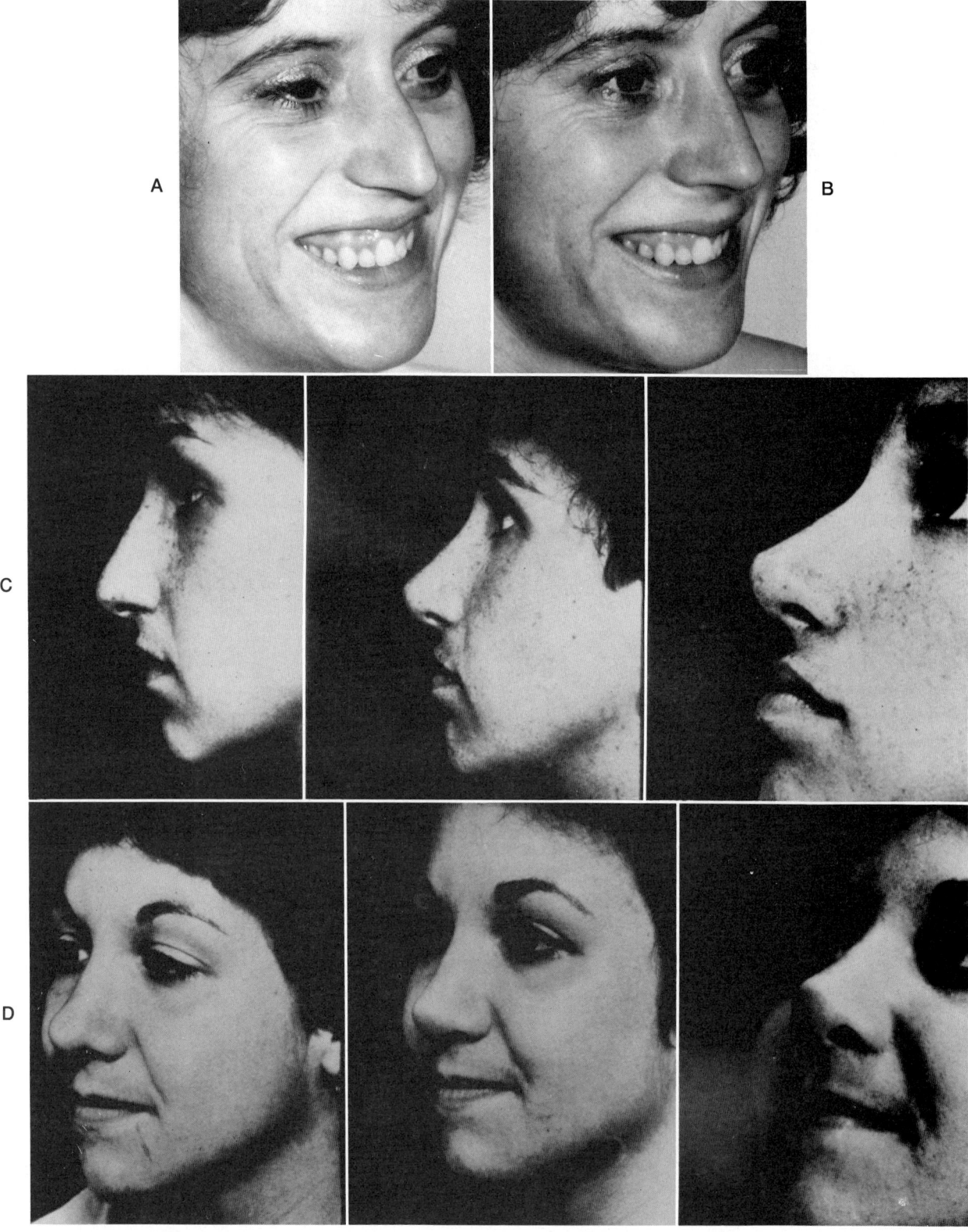

Figure 5-8. A and **B,** Division of the musculus depressor septi stops the pull on the nasal tip, prevents the hypermobile nasal tip, and may, on occasion, release the pull on the upper lip and be a factor in diminishing excess show of gum on smiling. **C** and **D,** It may be arguable as to whether a tip graft is a technique of finesse and produces of a refined tip, or produces an excessively "surgical" result on occasion.

TIP GRAFTS

Finesse in rhinoplasty is a term currently popular in nasal plastic surgery procedures. The tip graft popularized by Sheen was meant to give further refinement and definition to the tip of the nose. In primary rhinoplasty, however, I think this graft has a very small place; its role is mainly in revision rhinoplasty. A series of results with these grafts make me question its efficacy (Figure 5-8, *C* and *D*). The appearance of the nose may be surgical and the definition conspicuous and unnatural. Obviously individual taste is relevent; the surgeon must rely on his or her own judgment as well as the wishes of the patient to decide whether this type of tip definition is aesthetically pleasing.

SUMMARY

Over a decade ago Ralph Millard said, "Rhinoplasty is all take and no give." This remains a relevant aphorism, although clearly replacement of nasal tissue is now advisable in many cases, such as saddling and revision rhinoplasty. However, for primary routine rhinoplasty I think Ralph Millard's dictum is still generally valid.

6

Tip Projection—
Some Helpful Techniques

Thomas Rees

Achieving acceptable tip projection is the subject of much attention these days. Unquestionably more tip grafts fashioned from septal or ear cartilage are being performed, which can be attributed in large measure to the influence of Drs. Sheen, Ortiz-Monasterio, and Peck. Of course the problem has long been recognized, and various maneuvers, including tip grafts, have been proposed and practiced by many rhinoplastic surgeons. Goldman especially was interested in the topic and devised the so-called Goldman tip operation to provide both narrowness and projection. Personally, I believe there are more free-floating cartilage grafts being placed in the tip than are actually necessary.

Several traditional, well-tested techniques for achieving tip projection, or at least the illusion of projection, should be remembered (Figures 6-1 and 6-2). An important concept is that tip projection can

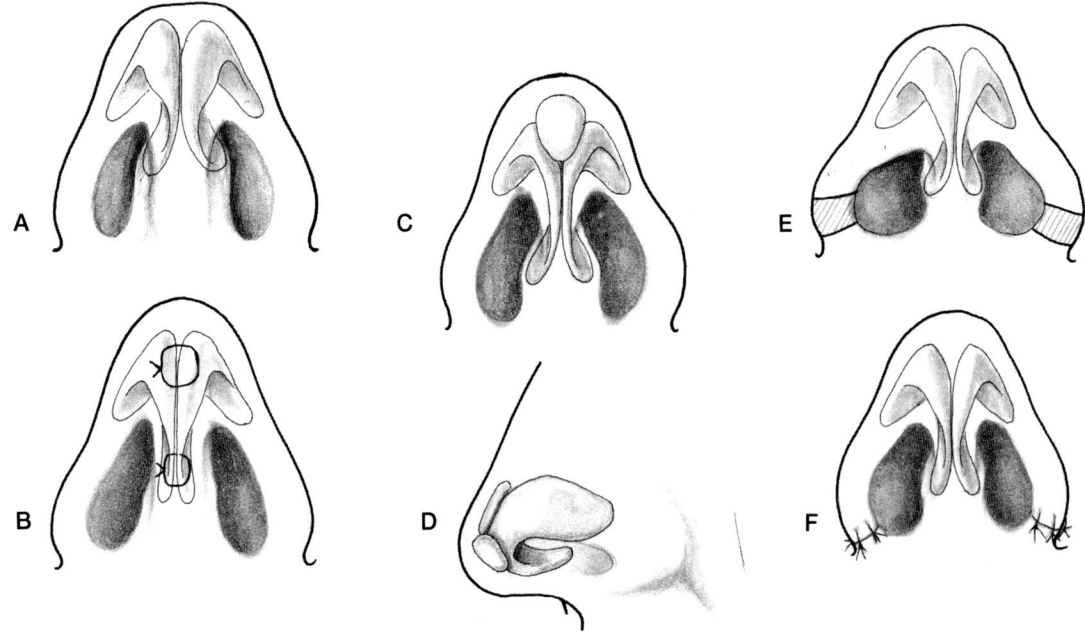

Figure 6-1. Maneuvers useful in providing tip projection. **A** and **B,** Increasing tip projection by overcoming diastasis of the alar cartilages. The spread cartilages are sutured together at the genu and at the feet of the medial crura. **C** and **D,** Graft augmentation of the tip. **E** and **F,** Alar base resections help to reduce width of the base of the nose and help achieve some forward thrust.

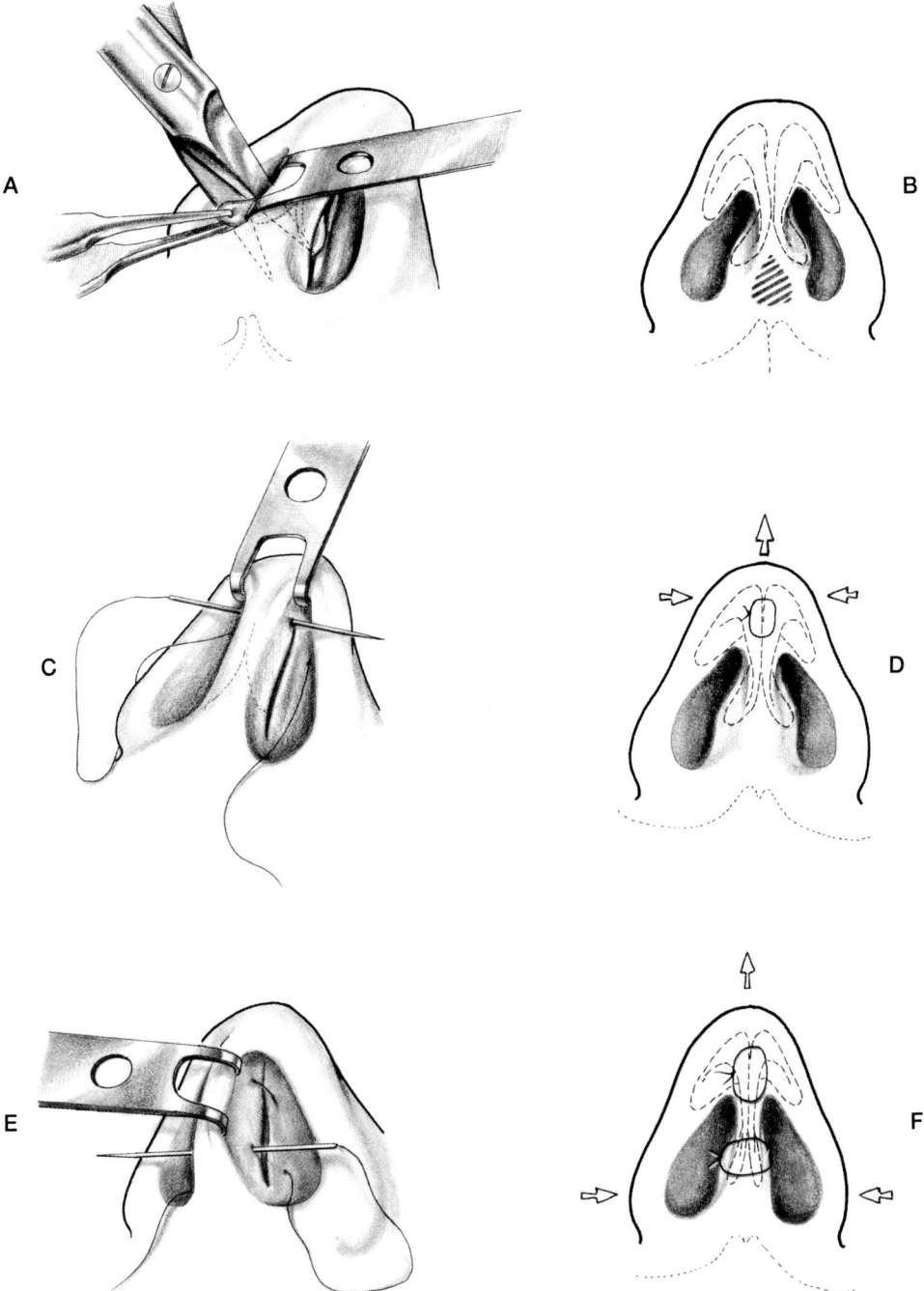

Figure 6-2. The base of the columella can be narrowed to promote tip projection by even 2 or 3 mm. **A,** The muscle and fibrofatty tissue is dissected from between the feet of the medial crura, which are often spread. **B,** Area of resection indicated. **C** and **D,** Mattress sutures approximate the alar cartilages at the tip. Arrows indicate narrowing and the forward thrust that occurs. **E** and **F,** Mattress suture at the base of the columella narrows the base and contributes to the forward thrust. These technical aids all add up to minimal but effective projection of the tip. Even 2 or 3 mm can be helpful.

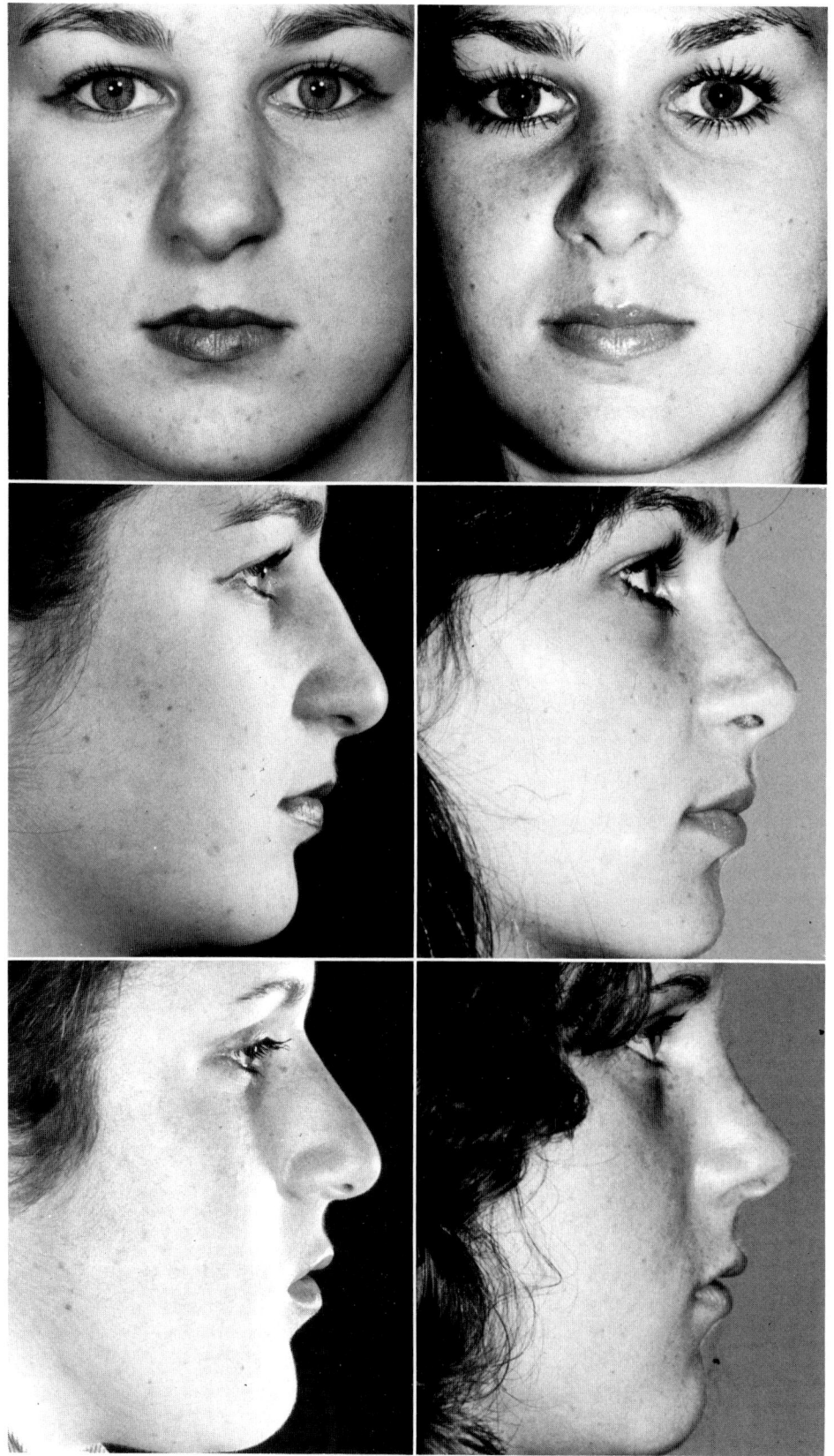

Figure 6-3. Both patients could be considered candidates for tip grafts. Adequate projection (in the author's opinion) was achieved in each by employing the techniques described in Figure 6-2, along with rotation of the tip.

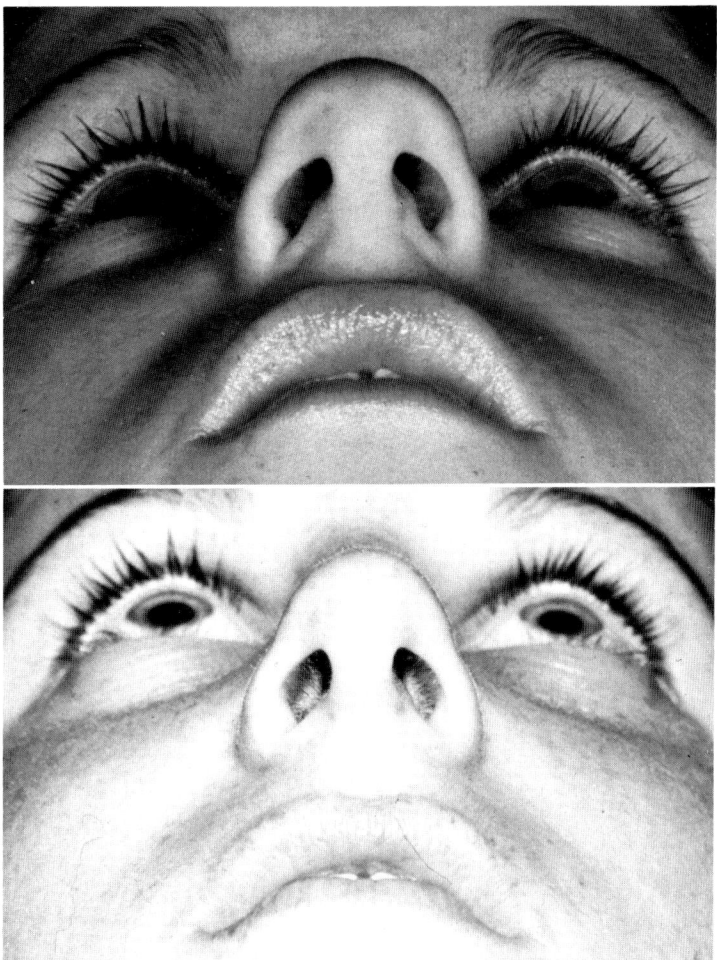

Figure 6-3, cont'd. For legend see opposite page.

be measured in millimeters. An increase of even 1 or 2 millimeters can, in certain instances, be significant. Simply narrowing the tip can also prove helpful by creating the visual impression of projection. Narrowing the boxy tip and approximating the medial crura by eliminating any diastasis also helps. Direct suturing of the medial crura at the genu as well as approximating and suturing the feel of the medial crura at the base of the columella also achieves a couple of millimeters of forward thrust to the tip. Undermining and medial rotation of the alar bases provides a medial shift of all tissues at the base of the nose, which is translated into a slight projecting force (Figure 6-3).

These maneuvers have been described in correction of the non-Caucasian nose, but are certainly applicable to Caucasian noses as well. Reshaping the alar tip cartilages by morcellation or weakening to decrease the angle formed between the medial and lateral crura is practiced frequently, possibly without any realization that this routine procedure is, in fact, increasing the apparent projection of the nasal tip.

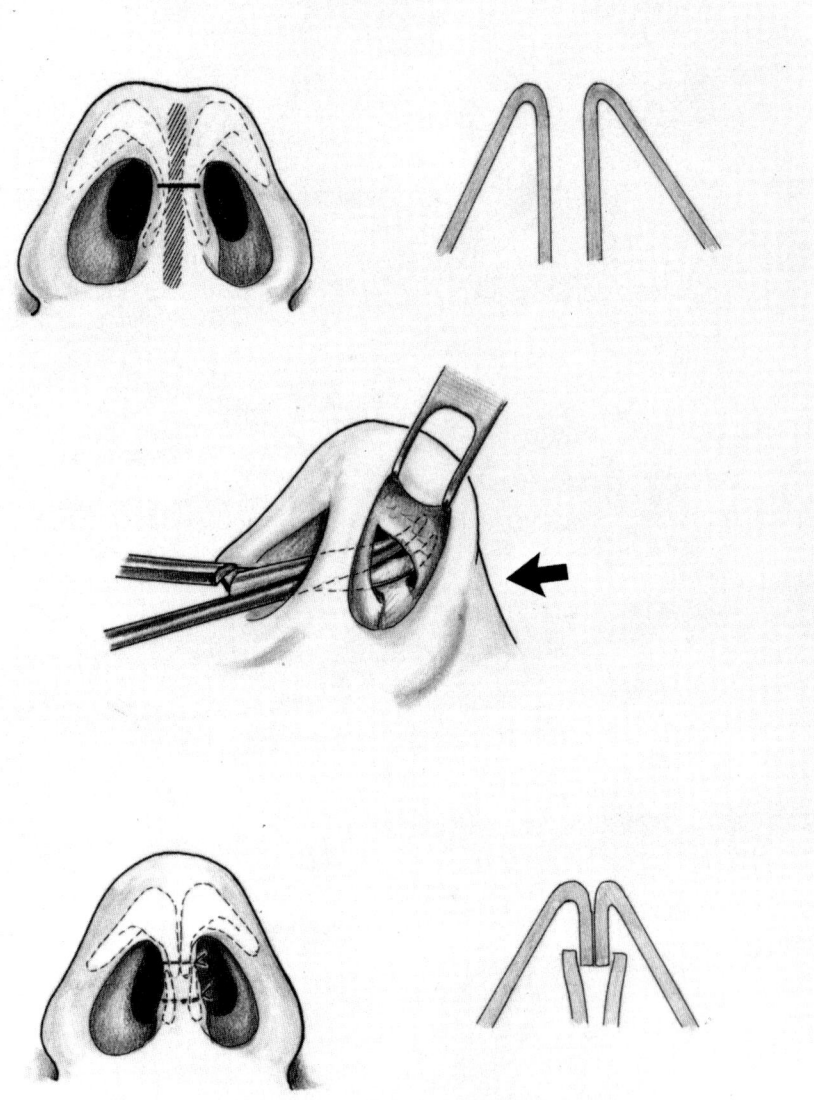

Figure 6-4. To achieve narrowing of the tip and slight recession, the alar cartilages are undermined completely to overcome diastasis that is promoted by fibrous attachments as shown by the large arrow in the center drawing. The medial crura can be transected well around the medial side of the genu. This combination permits medial displacement of the tips of the alar cartilages as well as slight recession if required. These forces are indicated by the small arrows.

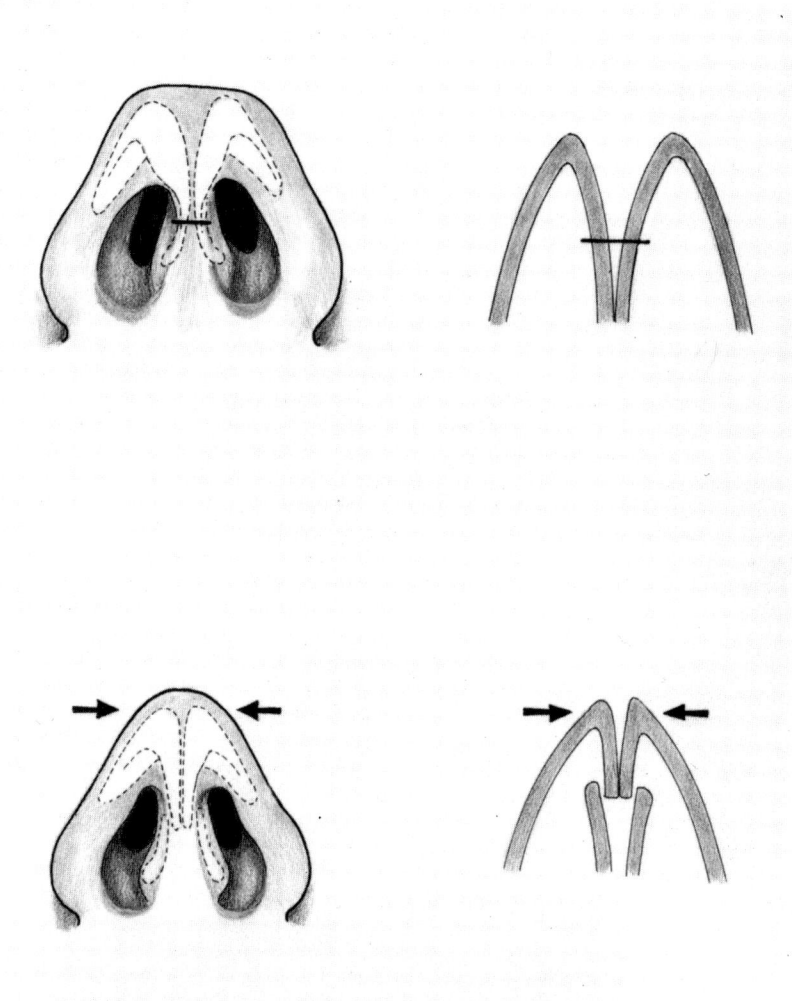

Figure 6-4, cont'd. For legend see opposite page.

Another problem, the reverse of increasing tip projection, is reducing tip projection. Reduction of the dorsal profile, even when performed conservatively, can create the impression that the tip is overly long. Frequently during routine rhinoplasty I recess the tip slightly and bring the domes together by the technique illustrated in Figure 6-4. The alar arch is visualized as a triangle (Figure 6-5). To recess the triangle it can be transected both laterally and medially. I emphasize the word *transection* rather than *resection,* since resection of a piece of cartilage from either the medial or lateral crus would result in a notch deformity, especially of the lateral nostril rim. Transsection permits a periscoping of the fragments and a "settling" of the tip (Figure 6-6).

Text continued on page 55.

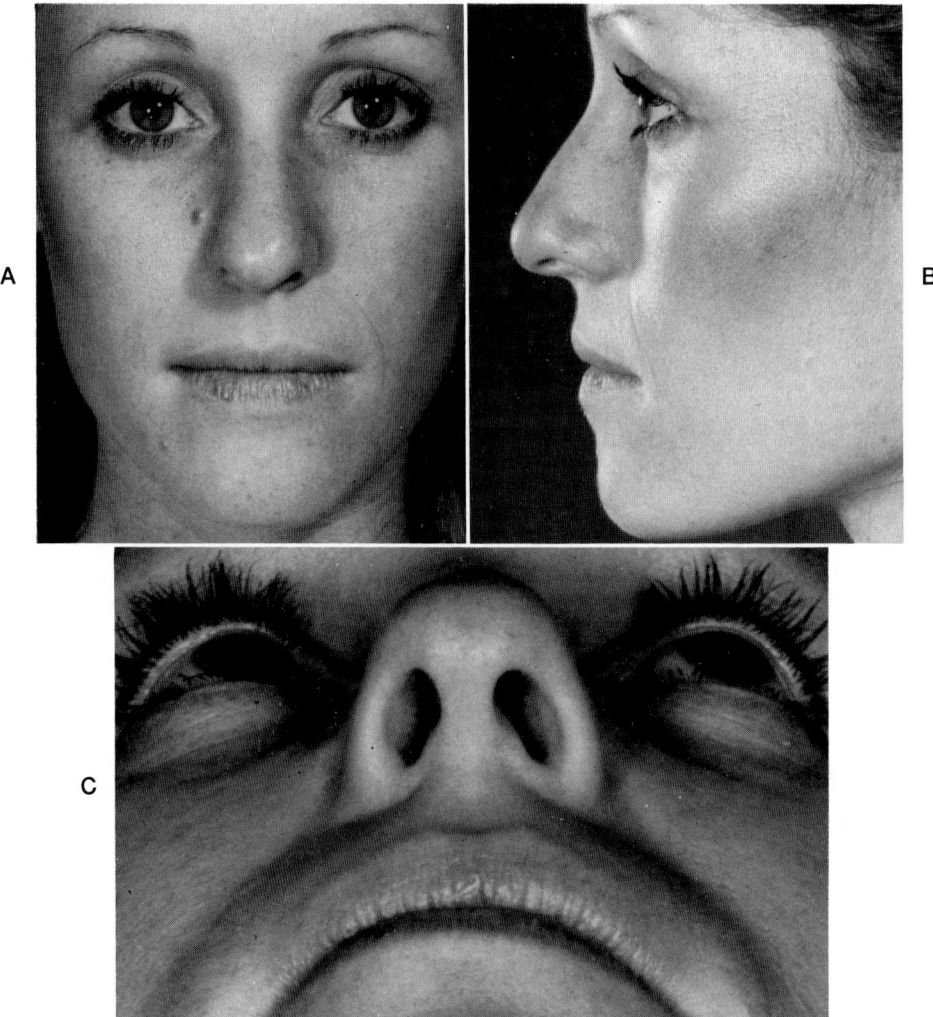

Figure 6-5. This patient has wide tip cartilages that are diastatic. She lacks definition and delicacy. The procedure described in Figure 6-4 provided medial shifting of the domes after resection of the excessive cephalic portion of the lateral crura. **A, B,** and **C** are preoperative photographs; **D, E,** and **F** are postoperative. Note in the inferior or "worm's eye" views that there is more apparent projection to the tip after this technique.

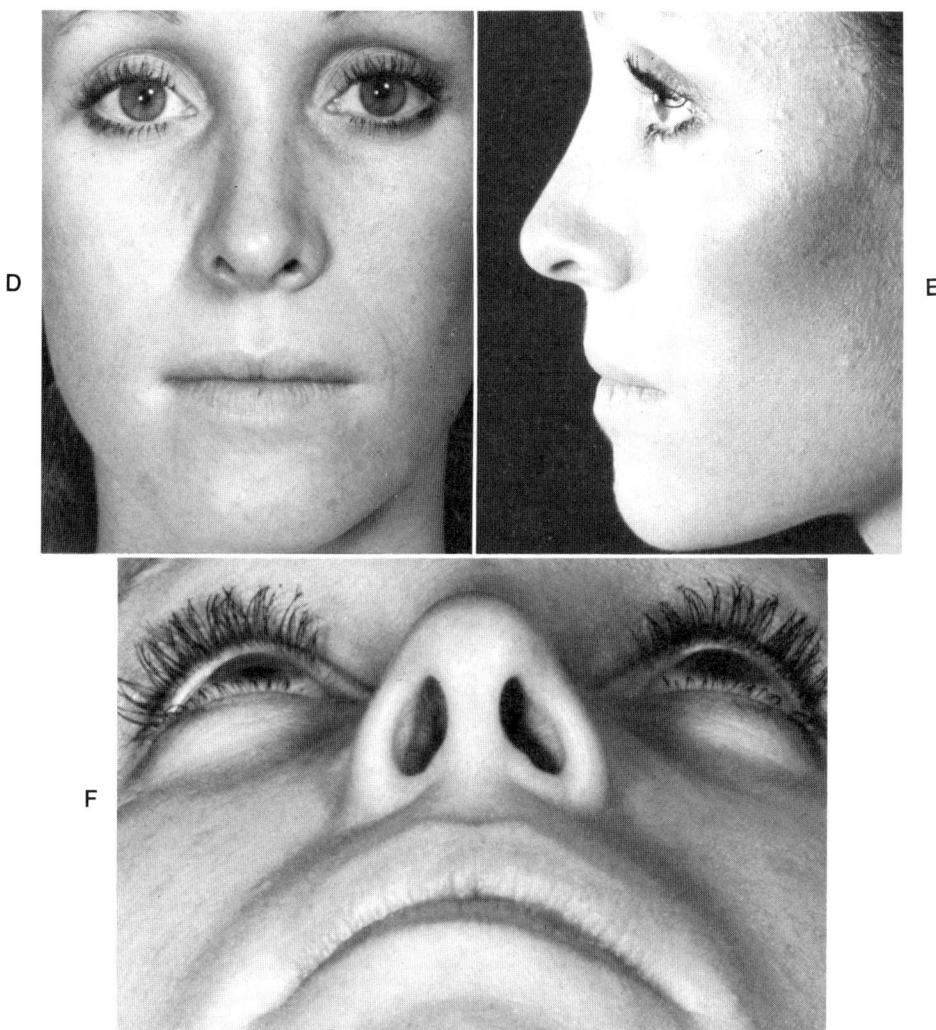

Figure 6-5, cont'd. For legend see opposite page.

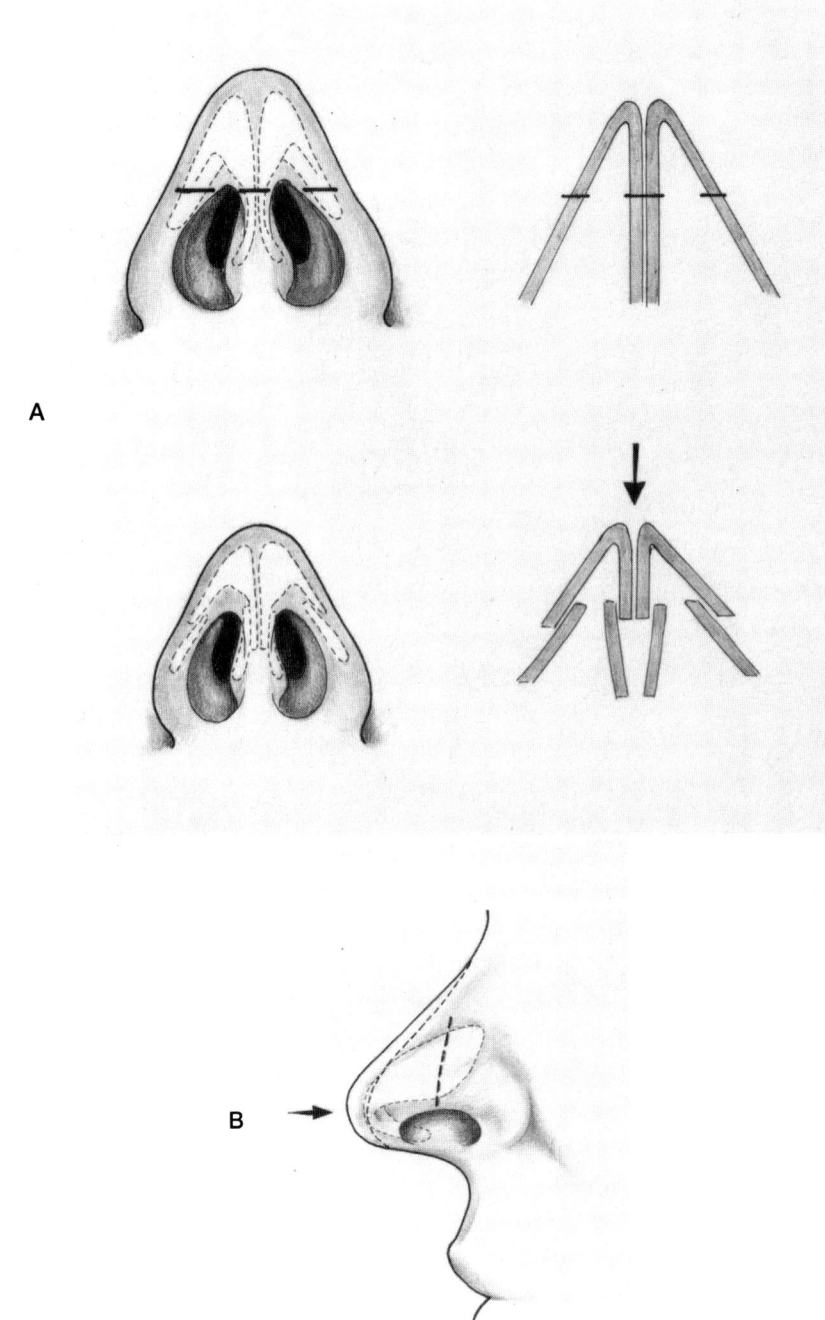

Figure 6-6. Excessive forward projection of the tip can be improved by recessing the alar cartilages. **A,** If one visualizes the alar cartilages as a tripod, then cutting through the legs of the tripod and allowing the cut ends to telescope permit recession of the tip of the tripod. This maneuver is especially helpful in setting back slightly prominent nasal tips, which are not so protuding as to require resection of the domes or genu. **B,** Transection of the lateral crus should be located near the flange.

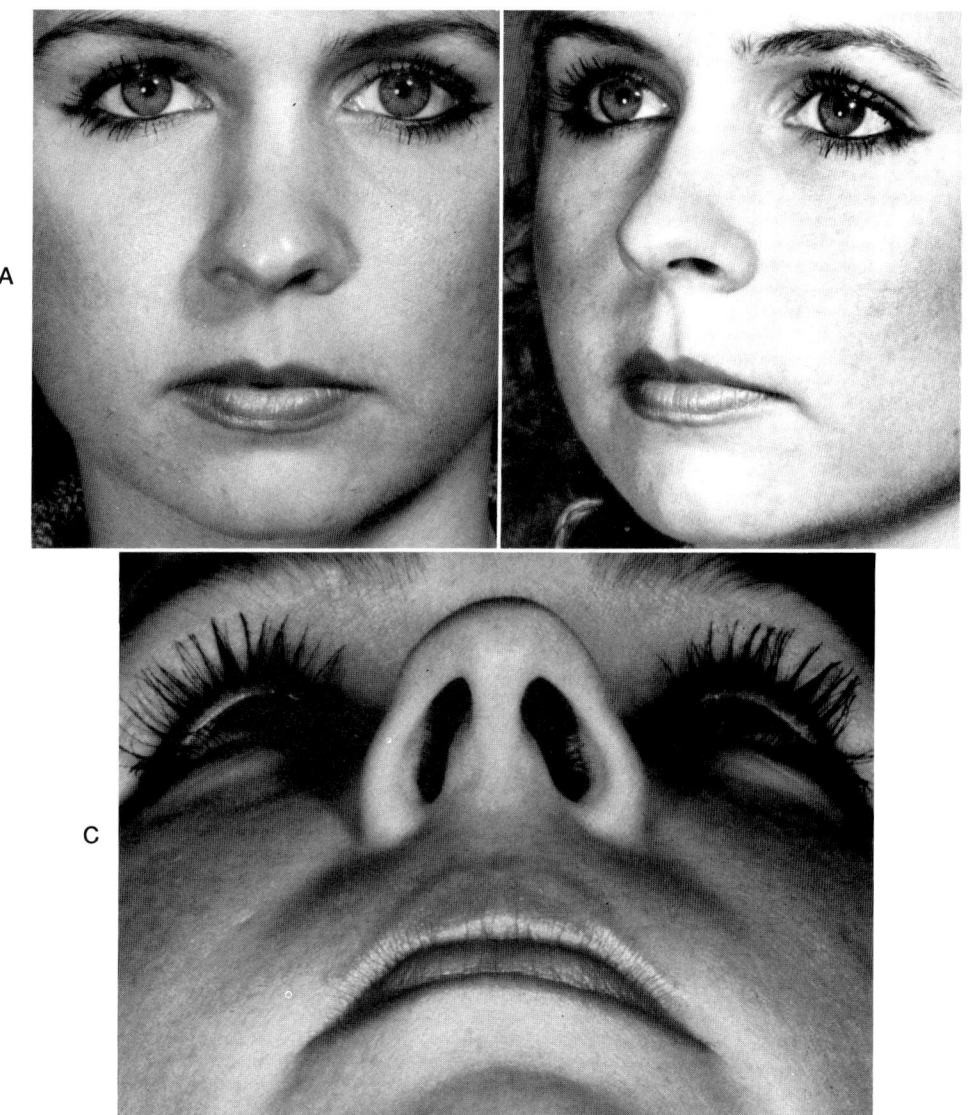

Figure 6-7. This patient posed a minor but difficult problem. Her main complaint was excessive projection of the tip of her nose. Examination of the preoperative photos (**A, B,** and **C**) revealed that the tip not only projected, but that there was also an excess of lateral crura and a flattening of the nose just above the genu.

Continued.

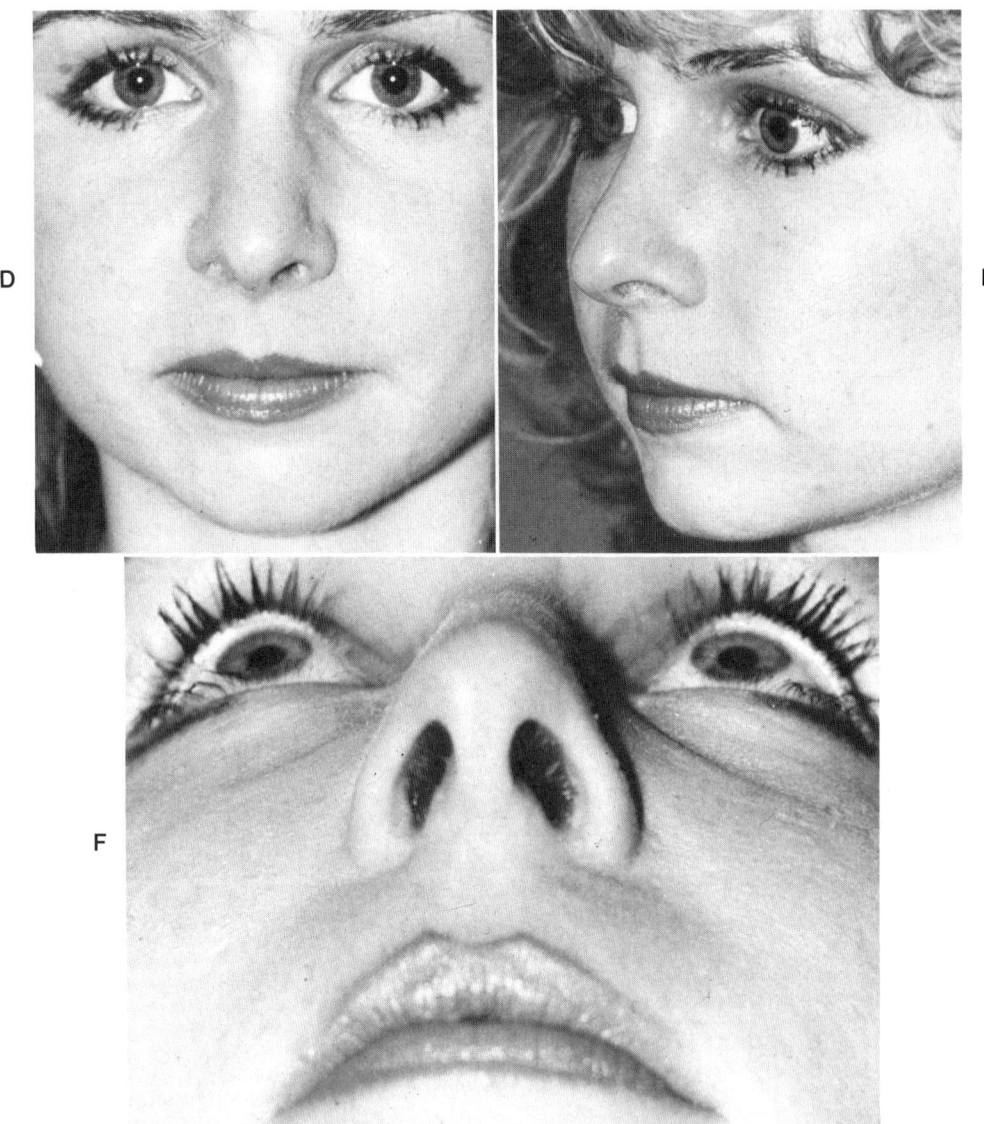

Figure 6-7, cont'd. Postoperative photos (**D, E,** and **F**). Correction was achieved by resecting the excessive lateral crura, and recessing the tripod as described in Figures 6-6 and 6-8. The result is a softening effect.

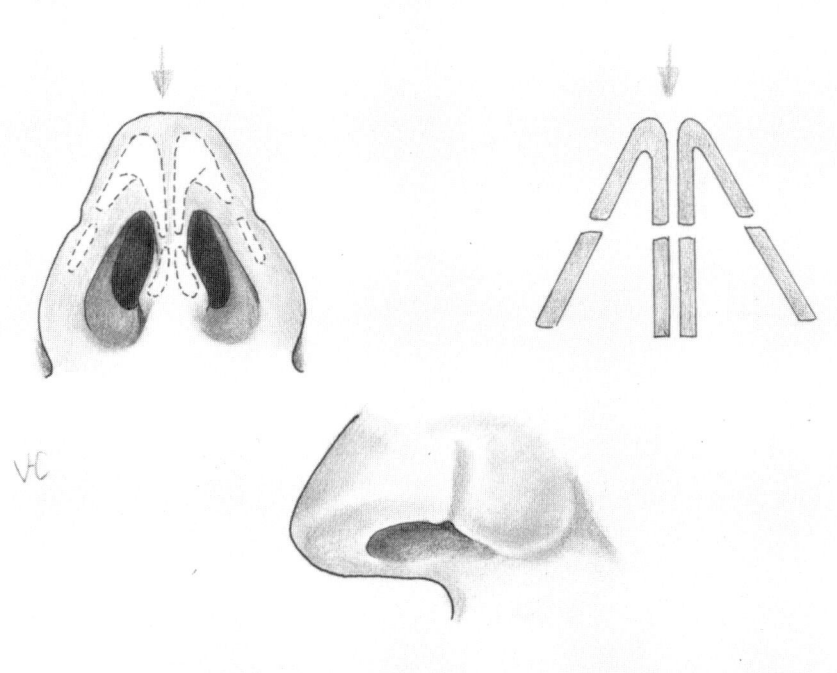

Figure 6-8. Transection of the lateral and medial crura is preferable to excising strips, because excision can result in a notching of the nostril at the point where lateral crus is excised. Allowing the cut end to overlap obviates the notching problem.

Transecting the cartilages proximal to the dome or genu maintains the natural arch of the tip and prevents sharp cartilage points from appearing after surgery. The patient in Figure 6-7 has a difficult tip problem with reasonably prominent forward projection. The recession maneuver (Figure 6-8) resulted in a softening of the tip as well as a very real recession. The transection technique is also useful as an adjunct procedure in correcting the extreme projecting tip in the so-called Pinocchio nose.

I reserve tip grafts for use in those patients in whom I cannot achieve tip projection by more traditional means. If in doubt as to whether a tip graft is needed or not, I prefer to wait a few months and see. A graft can always be performed as a secondary procedure.

Point & Counterpoint
Part I

Question: Is it necessary to make a complete transfixion incision?

Comment (George Peck): I have changed my technique in the last few years. If you make an intracartilaginous incision and carry it around into the transfixion, a horseshoe-shaped incision results that can heal as a constricting scar. If you look at these noses postoperatively you see many contracture scars that could have been prevented. The entire rhinoplasty can be done through bilateral cartilage–splitting incisions separating the transfixion incision completely so that there is an intact bridge of vestibular skin between the two incisions.

Comment (Jack Sheen): I like to limit the incisions as much as possible. I think it is extremely important to do so. There should be no routine incisions in rhinoplasty. Each cut, including the transfixing incision, should have a specific purpose. I disagree with Dr. Peck's statement about vestibular scar contracture caused by transfixing incisions joining intercartilaginous incisions. I join these incisions all the time and I don't get scar contractures in the vestibule. Scars in the vestibule result only when mucosa is resected. I think synechiae are usually caused by resection of the upper lateral cartilages, especially when the caudal edge of the upper lateral cartilages with mucosa is resected with right-angle upper lateral cartilage scissors.

Comment (Gene Tardy): There are times when I use a complete transfixion and there are times when I do not. I make that point only because I feel the supports of the nose are too often violated without purpose. If you maintain a complete attachment of the medial crura footplates to the base of the septum, why not limit the incision to a partial or limited transfixion? However, if you need to resect the nasal spine or gain access to the septum, a complete transfixion incision becomes necessary. There should not be a hard and fast rule.

Comment (Harvey Caplan): There are all degrees of transfixion incisions. I am intrigued by the so-called high transfixion incision, where the membranous septum is not detached, but a component of the inferior border to the septum, say about 2 to 3 mm, is contained in the lower segment by incising just cephalad to the caudal border of the septum. In this way the fibroligamentous crural attachments are undisturbed, yet the nose can be shortened if required. I do not object to a transfixion incision, but I do object to using large, heavy septocolumellar mattress sutures. I suture the mucous membrane to the vestibular lining with 5-0 catgut.

Question: What is tip rotation as contrasted to tip projection? Also, how do we recess the excessively projecting tip, the real Pinocchio nose?

Comment (Jack Sheen): Tip rotation is achieved by trimming the cephalic edges of the lower lateral cartilages, the caudal edges of the upper lateral cartilages, and to some extent, by the initial skeletonization. These maneuvers rotate the tip in a cephalic direction. Tip projection is the anterior-posterior dimension of the tip and is relative to the height of the dorsum. The tip can be projected by altering the arch of the lower lateral cartilages or by using tip grafts.

There are two ways to improve the appearance of the ultraprojecting tip. One is to raise the root of the nose if the nasion or the root of the nose is disproportionaely low. In such cases the tip of the nose appears to be overly projecting. Therefore, one can improve the balance by placing a graft to raise the dorsum at the root. The second way is to reduce the actual projection of the lower lateral cartilage. The easiest way, in my experience, is simply to resect the domes, taking a rather sizable segment of the medial and lateral crura at the domes. I find that I can reduce these about 2 to 3 mm. The soft tissues will settle down; you don't have to worry about spicules because as the tissues contract, they will thicken. If you overreduce the lower alteral cartilages, excessive thickening will occur, accompanied by loss of definition.

Comment (Wally Berman): I like to deliver the cartilages as a bipedicle flap in such noses, then create a unipedicle flap by incising through the medial columella and resection as many millimeters as I wish to decrease projection. The lateral cartilage is then rotated and becomes the new dome.

Comment (George Peck): I do exactly the opposite. This is a rare deformity. During the basic rhinoplasty, I leave a narrow rim of the lower lateral cartilage. In many patients that will correct the problem; however, if the tip is still projecting too much, I deliver the alar cartilage and weaken it with cross-cuts, especially the medial crura part of the dome, to create a new dome. I then excise a segment laterally from the lateral crura and this effectively lowers the domes.

Comment (Gene Tardy): The projecting tip is very difficult to correct, because many of these tips are under tension and have very thin skin overlying the skeletal structure. I try to determine what the cause of the excessive projection is, and then reduce these anatomical components. Sometimes it is the nasal spine that is at fault, and it must be reduced. I prefer to leave the domes intact whenever possible. Finally, I think that we should not try to make the nose too small. There is nothing wrong with a nose that is a little larger, as long as all of the lines and contours are proportionally large.

Comment (Tom Rees): The cardinal sin of trying to reduce a markedly projecting tip is to overly reduce the vault. I agree with Jack Sheen that we must frequently consider augmenting the dorsum in such problems. In severe degrees of projection, the domes must be excised and if the skin is very thin, it then becomes necessary to reconstruct the natural contours of the domes with a small crushed cartilage-onlay graft; otherwise one is left with sharp points in the tip. In lesser degrees of projection, I have found it useful to view the alar cartilages as a tripod that must be set back or recessed. I then cut through the medial crura on the medial side of the genu, and the lateral crura quite far laterally. The unsatisfied ends are then telescoped. This is a very useful maneuver.

Question: What about warping of the cartilage grafts? You are now using two, three, or even four thicknesses, but if you use a single thickness of graft from the quadrangular plate of the cartilage of the septum, do you have warping problems over a period of time, particularly with thin, tight-skinned individuals?

Comment (Jack Sheen): No, I have not had any problems with warping of the nasal cartilage. If you maintain the integrity of the cortical portion by scraping or contouring the graft just on the edges, the graft will not warp.

Question: Do you have any idea of the percentage of primary cases in which you use a tip graft today?

Comment (Jack Sheen): I use some type of tip graft, for either contour or projection in about 30% of my primary rhinoplasties.

Comment (George Peck): This is a difficult question to answer. It depends on the individual problem at hand. I would say that at the present time I am using some sort of onlay graft to the tip in about 40% of my patients, but then I am especially enthusiastic just now.

Comment (Gene Tardy): It is always very difficult to quote meaningful percentages because you may encounter three patients in a row who require tip grafts and then none for awhile. The need is infrequent in primary cases unless there is significant inadequacy of tip projection. Most patients that I see are Caucasian patients who are concerned about either a tip that is too wide or too bulbous, or who wish profile changes. Most such patients have satisfactory tip projection to begin with; therefore, it is my responsibility to preserve what is already there. I would estimate that I do tip grafts in less than 10% of my primary cases.

Question: Have you totally given up using vomer or ethmoid bone as tip grafts:

Comment (Tony Bull): I use bone as a filler in the nose, but I prefer to use cartilage. I don't like L-shaped struts. I think they invariably look surgically created, and you've got to have a pretty ugly nose to trade it for a surgical appearance. Cartilage is best, especially the patient's own septal cartilage, if you've got it, or that from the ear; both are preferable to bone. Bone is okay as a filler in saddle or perhaps a columella. I also like some plastics. All around the world people are saying, "Well, I am taking out other peoples' plastics; they don't work." Well, I had a registrar who said that, and of the last 63 we did, we didn't lose any. I use plastic a lot. The patients who do best with it are those with racial saddling. I don't think with augmentation there is one best choice. Plastics are not to be discarded. They are useful.

Comment (Ralph Millard): No, I think we all believe that bone does not stay in the tip, I believe that even Jack Sheen will admit that now. No question about it, a piece of bone in the tip is going to go.

Comment (Wolfgang Mühlbauer): I use bone. You need a good pocket and wide dissection so there is not so much strain and tension on the bone. Of course, it also must be revitalized; the blood circulation must be established in a limited amount of time.

Question: How is that done? Through the soft tissue? In contact with bone?

Comment (Wolfgang Mühlbauer): Contact with bone is only at the lower nasal spine and the inferior edge of the nasal bones. The rest is soft tissue.

Comment (Jack Sheen): I now use ethmoid or vomer as fillers only; that is, to improve contour rather than to provide support. I have found that vomer does not withstand stresses well: therefore, I will not use it as a primary supportive graft for the tip.

Comment (Gene Tardy): I do not use bone in the tip or columella. I use only autogenous cartilage in the nose in general. I sometimes use bone to correct other than tip deformities, and I also use fascia. It is my firm conviction that alloplastic implants have no place in nasal reconstruction.

Comment (George Peck): I would like to emphasize that I much prefer cartilage. I would not use anything except autogenous material, by the way, and I have seen some disastrous results after using other than autogenous material.

Comment (Rodolphe Meyer): I sometimes use iliac bone in difficult secondary cases, but I, too, prefer cartilage.

Question: While we are on the subject of cartilage grafts, is there any virtue in leaving perichondrium on the cartilage graft?

Comment (Gene Tardy): It depends on what you are using it for. In some children, I think perichondrial preservation may be a useful principle. I like to leave perichondrium on all grafts when extensive carving and sculpting are involved, since it contributes nicely to graft shape and stiffness. I prefer to use septal cartilage when it is available for grafting of the tip because I like the bulk strength and integrity of that cartilage; no perichondrium is employed with septal cartilage. I don't really think it makes a lot of difference in the adult. In a child I think it might, because of its neochondrogenic potential.

Comment (George Peck): I never leave perichondrium with the ear cartilage. I think that in his studies of cartilage grafts Dr. Lyndon Peer showed pretty well that it really did not make any difference for survival.

Comment (Jack Sheen): I do not leave perichondrium attached except with ear cartilage grafts, in which I leave it attached to the posterior side.

Question: Dr. Sheen, please explain your technique of using multiple grafts in the tip, rather than a single graft.

Comment (Jack Sheen): The multiple graft technique was developed because of some unsatisfactory results I had using a single graft. I now use additional grafts to stabilize the single graft and to fill out the tip lobule. By placing an anterior fill, I found that I could get a nice triangular look to the tip. I now use multiple long grafts and grafts anterior or posterior to the primary graft to create a softer, more natural-appearing tip.

Question: When grafts are placed in the nose from any source or donor site, after about 6 months or a year we often see little, sharp edges or small irregularities, especially along the borders of the graft. The nose looks wonderful until the last of the edema is resorbed, then these tiny defects show up even when the nose looks very good in general. There might be a little ridge, a depression, a small sharpness. Aside from the basic techniques we have all been talking about, what "tricks" might be used to obviate these small problems? How can these sequelae be prevented in the first place, and how can they be treated when they occur? "Knuckling" and "bossing" of the alar cartilages can of course occur without grafts. How do you prevent them?

Comment (Wally Berman): I like to deliver the cartilage whenever I can. I feel more secure when I see the problem firsthand and under direct vision. I can then morcellize it, or whatever else I wish. A little extra cartilage can be shaved off. For depressions, I admit to employing an occasional drop of silicone fluid.

Comment (Thomas Baker): I don't like to inject anything into the nose. Some surgeons advocate injection of droplets of silicone to fill depressions. If sharp edges or depressions appeared, I would use small autogenous grafts to cover them, usually cartilage. The only way I can approach the problem is to explore and see what is causing the defect and treat it accordingly.

Comment (Harvey Caplan): I call the small tip projections that occur "bosses." They are caused by buckling of the cartilage that has been weakened. I correct them under direct visual approach.

Comment (George Peck): I treat these problems if they are significant. In patients with thin skin and thick lower lateral cartilages, lines and edges will be seen. In one sense, that is exactly what makes a nice tip. If I have a small depression, I fill it with a small piece of cartilage, just a shaving. I also think that morcellization is an excellent means of softening the cartilage points.

Comment (Gene Tardy): I try to avoid sharp edges in my grafts by beveling the edges with a No. 15 blade. I sometimes abrade the sharp edges of the graft or morcellize it. I worry about morcellization, since there is some evidence that crushing of cartilage liberates chondroitin sulfate, which might lead to long-term absorption of the graft, even an autogenous cartilage graft. I usually try to avoid crushing, damaging, or otherwise injuring cartilage. I try to carefully carve the small wafer grafts, or layer them if necessary. Such grafts fill depressions very nicely.

Comment (Jack Sheen): I resect small irregularities under direct vision and often place crushed cartilage over defects if there is a depression. If one side of the tip is projecting and the other side flat, I treat the site opposite that which the patient seems to like. If the patient likes the pointed side, I create a point on the contralateral side. If the flatter side is preferred, I resect the point.

Comment (Tom Rees): I try to prevent points on my grafts with careful sculpting, shaving, crushing, morcellizing, or whatever I can do. Wrapping the grafts in fascia as suggested by Dr. Guerrero-Santos is also an excellent idea. For depressions, there is no question than a small drop or two of silicone fluid is excellent, but of course, the material is not available at this time. We are all wondering just what the newer and thicker collagen preparations might do to fill these small contour depressions.

Question: Before we get away from tip grafts, in the secondary case in which the tip is short, the skin nonelastic, and perhaps with thickened and scarred skin, is it possible to overcome this shortage of good soft tissue and obtain projection with a tip graft of free cartilage? In other words, can a tip graft overcome contracted soft tissue in terms of the aesthetic effect?

Comment (Frank Kamer): Yes, I think it can. The skin will give somewhat no matter how many times it has been operated on, as long as it has not been directly violated. Sometimes, it's difficult to get the graft in through thick scarring, but I know no other way to provide some projection except to replace tissue that has been removed.

Comment (Rodolphe Meyer): Yes, I think grafting helps, but it is best accomplished with septal cartilage if there is any available. If not, we must make ear cartilage do.

Comment (Tony Bull): Yes, tip augmentation helps, but the projection is an illusion. I think it is the mass caused by the graft that we are looking at and interpreting it as projection. If putting bits of cartilage in these revisional rhinoplasties provides the illusion of projection, then it is worthwhile, but I do not think that the cartilage is actually propping up the nose.

Comment (Wolfgang Mühlbauer): A solid bone graft in the middle of the columella or a composite graft can help, if the scar tissue can be loosened with a submucosal dissection. I think these free grafts of bone will survive in the columella, especially if it is iliac bone. Of course, I prefer a strong strut of septal cartilage, but in secondary cases there is rarely any septal cartilage left.

Comment (Guy Jost): I don't think real projection is obtained by putting any kind of graft into the col-

umella. If one measures from the nasolabial angle to the tip of the nose, the distance before and after inserting the implant in place is exactly the same. The tip of the nose does not participate in the shortening of the supratip area. I agree with Tony Bull that the projection of the tip noted in these cases is relative. It is relative at the same distance, but the nose is shortened a little bit.

Comment (Ralph Millard): I think obtaining projection depends on the case. When repairing the scarred tip, one must be aware of the position of the pocket and the platform base at the bottom of the pocket. It is the platform base that will support the graft and provide push to the tip, provided you have cartilage that is strong and will do the job. Septal cartilage is of course better in this regard than auricular cartilage. The thickness of the scar also affects the outcome. In some, we get actual projection and in others we get contour improvement, which picks up the highlight.

Comment (Tom Rees): I don't know if we have answered the question. I agree that grafts to the tip are often an illusion in that they pick up the highlights and do make the tip look higher and more projecting. I find them much easier from a technical point of view in the secondary case than in the primary. In the secondary case I can dissect the pocket exactly as I wish it, but in the primary after fully dissecting the nasal tissue, I have difficulty getting the graft to stay in position without wobbling back and forth. For this reason, I fix them transcutaneously with a suture.

Question: How many of you on the panel have used radiated cartilage allografts for the nose? How many use banked grafts that have been removed during routine SMR? Do you make a practice of banking cartilage from your submucous resections for possible use as allografts?

Comment (Ralph Millard): I used homologous rib grafts for chin implants years ago. Dr. Barret Brown convinced me of their usefulness during my training. After some experience and when I had a chance to evaluate them long term, I found that most of them absorbed.

Question: Does anyone use inert material of any kind as synthetic implants to the nasal tip, columella region, or lobule of the nose? Glass rods, tantalum, polyethylene, silicone, Teflon, and many others have all been used. Does anyone use them now?

Comment (Tony Bull): As I said earlier, I favor them for certain situations, but obviously not in the complicated or scarred tip. I use plastics sometimes, especially in non-Caucasian nose.

Question: We are considering alloplastic materials here for use in the primary, unscarred nose.

Comment (Frank Kamer): In primary cases no, I prefer autogenous materials. In secondary cases, I use plastic materials if I don't have enough material to harvest from the ear or the septum. I like Supramid rolled into a cylinder as a dorsal graft in the immobile portion of the nose.

Comment (Ralph Millard): I have used foreign body implants. They simply are incapable of supporting work. If you stress them in any way, they will come right through the tip or the dorsum. If they are lying quietly along the dorsum, without much motion, then the chances for success might be better.

Comment (Tom Rees): Dr. Dan Baker and I reviewed the non-Caucasian operations at Manhattan Eye, Ear, and Throat Hospital for a period of several years. We had very good luck with silicone implants in these patients, I suppose, because they had good soft tissue with excellent blood supply and no scarring. Under such conditions alloplastic implants are acceptable, but they should never be used to gain tip projection or as columella implants. The success rate in the tip is very low.

Question: How about the use of Supramid? Many nasal surgeons seem to support this material as acceptable for implantation into the nasal tissues.

Comment (Gene Tardy): I do not use Supramid mesh in the tip reconstruction. I use only autogenous cartilage.

Comment (Frank Kamer): I like Supramid for filling in dorsal saddling, but I do not use it in the tip. After many operations, I have only had one problem.

Comment (Jack Sheen): I never use Supramid in the nose, but I have often used it as an implant over the maxilla. I observed strict sterile technique and used it for years with absolutely no problems; then I had two problems in 1 year. So I have now become much more conservative in using Supramid over the maxilla. I use it only if there is a real indication for increasing the anterior arch of the maxilla.

Comment (Tom Rees): At this point I think it is advisable to point out that camouflaging defects of the maxilla, especially deficiency of the maxilla or an overly long one (the long face syndrome), may not be the optimal treatment. Surgery to the maxilla such as osteotomy or ostectomy should be considered. Patients having significant problems along these lines should be considered for a thorough maxillofacial workup to determine what is best. Simple onlay grafts or implants may not be the best remedy.

CORRECTION
OF UNUSUAL
TIP PROBLEMS

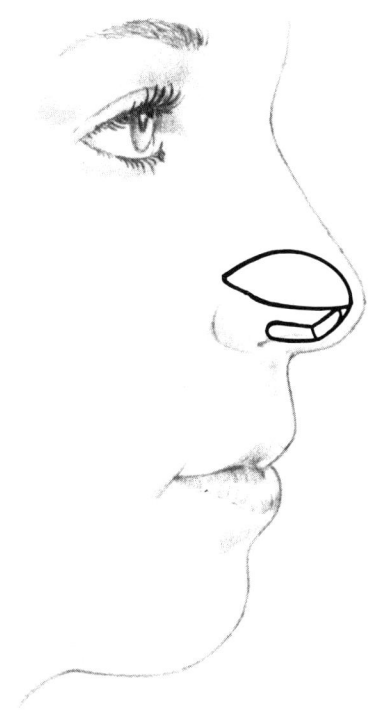

7

Correction of the Boxy Nasal Tip

Thomas J. Baker

The boxy nasal tip is usually large, amorphous, and bulky, and the dome is rounded in contrast to the more pyramidal configuration that is considered to be more aesthetic. The patient shown in Figure 7-1 presents a classic example of the boxy nasal tip. The postoperative view of the same individual (Figure 7-2) shows how the rounded tip has been converted into a pyramidal shape.

Patients often say they do not want "a pig-shaped nose." They are asking that the plastic surgeon not shorten the nose too drastically, and they especially do not want the tip turned up at an acute angle. It is not aesthetically pleasing to have the nose turned up to such a degree that other people are staring into the floor of the patient's nostrils when standing at a conversational distance.

Another example of the more rectangular tip is seen in Figure 7-3. In this individual the medial crura are widely displaced. The fibroareolar tissue between the medial crura needs to be exposed and removed so that the medial crura can be brought into apposition. The nasal tip of this patient can be narrowed somewhat but not to the degree shown in Figure 7-2, because the nasal skin is thicker and more difficult to alter. It is frequently impossible to produce a well-defined sharp nasal tip when the skin is thicker and less apt to contract. The result is seen in Figure 7-4.

Figure 7-5 shows the problem schematically. The diagram on the left demonstrates the boxy nasal tip, and the one on the right shows the more aesthetically appealing pyramidal shape. This alteration

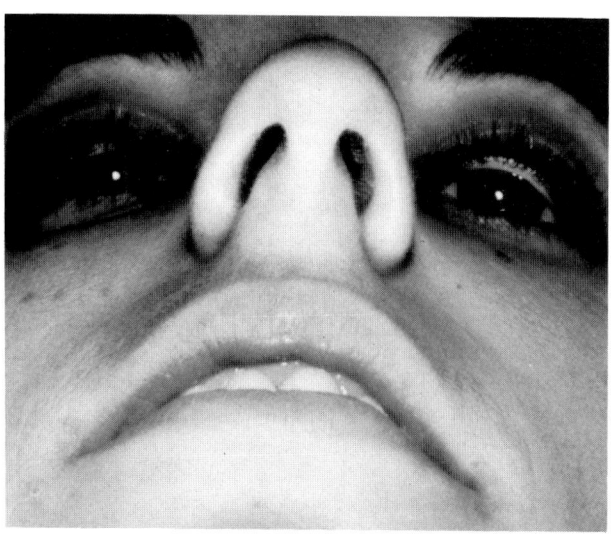

Figure 7-1

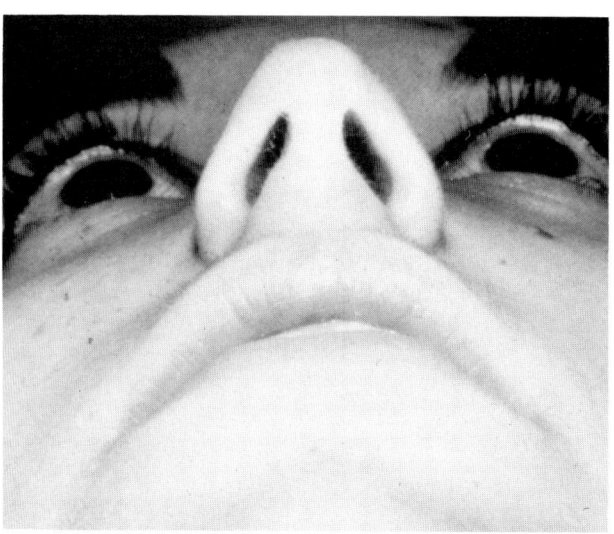

Figure 7-2

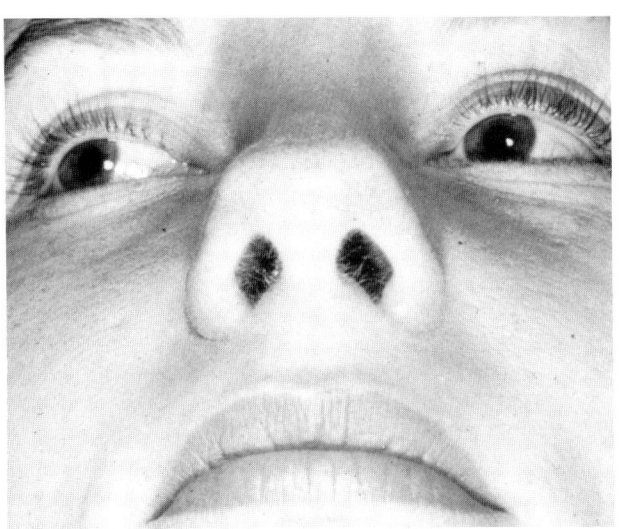

Figure 7-3

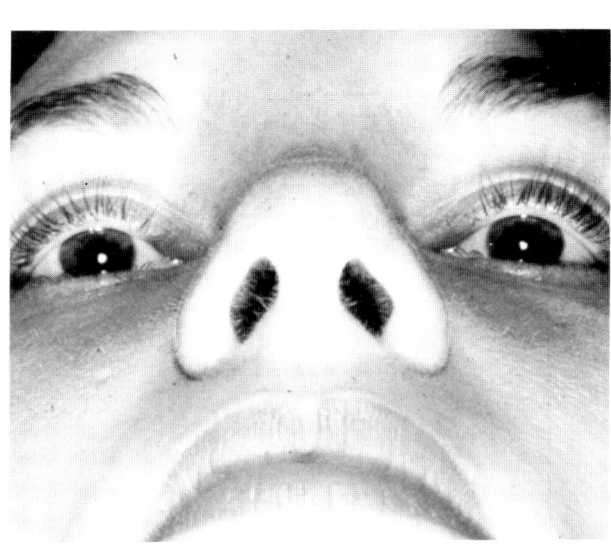

Figure 7-4

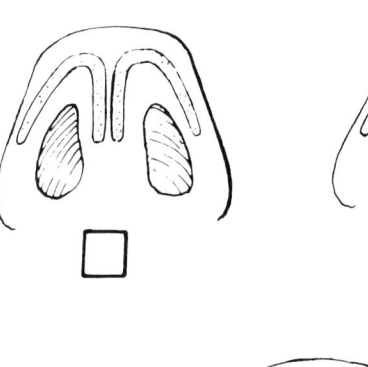

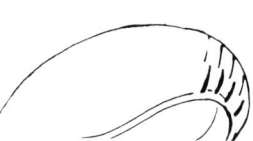

Figure 7-5. (From Sheen, J.H., and Sheen, A.P.: Aesthetic rhinoplasty, ed. 2, St. Louis, 1987, The C.V. Mosby Co.)

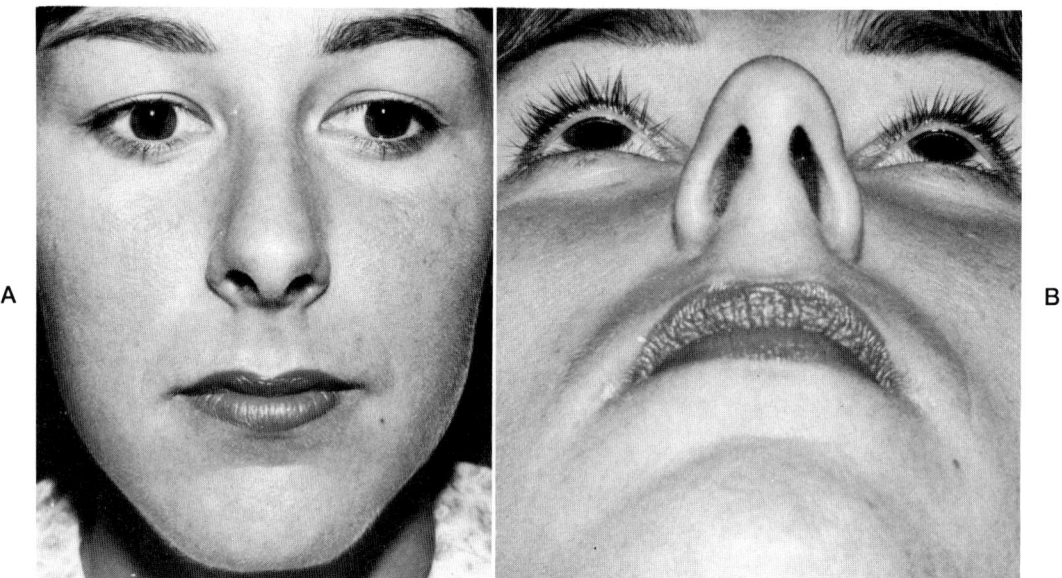

Figure 7-6

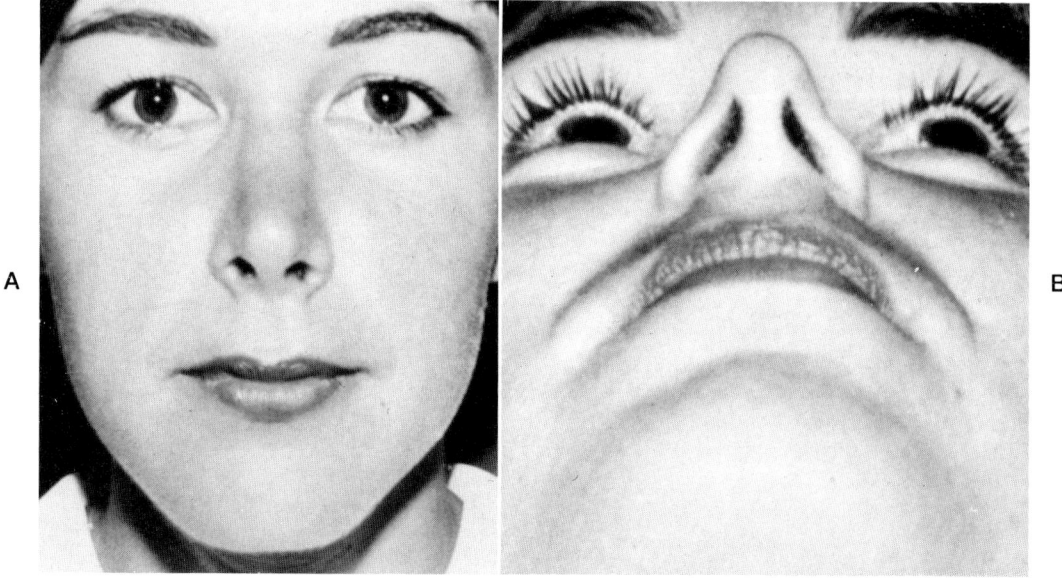

Figure 7-7

is brought about by appropriate sculpturing of the alar cartilages. The lower portion of the diagram shows that interdigitating incisions have been made in the cartilage, yet the continuity of the dome is preserved. These interdigitating incisions usually number from three to six, and care is taken not to incise all the way through the dome. I prefer interdigitating incisions to morcellation, since the incisions allow more precise control.

In the earlier years of my practice I frequently completely divided the alar cartilages in the apex of the dome. This all too frequently resulted in a nasal tip that was too pointed.

I did a rhinoplasty on the individual shown in Figure 7-6 20 years before this writing; the postoperative view (Figure 7-7) shows the result after 1 year. The alar cartilages were completely divided (Figure 7-8). This maneuver resulted in a tip that was too sharp. After 20 years the skin became more atrophic, and the nasal tip appeared pointed. A deformity created during the initial surgical procedure will persist and may even become less acceptable as time passes. Figure 7-9 shows the result after 20 years.

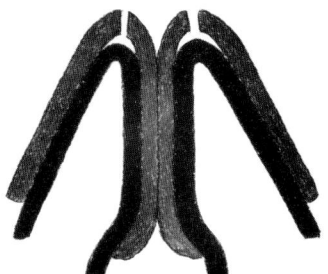

Figure 7-8

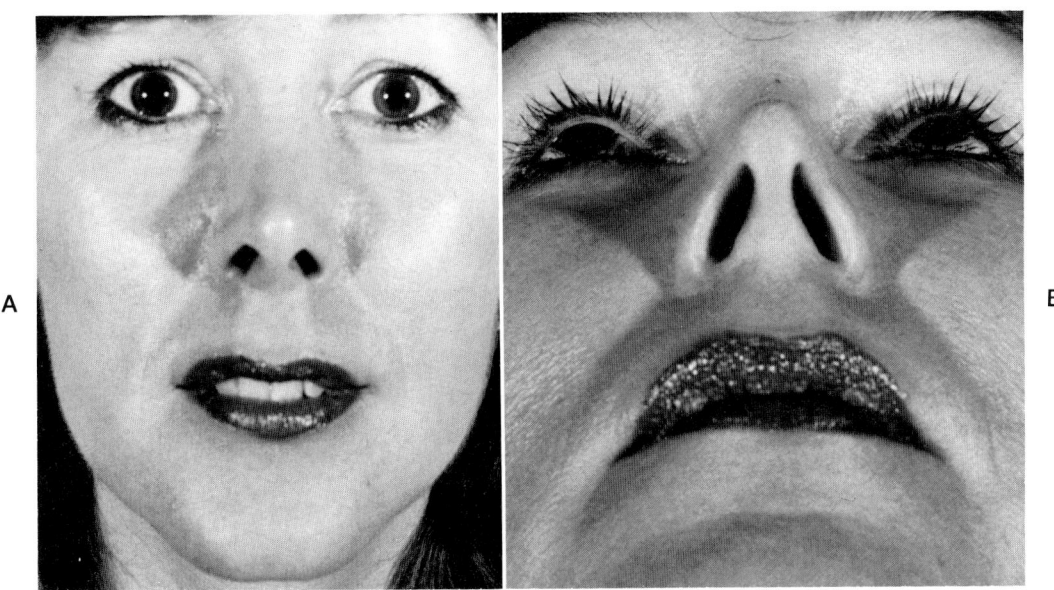

A   B

Figure 7-9

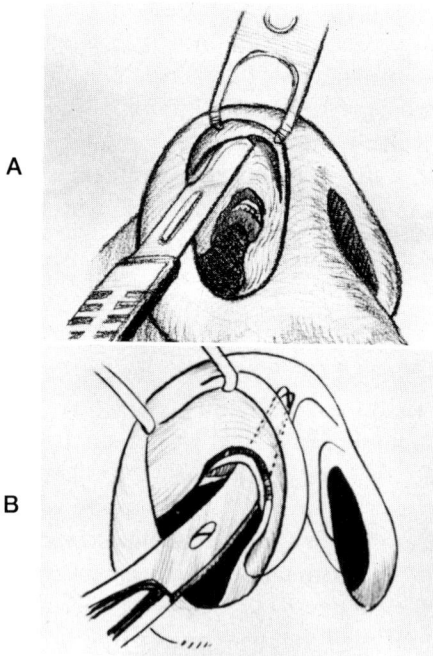

A

B

Figure 7-10

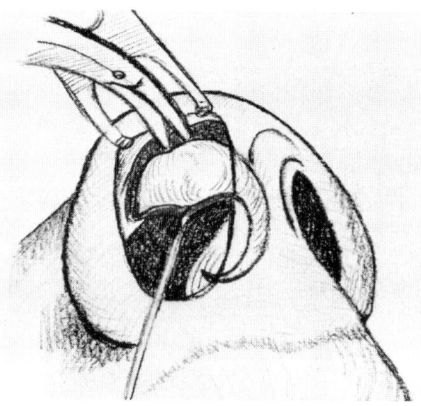

Figure 7-11

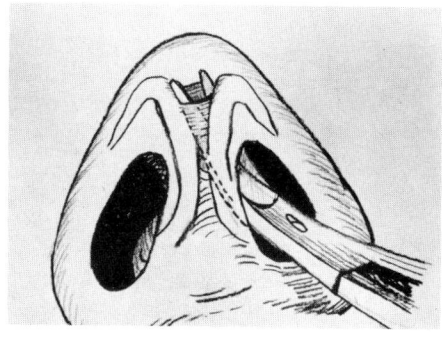

Figure 7-12

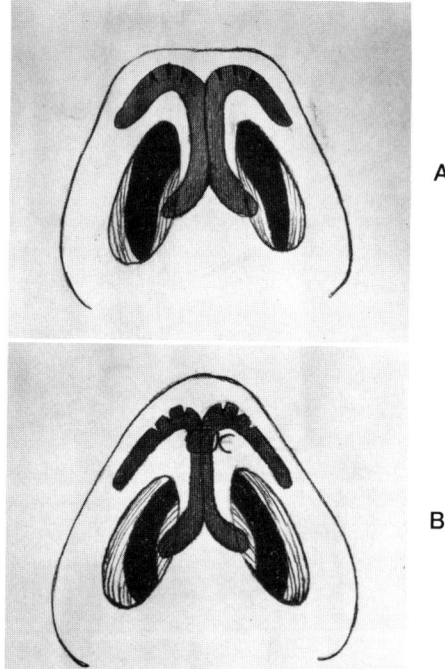

A

B

Figure 7-13

I prefer a rim incision for sculpturing large, boxy nasal tips (Figure 7-10), because the alar cartilages can be mobilized to allow the surgeon to obtain a good view of both cartilages, thus helping to assure symmetry. A skin hook is placed in the dome of the cartilage after adequate skeletonization has brought the alar cartilages into plain view (Figure 7-11). If the alar cartilages are visible the surgeon can more easily sculpture them into a preplanned shape. An attempt to do this blindly may result in assymetry. If there is any soft tissue between the medial crura, it should be removed so the medial crura can lie back to back (Figure 7-12). A mattress suture between the medial crura can bring this portion of the alar cartilages back to back and thus create a narrower nasal tip (Figure 7-13).

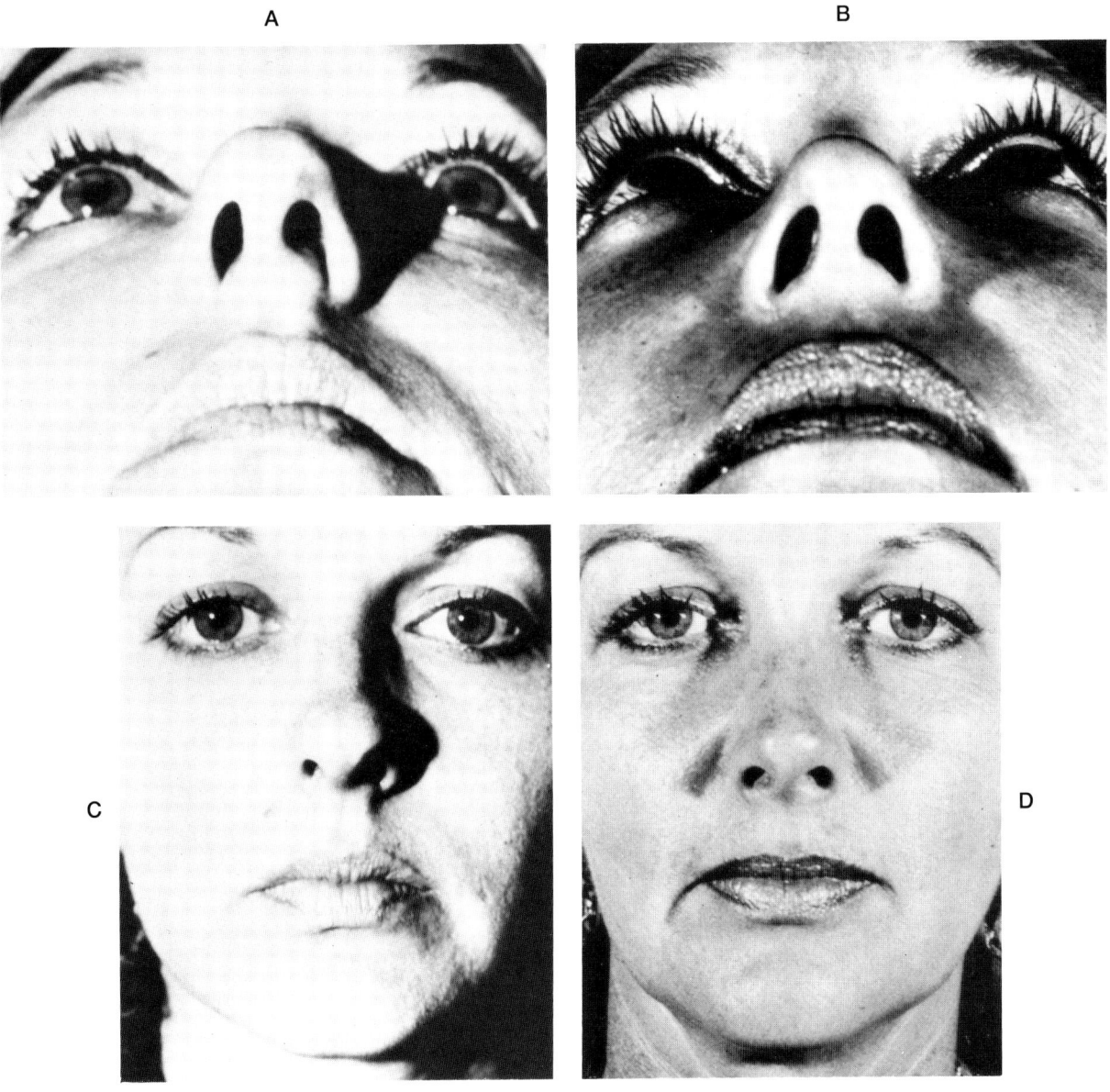

Figure 7-14

Figure 7-14 shows an individual 10 years after having had a rhinoplasty and demonstrates the result from such a procedure. Natural lines exist rather than a sharp nasal tip, which would have been the result had the domes been completely divided. The front view shows the double light reflection on the tips of the alar cartilages, indicating symmetry and a pleasant postoperative appearance.

There are many variations in handling the sculpturing maneuvers of the alar cartilages (Figure 7-15). The bucket-handle delivery of the cartilages is most suitable for full visualization. The cartilage occasionally can be everted through an intercartilagenous incision, which I use occasionally if the tip is not too bulky (Figure 7-16). A small triangle can then be removed from the dome (Figure 7-17), but

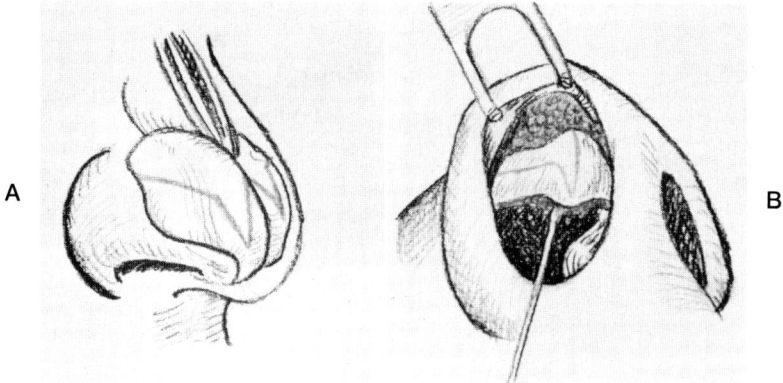

Figure 7-15

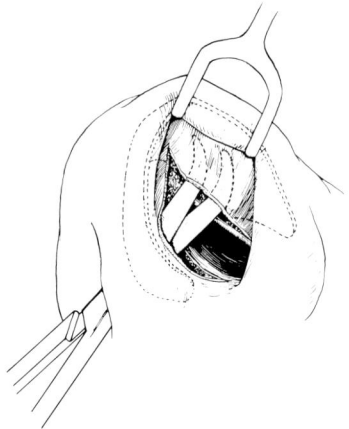

Figure 7-16

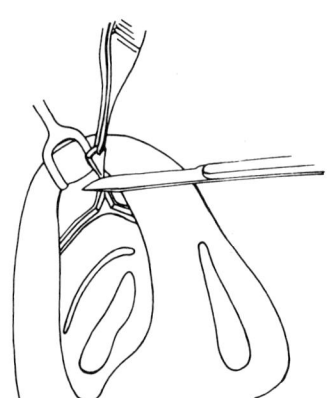

Figure 7-17

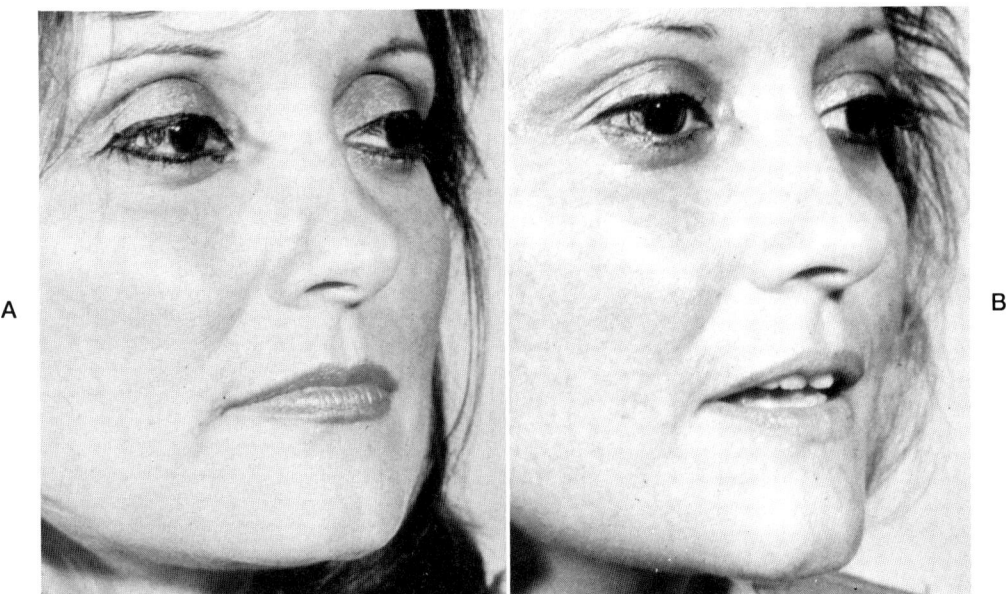

Figure 7-18

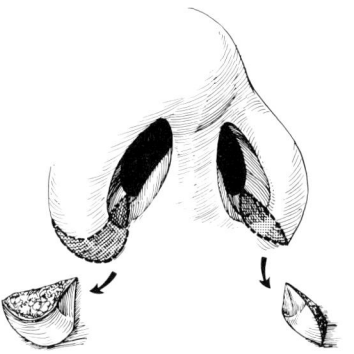

Figure 7-19

care should be taken not to remove the triangular piece all the way through the rim of the alar cartilage if continunity along the cartilagenous rim is to be preserved.

In the individual shown in Figure 7-18 a rhytidectomy was the primary procedure, but she also wanted the boxy nasal tip reduced. The only nasal surgery was done through an everting incision of the alar cartilages, and the tip was easily reduced by removing a simple triangle. No osteotomy or other procedure was carried out.

Alar wedges can be done in certain selected cases, as shown in Figure 7-19.

SUMMARY

The time-tested technique of interdigitating incisions in the dome of the alar cartilages produces consistently good results. In only rare individuals would I recommend complete transection of the alar cartilages in the dome because of the possibility of producing a nasal tip that is too sharp.

8

Correction of Unusual Tip Problems

Walter Berman

I believe, and I am sure many will agree, that rhinoplasty is probably the most intriguing and fascinating of all head and neck plastic surgery. The nasal tip sets the stage for rhinoplasty. Any surgical alteration of the nose causes compensatory problems. When some of the ligaments are cut to change the contour of the nose or when cartilage is removed, it should be recognized that there will be consequences. I will describe a few of the procedures I have found helpful in transforming the large, bulky tip into the thinnest tip possible.

Figure 8-1 shows a 20-year-old woman with an overly developed (wide bifid) nasal tip and skin that is thicker than usual in this area. The bifidity of the nasal tip results from separation of the nasal domes by intervening fibroadipose tissues. The figure shows how a fairly smooth and more aesthetically pleasing nose can be fashioned from such a large nasal tip.

Excellent visualization is of paramount importance in any surgical procedure to remedy this type of problem. Thus the lower lateral delivery is used. A bipedicle flap created over the medial and lateral crural tissues provides an excellent view (Figure 8-2). I therefore make an intercartilaginous incision, followed by marginal rim incisions along the course of the lower lateral and anterior parts of the medial crural cartilages. I then connect the two incisions by undermining, leaving intact 4 to 5 mm of the lower lateral, dome, and medial crural cartilages.

Certainly the same thing can be done in a number of other approaches to the nasal tip, but it is useful to eliminate all guesswork, particularly in view of problems with asymmetry or any secondary problems. A number of surgeons have chosen to use open rhinoplasty, but the delivery technique allows obviation of the columellar scar and maintains adequate visualization during the procedure. I remove a portion of the superior aspect of the lower lateral cartilage and, frequently, a portion of the medial aspect. With a very thick medial cartilage the surgeon must follow along the dome into the medial crura and remove some of that also; otherwise maximal thinning of the tip will be impossible. In doing this the surgeon is also rotating the tip and shortening the nose. Remember, however, that some noses should not be shortened. Only a triangle of cartilage is removed at the dome with short noses; the rest of the cartilage is morcellized.

Many of these patients have a large amount of fibrofatty subcutaneous tissue; I believe most surgeons remove this tissue from the lower lateral cartilages. This approach gives a sharp dissection and allows the surgeon clearer visualization during the procedure, permitting fibrofatty removal subcutaneously. Leaving excess fibrofatty tissue attached to the skin causes extra width in the nasal tip after the operation. I believe the key to a naturally smooth dome postoperatively is avoidance of incisions in the inferior (caudal) part of the dome or lower lateral cartilage near the dome. Any disruption of the inferior border, in this area, can cause irregularities months or years later.

Next, I completely morcellize the remaining nasal domes and lateral and medial cartilages to conform the cartilages to their new positions. I like the Rubin morcellizer a great deal and use it frequently to contour a nasal tip. The one-sided morcellizer is best, since there is no reason to morcellize vestibular skin. The fibrofatty tissues can be dissected from the cartilage, and everything remains intact. Thus the chances of abnormalities developing in the future are minimized. I remove no epithelial lining in this

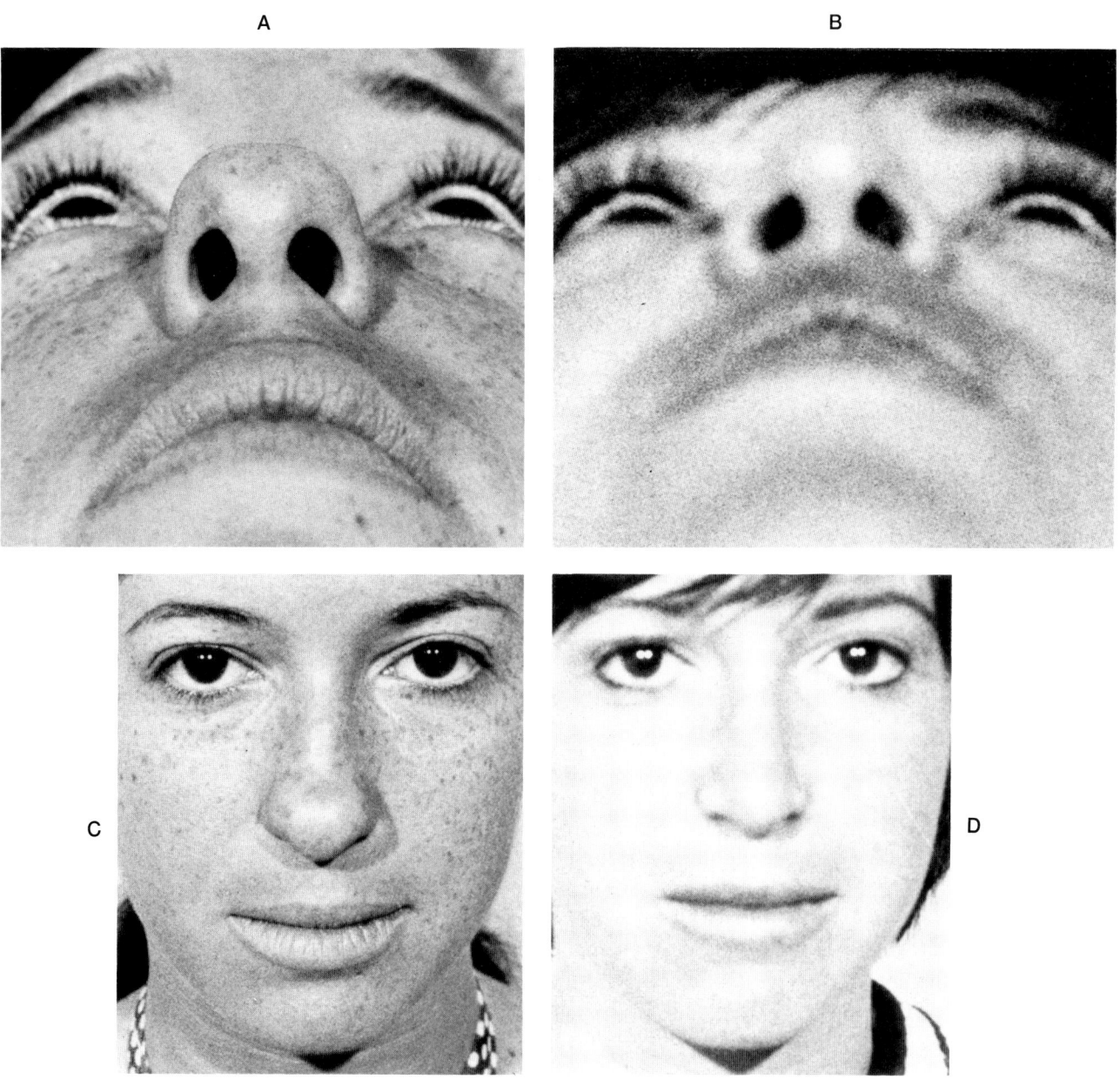

Figure 8-1. Preoperative and postoperative photographs of young woman with wide bifid nasal tip.

Superior portion of
lower lateral crus

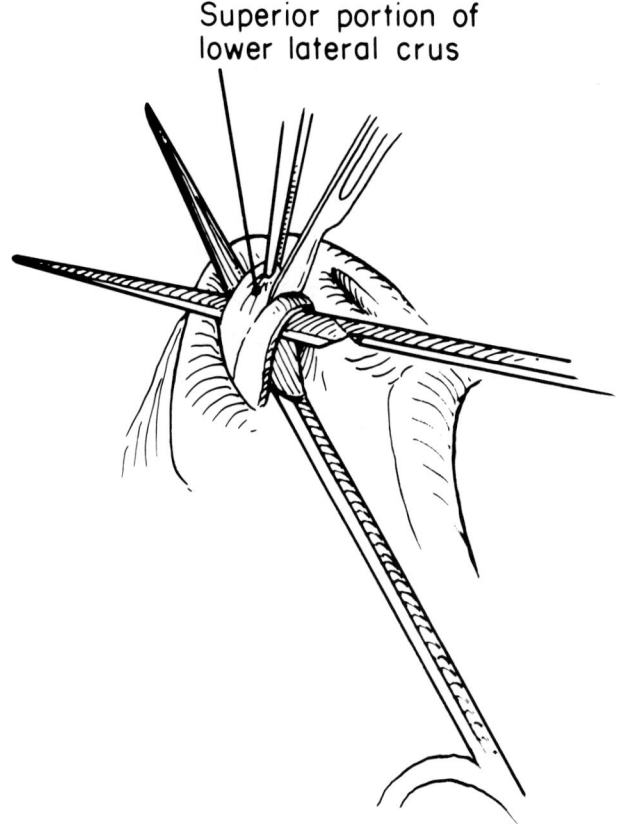

Figure 8-2. Delivery diagram. (From Berman, W.E.: Rhinoplasty, ed. 2, Washington, D.C., 1984, American Academy of Otolaryngology—Head and Neck Surgery Foundation, Inc.)

procedure. Excessive removal causes lining contractures postoperatively. Many years ago I began using permanent sutures, which I put directly through the epithelium at the domes. I found that use of a nylon suture at the domes and through to the vestibular skin worked very well; in my experience none have come out. Why is the suture not extruded? First, monofilament nylon suture has some elasticity. Second, some granulation and subsequent epithelialization occur over the suture. Third, the patient has difficulty getting a finger in position to manipulate the suture.

Figure 8-3 shows the double dome suture I use in practice. This suture must be placed with great care. I suture through the vestibular skin rather than internally, because internal suturing sometimes cre-

ates slight asymmetry of the domes. The two nasal domes are held together with a Brown-Adson forceps while I place a simple horizontal mattress through and through to obtain good approximation. This approach is of course based on the premise that any fibrofatty tissue between those two domes was removed before the suture was placed. I do not think it matters which suture is used; however, I use a 4-0 clear monofilament nylon as a horizontal mattress suture.

Another way of keeping that tip up, which may be a problem in these cases, is placement of a simple mattress suture that extends from the septum to the columellar cartilage. It is quite easy to bury this suture (Figure 8-4). It is preferable to keep the normal anatomy of the two domes and achieve projection

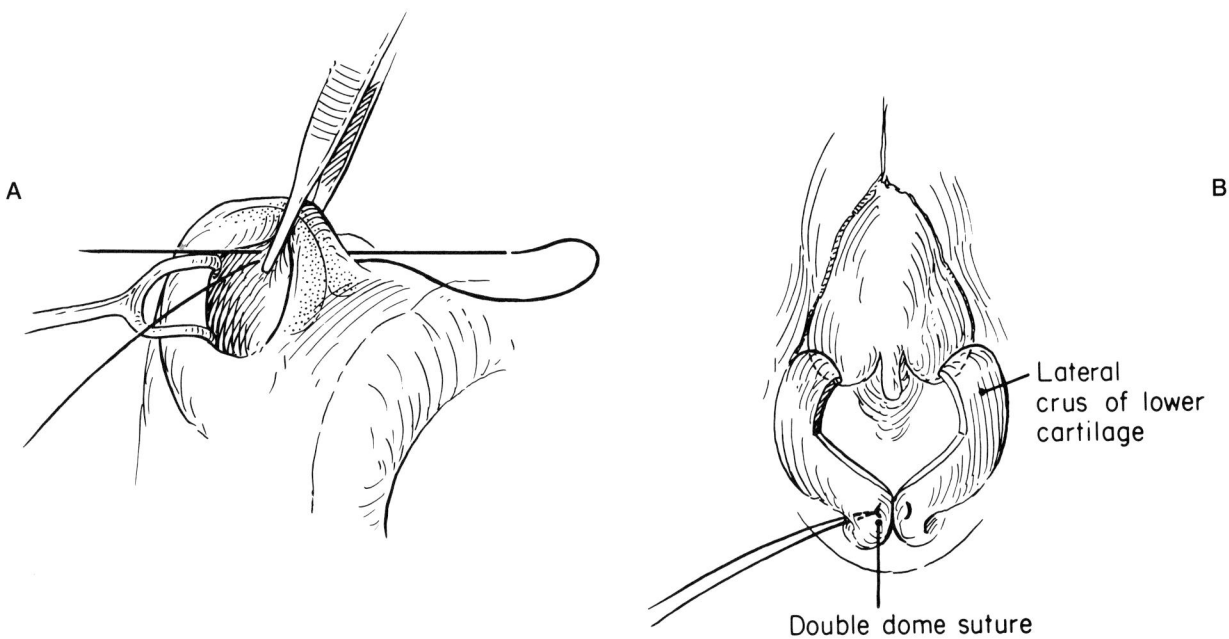

Figure 8-3. Diagram of double dome suture. (From Berman, W.E.: Rhinoplasty, ed. 2, Washington, D.C., 1984, American Academy of Otolaryngology—Head and Neck Surgery Foundation, Inc.)

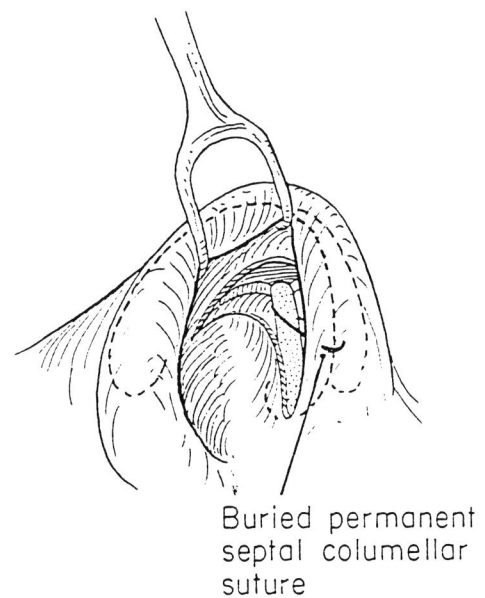

Figure 8-4. Buried permanent septal columellar suture. (From Berman, W.E.: Rhinoplasty, ed. 2, Washington, D.C., 1984, American Academy of Otolaryngology—Head and neck Surgery Foundation, Inc.)

without adding a graft over the domes whenever possible.

The mattress sutures are positioned near the septal angle, buried in the cartilage, and then buried at a lower angle, deep into the medial crura. The suture is placed at a slightly higher level in the septum, and then at a more posterior or lower level in the medial crura; this affords a good deal of projection. Although placement sutures provide an excellent solution for the mild problem, they are not a panacea for a severe problem in which much projection is needed. In addition, there is no reason the surgeon cannot do the same procedure while adding a cartilaginous graft for support from the nasal spine to the tip. This is a safe and simple method of treating loss of tip projection.

9

Correction of the Bulky and Boxy Tip

Harvey Caplan

In the hands of the skilled rhinoplastic surgeon correction of the bony dorsum and the lower cartilaginous dorsum does not pose an especially difficult problem; however, correction of the boxy tip is considerably more challenging and requires more advanced expertise. Many techniques are available for correcting deformities of the vault; saws, scalpels, chisels, or scissors, singly or in combination, are used. The results are usually quite predictable. In contradistinction, there is no single definitive procedure that will ensure predictable or completely satisfactory results with the boxy tip. Perfection in

surgery is always our goal; sometimes, however, we must accept a lesser objective in correcting the boxy tip—a goal to be achieved without the hazards of atresia, excessive scarring, valvular collapse, and other complications.

Thorough analysis of the problem is mandatory to arrive at an intelligent plan and to help avoid the untoward sequelae just listed. Careful study of preoperative photographs and anatomic features in each patient is of great importance in arriving at a safe plan.

In most patients I approach the nasal tip after

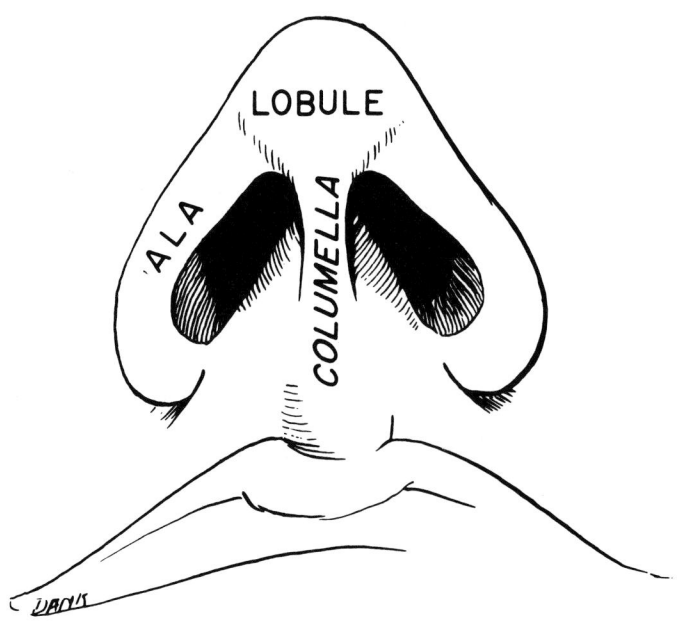

Figure 9-1. Areas of nasal tip.

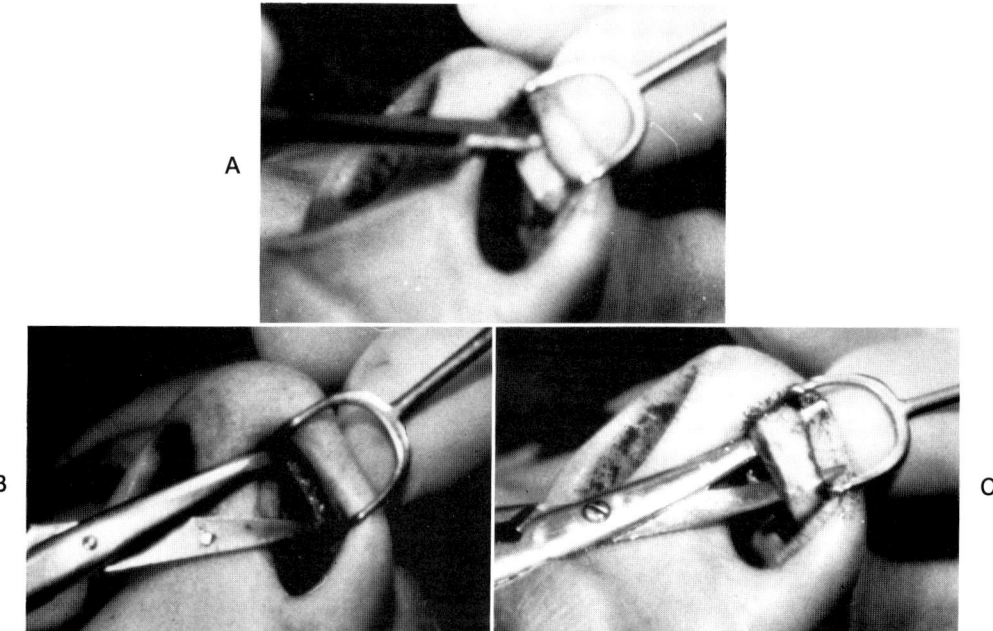

Figure 9-2. Modified rim technique.

undermining the dorsum and completing the transfixion incision, for the following reasons:

1. Tip surgery has limitations, and in the event that the dorsum is overcorrected before tip surgery is done, the task of matching the reshaped tip to the undermined dorsum becomes very difficult. The same thinking applies to the overshortened nose before the tip is corrected.

2. Performing medial and lateral osteotomies early in the procedure, before tip surgery, can result in considerable edema, which can disguise the tip problem. Therefore osteotomies are done after the tip is corrected.

I define the nasal tip as the inferior area of the nose, consisting of the alar cartilages, the membranous columella, and the inferior border of the cartilaginous septum (Figure 9-1). The lobule consists of the morphologic components of the nasal tip, extending above the ventral border of the nostrils, and should measure roughly one third of the length of the nasal tip in the aesthetically ideal nose.

The most commonly performed tip technique that I use is the transcartilaginous, or sandwich, tip.

There are many variations of this technique, which is also called the *intracartilaginous technique*. This method is ideal in most tip reductions, but should a greater degree of reduction be required—a real diminution of bulk—it may not suffice.

For these more difficult problems I use an adaptation of this standard operation, which I call the *modified rim technique* (Figures 9-2 and 9-3). This technical variation permits additional rotation, bulk reduction, or even a decrease in boxiness when required. I believe it provides me with the capability of adjusting my operation as I proceed. I am not locked into one maneuver that may not provide the result I seek (Figure 9-4).

I favor the delivery or bucket-handle dissection in difficult problems, because I gain complete access to the alar cartilage. The cartilage is delivered as a double pedicle flap, attached medially and laterally. All excessive fat and fibrous tissue can be removed, and the alar cartilages trimmed and remodeled to provide a smaller cartilage with a new shape. I again emphasize what has been pointed out by others: the vestibular skin must be preserved intact whenever a rim or modified rim incision is made.

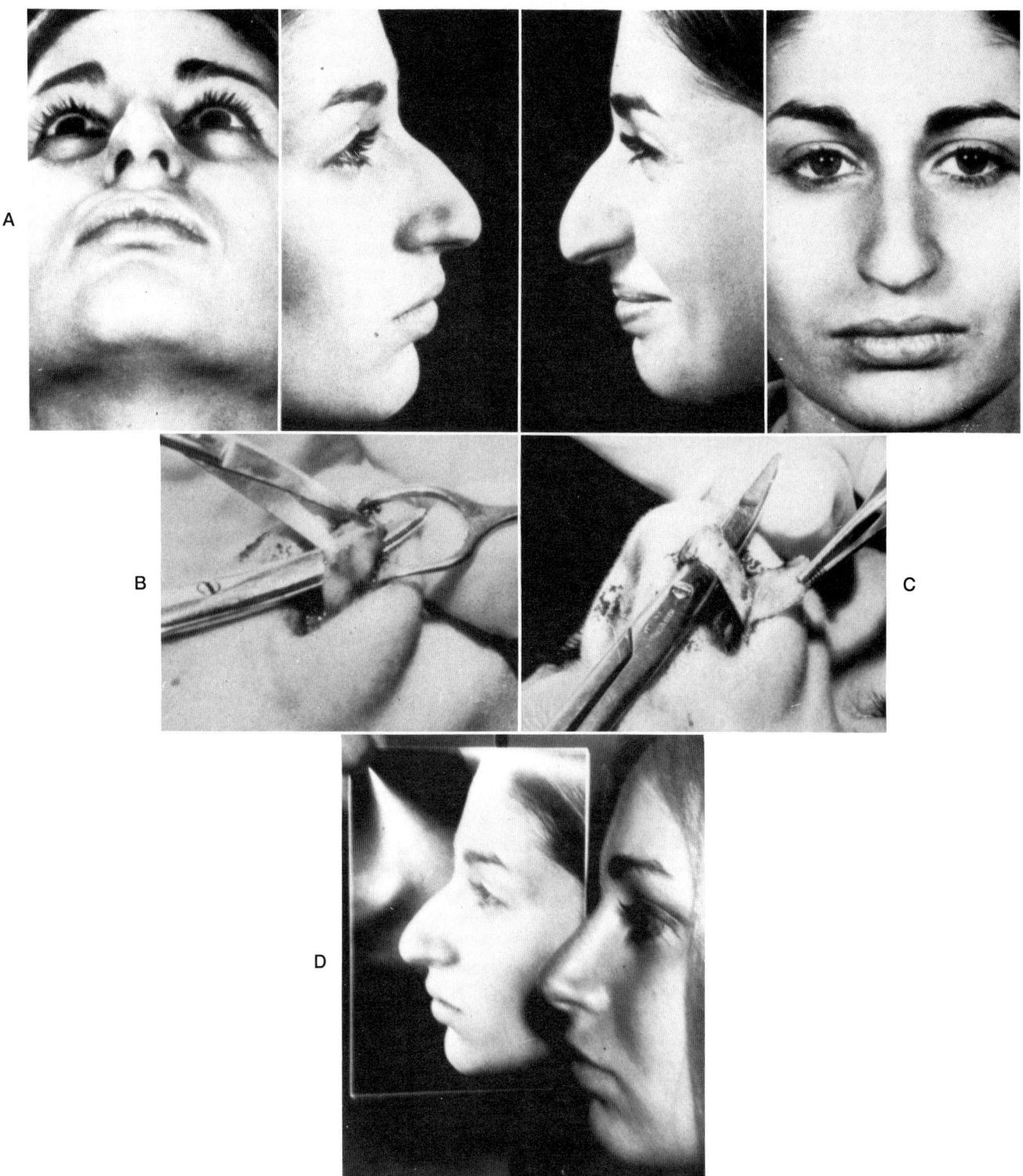

Figure 9-3. **A,** Patient required bulk reduction (basically cartilaginous) of nasal tip. Rotation and removal of nasal hump were also needed. **B** and **C,** Modified rim technique was used to remove 2 mm of alar cartilage. Circumferential nasal rim remained intact. **D,** Postoperative results were satisfactory.

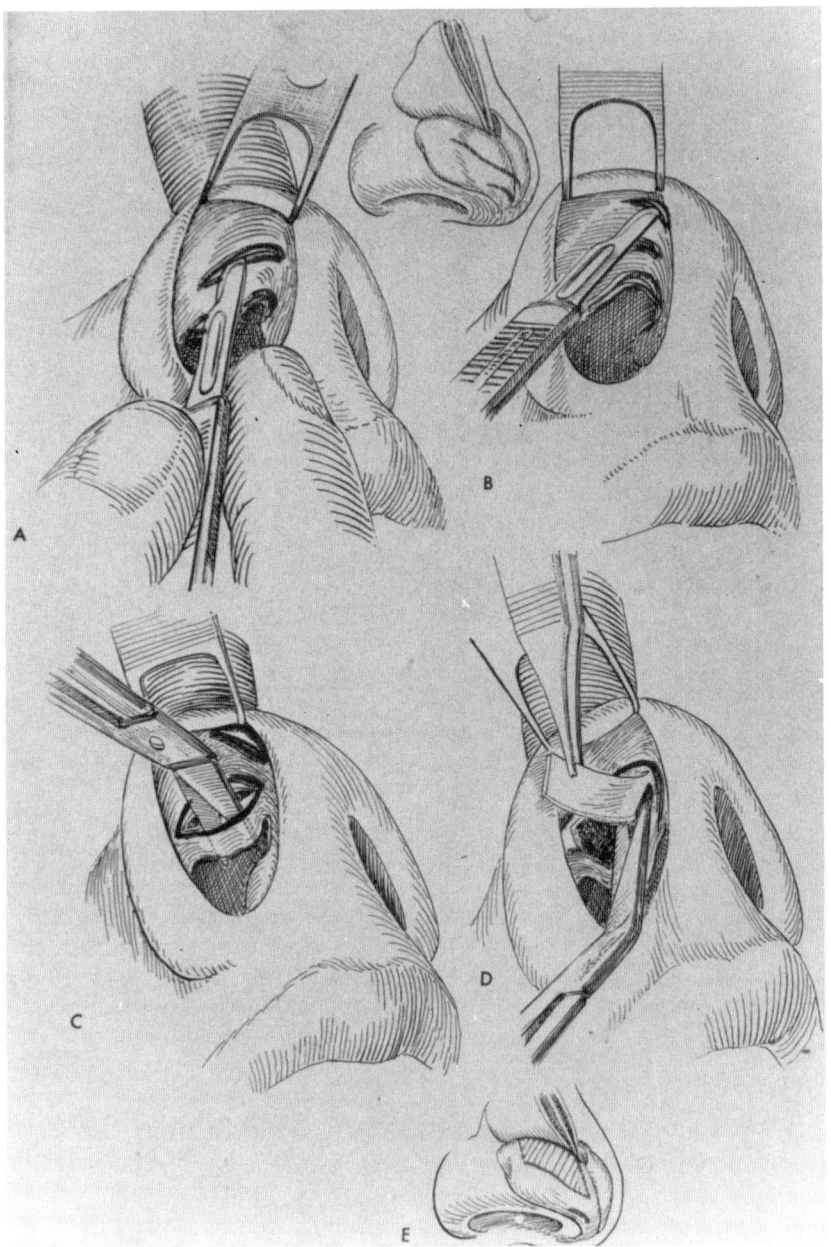

Figure 9-4. Patient had wide, bulky tip and very thick sebaceous skin. Modified rim technique did not provide sufficient bulk reduction, so concomitant Joseph maneuver helped to obtain satisfactory result (**A-L**). In this manner nasal tip procedure was staged. (From Rees, T.D.: Aesthetic plastic surgery, vol. 1, Philadelphia, 1980, W.B. Saunders Co.)

Continued.

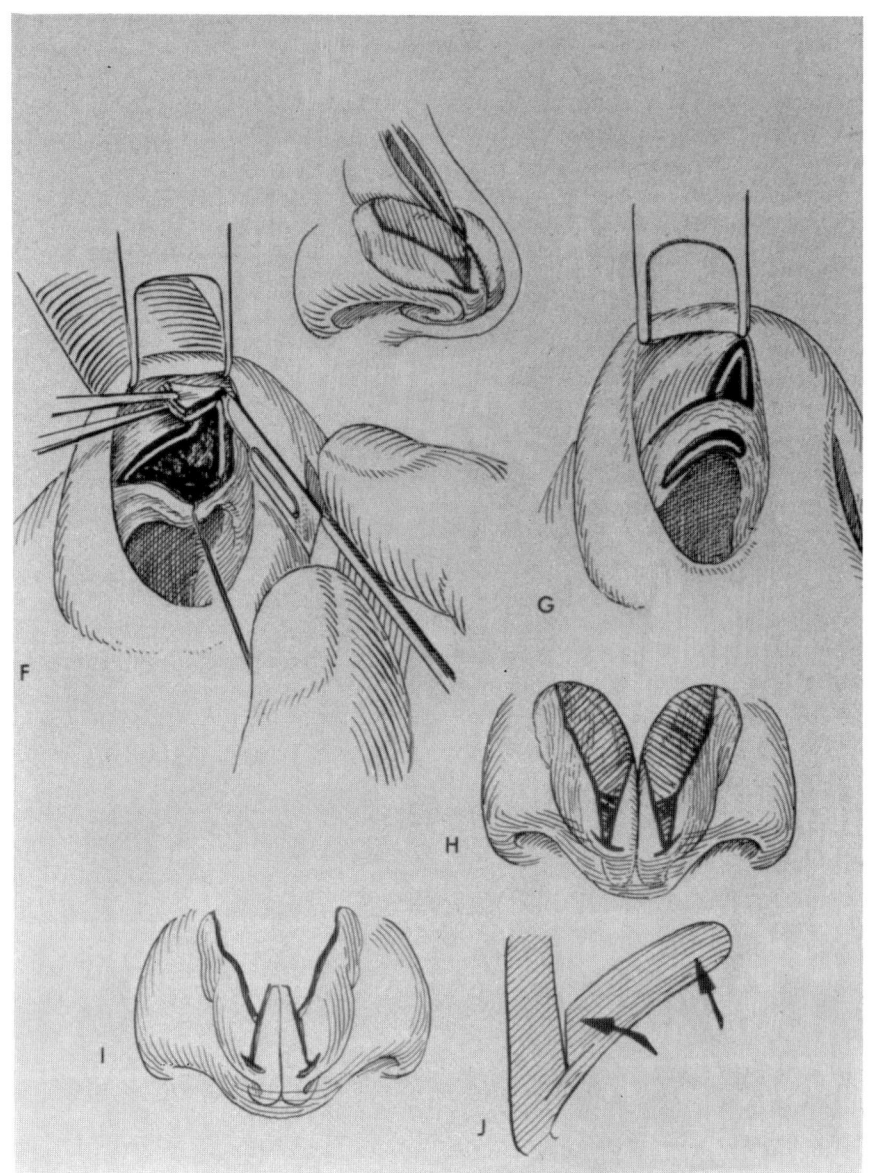

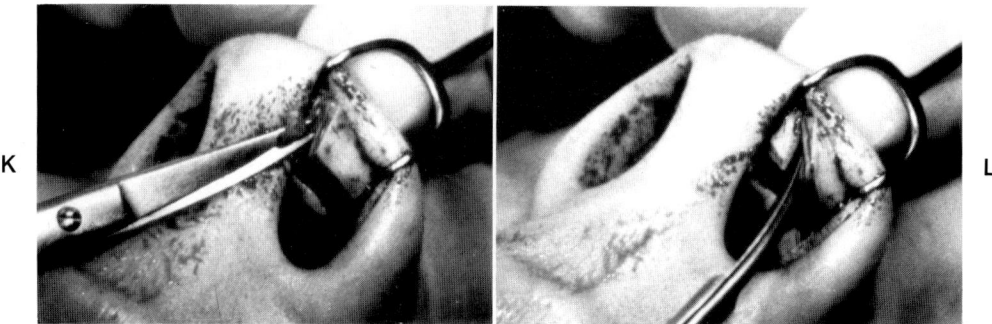

Figure 9-4, cont'd. For legend see p. 77.

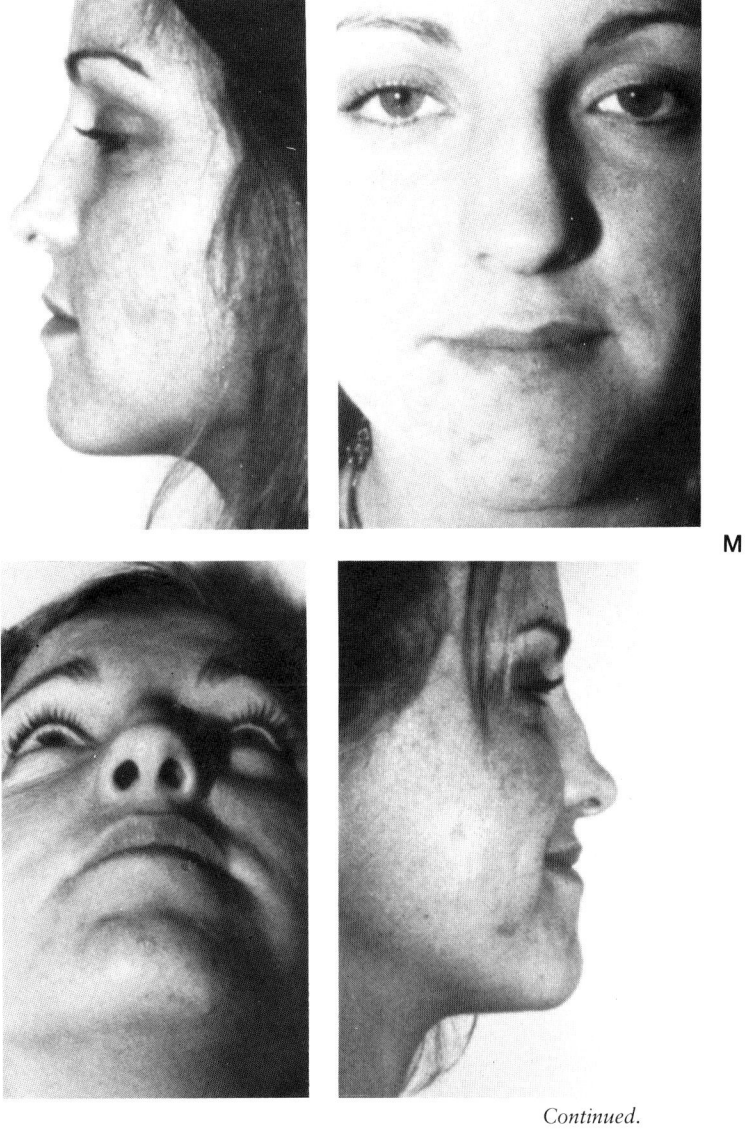

M

Continued.

Figure 9-4, cont'd. M, Preoperative views.

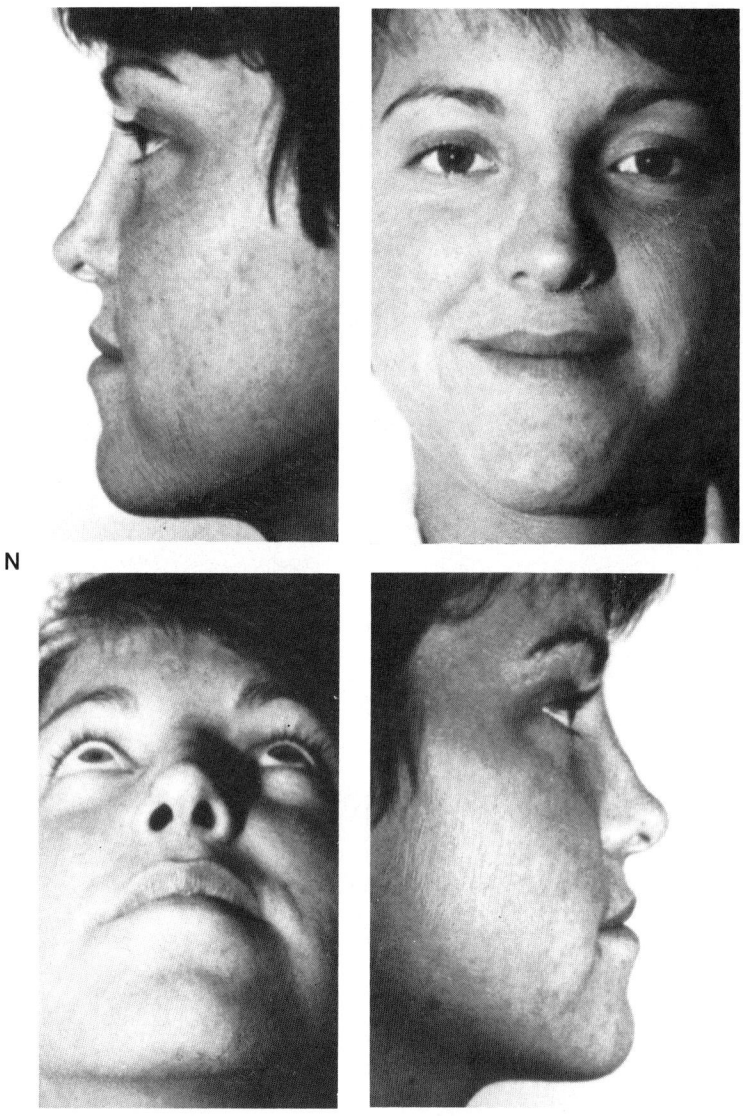

Figure 9-4, cont'd. N, Postoperative views of patient on p. 79.

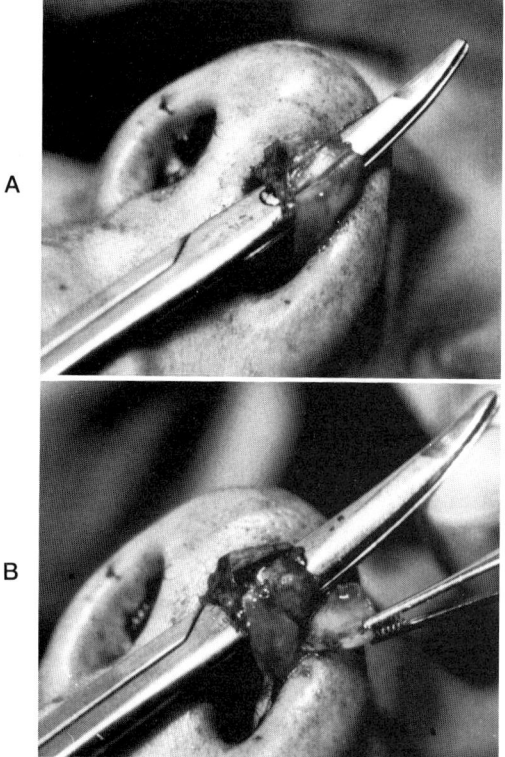

A

B

Figure 9-5. Preoperative assessment may determine that simple transcartilaginous incision would be inadequate to obtain adequate and aesthetically appealing results in nasal tip. Marginal incision can then be employed to provide good exposure of alar cartilage. Parallel track of cartilage is removed lateral to dome, and bulky cephalic portion is removed while vestibular nasal skin is retained (**A** and **B**).

Continued.

After the alar cartilage flap is delivered it is sculpted, and in the truly boxy tip a small track is excised vertically just lateral to the dome (Figure 9-5). In severely boxy tips it sometimes may be necessary to cut through the vestibular skin. Whenever the rim of cartilage or skin is completely transected, the tip must be reconstructed by suturing the medial crura together to provide stability and help prevent postoperative drooping of the tip with the inevitable supratip deformity as the end result. Should the medial crura be deficient in size or projection, I buttress the newly formed tip complex by inserting a cartilaginous strut from the septum.

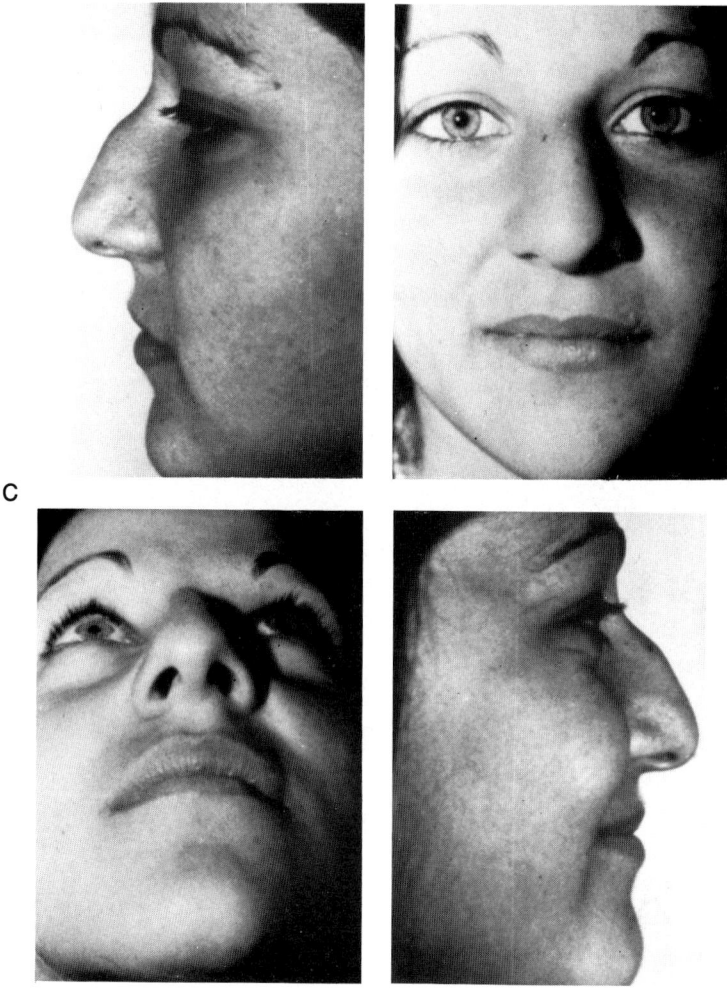

Figure 9-5, cont'd. C, Preoperative views.

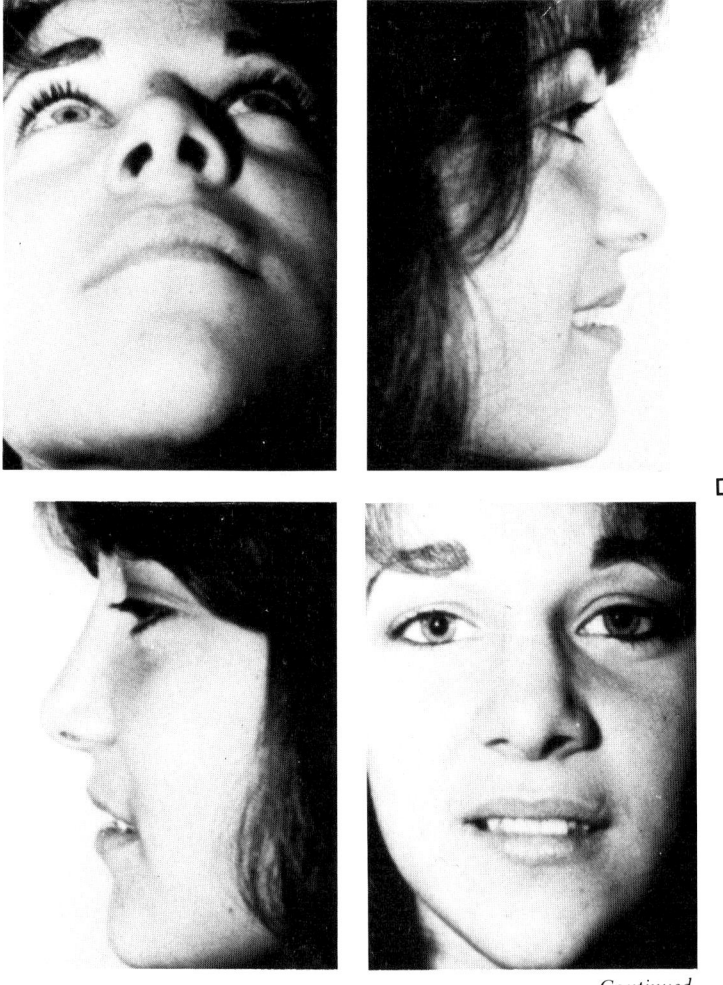

D

Continued.

Figure 9-5, cont'd. D, Postoperative views of patient on opposite page.

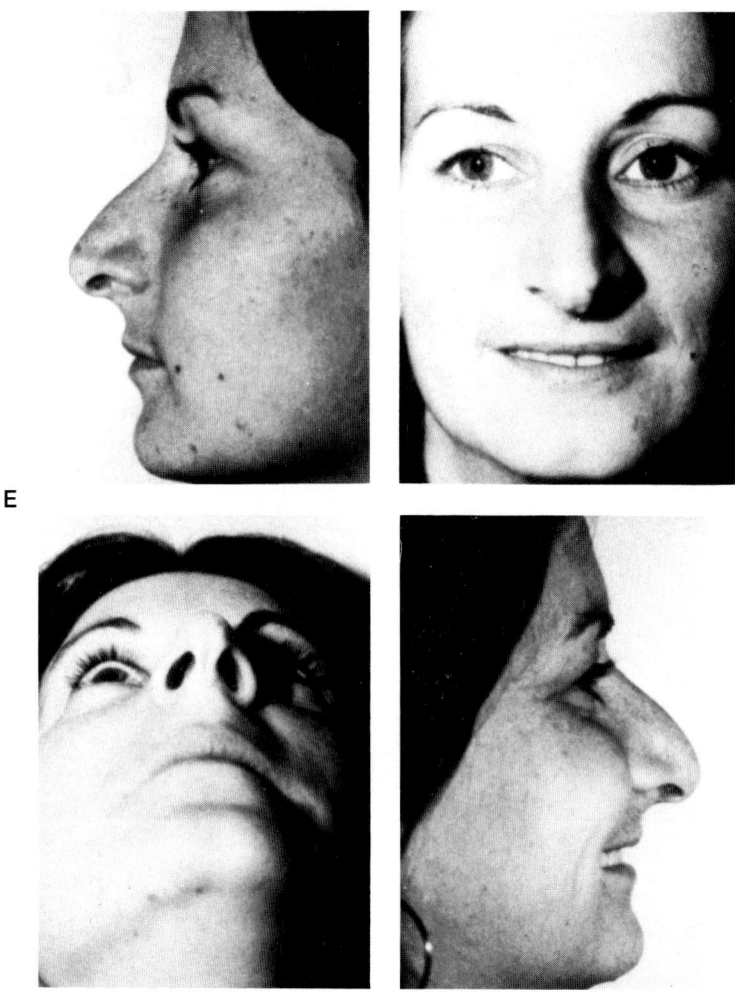

Figure 9-5, cont'd. E, Preoperative views.

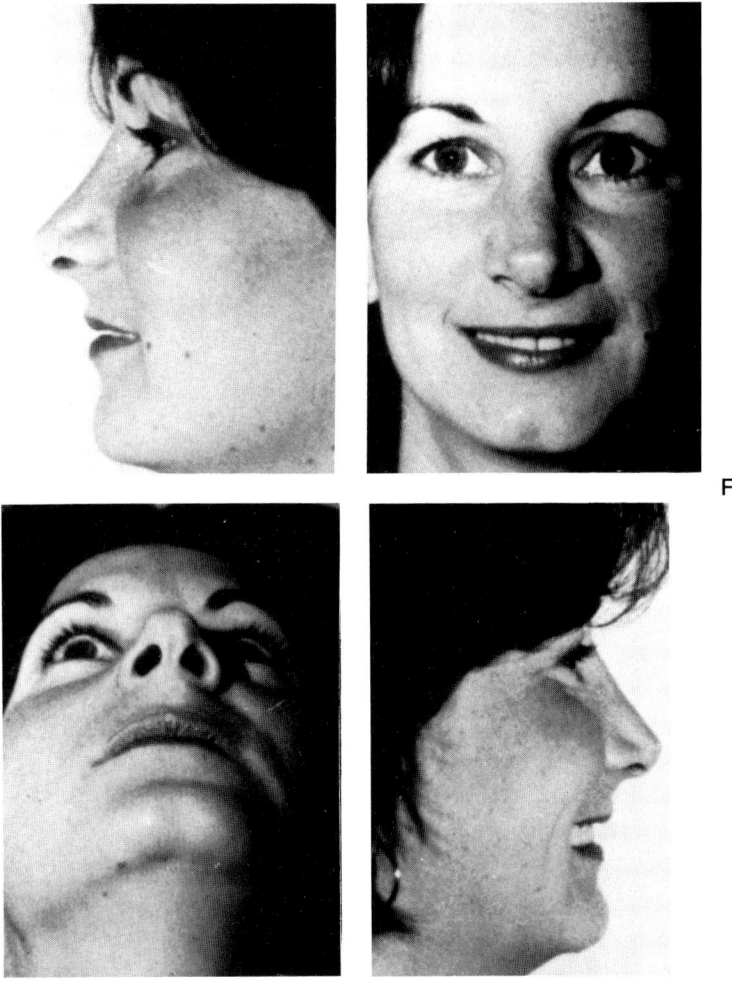

F

Figure 9-5, cont'd. F, Postoperative views of patient on opposite page.

10

Boxy Tip and Bulky Tip

Guy Jost

The tip of the nose is not built like a single column with the main support in the center. The principal supports are found on the sides, exactly like a gothic cathedral. It is important for the surgeon to understand this architectural anatomy, especially in dealing with tip surgery. Figure 10-1 shows that despite the absence of the columella in this patient, there is little or no loss of the projection of the tip, simply because the lateral supports maintain the forward thrust. The central column is simply not essential. In this case the lateral support is supplied by the lateral crura of the alar cartilages. Similarly, sometimes the lateral supports can be missing or can collapse, but if the central column remains, so does the projection.

The scheme of the nasal pyramid from the lateral side is presented in Figure 10-2. The strength of the lateral crus is obvious as a support structure, and there is a rather complex interrelationship of several anatomic structures, including the skin, fibrous tissue, and lining, as well as the cartilages, all of which are integral parts of the supporting system. Surgical alteration of any of these structures affects the whole, but it is mainly the alar cartilages that supply support and strength. It is important to understand that no gap exists between the superior upper lateral cartilage and the lower lateral cartilage. A gap can be created here only by the dissection and displacement of the skin, especially if downward traction on the skin occurs. There is no overlapping of the two cartilages, but there is an accordion-like articulation, and several small sesamoid cartilages placed strategically between the two almost separate them (Figure 10-3). If you stretch the skin with traction on the tip, the lateral wing triangle decreases in height, and the part overlapping the ala with the upper lateral cartilages decreases as a result of the gravitational pull. If the tip of the nose is pushed toward the face, the overlapping is increased because of the telescoping action and directional forces. This pulling on the tip, or pushing on it, especially affects the posterior prolongation of that lateral crura. In certain instances it becomes necessary to resect the posterior extension so that the length of the lateral crus is diminished, leaving a mini-alar cartilage. This step is frequently necessary to reduce an overly projecting tip, such as is found in the Pinocchio deformity, or a highly angular nose.

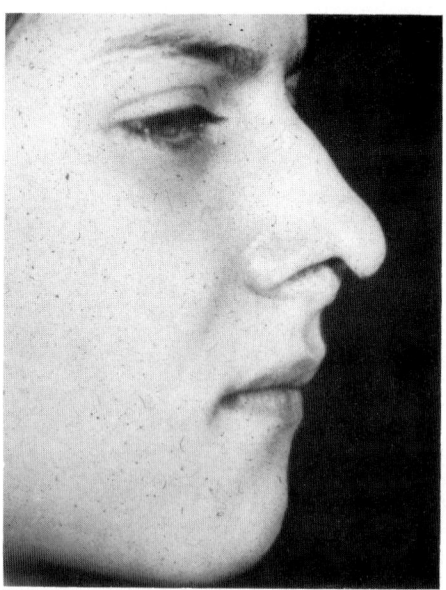

Figure 10-1. Columella is lost, but support from lateral walls provides projection.

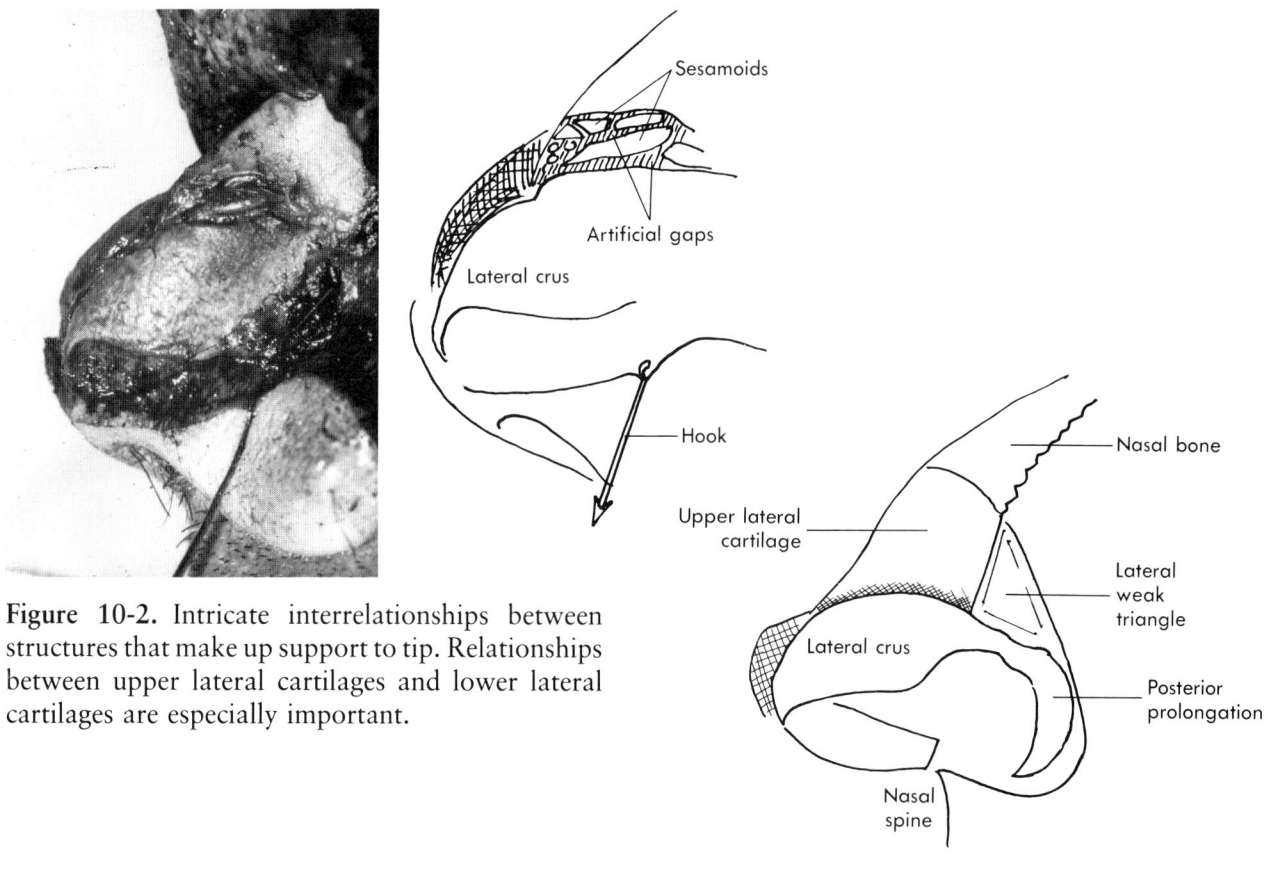

Figure 10-2. Intricate interrelationships between structures that make up support to tip. Relationships between upper lateral cartilages and lower lateral cartilages are especially important.

Figure 10-3. A, Role of sesamoid cartilages in the relationship of two nasal cartilages. **B** and **C,** Upward traction on tip results in "false overlapping" of cartilages.

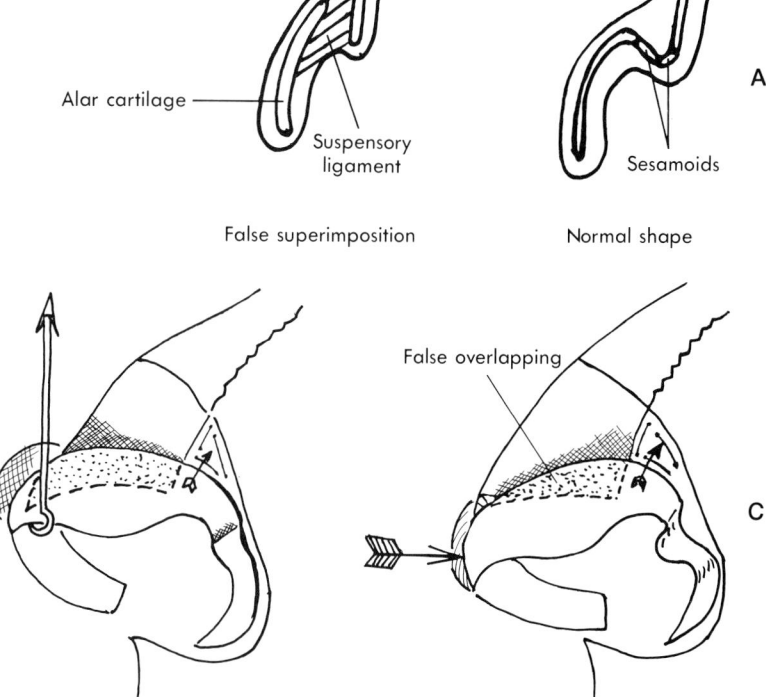

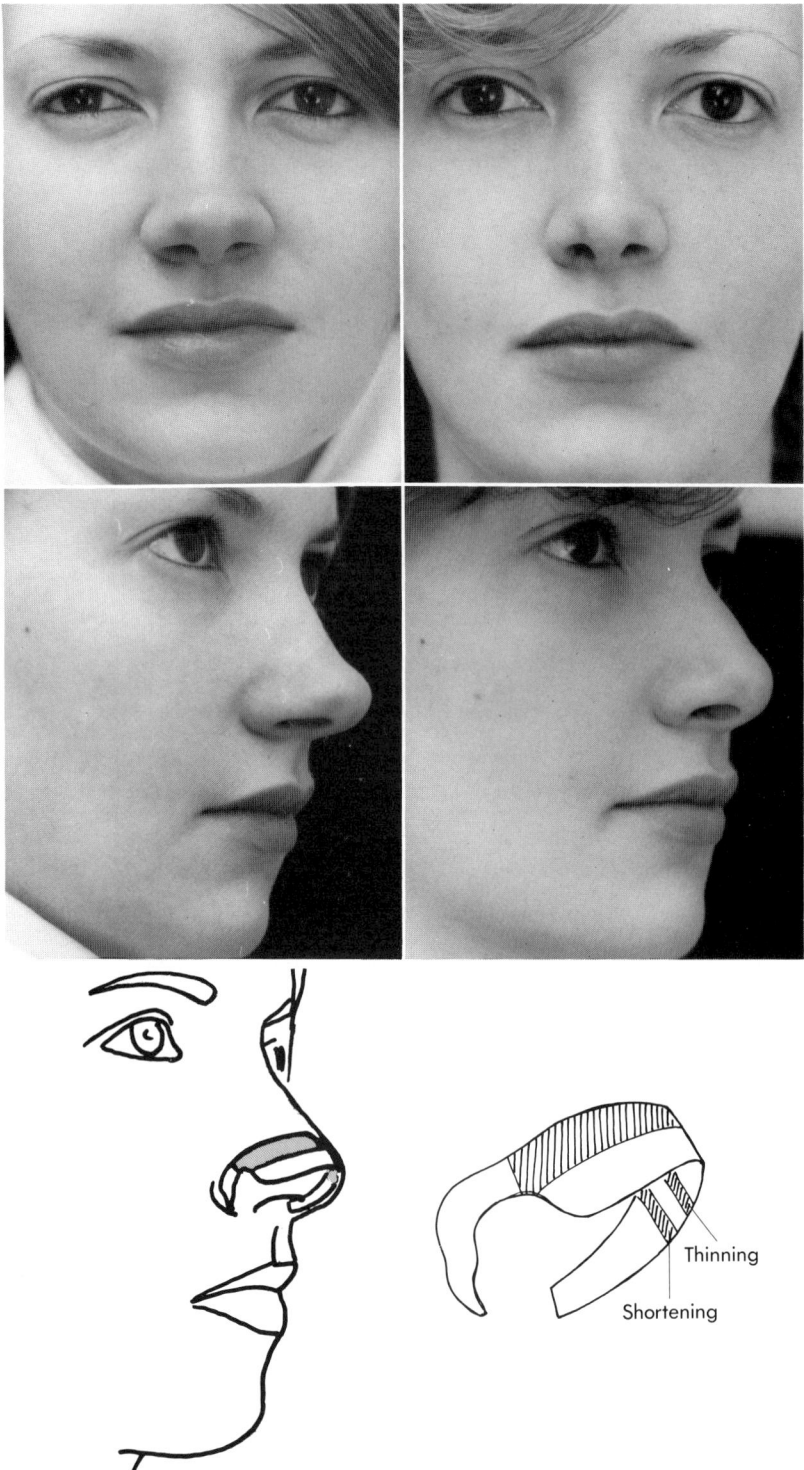

Figure 10-4. Correction of long, markedly projecting tip with strong supporting central column may require excision of strip of full-thickness cartilage from medial crus, preferably from medial side of dome.

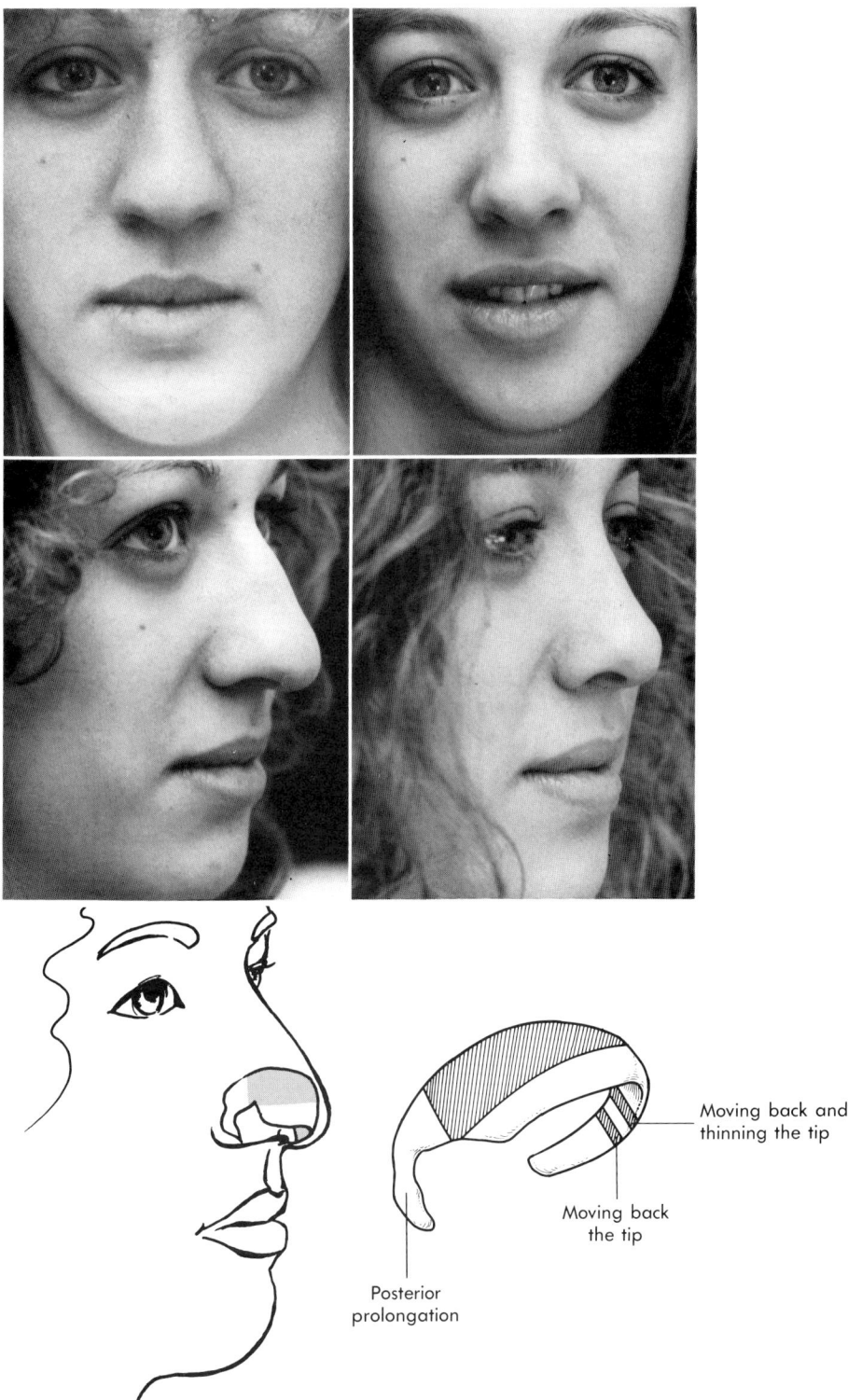

Figure 10-5. Reduction and refinement of thick, bulky tip in young girl. In such deformities it is especially important to maintain ample cartilaginous support to hold up thick, heavy skin.

In most cases one is obliged to retain intact the continuity between the lateral crus and the posterior prolongation to prevent overshortening of the nose. I dissect the cartilage in almost all cases so that I can control the surgery under direct vision in this area and can either cut the cartilage at the posterior prolongation, or not, as I find necessary.

The continuity between the lateral crus and the posterior prolongation must be respected in patients with long vertical faces and protruding chins. Overshortening the nose in such patients emphasizes the vertical length. Likewise, in patients with short columellae protection of the continuity prevents further shortening.

Sometimes the length and volume of the lateral crus are excessive, so that a full-thickness piece must be resected to permit backward displacement of the tip. At times it may be necessary to remove a full-thickness piece from both lateral and medial crura (Figure 10-7), although I dislike interrupting the cartilage in this way. Resection of more than 3 mm requires careful smoothing of the soft tissues to avoid deformity. I often employ this resection technique for correcting the so-called *boxy tip* where I have resected a full-thickness strip from the medial side of the dome of the alar cartilage (Figure 10-4).

In the patient with a very long columella that extends in a straight line, it may be necessary to resect more than 3 mm to adequately recess the tip. After such a large resection the angle must be smoothed to avoid a sharply acute double break. In such a situation the marginal incision is prolonged to permit exteriorization of the medial part of the lateral crus. A small triangle, which includes skin and cartilage, can then be trimmed, and the defect can be carefully repaired.

The bulky nose with thick skin is certainly one of the most difficult problems facing the rhinoplastic surgeon (Figure 10-5). Contrary to what seems logical, it is extremely important in such cases to leave behind more support in the form of retained cartilage to hold up the thick, heavy skin and protect the tip support. The cartilage acts as a shield. I virtually always retain more cartilage support in these thick and heavy-skinned noses than in thin-skinned noses with oversized cartilages. Such a preservative technique also applies to the acromegalic-type nose.

A special trap for the unwary is the boxy tip with posterior pinching. The cartilage seems to fade out at the posterior extension of the crura; this appearance is false, however, because the cartilage is present but is curved in the direction of the septum inside. In such patients aggressive resection of cartilage only aggravates the pinching effect, and the surgical result could be disastrous. It is preferable to allow the posterior part of the lateral crus to slip a little above the lateral walls, thereby maintaining spread and support. Such pinched noses often have an exaggerated lateral dimple. During surgery a pocket can be dissected beneath the dimple, and a small filler in the form of a plate of cartilage can be slipped inside.

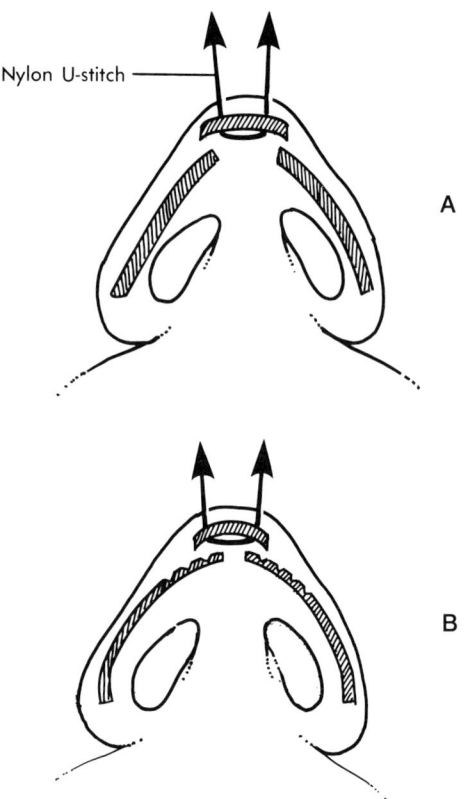

Nylon U-stitch

A

B

Figure 10-6. When it becomes necessary to resect significant amounts of full-thickness cartilage from lower lateral cartilage or to remove domes altogether, it is a good idea to prevent acute angulation by insertion of onlay graft to smooth contour. **A,** Shield graft smoothing the edges of the lateral crura. **B,** Shield graft and weakening of the lateral crura using the Lipsett technique.

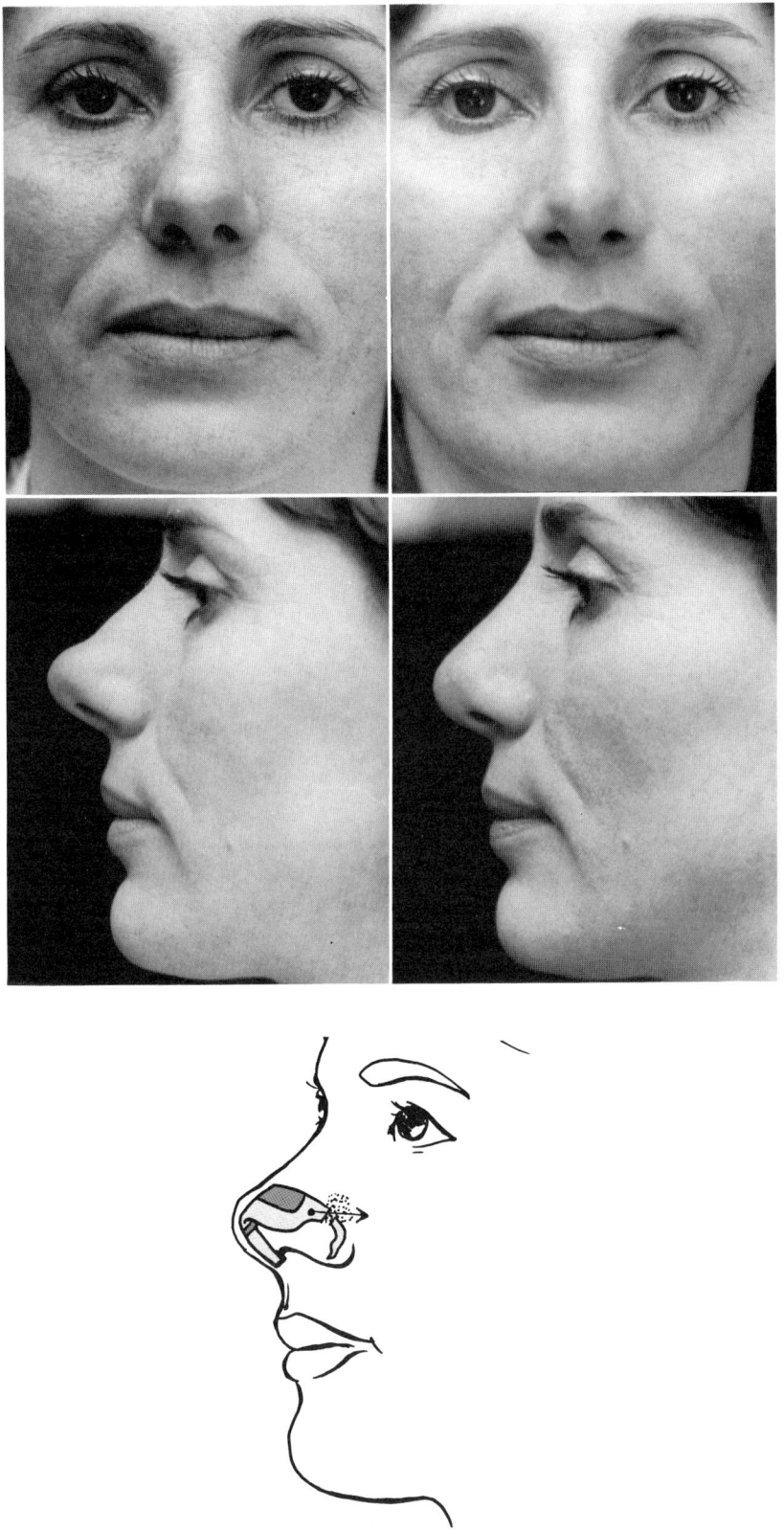

Figure 10-7. Bulky tip that is also markedly protruding requires not only reduction of cartilage (maintaining sufficient bulk for support) but also resection of medial and/or lateral full-thickness strip to permit retroposition of tip.

11

Unusual Tip Problems

Wolfgang Mühlbauer

HYPERTROPHIC ALAR CARTILAGES

The hypertrophic alar cartilage with a slightly or moderately prominent tip seems to be an easy problem to manage, but this perception is deceiving, because correction often can be achieved only with some difficulty. I usually plan to reduce and remodel the alar cartilages, preserving as much of the cartilage rim as possible. When two thirds of the cephalic portion of the lateral crura is resected, the tip is lowered by approximately 2 mm. If additional lowering is needed, the remaining cartilage rim can still be preserved but will be weakened by interdigitating incisions that extend incompletely through the width of the cartilage. These incisions weaken but do not break the spring (Figures 11-1 and 11-2).

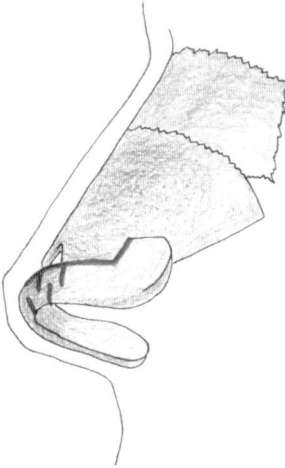

Figure 11-1. Pertinent anatomy in hypertrophic alar cartilage correction. Interdigitating incisions weaken the lateral crus to lower the tip.

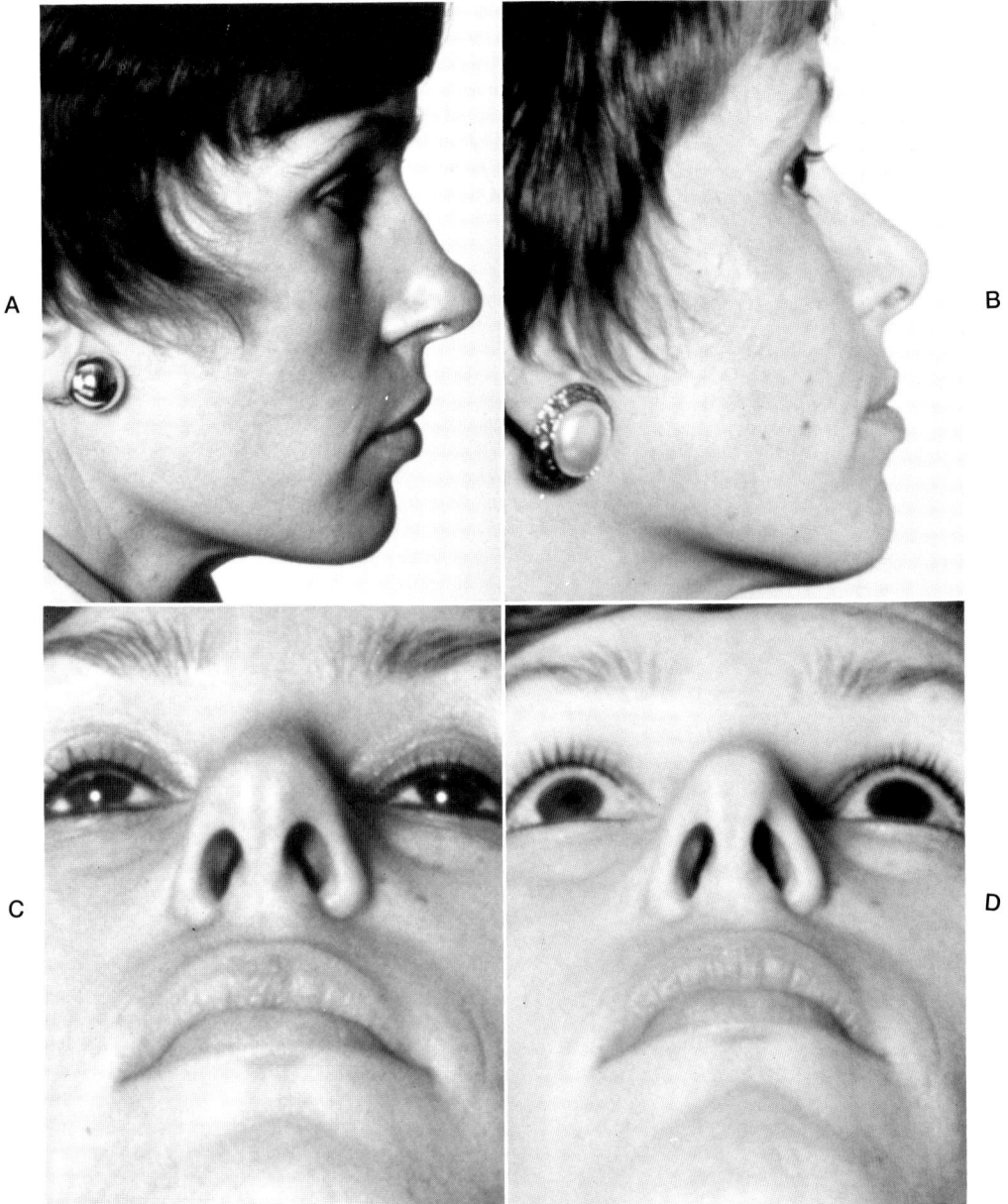

Figure 11-2. **A** and **B,** Lateral preoperative and postoperative views of patient with hypertrophic alar cartilages. **C** and **D,** Frontal views of same patient before and after surgery. Technique is shown in Figure 11-1.

BIFID TIP

The bifid tip is best handled by exposing the entire cartilage. Several options are then available for correcting this deformity. I often like to gain a full view of the lower lateral cartilages by exposing them completely to ensure precise resection. The entire cartilage must then be reconstructed; to achieve this I often suture the domes together (Figures 11-3 and 11-4).

BROAD TIP (Figure 11-5)

The patient in Figure 11-6 typifies the problem encountered in remodeling the broad tip. In this patient the lateral crura of the lower lateral cartilages are concave rather than convex. To correct this deformity I removed the cephalic three fourths of the lower lateral (alar) cartilage, then transected the remaining caudal part of the genu, reversing it by 180 degrees so that the concave shape became convex. I then replaced it in this rotated position. The dome was reconstructed with 6-0 absorbable sutures.

Of course, each case is different and requires a different strategy by the surgeon to solve the problem. The point I want to emphasize is that the cartilages must be reconstructed almost completely in many cases.

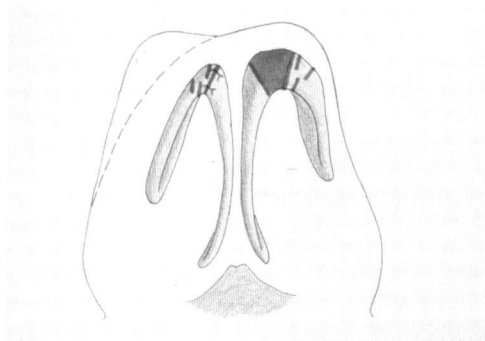

Figure 11-3. Pertinent anatomy in bifid tip.

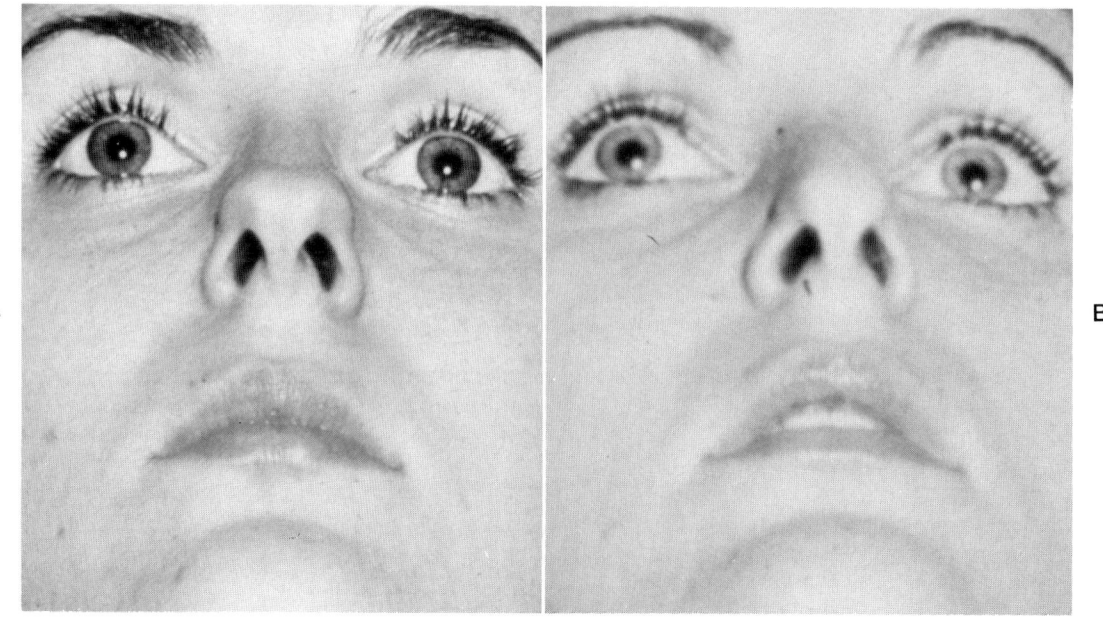

Figure 11-4. Preoperative (**A**) and postoperative (**B**) views of patient with bifid tip.

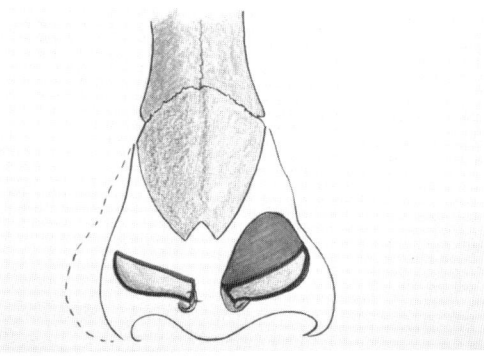

Figure 11-5. Pertinent anatomy in broad tip.

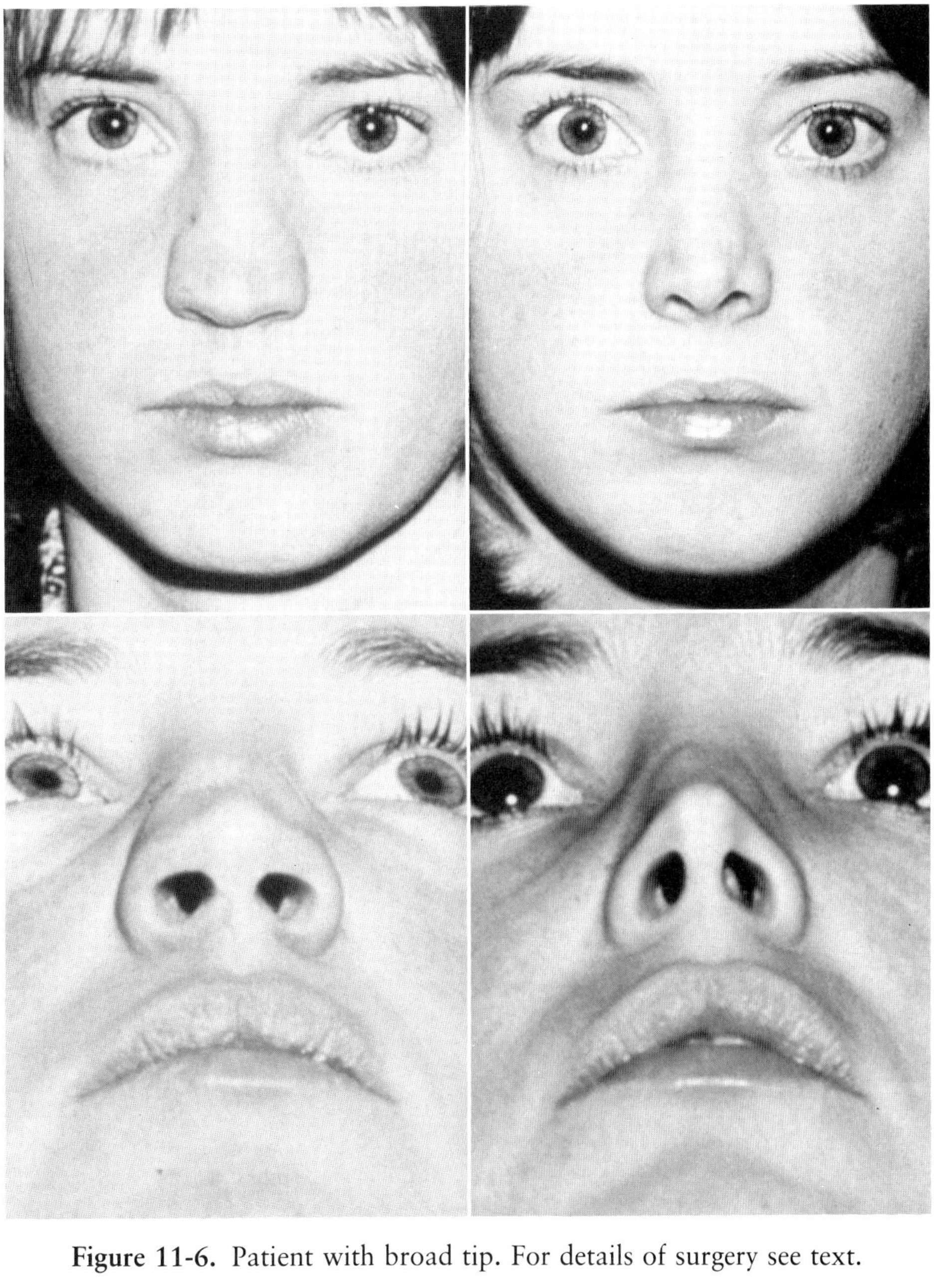

Figure 11-6. Patient with broad tip. For details of surgery see text.

PROMINENT TIP

I resect the domes in only about 10% of the cases I manage, but in truly prominent tips I think resection is necessary. I do no resection at the base of the medial crura and rely on the entire tip complex to slide downward. This maneuver is not precise but is often effective. When it is necessary to totally resect the domes in tips that project too much, I reconstruct them with interdigitating cuts so that the tip contour will round out and not be pointed. This technique and its variations are illustrated in Figures 11-7 and 11-8.

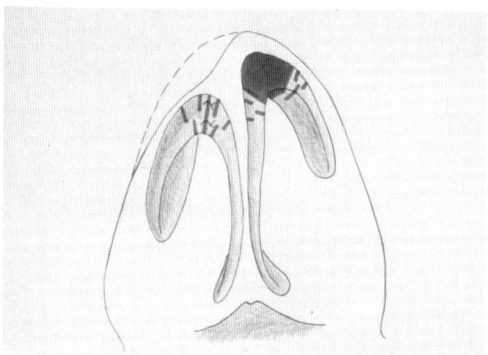

Figure 11-7. Pertinent anatomy in prominent tip.

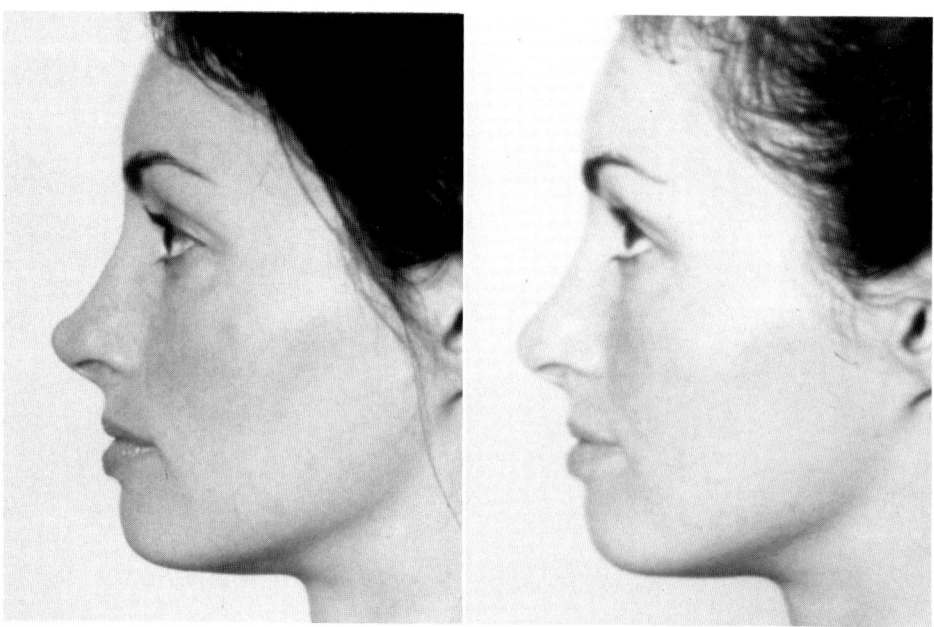

Figure 11-8. Patient with prominent tip. Projection was reduced by resecting domes and weakening the remnants of the lateral crura.

LONG NOSE AND HIDDEN COLUMELLA

In patients with this difficult problem I shorten the cartilaginous nose by resecting approximately two thirds of the lateral crura and then rotating the tip upward. To lower the tip projection I then resect the genua and reconstruct them. Once again, precise reconstruction of the dome is the key to success in treating these patients and is necessary for a predictable long-term result. Nothing need be done to the caudal septum; the shortening effect is achieved by the alar rotation alone.

Such a procedure was used to solve the problem in the patient shown in Figure 11-9. She also required a small amount of rasping of the dorsal hump.

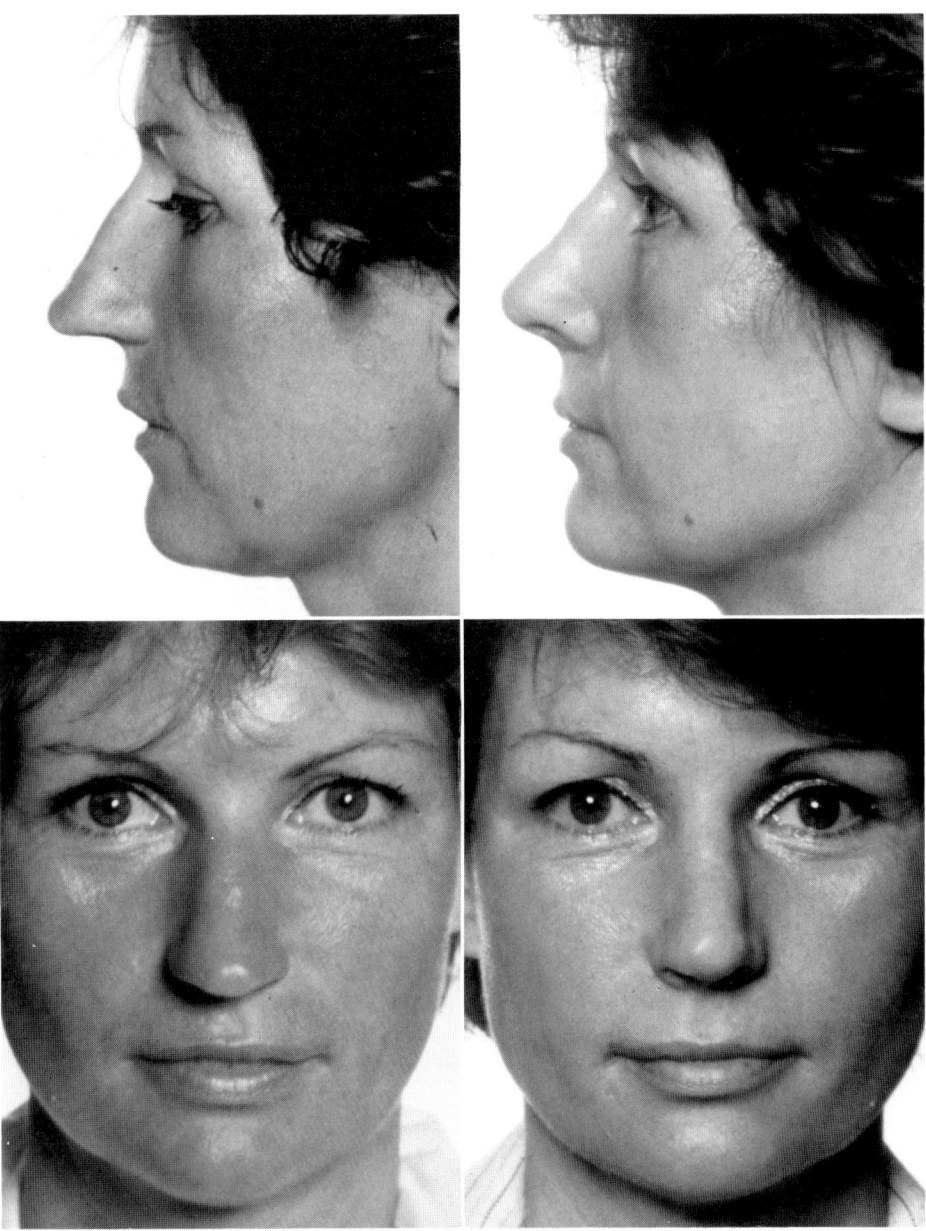

Figure 11-9. Preoperative and postoperative photos of patient with a long nose and hidden columella, treated by rotation of the reduced lateral crura and precise reconstruction of the dome.

DROOPING TIP

The tip that droops is at least partially the result of a hyperactive depressor muscle of the septum. This problem is illustrated in Figure 11-10. This patient also has a retrusion of the alveolus. In such situations strong support of the tip is required.

I usually denude the caudal part of the septum of its mucoperichondrium and then split the columella to ride over the denuded septum in a riding-saddle manner. Rees[1] has called this the *tongue-in-groove technique*. I suture the medial crura over the denuded septal edge with two mattress sutures to keep the tip firmly in its new position. To relieve the downward traction, the hyperactive depressor muscle of the septum is transected at two levels to prevent recurrence of the depressor action on the tip, which drags the tip down. This technique ensures strong support of the columella on the caudal septum even when the patient smiles or is otherwise animated. The technique is illustrated in Figure 11-11.

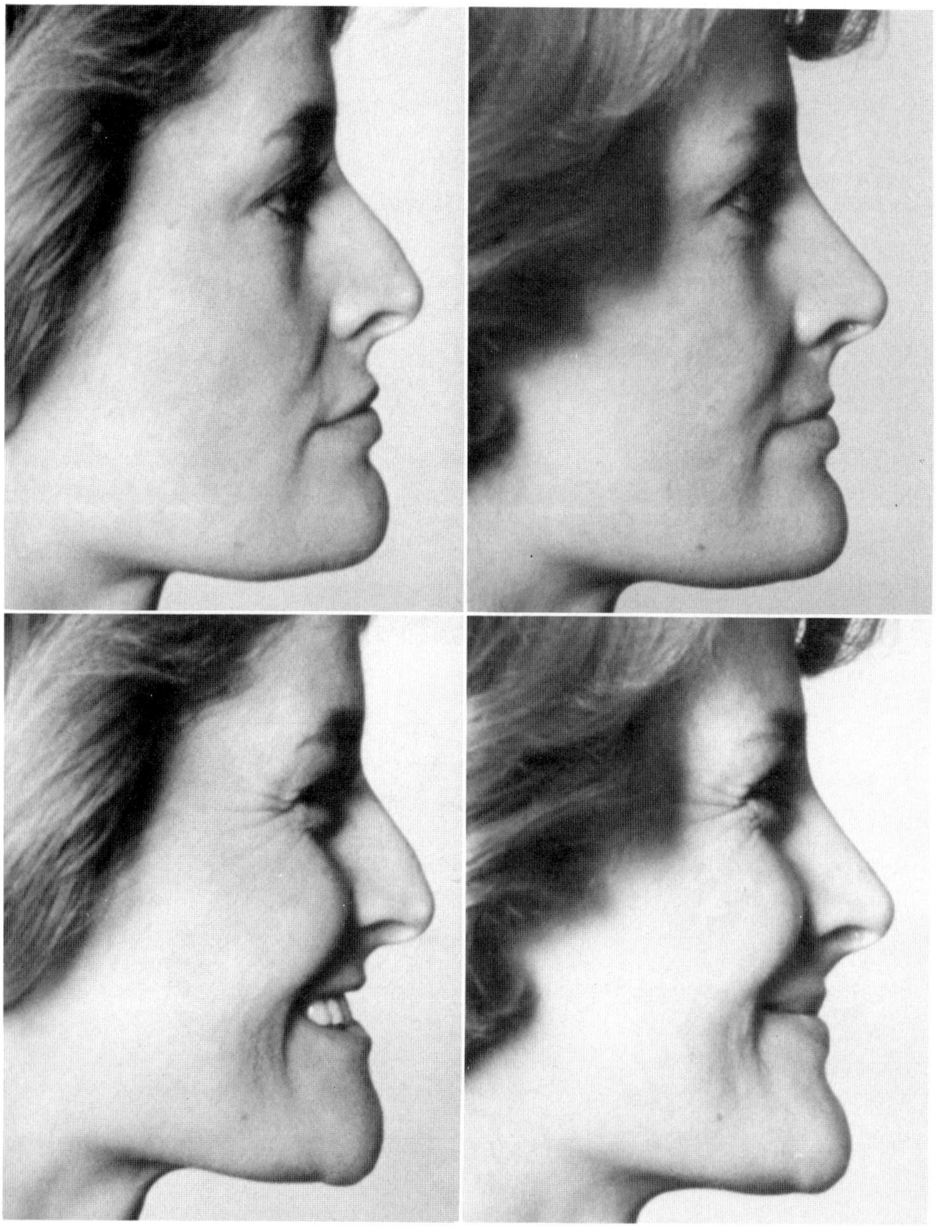

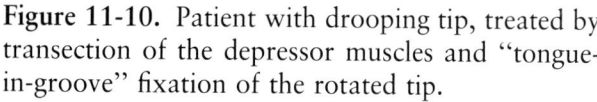

Figure 11-10. Patient with drooping tip, treated by transection of the depressor muscles and "tongue-in-groove" fixation of the rotated tip.

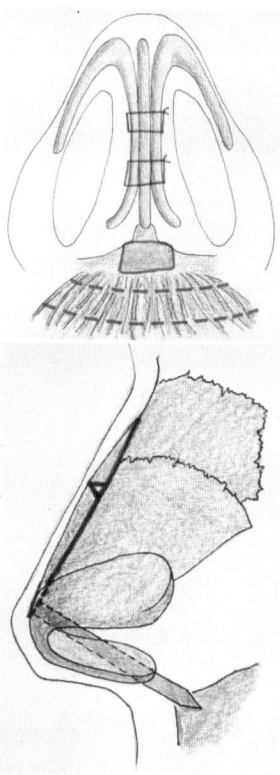

Figure 11-11. Technique for drooping tip.

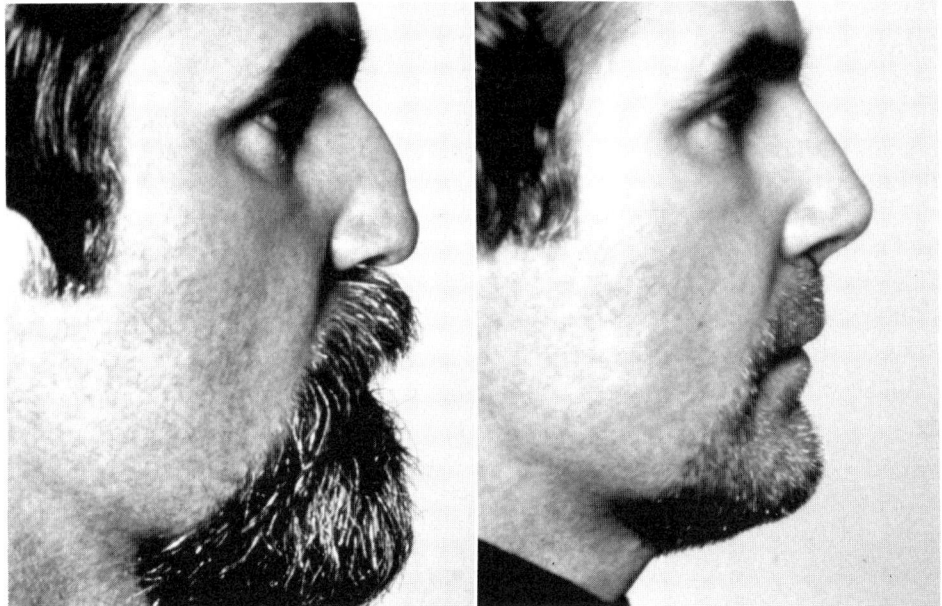

Figure 11-12. Patient with absence of tip support.

ABSENCE OF TIP SUPPORT

The patient in Figure 11-12 completely lacks tip support after radical submucous resection. Fortunately a pseudohump was still present, since a rhinoplasty had not been done. The problem was solved by shifting the pseudohump caudally about 1 cm, and then, for extra support, a Kirschner pin was placed to further hold the parts in position. The result shown has persisted for about 4 years, and the shape has been maintained (Figure 11-13).

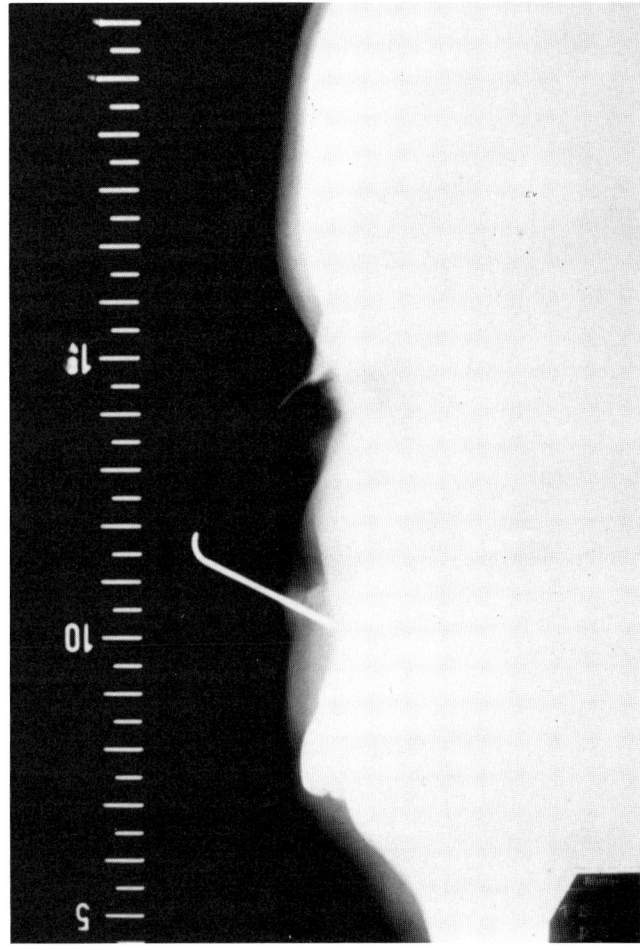

Figure 11-13. Radiograph shows Kirschner pin placed to provide tip support.

BULKY TIP

Management of the bulky tip with thick, oily, nonelastic skin can be very challenging. I often choose to reduce such noses in two stages. In the first stage a complete three-dimensional reduction is done, but little of the supporting structure of the tip is removed. The thicker the skin, the more support it requires. After the first procedure the nose is usually smaller in all dimensions. The patient in Figures 11-14 and 11-15 illustrates my approach to this problem. After the first procedure one can see that the supratip swelling was present because of the abundant subcutaneous tissue present. In the second procedure additional excessive subcutaneous tissue was removed, and an alar base resection was done. The final result (Figure 11-15, *D* and *F*) is far from ideal, but it is a definite improvement. I do not think the result in such a patient is ever ideal.

REFERENCE

1. Rees, T.D.: Cosmetic facial surgery, Philadelphia, 1973, W.B. Saunders Co.

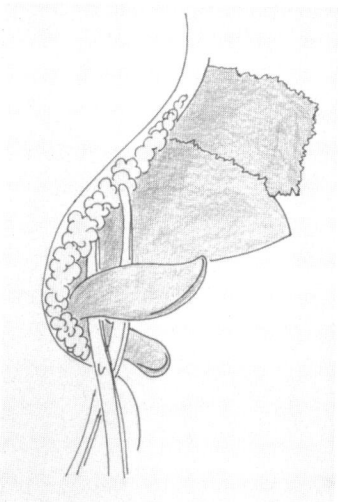

Figure 11-14. Technique for bulky tip.

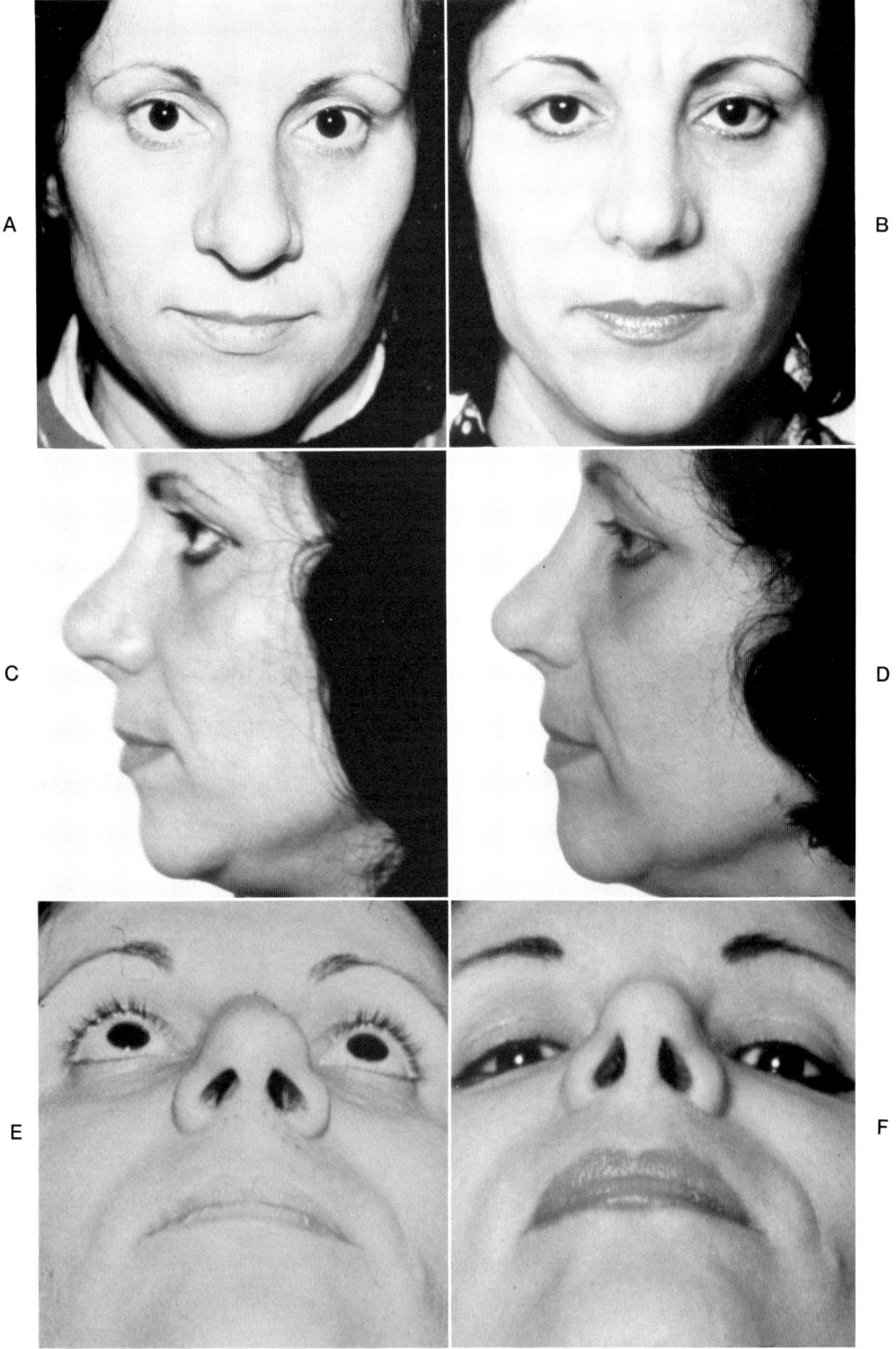

Figure 11-15. Patient with bulky tip.

12

Nasal Tip—Unusual Problems

Thomas Rees

In about 75% of operations I perform on the nose, I use the standard transcartilaginous or intracartilaginous (cartilage splitting) technique and strive to maintain intact a reasonable amount (3 to 4 mm) of caudal rim of the alar cartilages and to keep the spring uninterrupted. This technique is reliable in treating most patients. In fact, many surgeons prefer to use the intracartilaginous incision as the primary incision into the nose, obviating the intercartilaginous incision altogether. This technique is illustrated in Figure 12-1, and the patient in Figure 12-2 is an ideal candidate for this operation. The alar cartilages are moderately enlarged, and the aim of surgery is simply to reduce them and to allow them to assume a new position in the tip.

I believe that patients who have unusually shaped or distorted cartilages or who require reduction of projection, complete reconstruction of the tip angle, or any other nonstandard corrective procedure are best approached with the cartilage delivery or alar flap technique. This technique was probably first developed by Safian and further modified by many others, especially Lipsett. It can be performed safely by the beginning surgeon, since it permits complete visualization of the alar cartilage so that it can be carved, manipulated, and reconstructed as required. The cartilage is delivered by an incision made around the caudal edge of the alar cartilage—not truly a rim incision but a pararim incision. It is important not to violate the soft tissue triangle, as has often been emphasized by Converse and others. Injury to the soft tissues of the soft triangle results in notching, scarring, and distortion.

The alar flap technique creates a bipedicled flap that is delivered through the nostril for direct dissection by the surgeon. In certain patients, especially those in whom the projecting tip must be set back or reduced, the bipedicled flap can be converted to a single pedicle based laterally. The medial crus is transected through both lining and cartilage, the required carving is done, and any excess cartilage and lining is removed from the medial crus to recess the tip. Careful suturing and reconstruction are required. Altogether this technique is more painstaking and requires more time than do standard approaches.

Safian[2] has pointed out that the caudal margin of the alar cartilage can also be reduced by the alar flap method, with elevation of the nostril rim in patients in need. The procedure is shown in Figure 12-3. An important part of this technique is weakening or cross-hatching of the cartilage so that the remaining portion will bend to its new configuration. The cartilage can also be weakened by morcellizing or crushing it, although this is a somewhat less refined maneuver. Staggering the crosscuts so that none is carried completely across the width of the cartilage, as suggested by Sheen, has proved to be an important refinement in the technique that has to a large extent avoided much of the knuckling and distortion of the tip seen postoperatively when the original Lipsett[1] technique was carried out.

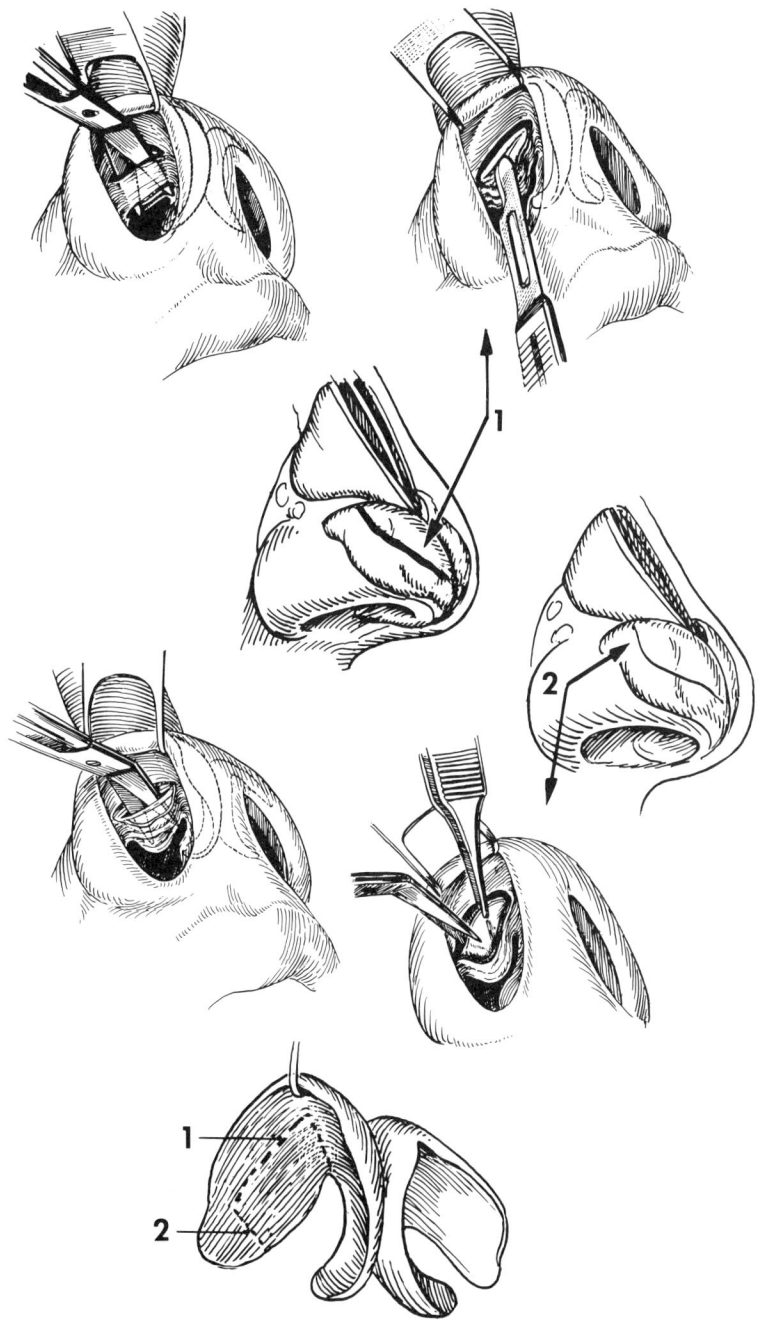

Figure 12-1. Intracartilaginous technique of tip reduction. Steps in procedure are shown beginning in upper left corner. Incision is made longitudinally, splitting lining of undersurface of lateral wing of alar cartilage, after which cartilage itself is incised within its borders; hence word *intracartilaginous*. Actual amount of cartilage to be removed from cephalic portion of lateral crus depends on size and shape of wing and can be determined by surgeon. In most patients spring, or lower border of wing, is kept intact, and at least 3 to 4 mm of alar width is preserved. (From Rees, T.D.: Aesthetic plastic surgery, vol. 1, Philadelphia, 1980, W.B. Saunders Co.)

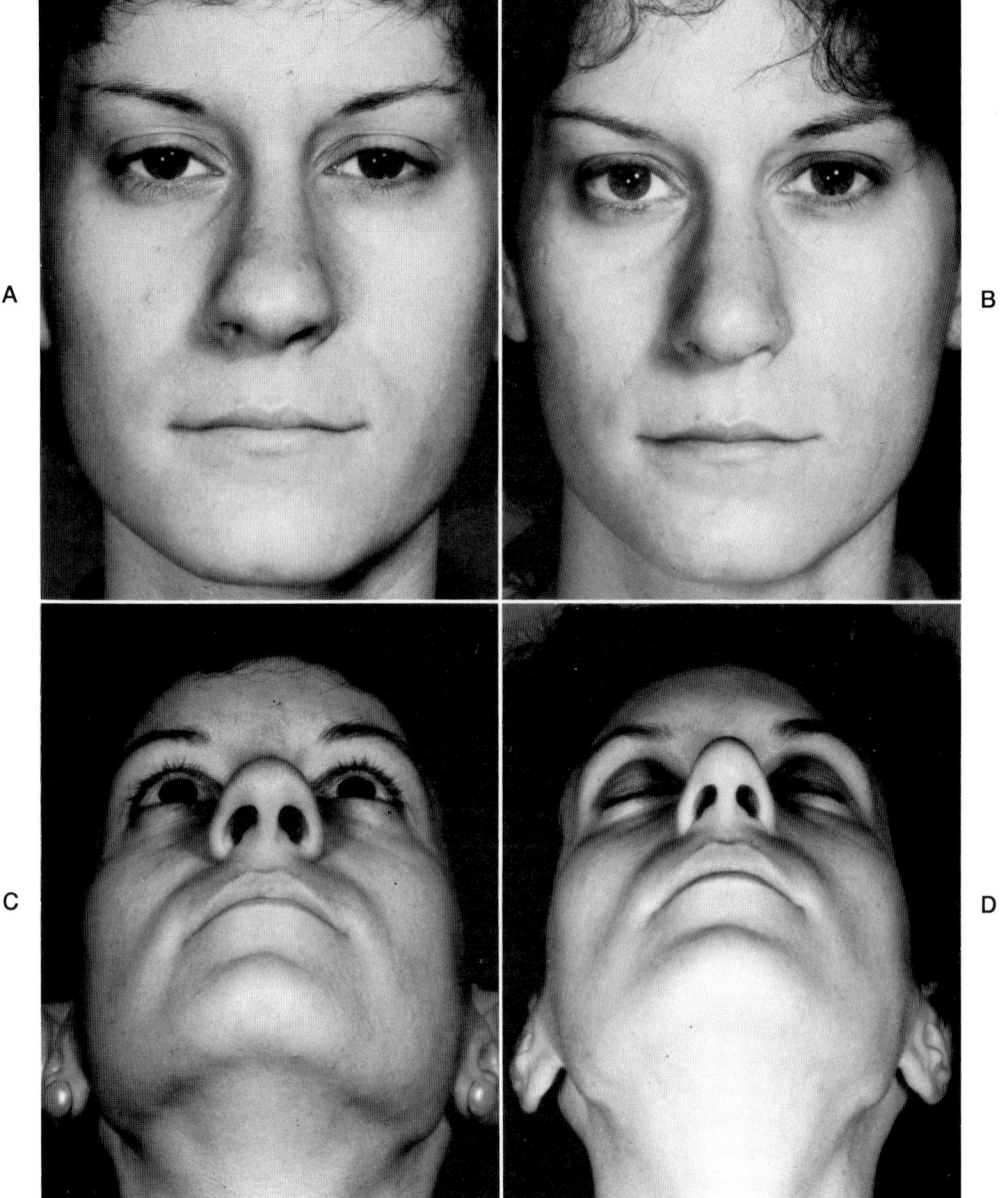

Figure 12-2. Excellent candidate for tip reduction by intracartilaginous technique (standard technique). Alar cartilages were quite hypertrophic, but shape of cartilages and angles formed between medial and lateral crura were not excessively acute or obtuse. Only complaint this patient had was large size of her tip; accordingly, only tip underwent operation, and alar base wedge was resected to reduce nostril size and flare. Osseocartilaginous vault was not surgically invaded. Result is certainly not small delicate tip but one that is much more in keeping patient's with general facial features and size of her nasal bony vault. **A** and **C,** Preoperative views; **B** and **D,** postoperative views.

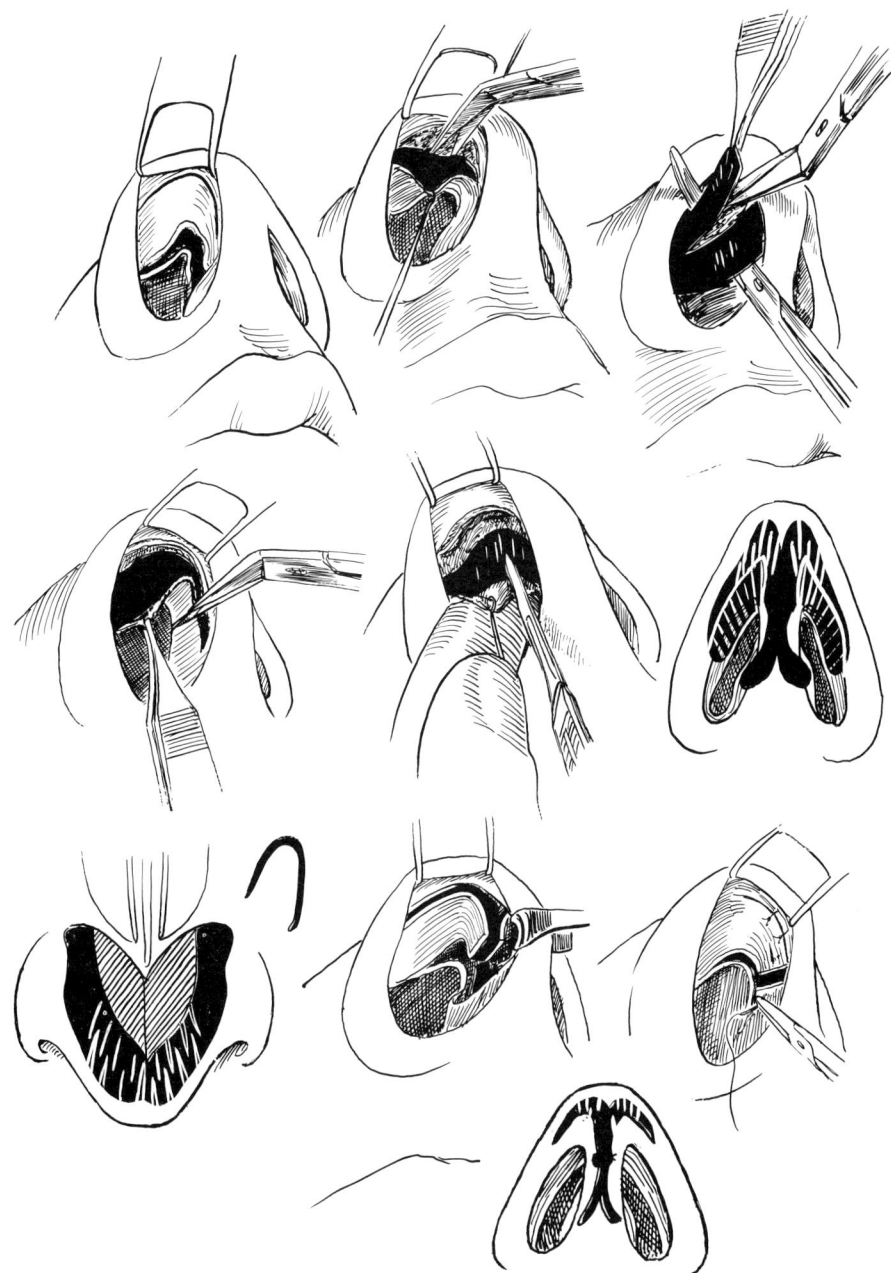

Figure 12-3. Various steps of technique involved in alar flap or "delivery" technique. Alar cartilages can be delivered as a bipedicled or single-pedicled flap based medially. Several variations of this technique can be selected for individual problem at hand. Cartilage is usually weakened by crosscuts or morcellation. Staggering of crosscuts is helpful in preventing postoperative "knuckling," which can follow multiple crosscuts through full width of remaining rim of alar cartilage. Section of cartilage is sometimes removed, usually from medial side of the genu or directly from genu or dome. All incisions must be meticulously repaired. (From Rees, T.D.: Aesthetic plastic surgery, vol. 1, Philadelphia, 1980, W.B. Saunders Co.)

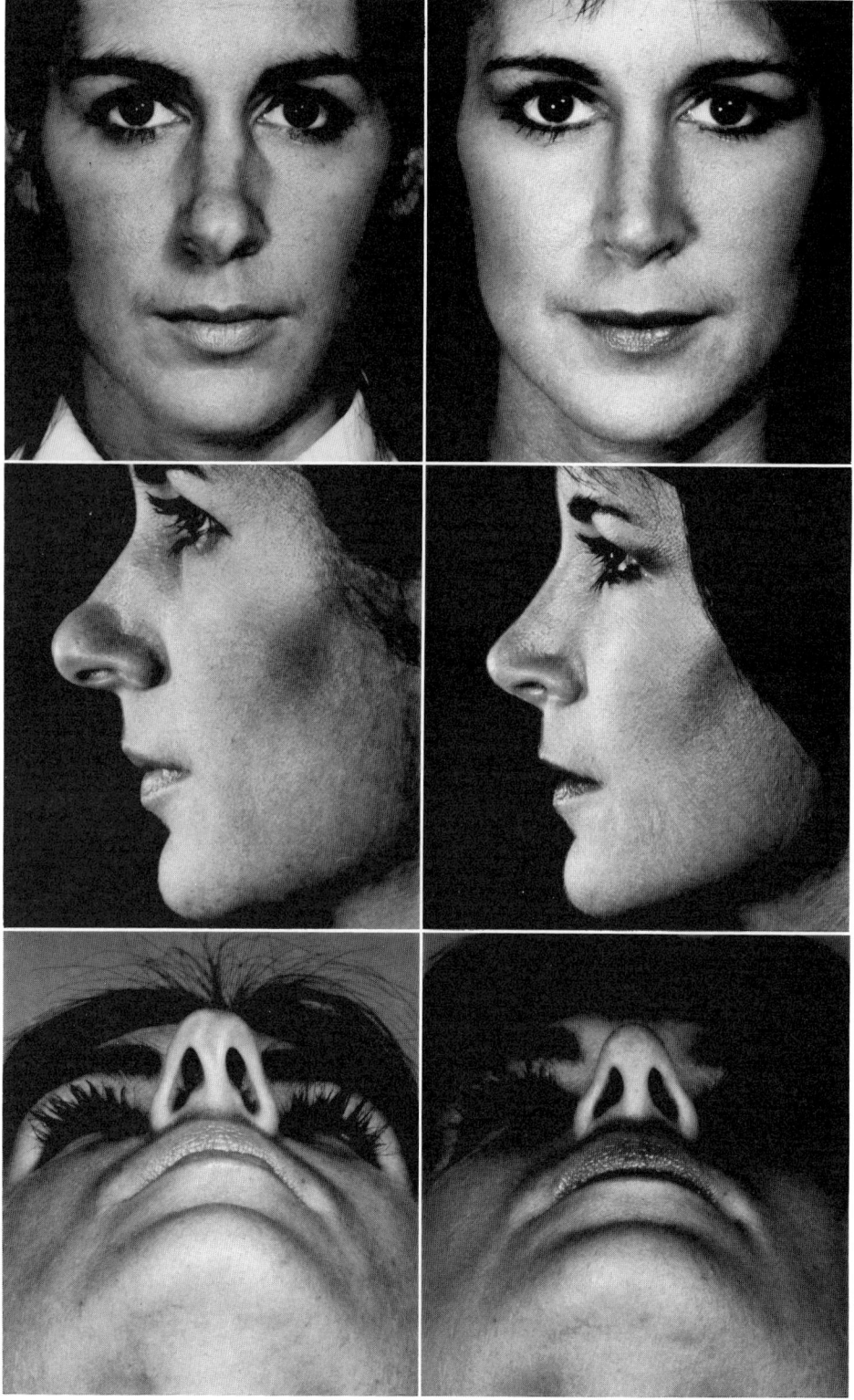

Figure 12-4. Ideal patient for tip reconstruction by alar flap technique. Tip cartilages are very large and asymmetric. Note that the right alar cartilage rides above the left in a more cephalic position, and the genua of the two cartilages are at different levels. (From Rees, T.D.: Aesthetic plastic surgery, vol. 1, Philadelphia, 1980, W.B. Saunders Co.)

The patient in Figure 12-4 is an ideal candidate for the alar flap operation. Her alar cartilages are huge and asymmetric. Simple reduction of the cartilages would not suffice; reduction and reconstruction were required. A single pedicled flap based laterally was used, and about 5 mm of full thickness was removed from the medial crus, along with the lining, to set the tip back.

All tip procedures are used to reduce the thick, bulky tip that grossly resembles a potato; however, an operation I prefer is the eversion technique. The procedure has been especially popular in England, where I learned it years ago. The lateral crus is undermined on the skin side, with every attempt made to include all subcutaneous fat with the cartilage. The entire wing is then everted, and a significant "chunk" of tissue, including lining, cartilage, and

subcutaneous tissue, is resected. A rim of cartilage is preserved to maintain projection and provide support. The raw area that results from removal of lining is partially covered by the upper lateral cartilage, which must be preserved virtually in its entirety to protect the integrity of the internal valve. A portion of the raw surface is permitted to heal by contracture, which partially explains the efficacy of this somewhat rough technique. Wound contracture is being used to advantage here to create a narrower tip. I emphasize that the eversion technique is used only in patients with large, beefy, and "difficult" tips. Sometimes, however, the results are striking. The technique is shown in Figure 12-5, and Figure 12-6 provides an excellent illustration of what often can be achieved.

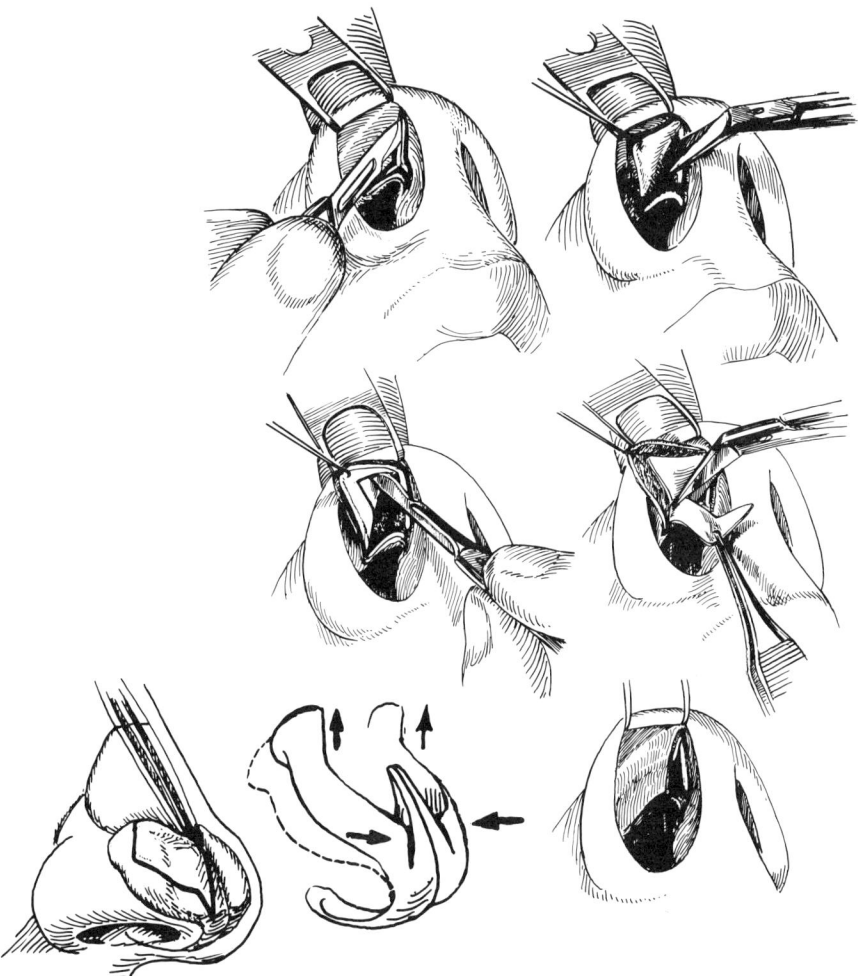

Figure 12-5. Eversion technique of tip reduction for large, bulky tips. Technique is often referred to as *retrograde technique*, since cartilages are undermined from above, inverted, and held with hook in retrograde position. (From Rees, T.D.: Aesthetic plastic surgery, vol. 1, Philadelphia, 1980, W.B. Saunders Co.)

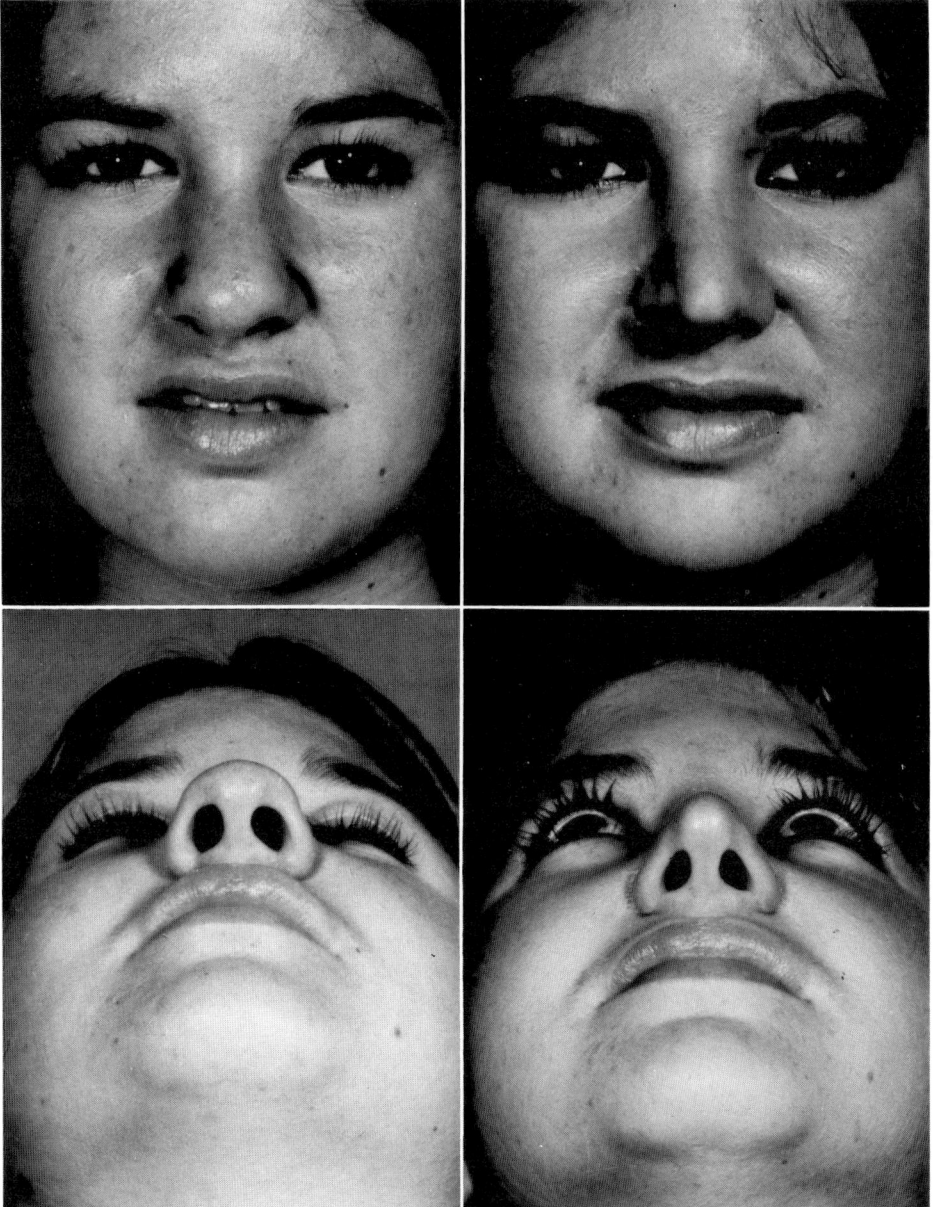

Figure 12-6. Patient presents very difficult problem in tip reduction. Cartilages are large and boxlike, with open angle between medial and lateral crura; however, aspect of this surgical challenge most difficult to manage is thickened skin and subcutaneous tissue, which always makes result problematic. Eversion technique is often effective in such patients, since subcutaneous fat is reduced, as is cartilage. Lining is also purposefully sacrificed to increase overall reduction of tip tissues, and even small area of unsatisfied lining is left inside nose to heal by contraction. Full reconstruction or maintenance of upper lateral cartilages is of course mandatory to protect internal valve when eversion technique is used. Result in this young woman was achieved without use of tip grafts or any form of tip augmentation whatsoever.

I use many small crushed pieces of cartilage to fill small defects of the tip during rhinoplasty; they can effectively augment the deficient tip and the inwardly curved lateral crus to fill the unwanted cleft or dimple between the medial crura and also to fill out the base of the columella.

I am not as enthusiastic as some other surgeons about primary tip grafts to provide tip projection. I use primary tip grafts in less than 15% of my patients, and when I sincerely doubt whether a tip graft is necessary, I wait several months and perform it as a secondary procedure. At that time I find it much easier to control the pocket size exactly and to place and fix the graft where I wish. It is difficult to stabilize a tip projection graft when the nose has otherwise been almost completely dissected, especially when the alar cartilage has been reduced during primary surgery. Therefore, I do not hesitate to immobilize the graft by transcutaneous sutures; I use double-armed plain catgut sutures. In about a week, when the cast is removed, the sutures are cut where they penetrate the skin. I have had no problems or complaints with this suture.

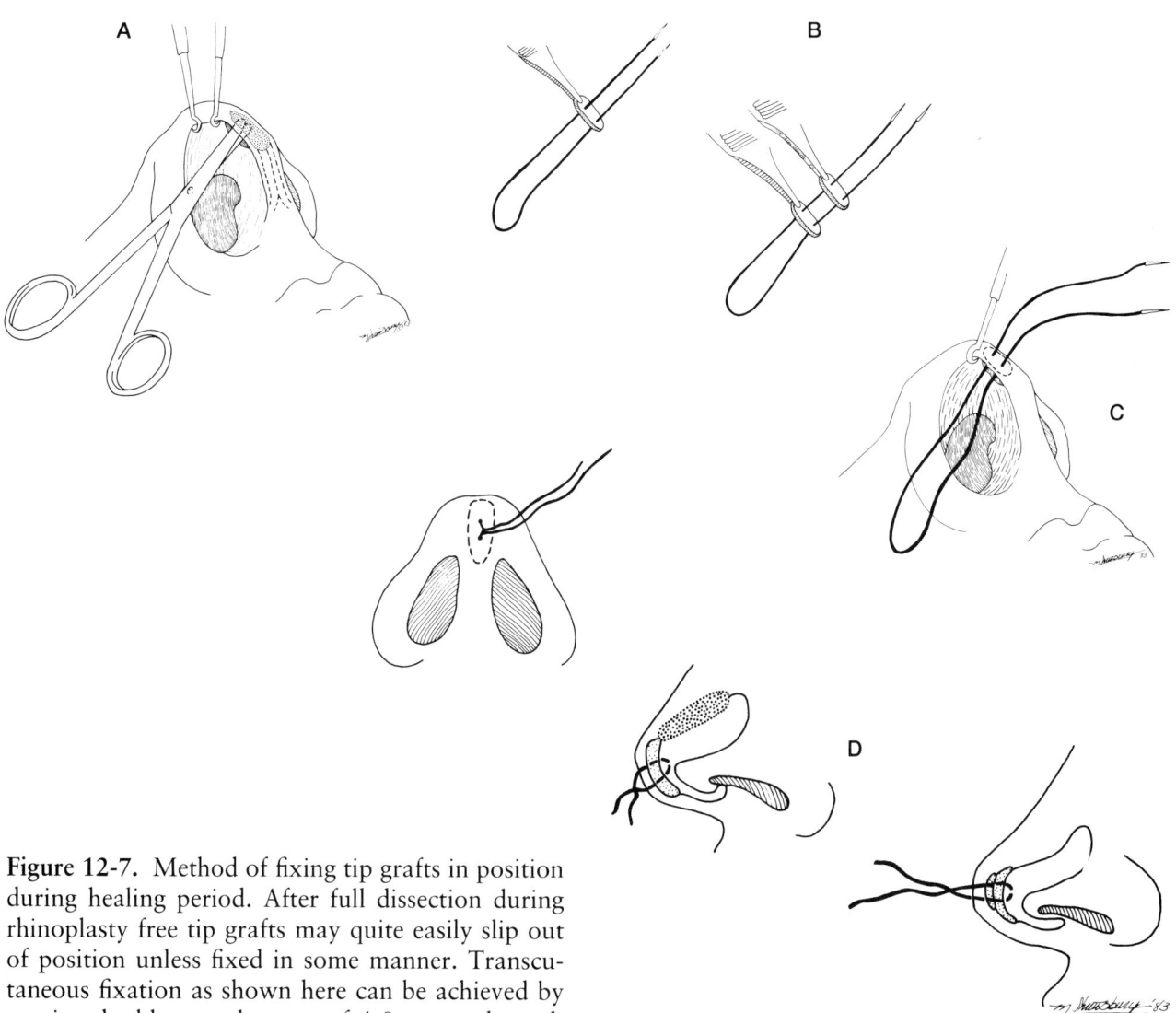

Figure 12-7. Method of fixing tip grafts in position during healing period. After full dissection during rhinoplasty free tip grafts may quite easily slip out of position unless fixed in some manner. Transcutaneous fixation as shown here can be achieved by passing double-armed suture of 4-0 catgut through graft (which can be one, two, or even three tiers in thickness) and then through the skin exactly where surgeon wishes. Suture is tied loosely to avoid cutting into skin, and ends are clipped in about 1 week, allowing ends to retract into skin. No permanent suture marks have been encountered in large number of patients. Grafts remain in position. **A,** Pocket is dissected through small rim incision. **B,** Double-armed suture is passed through one or two layers of graft, which can be alar cartilage or septal cartilage. **C,** Needles are passed through skin, holding graft in position. **D,** Sutures are tied loosely.

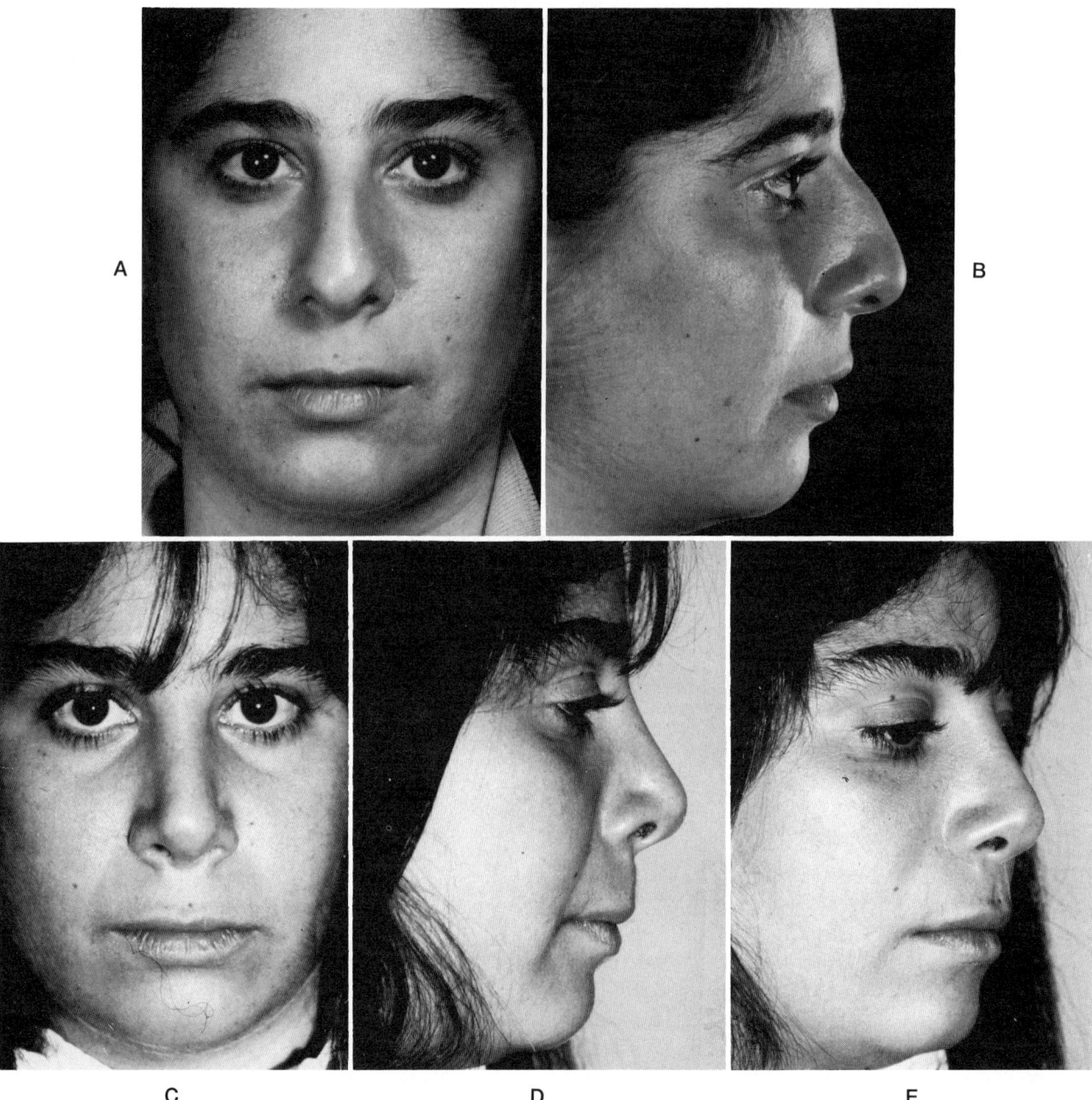

Figure 12-8. This patient demonstrates tip augmentation for increasing projection by transcutaneous graft suture fixation technique. **A** and **B,** Note flat, boxy tip with insufficient projection. **C, D,** and **E,** Note result achieved. Postoperative photographs were taken after 6 months.

The technique for graft fixation is depicted in Figure 12-7. I use one or two tiers of alar cartilage as graft material, provided the alar cartilages are firm and thick. If they are substantial, they provide excellent graft material, certainly as good as auricular cartilage. If the alar cartilages are flimsy or attenuated, I then prefer a carved septal cartilage graft, or I prefer auricular cartilage if the septum has been removed. I would stress that a tip graft is frequently visualized through the skin in thin-skinned patients and should be used with great care in such patients. Every effort must be made to trim the graft and soften the edges to avoid unsightly sharp lines. In very thick-skinned patients the opposite is true; that is, the problem is in seeing the grafts and maintaining projection of the tip despite the thick, nonyielding skin. A patient with a flat, boxy tip, as shown in Figure 12-8, is ideally suited to a primary tip graft. In such patients it is difficult to achieve tip projection by any other technique.

REFERENCES

1. Lipsett, E.M.: A new approach to surgery of the lower cartilaginous vault, Arch. Otolaryngol. 70:42, 1959.
2. Safian, J.: Corrective rhinoplastic surgery, New York, 1935, Paul B. Hoeber, Inc.

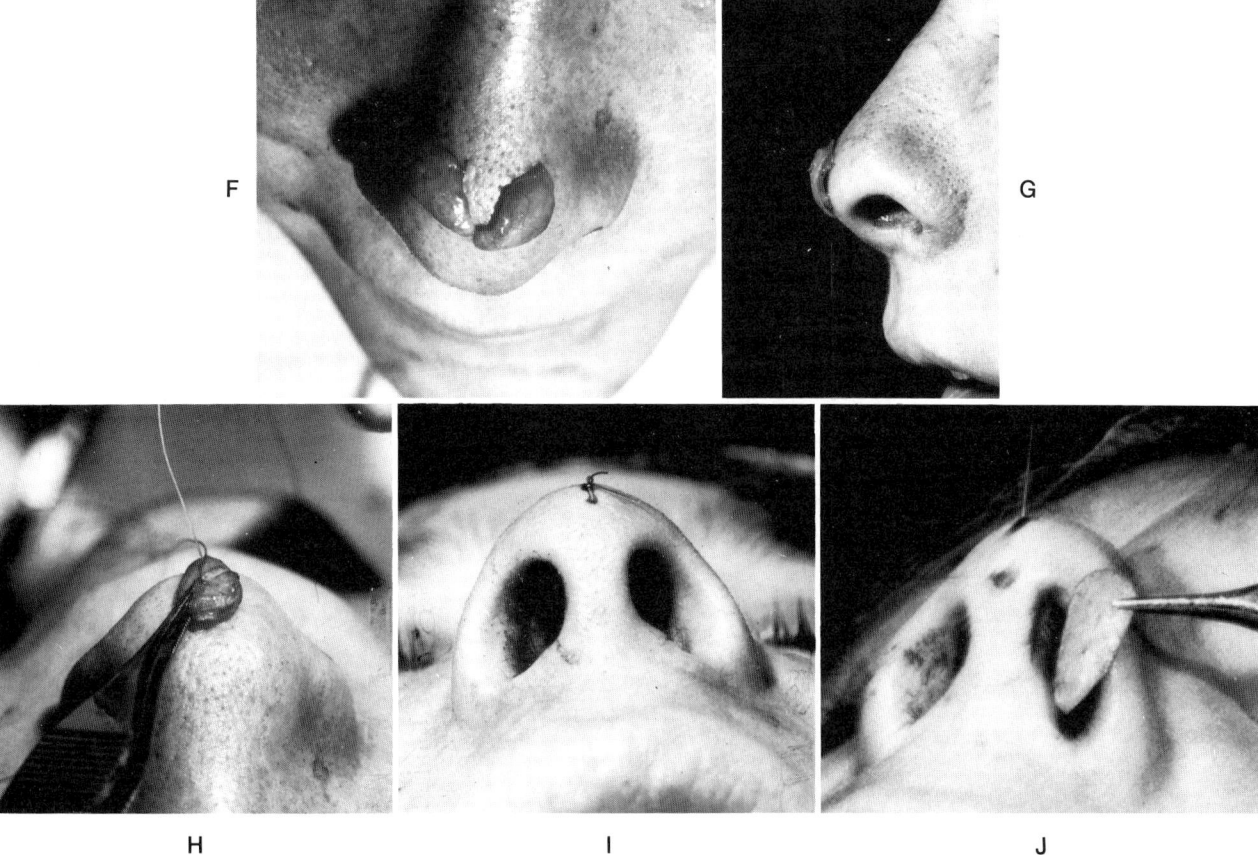

Figure 12-8, cont'd. F, G, H, and **I,** Intraoperative photographs of patient. Alar cartilages were quite thick and suitable for graft material. Resected cartilages were not discarded; rather, it appeared that they would suffice as graft material for projection (**F** and **G**). Two-tiered graft was carved, and tiers were sutured together, as illustrated in Figure 12-7 (**H**). Sutures were passed through skin and loosely tied (**I**). If alar cartilages are not of sufficient caliber sturdy septal cartilage graft can be fixed by same technique, as shown in patient in **J.**

Point & Counterpoint
Part II

Question: Is it necessary to make a complete transfixion incision?

Comment (Gene Tardy): There are times, such as in the recession of an overprojecting tip, when obviously a complete transfixion incision is preferable. I make this point only because the tip supports of the nose are often violated without purpose when projection is satisfactory and simply needs to be preserved. Too often we do things in rhinoplasty without thinking them out. If you can maintain the attachment of the medial crural footplates to the caudal margin of the septum, thereby preserving a major support mechanism, why not do that by limiting the incision to a partial or limited transfixion incision? However, if for some reason you require access to the nasal spine or to the caudal nasal septum, or if there is a caudal subluxation of the septum, a complete transfixion incision is useful. It is not, however, an absolute necessity, since other more limited incisions provide satisfactory access.

Comment (George Peck): I have changed my technique in the last few years. If you make an intracartilaginous incision to begin with and carry it around into the transfixion incision, a horseshoe-shaped incision results that will heal as a horseshoe-shaped scar. We know that a circular scar tends to contract as a straight line. If you will look at these noses postoperatively you will see contracture scars that can be prevented by making two incisions. You can do everything through both incisions. In other words, separate the transfixion incision completely from the transcartilaginous incision so that you have intact vestibular skin between the two incisions.

Comment (Harvey Caplan): There are all degrees of transfixion incisions. I have often been intrigued by the high transfixion incision where the membranous septum is not detached, but a component of the inferior border of the septum, say about 2 to 3 mm, is contained in the lower segment by transection above the caudal margin of the septum. The septum can be shortened, but in this way the fibroligamentous crural attachments are undisturbed, yet the nose can be shortened if required by trimming the posterior segment of the septum. I have no objections to the transfixion incision. I do object to use of strong septocolumella sutures. I don't overcorrect the tip

afterward or expect the nose to drop. I suture mucous membrane vestibular skin with fine 5-0 sutures.

Comment (Jack Sheen): I would like to second Dr. Tardy's comment about limiting incisions, which I think is extremely important. No cut is made in rhinoplasty without purpose, not only the transfixion incision. I disagree with Dr. Peck's statements about the cause of vestibular scar contracture being the joining of transfixion incisions with intercartilaginous incisions. I don't think scar contracture in the vestibule will result from joining those two cuts, because I see the proof every surgical day in my life. I never see scars in the vestibule. Scars in the vestibule result only when mucosa is resected. I think synechiae are primarily due to resection of the upper lateral cartilages, usually an exaggerated excision of the cephalic edge of the lower lateral edge of the cartilages.

Comment (Tom Rees): I have to agree with Jack Sheer. I almost always make a complete transfixion incision, because I like access to the whole caudal septum. I like to free the tip. Accurate anatomic repair of the tissues is what is important.

Question: How many years do you think it takes to see the final result in rhinoplasty? Do you think 1 year is long enough?

Comment (Wally Berman): I think it all depends on the thickness of the skin and other factors, but I have seen patients who noted changes after 10 years. This is rather common in my experience.

Comment (Gene Tardy): I think a nose that has not undergone operation goes through rather systematic changes from perhaps age 10 through age 70 years. We in rhinoplasty have not yet defined our endpoints. We are all trying to achieve the aesthetically pleasing nose but may not have the same endpoints in mind.

Comment (Tom Rees): I have always been amused by some of the earlier articles that showed all the angles and the measuring devices, calipers, and protractors, all of which I thought were fascinating. But at the operating table all this made no sense at all to me. These things were useless in practice.

I think we have established now that most surgeons don't care to use alloplastic material except for the occasional bit of mesh or maybe a strut now and then. A few years ago it was popular to use

112

cartilage from oxen, and a number of homograft materials were available for the nose.

Question: Do you use any homograft or heterograft materials in the nose?

Comment (by all): None.

Question: Does anyone use sclera in the nose? Banked sclera is almost an inert material. Some have used it to fill in little gaps and defects in the nose. I have seen some patients with quite interesting results.

Comment: No.

Question: When grafts are placed in the nose, whether from the ear or the septum or the alar cartilages, after 6 months or a year goes by we sometimes see small sharp edges or small irregularities. The nose looks wonderful while there is edema, and 6 months or a year later (or even 2 years) the edema is gone and the results are still good, but there is a little ridge, a depression, a slight sharpness. Aside from basic technique, what tricks might you suggest to obviate these minor problems? How can such sequelae be prevented in the first place, and how can they be treated when they do occur?

Comment (Tom Baker): I don't like to inject anything into the nose. Some surgeons advocate injection of droplets of silicone to fill depressions and gaps. I would use autogenous material if depressions exist and if there are sharp edges. I believe the only way I can approach the problem is to explore, see what the projection is, and try to correct it under direct vision.

Question: How do you deal with secondary points of cartilage that appear in the tip some months after the operation?

Comment (Wally Berman): I like to deliver the cartilage whenever I can. I feel more secure if the problem can be seen and if under direct vision morcellation or whatever can be done. A little extra cartilage can be shaved off. Also, old mature scar tissue, as exists in these cases, can be treated like cartilage. It can be morcellized too. Once in a great while, I admit, I do use a drop of silicone fluid.

Comment (Harvey Caplan): I call the small tip projections that occur *bosses*. They are caused by buckling of the cartilage that has been weakened. My treatment is to correct them under direct vision.

Comment (George Peck): I think you have to balance the scale here and indicate the level of significance of the deformity. In anyone with thin skin and thick lower lateral cartilages, lines and edges will be seen. In one sense that's what makes a nice tip. If the case of a slight depression that needs to be filled, I'll use a shaving of cartilage. I also think that morcellation is an excellent means of softening up cartilage points.

Comment (Tom Rees): The Selzer cartilage crushing box is an excellent instrument. Cartilage can be crushed almost to the consistency of fascia.

Question: What do you do to prevent these little edges?

Comment (Gene Tardy): At the risk being academic, one would like to avoid them. I try to reduce their occurrence by beveling the graft's edges with a No. 15 or smaller blade. I occasionally dermabraid the sharp marginal edges of a graft and also gently morcellize the margins with the delicate teeth of a Brown-Adson forceps, if you wish, to avoid palpable step deformities. Let me gingerly suggest that there is some evidence that morcellation or crushing of cartilage liberates chondroitin sulphate, which could conceivably lead to long-term absorption of autogenous cartilage. The fate of noncrushed autogenous cartilage is well known. I try to avoid crushing, damaging, or otherwise injuring cartilage. I'd rather have a nice cartilage "wafer" that I have carved, and, in addition, I strongly recommend the temporal fascia filler graft. It will persist, will remain viable, and can be layered. Fascia can efface little depressions very nicely.

Comment (Jack Sheen): I try to resect the little irregularity under direct vision and either put crushed cartilage over it or leave it if there is enough projection. If one side is projecting and the other side is flat, there will be two different obliques. If the patient does not object to the pointed side or likes that side, I will create another pointed side or projecting side on the opposite dome to provide balance.

Comment (Tom Rees): I will add a couple of considerations. I have had a lot of experience with minute droplets of liquid silicone. It is very useful in minute amounts to fill in very small depressions created by rhinoplasty. Unfortunately, the experimental protocol forbids the use of silicone fluid for anything but gross deformities, such as hemifacial atrophy, so some of these small uses will probably be denied to all of us forever.

We are now looking at collagen for the same purpose; the long-term efficay is, however, not known. But if collagen were to work it would probably be used most successfully in treatment of small contour deformities in the postoperative nose, because scar tissue is, after all, primarily collagen.

Question: Do tip grafts affect the lip in any way? Does the graft lift the lip or cause any problems by changing the posture of the lip?

Comment (Jack Sheen): The inferior part of the graft stops at the columella-lobule junction, so it should not in fact have any influence on the lip.

Question: Do you ever remove the entire lateral crus of the alar cartilage? Does that provide a pinched tip?

Comment (Harvey Caplan): Never.

Comment (Gene Tardy): I have never removed the entire lateral crus, nor can I conceive of any anatomic variant where such extreme resection might be useful. To the contrary, I find myself increasingly preferring to preserve a greater portion of the lateral crus in an attempt to weaken or reorient the excessive cartilage.

Comment (Tom Rees): It has been said by some that you can remove it with impunity. The only cases in which complete removal might be considered are in those fat, bulky tips. This would produce a totally unsupported tip and would make no sense at all physiologically.

Question: Would you please explain your technique of using multiple grafts in the tip, rather than a single graft?

Comment (Jack Sheen): The multiple-graft technique was developed because of my unhappy results with a single graft. I put more material in the tip to stabilize the single graft, because the tension at either end of the graft created a flatness to the tip lobule. By placing an anterior fill I found I could fashion a very nice triangular shape for the tip lobule. As a result I put in multiple long grafts, posterior fills, and some anterior fill.

Question: What is tip rotation versus tip projection? Also, how do you reduce the excessively projecting tip—the real Pinocchio tip?

Comment (Jack Sheen): There are two ways to reduce the ultraprojecting tip. First, pay attention to the root of the nose. In other words, if there is a disproportion of the root of the nose or if the nasion is very low, the tip of the nose will appear to overproject, so you can achieve some degree of balance by raising the dorsum with a graft. To reduce the projection of the tip in an anteroposterior direction absolutely, the projection of the lower lateral cartilage must be reduced. The easiest way in my experience is simply to resect the domes along with a rather sizable segment of the medial and lateral crura at the dome. The soft tissues will settle down; you don't have to worry about spicules, because as the tissues contract they will thicken. I find that I can reduce the crura perhaps 2 mm or so. If they are overreduced excessive thickening occurs and definition is lost; you have reduced the anterior projection of the lower lateral cartilages.

Comment (Wally Berman): One technique that I have found useful keeps the dome intact. A bipedicle flap is delivered first. Then a unipedicle flap is created by incising through the medial columella and taking off as many millimeters as you care to, to decrease projection. The lateral cartilage is then rotated and becomes dome. The dome then becomes part of the medial cartilage. This technique prevents widening of the base of the nose.

Comment (George Peck): I do exactly the opposite. This is an extremely rare deformity. The first step is a basic rhinoplasty, and I leave a narrow rim of lower lateral. In many instances this will correct the problem. If the nose is a little bit large but has good lines, it will still look good. However, if the tip is still projecting too much I deliver the alar cartilage as a flap, and by crosscutting on the medial crura area of the dome, I create a new dome, lower down on the medial crura. I then excise a segment laterally from the lateral crus to effectively lower the dome.

Comment (Gene Tardy): I consider the projecting tip a difficult problem, because many of these tips are under tension and have only delicate, thin skin overlying the skeletal structure. Very careful analysis is necessary before the dome is transected, although with thicker skin transecting and reducing the dome is certainly useful and safe. It is essential to determine exactly what is causing the excess projection and then to reduce those abnormal anatomic components. Alternatively, overprojection may be the consequence of an enlarged nasal spine. Hypertrophy of the caudal or dorsal quadrangular cartilage or combinations of these component hypertrophies may exist and therefore may require individual reduction. I prefer to leave the alar domes intact whenever possible, maintaining a complete strip of alar cartilage.

Finally, I think we should not try to make noses too small. There is nothing aesthetically wrong with a nose that is a little large as long as all of the lines and contours are in proportion. Therefore augmentation of the disproportionately small dorsum may be helpful.

Comment (George Peck): I see many secondary noses and find a lot of scarring intranasally. I disagree with Jack Sheen's position that contracture of a scar caused by incision into the vestibule never occurs unless lining is removed. I have seen this scarring many times. As a matter of fact, one of the things that I have done in recent years is to completely eliminate the intercartilaginous incision, because the intercartilaginous incision is made at the internal valve. This incision is absolutely unnecessary. You can preserve that valve in all instances without making an incision there. As far as the upper lateral is concerned, you rarely have to remove any of the caudal ends or the upper ends, and if you do the amount is minimal. So I make a plea; look into the nose to decide for yourself whether there are contracture scars and what may have caused them.

Comment (Tom Rees): I have to side with Jack on this. First, I have almost always done a complete transfixion incision and carried it around, and unless I have removed lining, I do not have trouble with scars there. Mucous membrane does not heal with scar contracture, not the same way that skin heals, anyway. It is all a question of repair. I make this incision in almost every case, and I simply don't see scar contracture problems. Second, it becomes a case of six of one and half a dozen of another; by the time an intercartilaginous incision is done and an attempt is made to bring it around the corner and another is made for the transfixion incision, most of the time the incisions are joined. There is no way one can work on a caudal septum, the septal angle, and everything else through two peepholes without great difficulty.

Comment (George Peck): My technique may be a little more difficult, but the vestibular skin at the septal angle is preserved.

Question: What do you do with the bridge of lining hanging across the septal angle?

Comment (George Peck): It serves the purpose of breaking the circular scar.

Question: But what if you want to rotate the tip? I assume you never rotate the tip?

Comment (George Peck): Yes, you are rotating the tip by trimming the septal cartilage and creating the obtuse angle.

Question: What do you do with that piece of cartilage as you go around the septal angle?

Comment (George Peck): You trim that without cutting the vestibular skin.

Comment (Tom Rees): Some people have to make things difficult. I would like to introduce one more technical means of reducing the projecting tip. If you look at the projecting tip as a tripod that you wish to recess slightly, yet you want to maintain the angle of the tripod, which is the natural dome, it is permissible to transect through the lateral crura quite far laterally and allow edges of the cartilage to overlap a bit. I emphasize that cartilage is not excised, simply overlapped. The medial crural sides are also transected completely approximately 3 mm below the domes. The whole tripod complex then recesses toward the maxilla. Sometimes a couple of millimeters is a lot and will let the whole tripod sit down.

PART
III

MANAGEMENT OF THE LIP-COLUMELLA-TIP COMPLEX

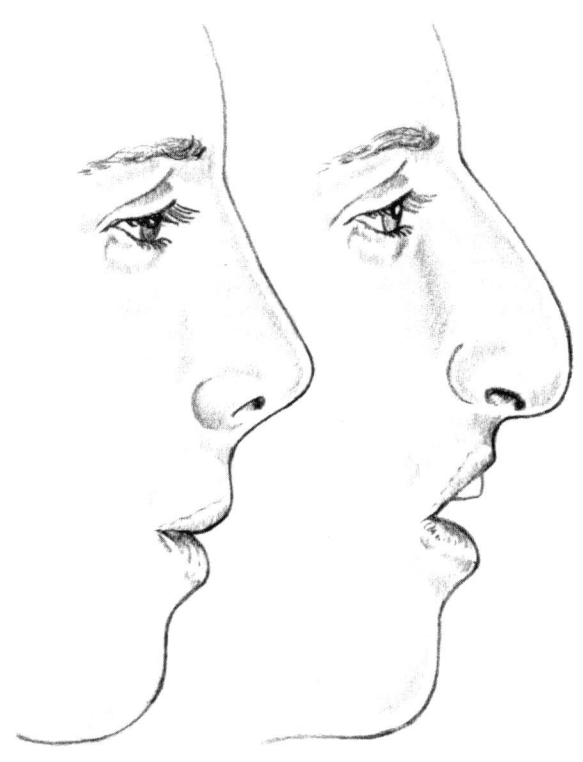

13

Unique Problems Associated with the Lip-Columella-Tip Complex

Thomas Rees

Rhinoplasty consists of a series of harmonious maneuvers aimed at achieving a total effect. There are certain unique problems associated with the lower nose, the lobule, and the lip that need to be addressed separately; therefore the lip-columella-tip complex cannot be considered as a single topic. The whole lower nose and lip can be viewed as a complex that is interrelated anatomically. The muscles of the face, particularly the nasalis, the zygomaticus, the depressor nasi septi, and the levator labii superioris, all act in synchrony to achieve some of the effects that surgeons plan to correct during surgery, such as plunging of the tip on animation.

As Gillies said many times, "There are no straight lines in nature"; nature abhors straight lines. Therefore we as surgeons should avoid chopping the septum or columella so that a straight line results; Figure 13-1 illustrates the preferred procedure for transfixation. The nasal spine is the subject of considerable interest and some controversy. I remove it only in about 5% of my patients and then only when it is severely crowding the upper lip. If it can be chiseled loose it often can be somewhat free-floating and still provide the bulk necessary to prevent columellar retraction at the labiocolumellar angle.

The "hanging columella" distresses many patients and can mar the otherwise excellent results of rhinoplasty (Figure 13-2). It is caused by one or both of two anatomical situations: (1) the curving caudal margin of the septum or (2) marked convexity of the caudal margin of the medial crura. If the septum

is at fault trimming the caudal edge will suffice. The medial crura can also be corrected directly by resection.

A pararim incision runs down the edge of the columella. The leading edge of the medial crura (not necessarily the whole cartilage) can be delivered, and resection of the offending curving lower portion of the cartilage, alone or in conjunction with the lining, can be done. Fine No. 6 nylon sutures are used to close the incisions. I reserve this step until the end of the procedure (about the time I begin thinking about resection of the alar base, after I have trimmed the caudal septum appropriately and rotated the tip. A curvature of the medial crus must be attacked by a direct excision but, again, not as a straight-line resection. I leave a little curvature on the columella.

Another problem I personally find challenging is the "Bugs Bunny" syndrome, an eponym created by Dr. John Williams. The patient is usually one who breathes through the mouth. This syndrome has several causes, and the surgeon needs to determine the cause before deciding on a surgical course of correction. The retracted upper lip often goes along with a "gummy smile," in which the patient shows excessive gingiva, creating an unattractive facies. If the cause of the problem is an elongated facial skeleton, where the soft tissues of the face are simply too short to stretch over the elongated maxilla (so-called *long-face syndrome*), the standard maneuvers presented here will not correct the problem but will improve it.

Figure 13-1. Transfixion incision is completed in most patients to permit mobility of soft tissues during operation. **B,** Note curving caudal edge of septum and its articulation with nasal spine. Line is curved, not straight. **C,** Some muscles that act on tip of nose during animation are seen with portion of anterior muscles cut away. **D,** Incision is frequently made at base of spine through muscle groups to help overcome their adverse affect on plunging of tip. **E,** Incision in muscle is shown. Excision of portion of muscles involved is probably more effective. **F** and **G,** Redundant caudal septum is excised, again with curving line. **H** and **I,** Excision of overhanging cartilaginous septum leaves projecting nasal tip so that accurate assessment can be made as to whether this structure should be excised or simply fractured.

Continued.

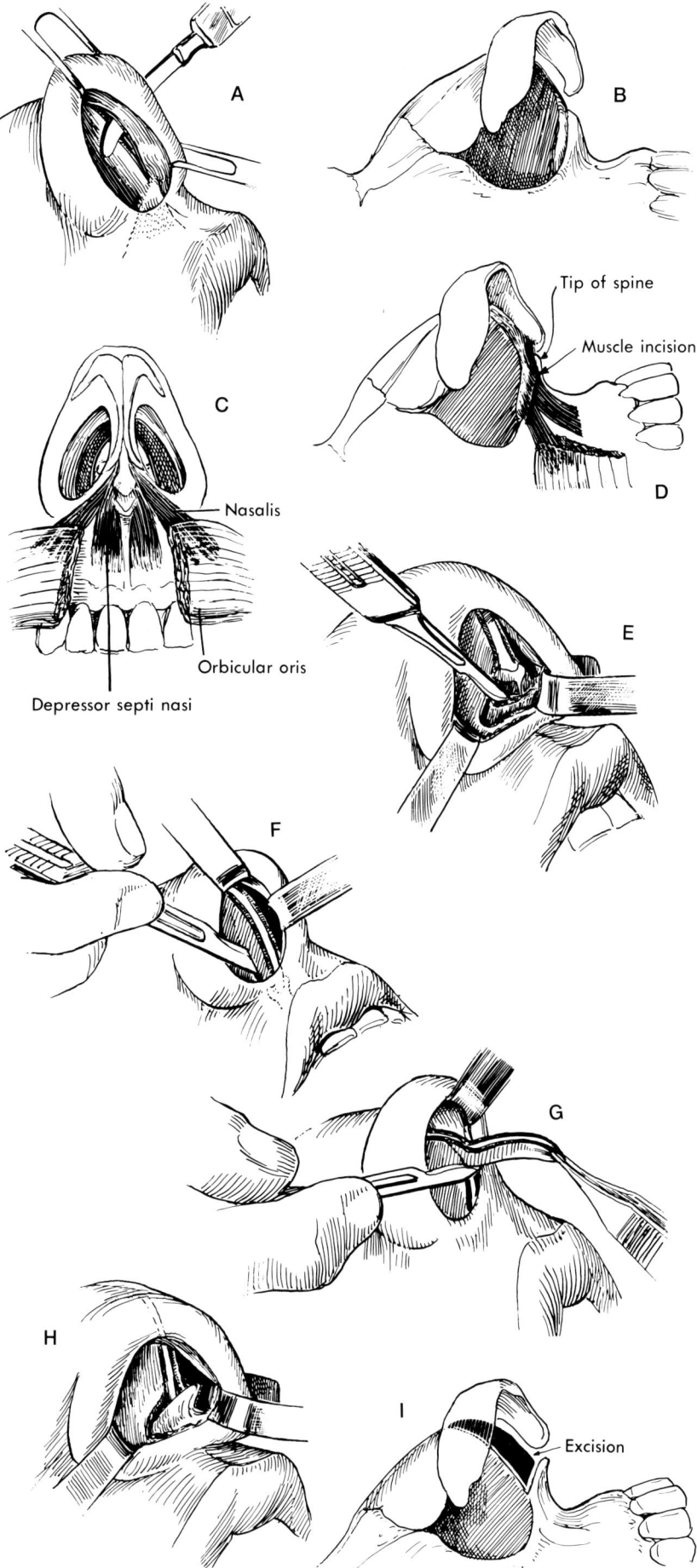

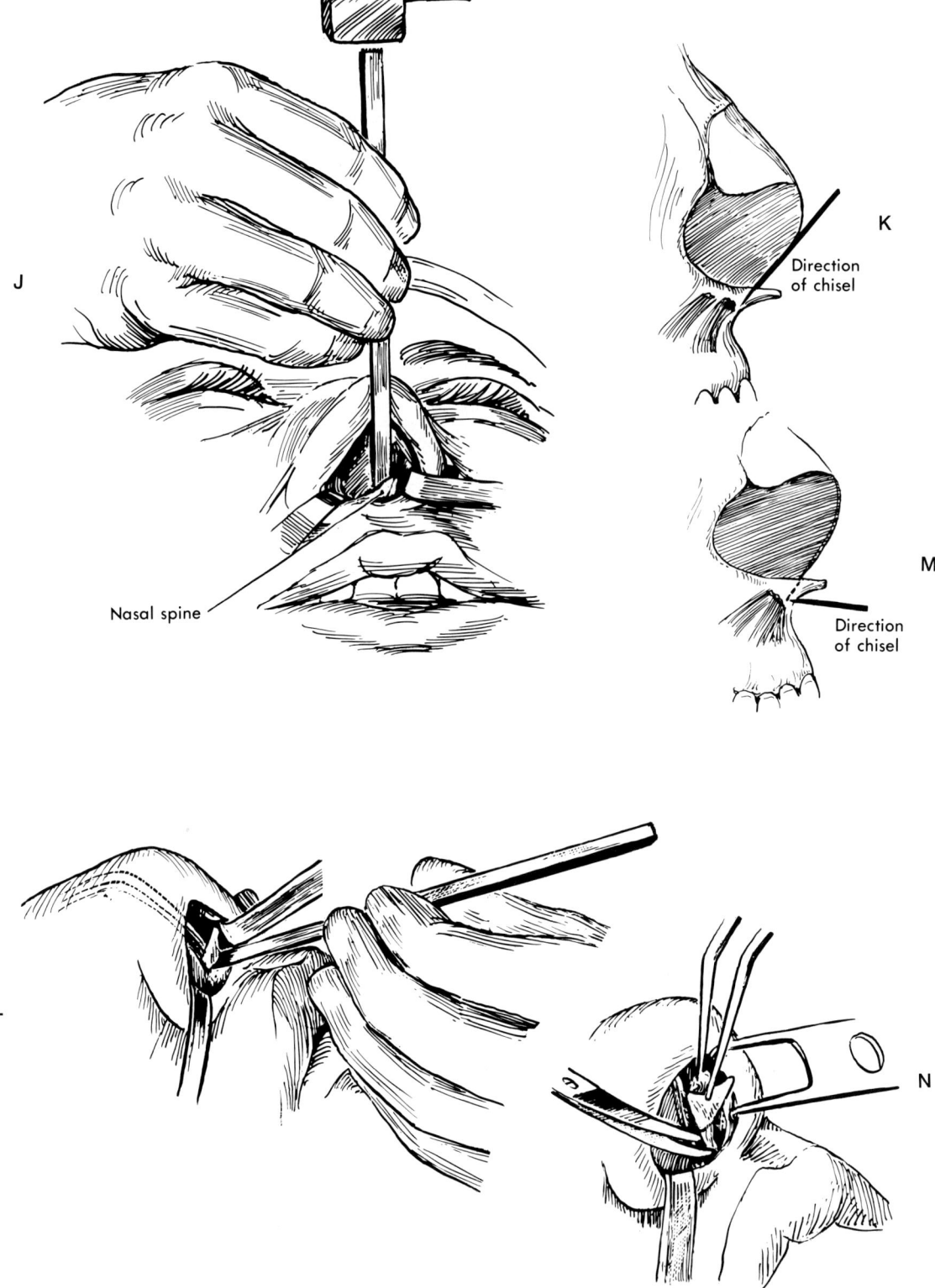

Figure 13-1, cont'd. J, K, L, M, and **N,** Small osteotome can be used to fracture nasal spine and remove it. It is often better to fracture spine and leave it in place, attached to soft tissues as contour filler at the columella-lip angle. In this way retraction of columella is avoided.

Figure 13-2. A-H, Technique of reducing "hanging columella," which is result of redundant and curving inferior border of medial crura. Reduction of caudal margin of septum often suffices; however, when primary problem is related to medial crura, trimming must be done. Incision is made just inside columella on each side, and medial crura are delivered. Appropriate amount is trimmed from inferior portions of each side with or without lining. Defect is sutured with fine interrupted sutures. **I and J,** Patient shows salutory effect of such surgery. Hanging columella in this patient required reduction of both caudal septum and medial crus to achieve result. (From Rees, T.D.: Aesthetic plastic surgery, vol. 1, Philadelphia, 1980, W.B. Saunders, Co.)

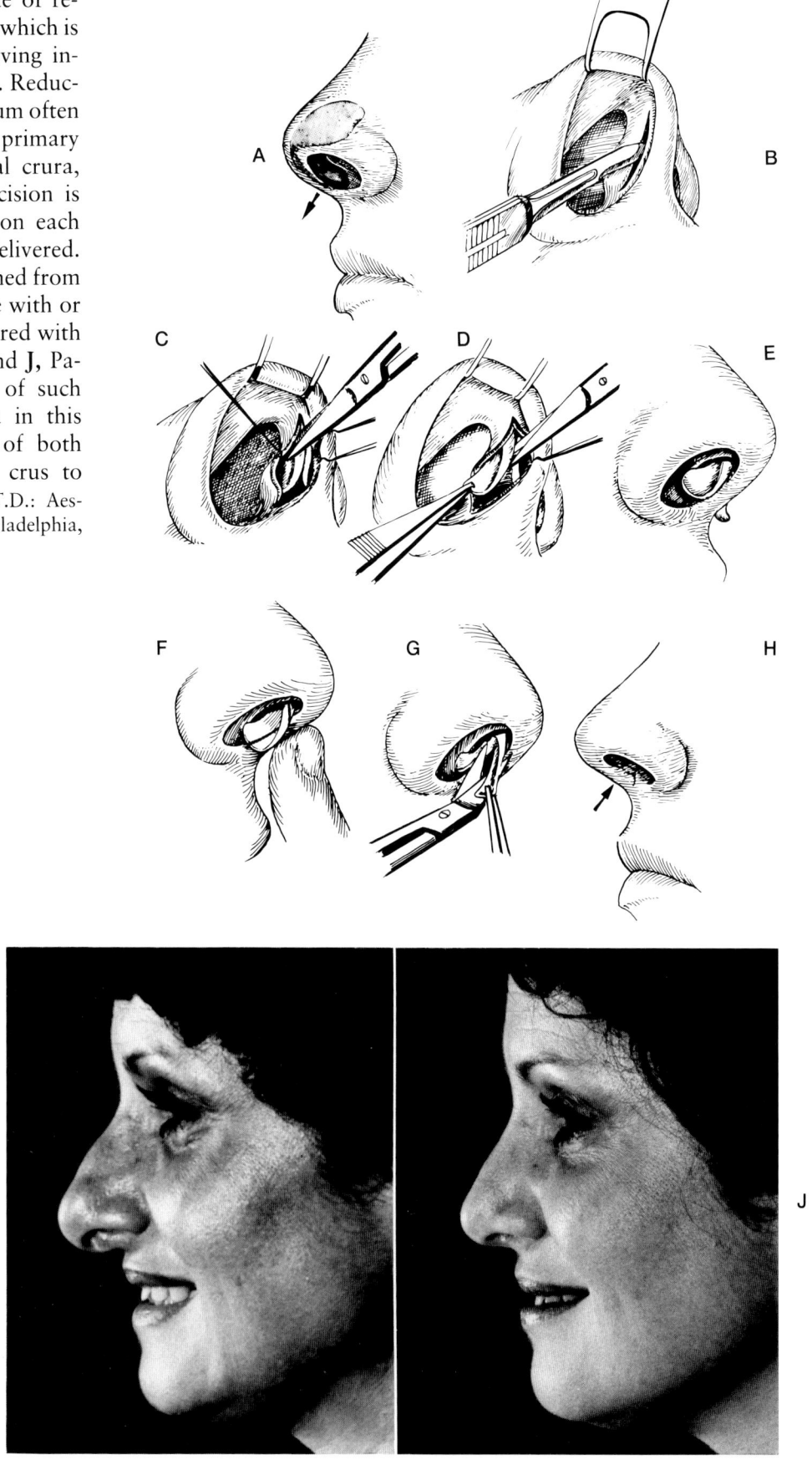

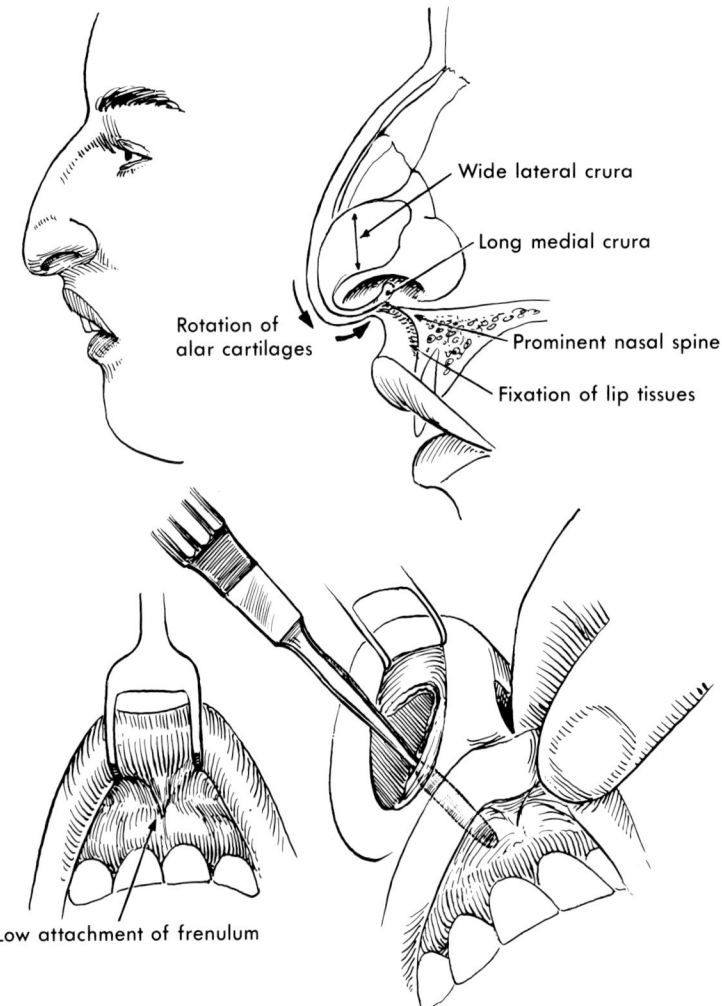

Figure 13-3. Tethered upper lip ("Bugs Bunny" syndrome) is result of one or combination of several anatomic problems. These include prominent dorsal profile of nose, high attachment of gingiva on maxilla, and, in some cases, true elongation of bony maxilla (so-called *long face syndrome*). Gummy smile may accompany this set of morphologic circumstances. Correction is achieved by reducing nasal skeleton, releasing soft tissues from anterior face of maxilla (alveolus) so they can be displaced in more caudal position, transecting frenulum, and, in appropriate cases, performing maxillary osteotomy. Gummy smile can be further improved in selected patients by inserting small cartilage graft along alveolus.

If the retracted upper lip results from a high attachment of the sulcus on the anterior face of the maxilla, the soft tissues can be released so that at least half, if not all, of the upper central incisors will be covered by the lip (Figure 13-3). The soft tissues can be released simply by passing an elevator or a pair of scissors through the base of the transfixion incision, dissecting the gingiva subperiosteally from the alveolus, and dropping the level of the sulcus like a curtain being lowered. Sometimes this effect is accentuated by muscle action and therefore requires transection or excision of a small piece of the musculature, the depressor nasi septi in particular, through the base of the transfixion incision in the columella. The upper lip can be relaxed by a combination of performing of a conservative rhinoplasty (lowering the profile), freeing up the soft tissues, and

simply letting the lip drop down. Sometimes the frenulum may have to be transected; I do not use a z-plasty when I cut the frenulum.

When severe lip retraction coexists with a high fixation of the soft tissues, true elongation of the maxilla is often present. For optimal correction of the problem one must consider performing maxillary osteotomy and shortening the maxilla. This approach involves a somewhat more complicated surgical procedure, and many patients find it hard to see the necessity of it all. However, even in patients with markedly elongated bony structure and relatively short soft tissues, a much more relaxed expression can be achieved with direct intraoral incisions along the sulcus. The incisions allow all the soft tissues to drop, and a more relaxed expression and correction of the gummy smile can thereby be achieved (Figure 13-4).

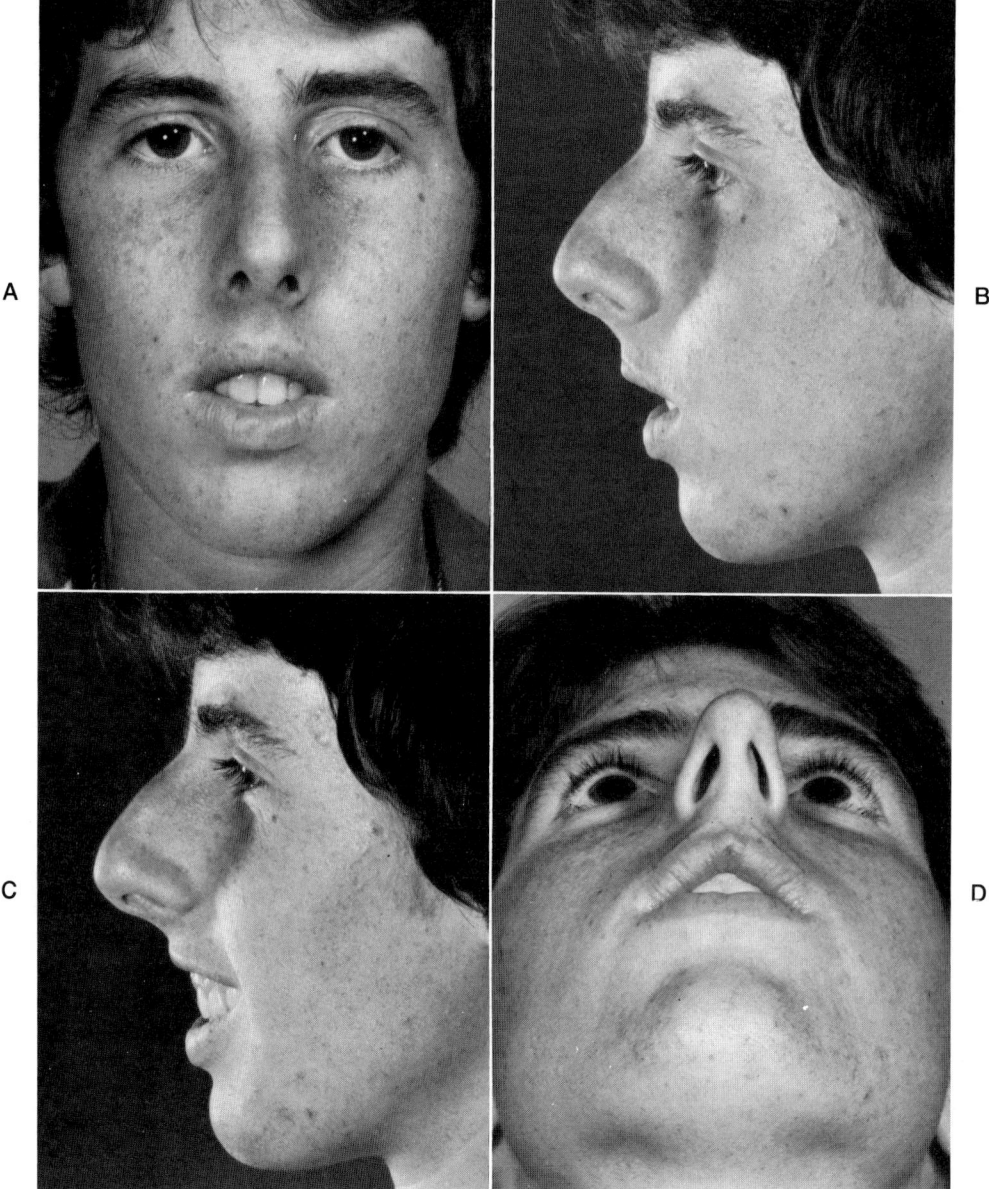

Figure 13-4. This patient is typical of "Bugs Bunny" syndrome. He appeared to have typical facies of "mouth-breather," which in fact he was not. He has true elongation of maxilla, constituting long-face syndrome; however, suggestions of direct bony surgery on maxilla were refused by patient and his parents. **A, B, C,** and **D** are preoperative photographs showing different views of problem. Very high dorsal profile contributed significantly to deformity. Patient was unable to force his lips to seal except with great and unnatural effort. Operation was carried out according to technique described in Figure 13-3.

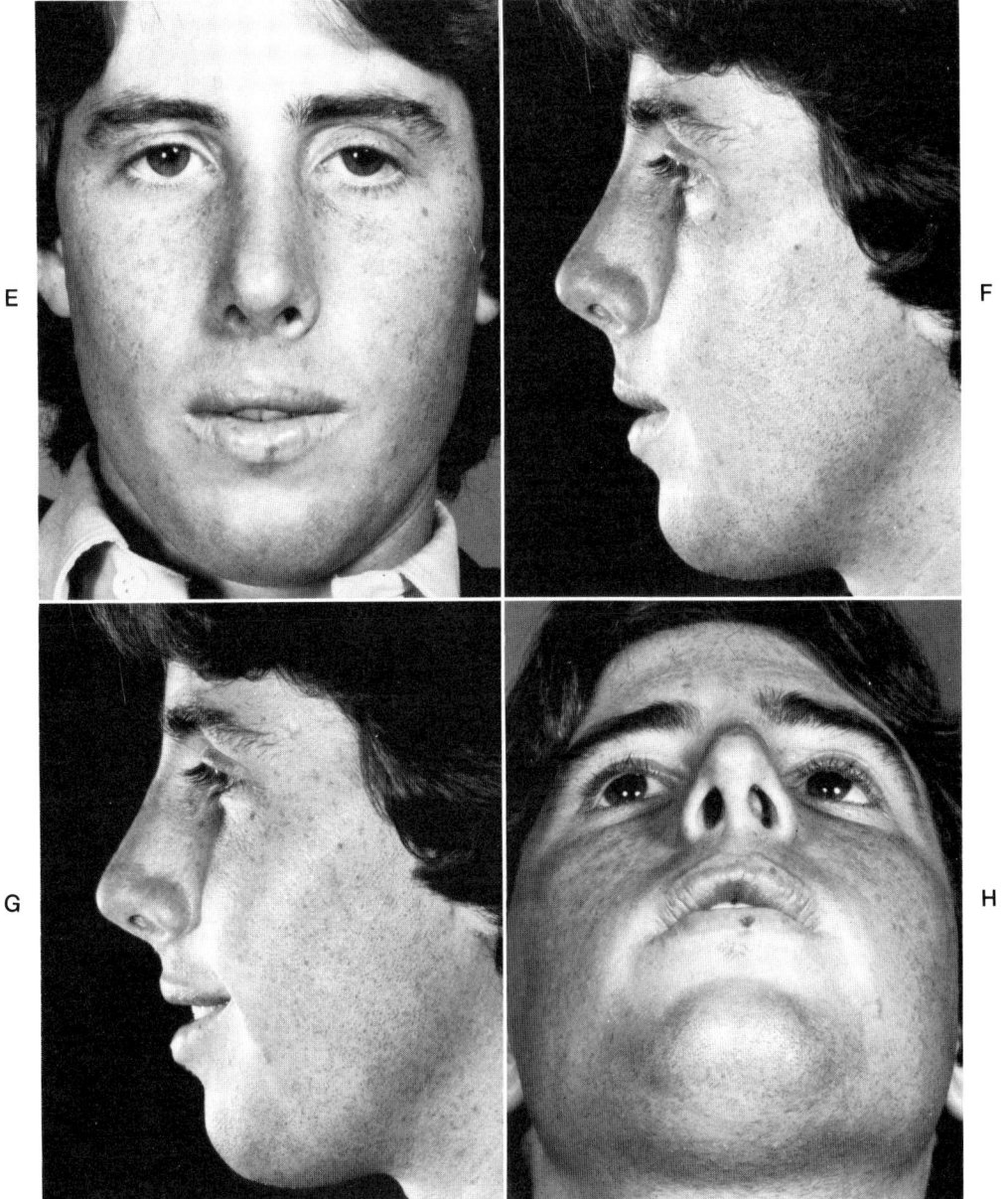

Figure 13-4, cont'd. E, F, G, and **H** show postoperative results. Whereas maxillary ostectomy undoubtedly would have been preferred method of treatment, along with rhinoplasty, result was nevertheless marked improvement. Lip seal is not complete but nearly so.

The hidden columella is difficult to correct. It can be a genetic problem with practically no columella showing on the profile view, or it can result from trauma or surgery. I will present various classical ways of dealing with this problem, but I feel that most of them produce results that are very disappointing (Figure 13-5). Use of the cartilage graft in the columella has yielded unimpressive corrections in my hands. If sufficient soft tissues are present an autogenous cartilage graft can distend them cau-

dally, although the results may not be permanent. Other techniques, such as the septal flap technique, can also be used to augment the columella. The septal flap technique looks very nice in illustrations but is difficult to execute.

The use of a transposition flap of alar cartilage complete with lining attached, a technique ingeniously worked out by Millard[1] (Figure 13-6), has proved to be a very useful maneuver for various types of defects of the nose. This procedure is quite

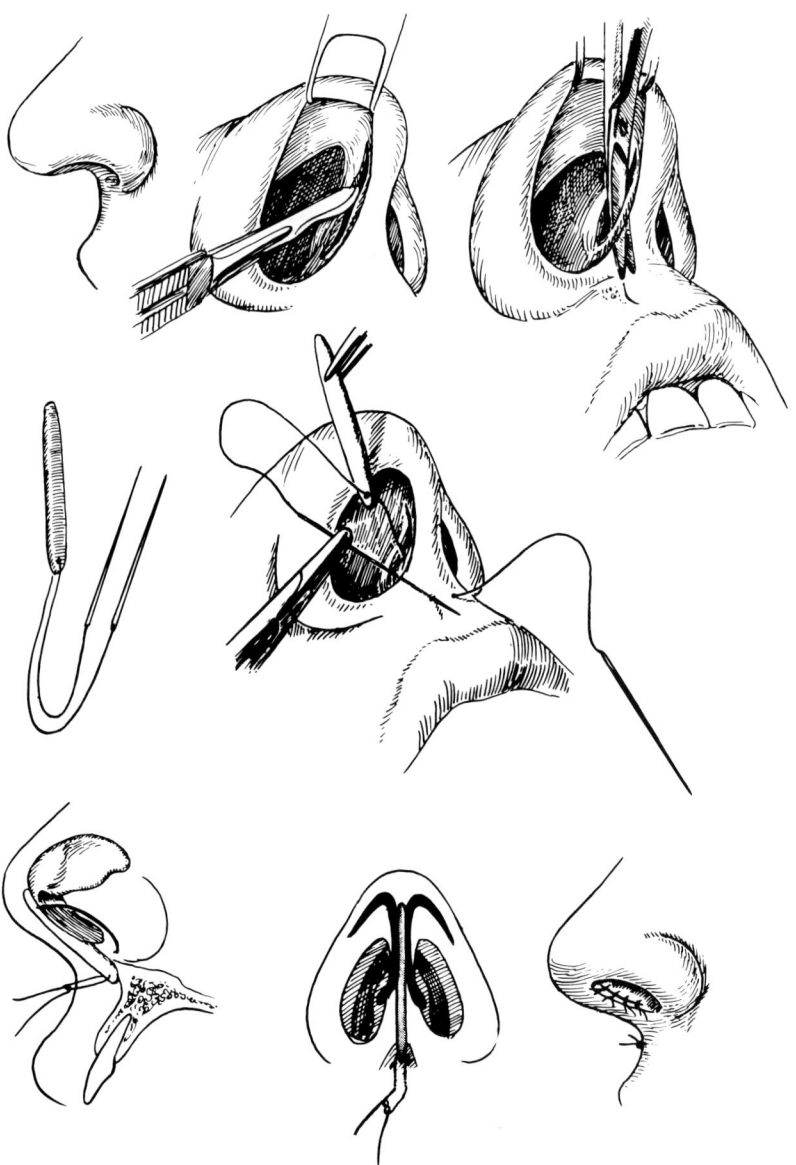

Figure 13-5. Well-accepted technique for improving hidden columella is use of cartilage strut graft. This graft is frequently of some usefulness, but long-term results are disappointing in my experience unless marked overcorrection is accomplished. Certainly, cartilage grafts are usually used successful in lesser degrees of deformity. (From Rees, T.D.: Aesthetic plastic surgery, vol. 1, Philadelphia, 1980, W.B. Saunders Co.)

simple. Success in its use requires a nose that has not undergone operation. With this procedure a transfixion incision is made and the columella completely released; a flap of the cephalic half or more of the lateral crus of the alar cartilage along with lining is dissected and interpolated into the columella, back to back with a flap from the opposite side. The flaps must be sewn together very precisely. I usually put one or two mattress sutures through and through to approximate the cartilages back to back. This alar flap has been quite useful in the "Miss Piggy" nose with a thick, hanging lateral nostril margin that often shows no columella whatsoever.

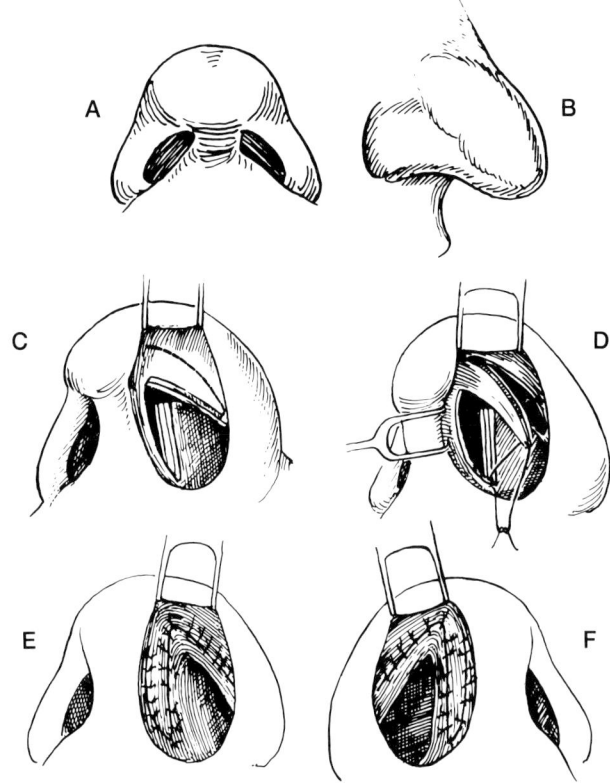

Figure 13-6. A to F, Millard's method of reconstructing hidden columella with interpolated flaps of lateral crura of alar cartilage. These flaps are sutured back to back in the space of the transfixion incision. In primary noses with no previous surgery to alar cartilages, considerable amount of tissue can be shifted by this method. Flaps are long enough to reach well down to inferior angle of transfixion incision. G and H, This male patient had as his only complaint absence of columella, as shown on profile, giving his nose short "snubby" look. Only surgical correction consisted of maneuver shown in illustration. Hidden columella was improved postoperatively, and more natural length of nose was established. (From Rees, T.D.: Aesthetic plastic surgery, vol. 1, Philadelphia, 1980, W.B. Saunders Co.)

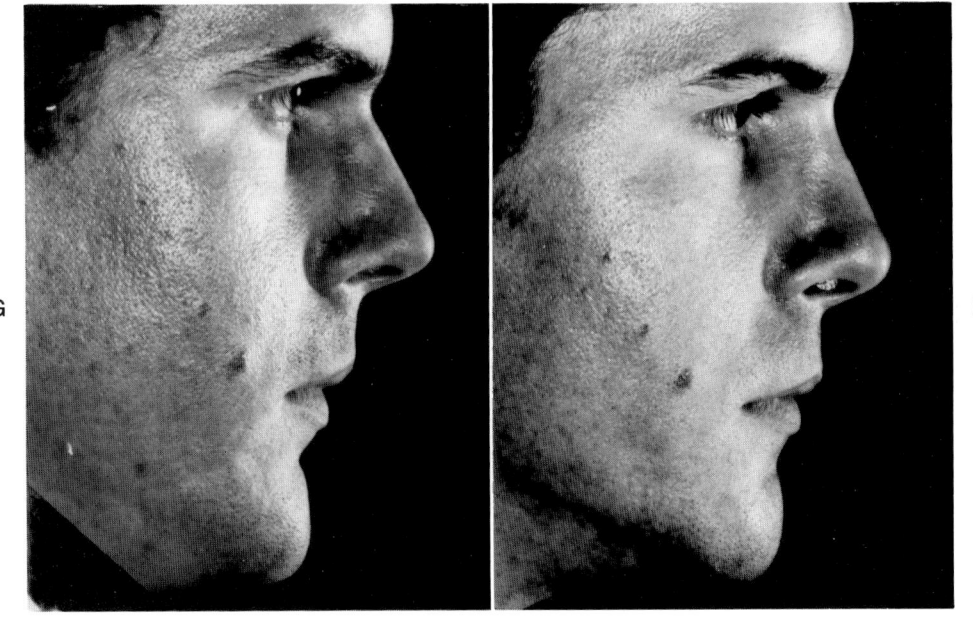

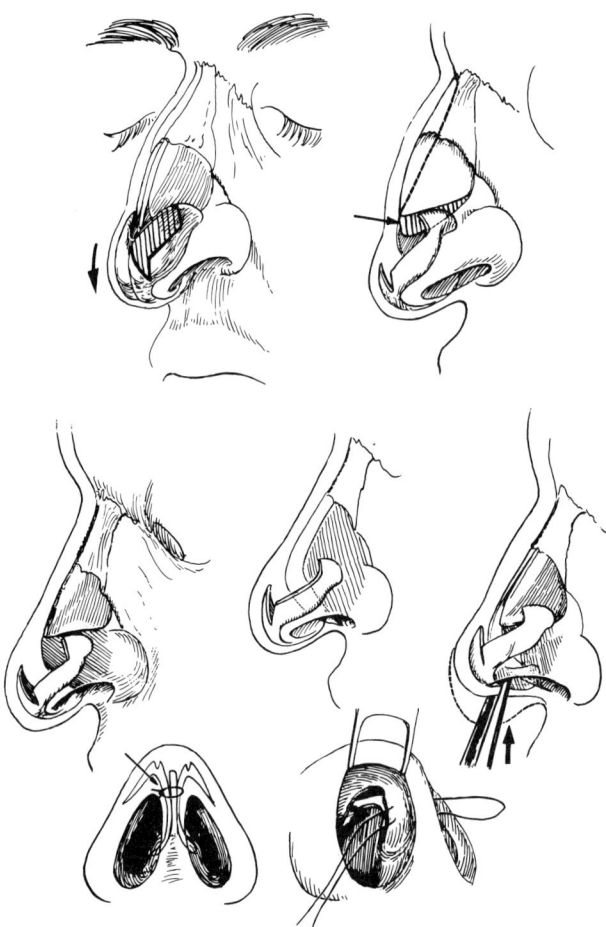

Figure 13-7. Severely plunging tip with acute labiocolumellar angle is challenging problem. Series of surgical steps may be required to improve contour and overcome plunging. These include tip rotation; excision of cephalic portion of lateral wing of alar cartilages; occasionally, transection through genua of alar cartilages; minimal shortening of septum; tongue-in-groove fixation of denuded caudal septum into pocket between medial crura; and fixation of septum in its new position with mattress suture. These steps are often further enhanced with free-floating, tip graft. (From Rees, T.D.: Aesthetic plastic surgery, vol. 1, Philadelphia, 1983, W.B. Saunders Co.)

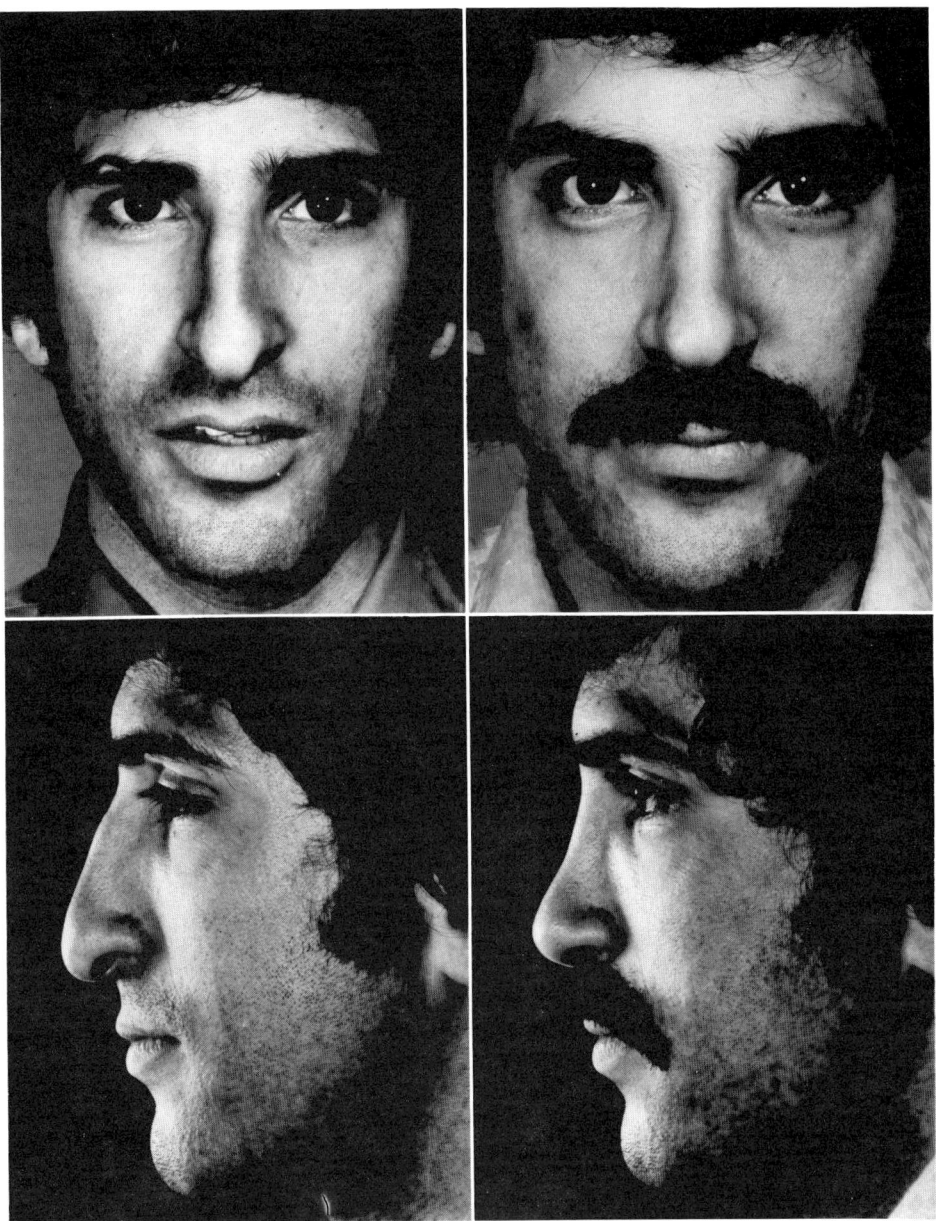

Figure 13-7, cont'd. For legend see opposite page.

The tip that points caudally with an arching nostril, curving columella, minimal tip projection, and minimal hump presents an exceedingly difficult problem. Today I undoubtedly would use some type of ala-only graft in addition to the procedures that follow (Figure 13-7). First, the entire alar spring is rotated in a cephalic direction. Often a bit of medial crus must be trimmed away and the rotated tip fixed in its new position with a tongue-in-groove maneuver, in which the denuded caudal margin of the septum is inserted between the two medial crura. A disadvantage of this method is that the membranous septum is eliminated so that the tip is no longer immobile. Second, the entire complex is fixed in position with a strong mattress suture. The alar cartilages may need to be weakened to permit rotation of the tip. I usually cut the muscles on such patients to eliminate some of the stresses that can pull the tip down again.

REFERENCE

1. Millard, D.R.: The versatility of a chondromucosal flap in the nasal vestibule, Plast. Reconstr. Surg. 50:580, 1972.

14

The Nasolabial Angle

Claus Walter

The aesthetic appearance of the nasolabial angle is influenced by age, sex, and ethnic group. In discussing surgical problems related to this angle or other structures in the area, we must differentiate whether the columella is long and hanging or suffers from retraction or shortness of tissue. Treatment should then be directed toward achieving our goal in rhinoplasty—a pleasing nasolabial angle.

Except in the case of congenital malformations or injuries, there is great potential for surgical damage in this area, specifically in resection of the caudal portion of the septal cartilage. This procedure was widely advocated in the past, but the results were often marked retraction of the columella, drooping of the nasal tip, and consequent impairment of nasal breathing. Appropriate therapeutic measures are divided into the following areas:

1. Resection of redundant tissue
2. Correction of columellar position in relation to the upper lip
3. Augmentation where tissue is missing
4. Tissue transplantation where substance has been lost

RESECTION OF REDUNDANT TISSUE

The so-called *hanging columella* gives the nose-lip complex an unattractive appearance. Two causes are possible: an overgrowth of septal cartilage, which pushes the medial crura down, or enlargement of the medial crura themselves, resulting in a less than aesthetically pleasing relationship between the medial and lateral portions of these cartilages.

Treatment consists of resection of tissue from the caudal border of the septum or a more sophisticated procedure performed on the medial crura. Simply resecting a portion usually does not suffice. The tissues must be freed from their cutaneous bed and the cartilaginous continuity severed at or near the junction of the lateral crura to eliminate the spring effect of cartilage, which can propel itself forward again.

I prefer the rim incision to free the cartilage. With this method of mobilization I can also shorten the caudal ends of the medial crura if they flare out and distort the columella's lower end. However, the surgeon must guard against overresection, which invariably results in skin retraction and an unwanted lengthwise columellar retraction months after surgery.

CORRECTION OF COLUMELLAR POSITION IN RELATION TO THE UPPER LIP

The transfixion incision can alter the relationship of the lip-tip-columella complex. In particular, the position of the upper lip depends markedly on the extent of the cut into the floor of the nose and beyond the nasal spine. A deep transfixion incision may be needed to relieve tension and allow free rotation of the nose tip and upper lip up or down. The surgeon may also resect part of the depressor nasi septi muscle and subcutaneous tissue or borrow septal tissue to augment the base of the columella, further altering positions. Final suturing can support the surgically altered relationship and retain the corrected parts in their new positions. In particular, the horizontal mattress and triangular retraction sutures help fix the lip-tip-columella complex.

In areas of retraction where the caudal end of the septum is intact, the Cinelli operation can be useful. This consists of dissecting a strip of cartilage three fourths of the length from the caudal portion of the septum, creating a pocket between the medial crura, turning the cartilage, still attached to the septum, downward 90 to 110 degrees, and lodging it in the pocket at the caudal septal end. The resultant small deficiency of cartilage in the septum is negligible and adds to the pleasing effect created by a more obtuse nasolabial angle (Figure 14-1).

The transfixion incision is not used in these cases, because the goal is to achieve as much intact mucosa and vestibular skin as possible. Therefore smaller incisions are preferable. The oral approach through the frenulum into the columella and caudal septal end is often preferred. One definite advantage is the ability to then dissect the mucosa and distribute equal tension when the columella is pulled or pushed forward.

The Cinelli principle cannot be applied to cases where there has been previous nasal septal surgery unless enough cartilage remains to support the increased deficiency. If there is sufficient cartilage the Cinelli procedure is excellent in preventing recurrence of the retraction caused by the fixed connection of the residual cartilage to the columella.

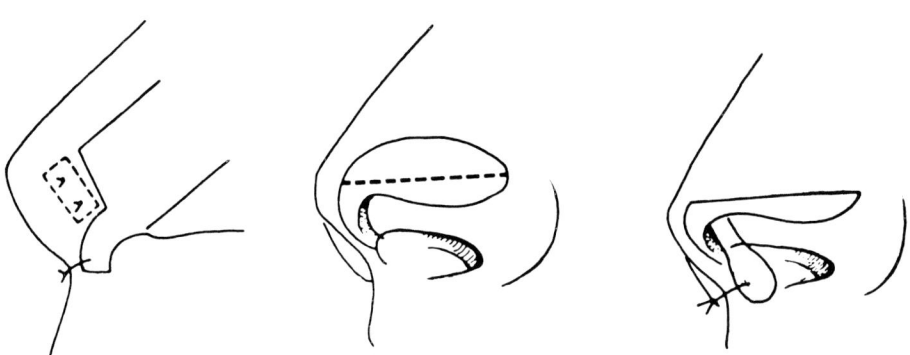

Figure 14-1. Modified Cinelli method. Area void of cartilage is filled by cartilage transplant. (Redrawn from Walter, C.: HNO 13:104-105, 1965.)

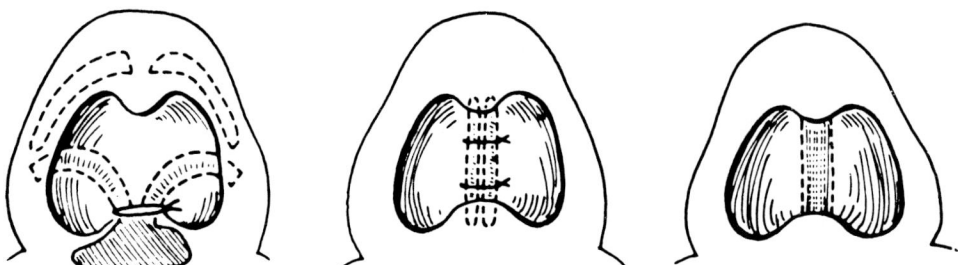

Figure 14-2. Creation of alar flaps based laterally for reconstruction of columella or correction of hidden columella. (Redrawn from Walter, C.: HNO 13:104-105, 1965.)

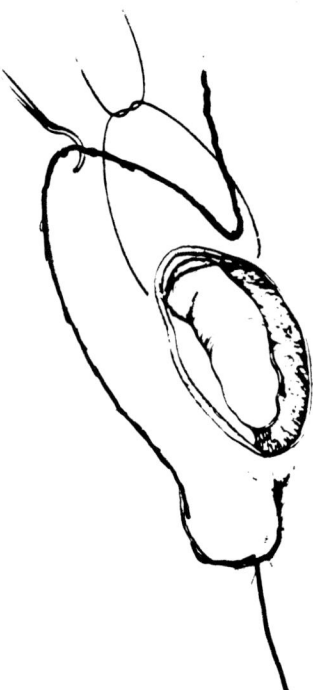

Figure 14-3. Outline of island flap on postauricular mastoid skin. This island flap is pulled through incision in postauricular skin and is sutured to anterior skin. Postauricular incision is closed by direct approximation. (Redrawn from Walter, C.: Arch. Otolaryngol. 90:622, 1969.)

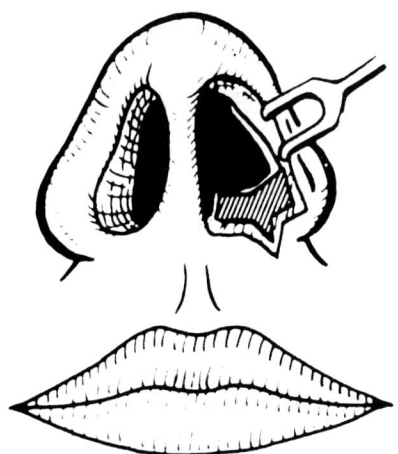

Figure 14-4. Composite graft in place to correct anterior stenosis. (Redrawn from Walter, C.: Arch. Otolaryngol. 90:622, 1969.)

AUGMENTATION

I prefer autogenous rib cartilage for replacement of missing cartilage and favor a large piece rather than several small ones, which may overlap and collapse under the forces of retraction at the nasolabial angle. Autogenous cartilage works quite well for dorsal saddle deformities but dissolves under nasolabial pressures. For either graft several mattress sutures should be applied over the caudal septal area to securely fasten the cartilage.

If the Cinelli procedure is used and the pocket between the mucosal sides is large enough, the cartilage can be pulled up to the center of the septum and extended to the dorsum and can also correct a saddle defect. Another modification of this procedure has found use in repair of congenital malformation of the nose with a very short, thickened columella. To lengthen the columella several Z-plasties have been applied to one or both sides.

Severe scarring of the upper lip can cause retraction and narrowing of the nasal entrance. The major problem is with breathing, because when the mouth is opened the upper lip scars retract the nose and close the nostrils. To correct this problem I recommend numerous Z-plasties and tissue shifts and/or composite grafts inside the nose. In excessive scarring after rhinoplasty removal of the nasal spine will allow the fibrous tissues to reset and will provide a more pleasing nasolabial angle.

In general, the nasal spine should be preserved to maintain the patient's ethnic characteristics. In addition, care should be taken when operating on the caudal septal end that a man's masculine nose is not feminized by overshortening.

TISSUE TRANSPLANTATION

Tissue loss can be overcome only by transplantation. Skin transplants alone are not sufficient, because the skin retracts. I have noted good success with composite grafts in conjunction with rib grafts.

It is possible to lengthen the columella by inserting an auricular composite graft into the horizontally severed columella. Such a composite graft should be reinforced by a cartilagenous strut inserted through it to provide tip projection. Without this reinforcement the composite graft will contract and may be slow to heal.

To bring the columella forward the membranous septum must be enlarged with cartilage and skin throughout its length. I use a flap that is based laterally and composed of cartilage and vestibular skin. A bridge of tissue that divides the nasal entrance is created from the lower lateral cartilage. Then the cranial portion of the dome is sutured downward into the caudal membranous septal gap (Figure 14-2). Two weeks later the lateral attachment is severed and turned into the cranial half of the membranous columella (Figure 14-3). If necessary, the defect in the cranial portion of the nasal dome left by excision of the flap is covered by an auricular composite graft (Figure 14-4).

15

Variations in Primary Treatment for the Lip-Columella-Tip Complex

Rodolphe Meyer

As part of any rhinoplasty the tip-columella profile is checked to be sure it shows an aesthetically pleasing double angle. If the profile line is too straight the surgeon can produce a second angle between the lobule and the columella by inserting a cartilaginous graft in addition to the lobular one of Eitner (later reintroduced by Meyer and Sheen). Figure 15-1, *A* to *C*, shows a tip-columella profile that was a straight line preoperatively. After the line is corrected (Figure 15-1, *D* and *E*) a double break can be seen.

Battens are not used alone for retracted columella. Instead, the columella is augmented by transferring a graft from the posterior part of the septum into the transfixion wound or by introducing the cartilaginous strut between the anterior septal border and the medial crura of the lower lateral cartilages. More rigid support of the columella can be provided by a rolled cartilage graft from the ear.

This strong graft is usually combined with the two grafts in the lobule. The lobule-columella junction helps to shape the tip-columella profile.

A marginal alar resection is sometimes indicated. This can be done along the entire length of the nostril or in only the posterior or anterior portions. If a circumflex accent–shaped alar border is encountered, short anterior and posterior marginal resections are used, with the middle of the rim left at its original level. It is fixed with a 6-0 over-and-over running suture. When columellar width also must be reduced the rim can be removed nearly all around the columella and alae. Closure is achieved by a 6-0 over-and-over suture around the nostril. The alae are occasionally defatted according to the technique of Fomon, but subtle cauterization with the scalpel blade between the two skin layers after marginal resection may also suffice. The interstitial cellulofatty tissue can also be removed by direct dissection.

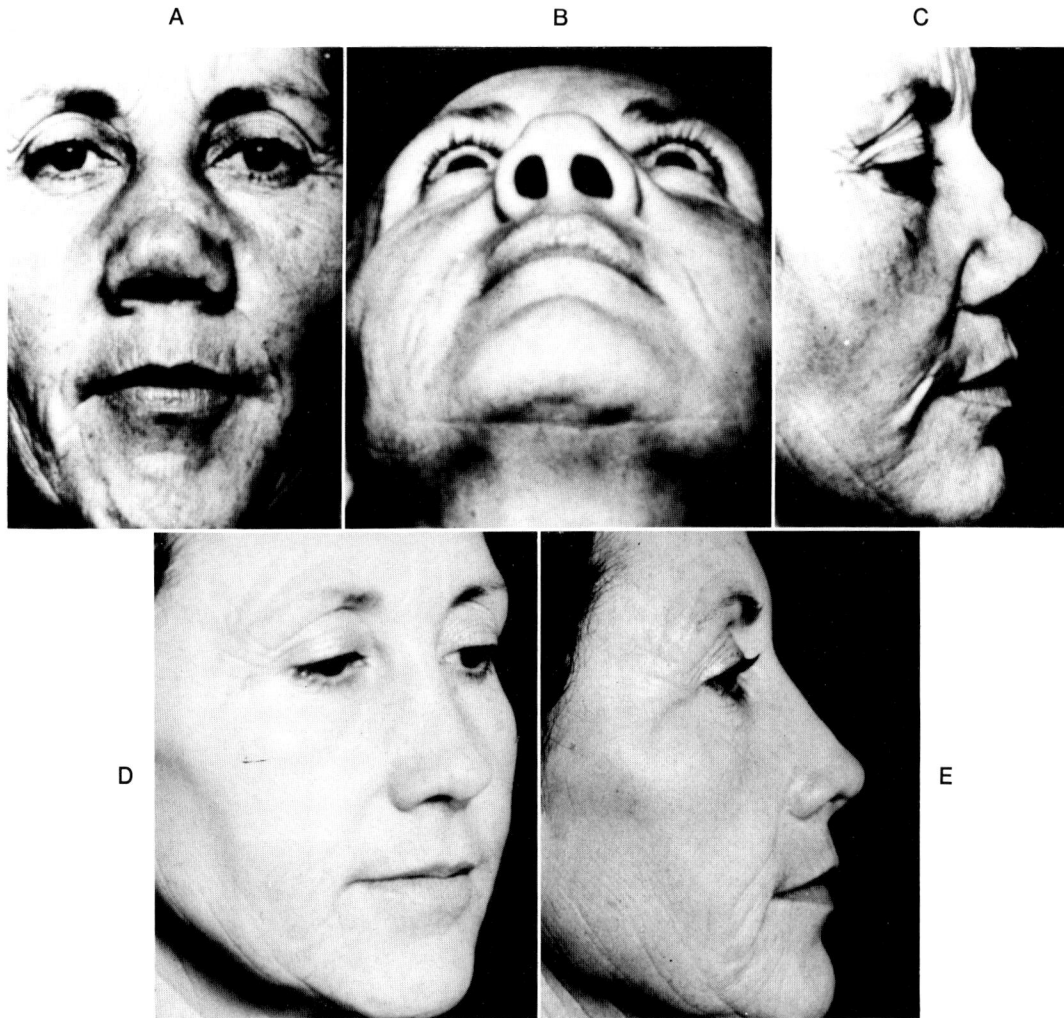

Figure 15-1

Aging lips frequently require augmentation of the vermilion and reshaping of Cupid's bow. The preferred procedure in young women is lifting of the vermilion border in combination with correction of the nasolabial angle by skin excision at the sill of the vestibule. This buffalo horn–shaped excision allows the surgeon to enter the floor of the vestibule as much as needed and lift the pit bilaterally. The lip can also be shortened to obtain a beautiful, high Cupid's bow without resorting to a skin strip resection along the bow. Sometimes only downward displacement of the columellar base is needed.

In patients with a high vestibule sill a small incision is made in the vestibule floor, and the sill is defatted, which helps obtain a more aesthetic entrance to the nasal vestibule. To widen the vestibule, as in cases of stenosis of the floor, a tiny myocutaneous island flap is used with a half-moon–shaped cutaneous patch, which is transferred into the vestibular floor. This can be done through a more lateral tunnel under the alar base. Figure 15-2 shows the correction of a very narrow vestibular floor along with a very narrow cavity. The problem was associated with a tethered lip. The procedure involved the combination of widening the vestibular floor and correction of the "Bugs Bunny" appearance described by Rees. The gingivolabial fold was lowered, with interposition of the nasal hump below the nasal spine, and the lip was fixed in the lower position with gingival and mucosal mattress sutures. After the gingiva was extensively dissected the hump was transferred as a bone graft. If the nasal hump is unavailable a bone graft from the iliac crest or chin can be used. The narrow entrance to the vestibule can be seen in the axial view (Figure 15-2, *A*). The outline of the island myocutaneous flap is seen on both sides; this will be transferred into the vestibular floor through a tunnel without sectioning the alar base. Figure 15-2, *B*, shows the enlarged vestibule.

The patient in Figure 15-3 had a narrow vestibule in which the upper lip was too long. The approach in this case involved the combination of widening of the vestibules with bilateral island flaps and shortening of the lip by resection of a buffalo horn–shaped strip of skin. In this case the alar base was sectioned and resutured after the flap was transposed.

Posttraumatic stenosis of the nasal cavity is difficult to treat. The method I recommend consists of displacing the lateral wall of the cavity a few millimeters into the maxillary sinus. The antronasal wall can be displaced either medially or laterally; medial displacement is chosen in cases of ozena, and lateral displacement is the method of choice in patients with a cavity that is too narrow. This method can also be used in patients with stenosis not only of the vestibule but also of the cavity. For surgical treatment of ozena the overly enlarged cavity is narrowed by a median repositioning of the lateral wall. Then the wall is fixed in the new position by interposing a piece of rib cartilage between its anterior border and the piriform crest.

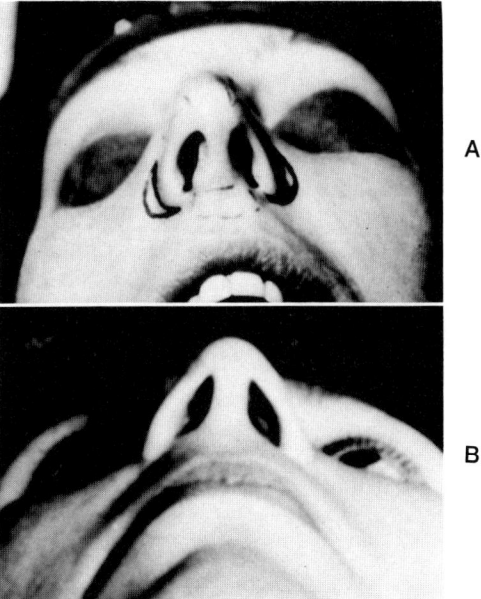

Figure 15-2

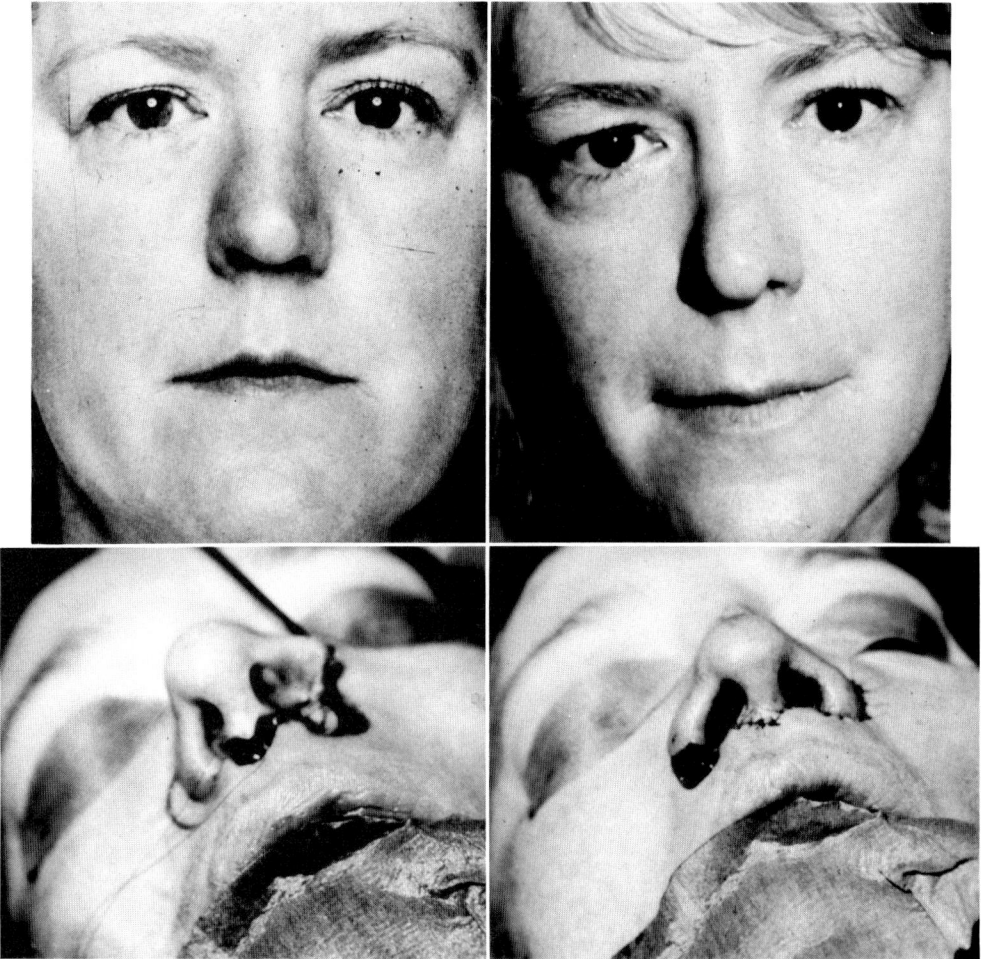

Figure 15-3

TECHNIQUES FOR THE OSSEOCARTILAGINOUS VAULT

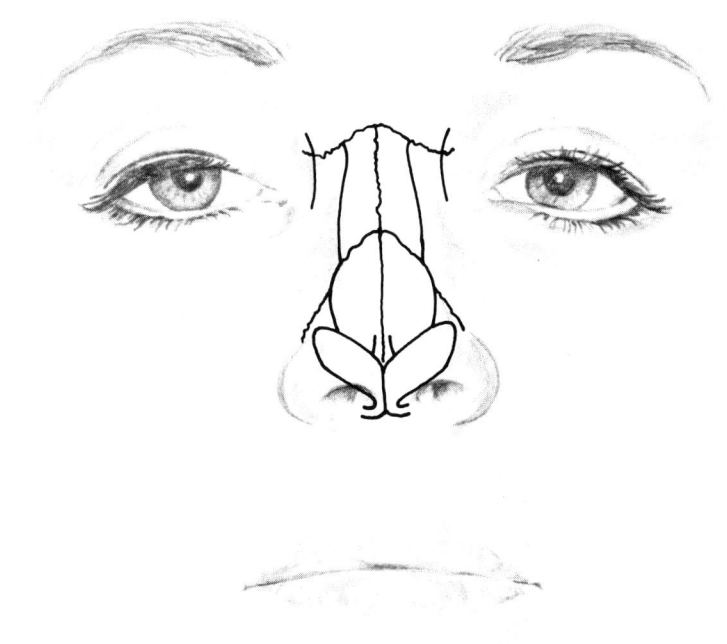

16

Personal Technique

Wolfgang Mühlbauer

GOALS IN RHINOPLASTY

My goal in rhinoplasty is to achieve an individualized nose that blends into the rest of the facial features. Most important, it should be a nose that is desired by the *patient*, which is not always the nose the surgeon thinks the patient should have.

Patient selection

Patient selection is extremely important. It is the first and most important step in rhinoplasty. I do not believe psychologists need to tell us how to choose candidates for operation; the surgeon must make this decision. I do not operate on patients with a bizarre appearance, even though the nose can be improved. Truly psychopathic personalities can often be recognized. A certain number of patients asking for rhinoplasty are overly narcissistic, insecure, neurotic, or a combination of all of these. They may well benefit from "psychotherapy with the scalpel."

Preoperative analysis and marking

I prefer to analyze and mark as exactly as possible all of the nasal structures before surgery is performed. The supportive structures are of utmost importance to me (Figure 16-1). In looking at a patient such as the one in Figure 16-1, it is important to try to visualize what is underneath the skin. For this purpose cadaver dissections are most informative (Figure 16-2). There are great variations in the supportive structures. For example, the girl in Figure 16-1 has extremely long nasal bones and bony sidewalls and very minimal upper lateral cartilages. Without a dissection it is difficult to see structures through the skin. Fiberoptic light in a darkened room can help the novice surgeon better delineate these structures. With experience the surgeon can derive the necessary information by inspection and palpation of the nose. For precision and teaching purposes I paint the skin over the structures I will resect, as shown in Figure 16-1.

The tip. Figure 16-3 shows the amount of alar cartilage I plan to remove in this type of nose. I always leave a sizable portion of caudal alar cartilage, and to be absolutely sure of symmetry I insert two pointed cantilevers and continue the marking inside the vestibule (Figure 16-4).

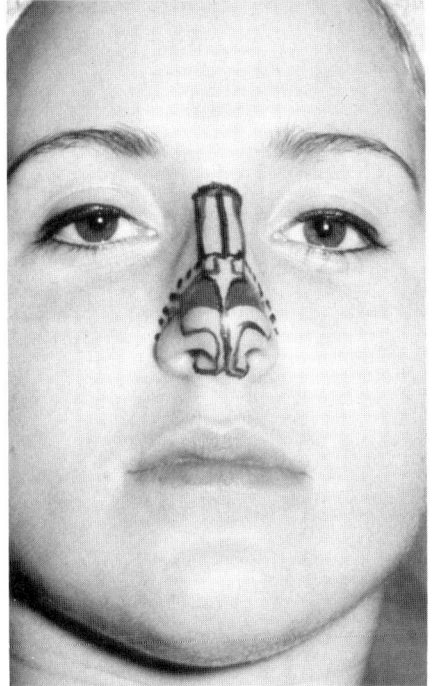

Figure 16-1

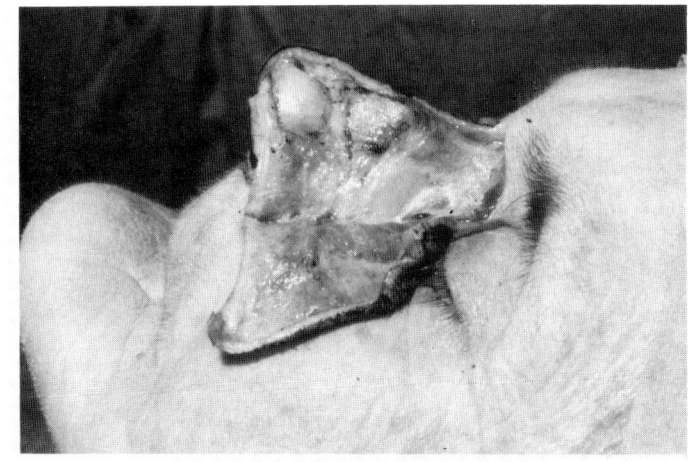

Figure 16-2

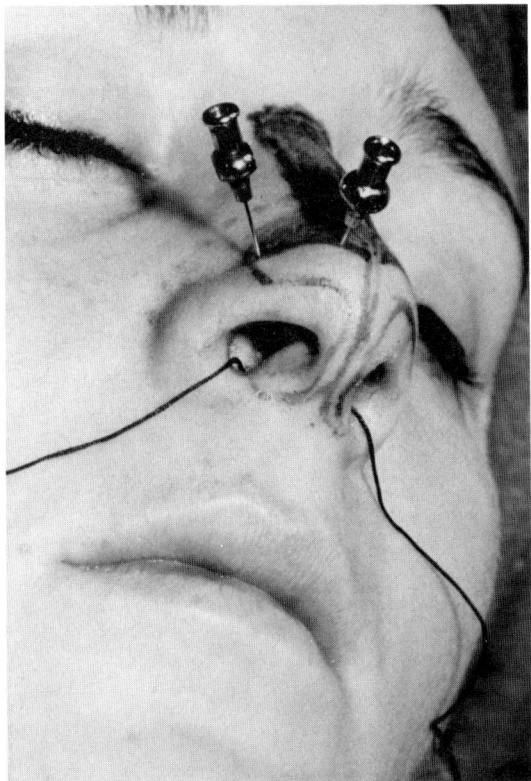

Figure 16-3

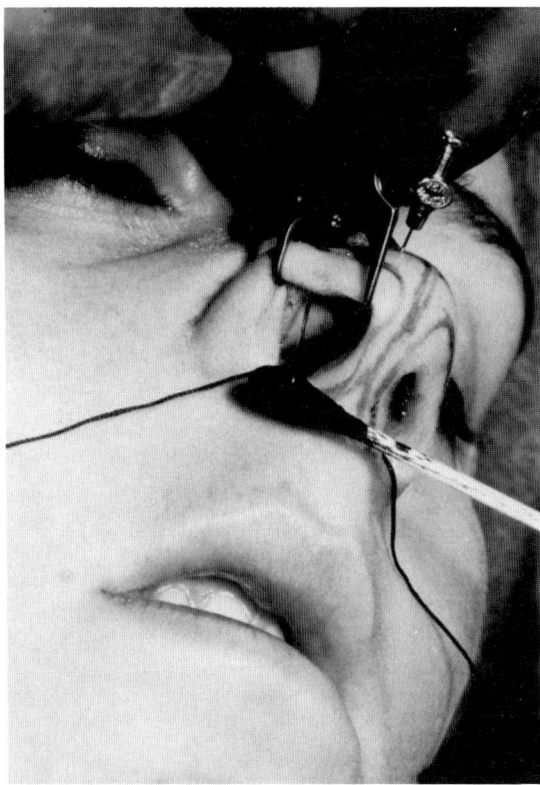

Figure 16-4

For routine cases I use a transcartilaginous incision, because minimal trauma to the nose provides better healing. This incision can be extended down to the transfixion suture. The various incision sites inside the vestibule that I favor are shown in Figure 16-5. The incision is chosen on the basis of what I want it to accomplish. Figure 16-6 shows the amount I usually hope to remove; note that this resection of the cephalic portion of the alar cartilage somewhat reduces the projection.

I agree with others who stress the importance of removing as much fatty subcutaneous tissue as possible along with the cartilage, as shown in Figure 16-7. I find in advantageous to expand the vestibular lining with a local solution, which has been called *hydraulic dissection,* to assist in dissecting in the right plane. I also usually put the resected pieces back on the skin so I will know exactly how much I have resected.

Preservation of character

Preserving the character and individual nature of each nose is important. The patient in Figure 16-8 had an aquiline nose, not uncommon in a man. This man should not be made feminine by a standard reduction. His nose was like his father's and he expected that his nose would droop even further as he aged. I carefully rasped the osseous dorsum, shaved the cartilaginous dorsum, and implanted the alar cartilage pieces from the acute nasolabial angle (Figure 16-9). I also softened the rather deep angle at the radix. The preoperative view and 10-year postoperative results are shown in Figure 16-10, *A* and *B,* respectively. The nose reconstruction remained stable, and character was preserved without feminization. No lateral osteotomy was performed in this patient.

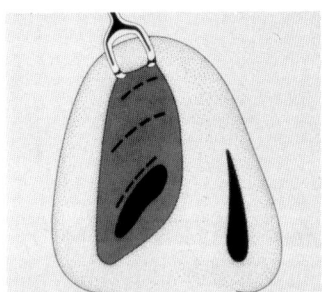

Figure 16-5

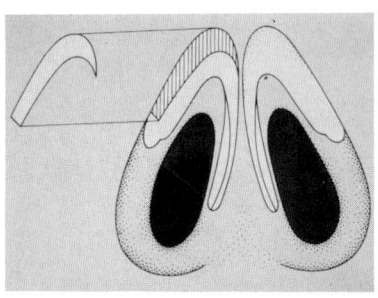

Figure 16-6

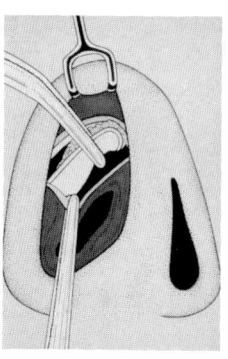

Figure 16-7

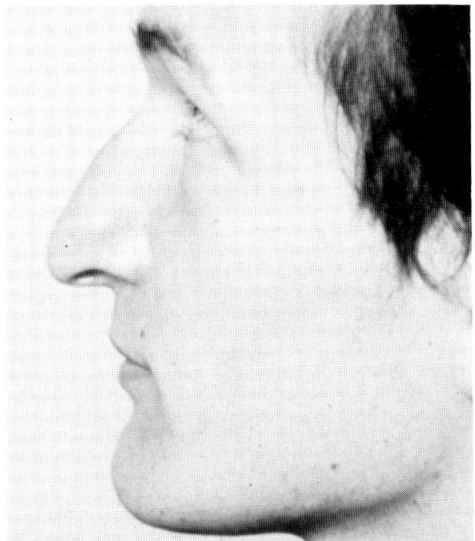

Figure 16-8

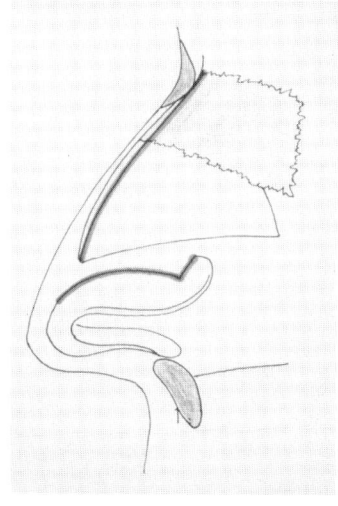

Figure 16-9

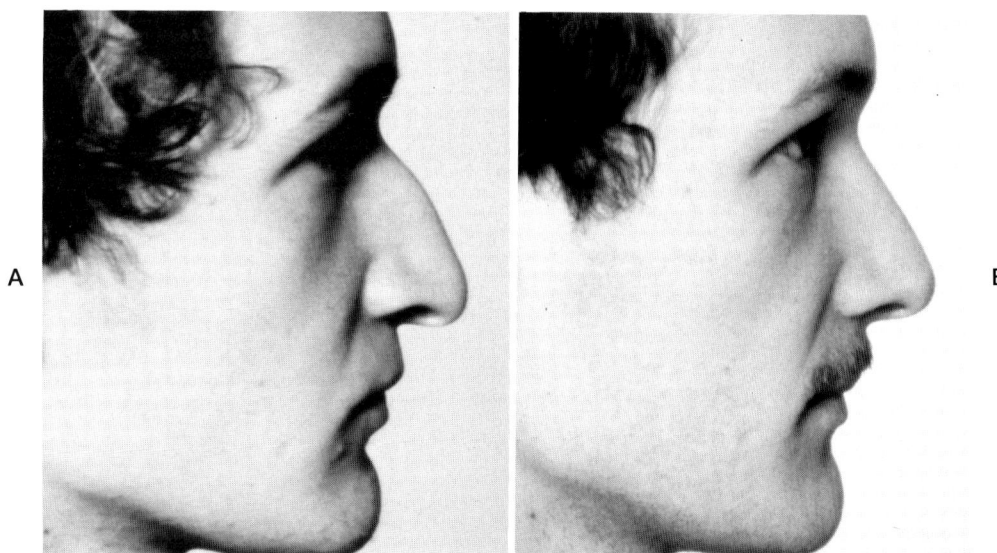

Figure 16-10

The minimal hump. Figure 16-11 shows a patient with a minimal hump and a narrow nasal pyramid. I shaved the cartilaginous dorsum and rasped only the osseous dorsum. Refinement of the tip was necessary, but there was no need to narrow the pyramid. I shaved the cartilaginous portion, because I have never been able to rasp such a resilient structure as the upper lateral area; I always use a sharp scalpel and achieve more precision without creating debris as a result of the shaving. The shaving is shown on a cadaver in Figure 16-12, *A*, and the rasping is shown in Figure 16-12, *B*. The preoperative photographs are shown in Figure 16-13, *A* and *B*, and the 2-year postoperative views are in *C* and *D*. Postoperatively the patient *appears* to have a widening of the nasal pyramid, although nothing was done to the pyramid. An infracture was not performed. Shaving and rasping must be confined to narrow nose if infracture is to be avoided.

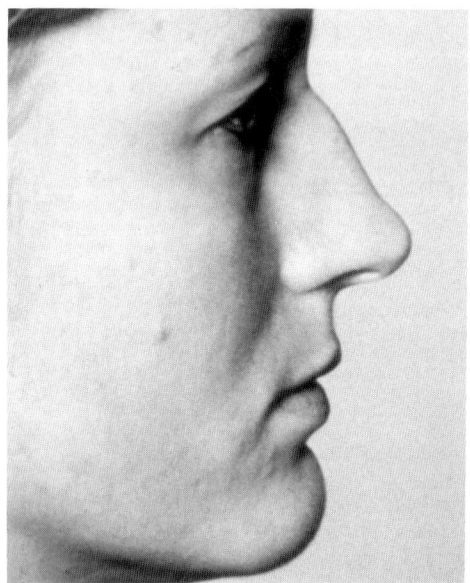

Figure 16-11

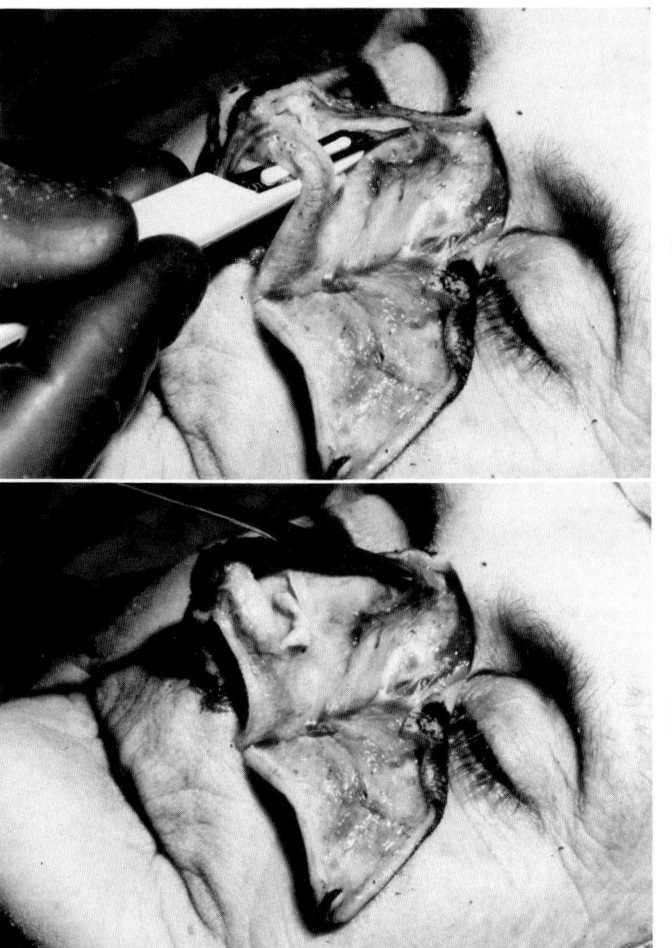

A

B

Figure 16-12

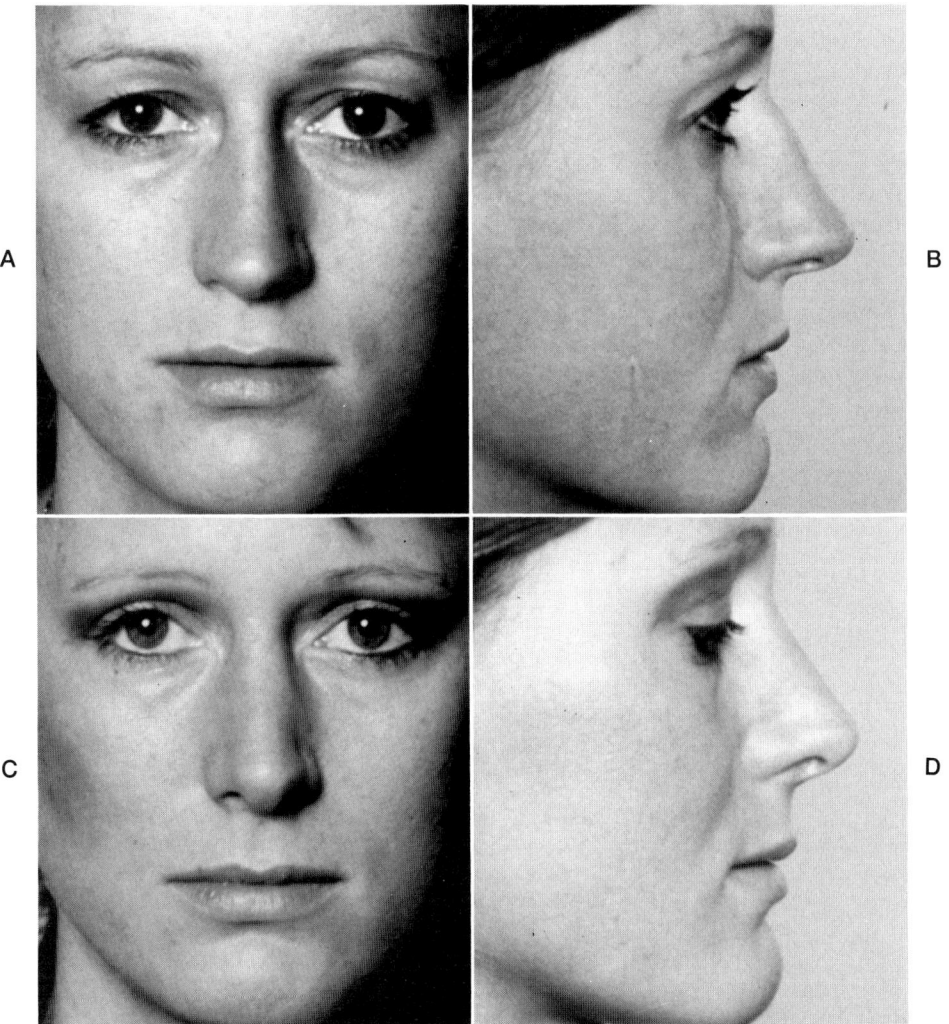

Figure 16-13

The moderate hump. In the patient with the moderate hump and a wide nasal pyramid, I try to do a subperiosteal dissection, especially if the patient has thin dorsal skin, because any remaining irregularity or spicule will show later. The subperiosteal dissection may also prevent telangiectasis. I also prefer a submucosal dissection in such patients, not to the extent Jost recommends but only under the part of the dorsum to be removed. I use a periosteal elevator and detach only as much lining as necessary, avoiding the creation of unnecessary dead space. I often use the hump for replantation, so I resect the cartilaginous portion in one piece with a scalpel. Then I continue at the same level with a guarded osteotome high up into the radix, much higher than most other surgeons attempt. As a final check I put everyting back to be sure I have removed the pieces completely, as marked beforehand.

In a wide hump the nasal bridge is also wide, and I remove a portion of bone between the osseous septum and the lateral walls to provide narrowing. I prefer a chisel for precise excision of these bony fragments. Removal of these pieces allows narrowing of the nose. Then lateral osteotomy and infracture can be performed to achieve a closed dorsum. I doubt whether thick noses can be infractured completely without a resection of paramedian bone. There may be a slight open roof remaining.

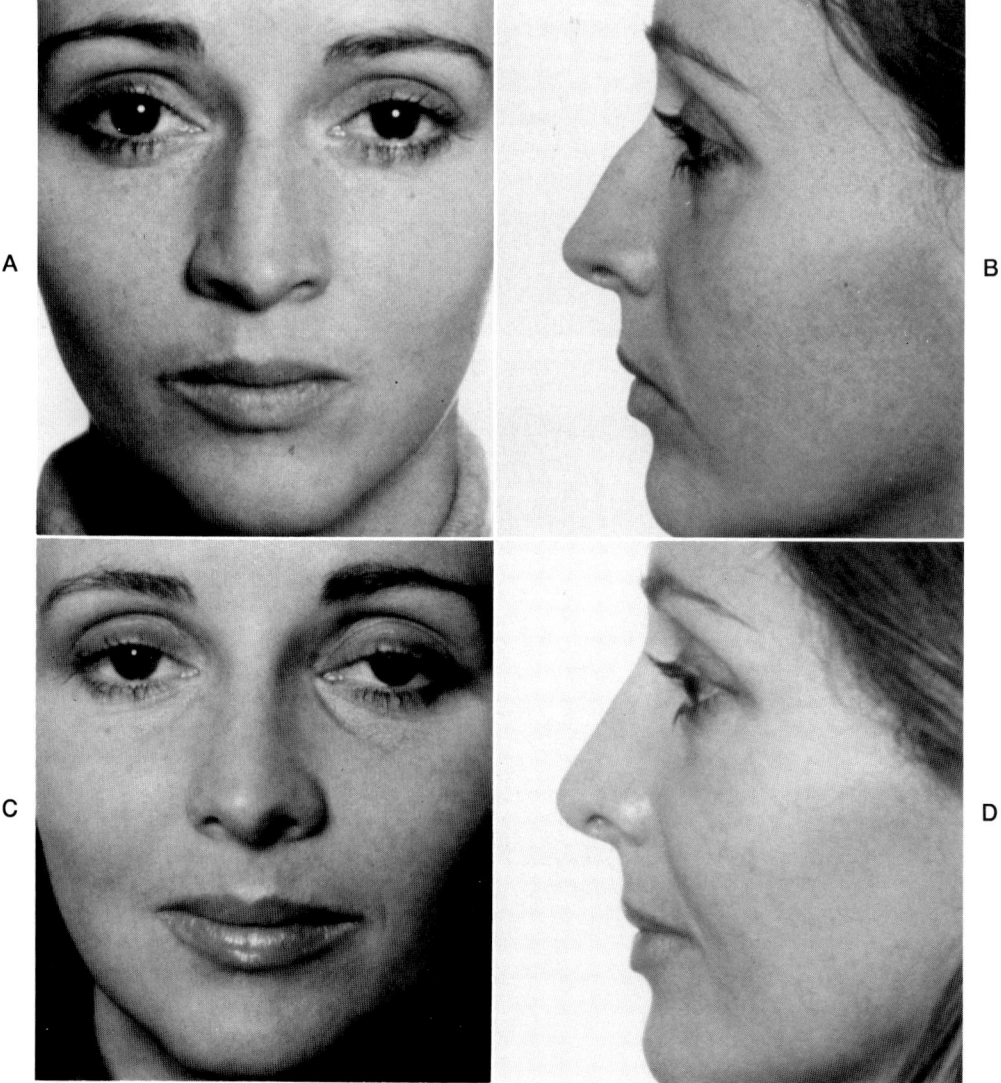

Figure 16-14

For the lateral osteotomy I reach high up into the nasal root at a low level in the maxilla. I also perform a submucosal elevation for the lateral osteotomy.

The patient in Figure 16-14, *A* and *B,* has a wide pyramid with a moderate hump, which was treated in the manner just described. The postoperative result after 1 year is shown in Figure 16-14, *C* and *D.*

The large hump. In the hypertrophic nose with a wide and projecting hump, in addition to all of the steps previously discussed, I recreate a natural dorsum using the straightened hump material, as described by Skoog. A sizable hump is removed with a sharp, curved osteotome after the lower cartilaginous nose is incised. Figure 16-15 showed the essential steps in this maneuver. In *A* the amount of hump to be resected is shown on the profile, with the osteotome in place. In *B* the open roof is considerable after removal of such a large hump, often necessitating excision of spicules of bone from the radix. In *C* a lateral osteotomy is performed, keeping well down on the maxilla as described previously. In *D* the hump is replaced to fill in the dorsum after it is reduced and shaped. The underlying septal portion is trimmed away, and the joint between the remaining cartilaginous and osseous portions then becomes mobile, like a hinge, facilitating its adaptation to the dorsal contour. After replantation is completed, use of fibrin adhesive (Tissuecol; Immuno GMBH) will stabilize the parts in precise positions.

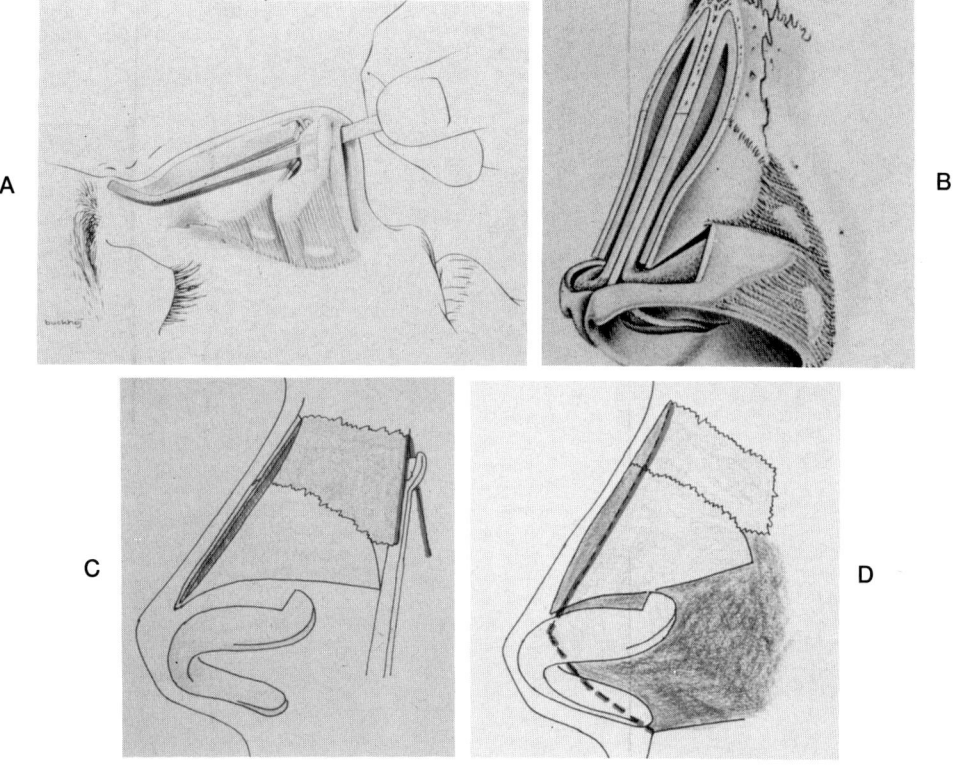

Figure 16-15

The replanted osseocartilaginous dorsum looks and feels more natural than a cartilaginous cover alone. I have not found absorption to be a significant problem. The hump should be reinserted into a subperiosteal and submucosal pocket to minimize infection. The patient in Figure 16-16 was treated in this manner, with reinsertion of the sculpted hump. The view in Figure 16-16, *A*, is preoperative and in *B*, postoperative.

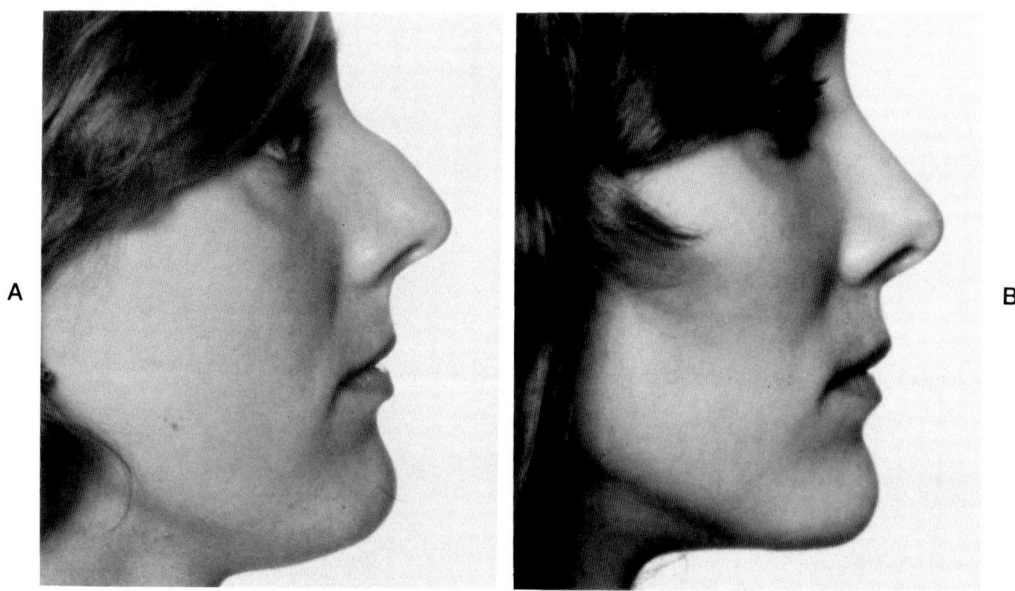

Figure 16-16

17

Lateral Osteotomies: Considerations and Problems with Midnose Torsion

Walter Berman

The least surgery is the best surgery. Following this maxim, I have found that knowledge of when to use what instrument is invaluable. For example, to remove a small amount of tissue and eliminate a minimal anterior or dorsal bony protuberance, I have found a small, curved gouge helpful. But if I want to remove some of the nasal bone at the nasofrontal angle, a straight osteotome is the best instrument; a gouge would remove more of the perpendicular plate of the ethmoid of the bony septum as well as the two nasal bones and would cause an open-roof deformity.

Extending the maxim one step further, choice of procedure is also important. For example, to narrow the nasal pyramid in a person less than 35 years of age, the lateral osteotomy is most effective. This al-

lows the use of the suture line between the nasal bone and maxilla, which lies halfway up the lateral bony nasal wall (Figure 17-1), as a hinge; if some of the bony anterior or dorsal hump has already been removed all the way up, a medial osteotomy is a wasted maneuver.

The requirements for lateral osteotomies differ from those for medial osteotomies. The lateral osteotomy does not have to extend the full length but can be moderated to the length needed to produce an infracture. Sometimes a small triangular piece of bone may be left (Figure 17-2). I prefer to carry the

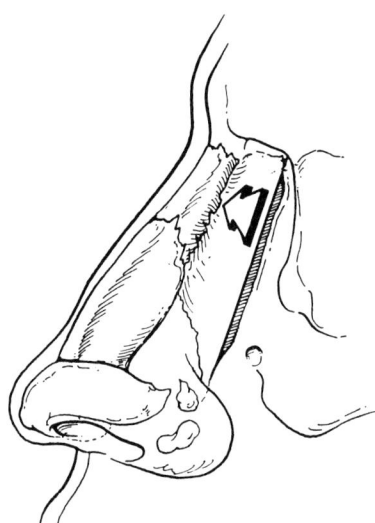

Figure 17-1. The arrow points to the hinge between the nasal bone and the nasomaxillary process.

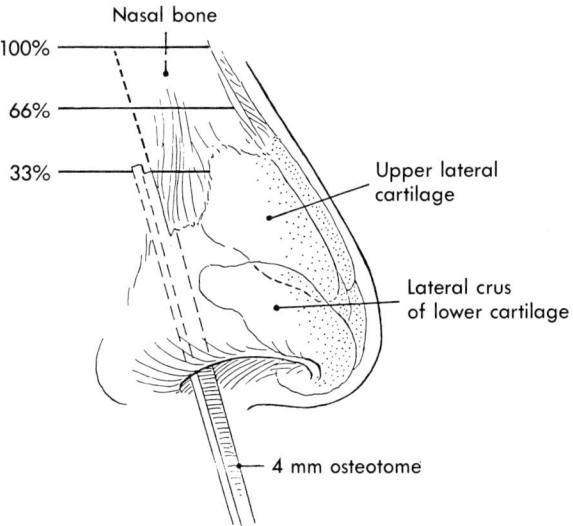

Figure 17-2. Various extents of lateral osteotomies as necessary. (From Berman, W.E.: Rhinoplasty, ed. 2, Washington, D.C., 1984, American Academy of Otolaryngology—Head and Neck Surgery Foundation, Inc.)

incision posteriorly or near the face of the maxilla. If it is left too high or too far anteriorly, a noticeable shelf may be produced.

If the bone is curved as a result of posttraumatic or congenital deformity or if the nasal bone is curved on one side, a double osteotomy is the treatment of choice. The anterodorsal osteotomy is done first, then a more posterior osteotomy finishes comminution of the bone. The triangular piece that is sometimes left over can also be included (Figure 17-3).

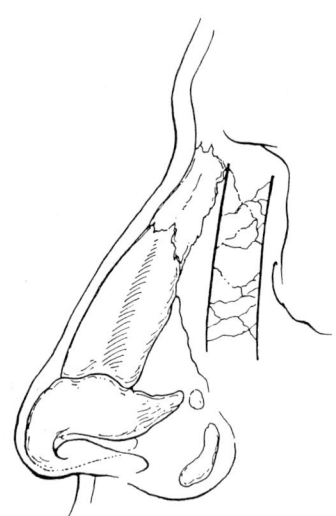

Figure 17-3. Double lateral osteotomies to comminute the bones to straighten the boney pyramid.

Figure 17-4, *A* and *B* shows a patient with Crohn's disease who had lost both supporting cartilage and lining epithelium. The resulting nasal collapse interfered with nasal respiration and caused external distortion of his nose. Structurally he needed replacement of both the lost cartilaginous framework (upper and lateral) and the lost epithelial lining. Before surgery a complete diagnostic workup was done, including multiple biopsies to detect a Wegener's or midline granuloma; none was found. When the patient was maintained on low-dose cortisone for Crohn's disease, the degenerative effect on the nasal cartilage ceased; it resumed when the cortisone was discontinued.

A large composite postauricular graft consisting of conchal cartilage and overlying medial skin was taken and an intercartilaginous incision performed. Extensive undermining of adjacent tissue was done to achieve tissue relaxation.

Inferior (caudal) traction was supplied by traction sutures through the lower lateral third of the nasal framework. This left a large epithelial and framework deficit on the nose's internal aspect; this was repaired by the postauricular graft, which replaced the epithelial lining on the internal nasal surface (Figure 17-5). One-sided morcellation of the cartilage allowed the surgeon to curve the graft to the patient's specific needs. This repair created a better nose physiologically, with a good external appearance.

The traction sutures were left in place for 5 days by means an external traction device. Currently the patient has no difficulty breathing, and his nose is externally straight. He has decided against further surgery to correct his columellar retraction.

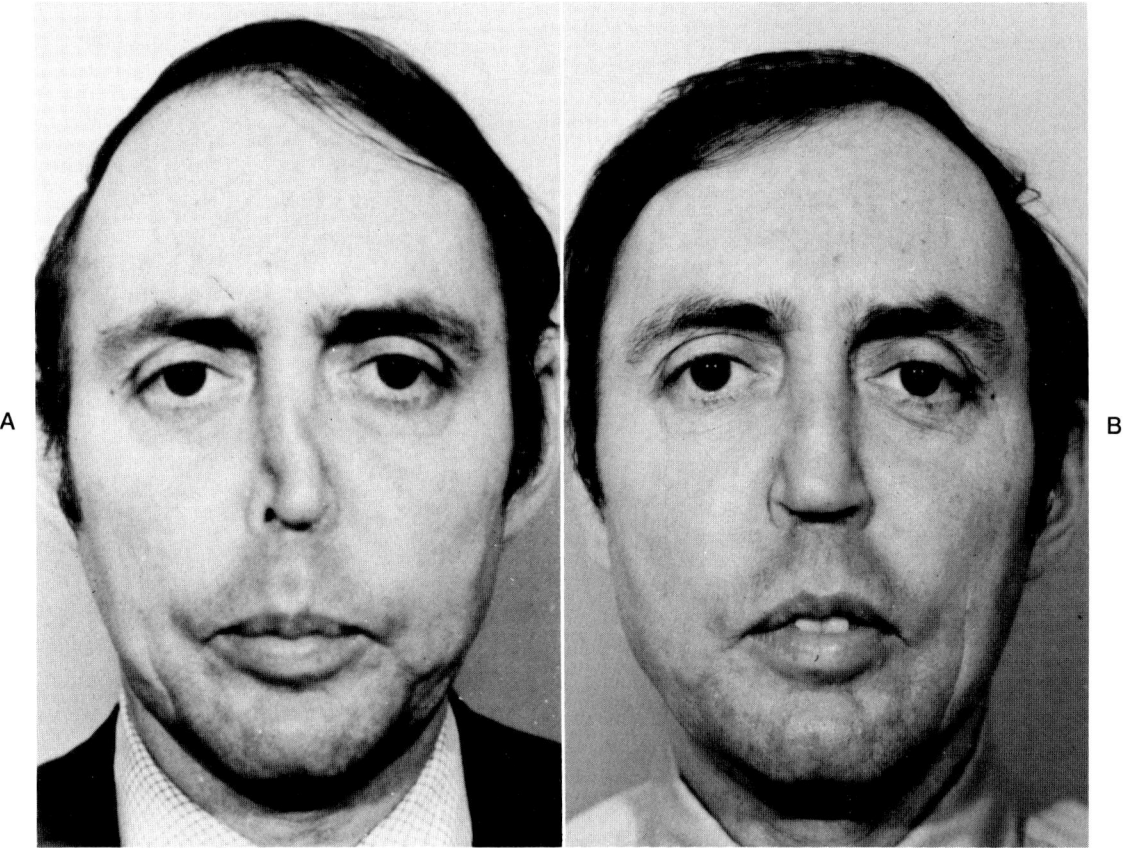

Figure 17-4. A, Middle third torsion of the nose, preoperative view. **B,** Middle third torsion of the nose, reconstructed with composite postauricular graft placed internally, postoperative view (4 cm septal perforation).

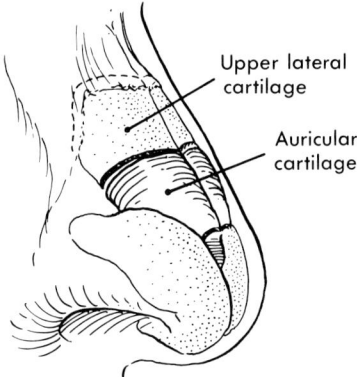

Figure 17-5. Diagram of postauricular composite graft using epithelium as lining. (From Berman, W.E.: Rhinoplasty, ed. 2, Washington, D.C., 1984, American Academy of Otolaryngology—Head and Neck Surgery Foundation, Inc.)

18

Correction of the Osseocartilaginous Vault

Eugene Courtiss

Although most rhinoplastic surgeons agree that an excellent result in surgery of the nasal tip is required for technical success, patient happiness more accurately reflects the success achieved in the osteocartilagenous vault. Unfortunately, obtaining desired results in the osteocartilagenous vault is taken for granted; it should not.

I will identify those considerations that result in the aesthetic objective; that is, a nose that appears *natural*. A natural nose varies with the individual patient's ethnic background, sex, physical stature, age, occupation, social status, and personality, which are reviewed elsewhere.[1] To obtain a natural result do *only what* has to be done and *only as much* as has to be done. Phrased differently, tailor the operation to the individual patient and be conservative.

This chapter concerns only the osteocartilaginous vault. However, that vault does not exist unto itself; it must be considered in relation to the other components of the nose.

Anesthesia

No matter how anesthesia is accomplished the patient must be free of pain. A patient who is agitated, crying, or moving will at best tax the surgeon's patience, and at worst a poor result will be obtained. As a result, anesthetic technique is important, albeit neglected, in rhinoplasty surgery.

Some surgeons prefer general anesthesia. Its advantages are that the patient is free of pain and usually still, and someone else is worrying about the patient's essential body functions; the surgeon's only concern is performing the operation. On the negative side, the endotracheal tube makes instrument use awkward, and facial relationships cannot be seen. If a chin implant is being inserted coincidentally, the jaw cannot be closed; therefore facial balance is difficult to assess. Finally, unless the same anesthetist is always present, the surgeon may suffer frustration, because the constantly changing anesthesia personnel frequently have different philosophies.

I prefer local anesthesia with intravenous sedation, despite its disadvantages, and continuous monitoring, usually provided by the same anesthesiologist. No medication is given before surgery unless the patient is extremely nervous, in which case diazepam (Valium) (10 mg by mouth) is given 2 hours before operation. In the operating room an intravenous line is started, and the patient is given 10 to 20 mg diazepam. The exact dose is determined by the degree of sedation obtained. Then 1 to 2 ml of fentanyl (Sublimaze) is given intravenously. In most patients these medications allow by objective: *the painless injection of the local anesthetic*. Those patients who experience pain at the time of the injection are given low-dose ketamine (1 mg/kg body weight). Even if ketamine is preferred to fentanyl, diazepam should be given. These medications and local anesthesia are usually all that are used during the operation; however, during turbinate resection or at the time of the lateral osteotomy, additional medication (diazepam/fentanyl) may be required.

Several local and topical anesthetics are available. Most commonly, lidocaine is used for injection and cocaine is used topically. Because it provides a longer period of anesthesia, I prefer 0.25% bupivacaine (Marcaine) to which *fresh* epinephrine is added to make a concentration of 1:200,000 and 300 N.F. hyaluronidase is added to lessen edema. For topical anesthesia my choice is 2% pontocaine mixed half and half with 1:1000 epinephrine. The mixture obviates use of cocaine, a drug that has found nonmedical uses. One-inch selvage-edge gauze is a satisfactory pack.

The injections should be made slowly, starting at the bony radix and then fanning down the nose to the lateral walls and tip. Then the base of the columella and the sites of the incisions should be injected with anesthetic. Last, the anesthetic is injected into the lateral osteotomy sites.

The vibrissae are trimmed. Then I scrub, following which the patient is prepared and draped. The reader should note that the anesthetics are injected and packs placed *before* I scrub. This permits the agents time to work.

Sequence

Some surgeons *always* do the hump first; others *always* do the tip first. My philosophy is to do what is *worst* first. Even partial correction of the worst defect improves the nasal relationships. When the worst is no longer the worst, the overall nose looks better; as a result, less is removed and a more conservative procedure is performed.

Incisions

Bilateral intercartilaginous incisions are made *caudal* to the internal valve with a No. 11 blade. If the caudal septum requires alteration the intercartilaginous incisions are connected with a through-and-through (transfixion) incision in the membranous septum. If the caudal septum is satisfactory the transfixion incision is omitted.

Dissection

A Foman scissor is used to elevate the soft tissues over the nasal dorsum. The periosteum is not elevated separately. However, the desired plane is just above the periosteum. As much soft tissue as possible is left on the side with skin.

Bony hump

Although some surgeons use saws and others advocate an osteotome or chisel, I prefer *sharp* rasps. They must be sharp lest they tear rather than cut. I prefer rasps because the bony profile is lowered gradually and the effects can be constantly reassessed. Saws take too much tissue, and osteotomes are too difficult to control. Both draw rasps, honed after each use, and the Rees rasp are satisfactory instruments for this use.

Cartilaginous hump

After the cartilaginous hump is visualized with an Aufricht retractor, it is reduced with a No. 15 knife blade. The upper lateral and septal cartilages are trimmed simultaneously. The upper lateral cartilages need not be divided from the septum. In most cases lowering the upper lateral and septal cartilages does not cut through the lining. However, if the lining is divided no harm is done.

Nasofrontal angle

Deepening the nasofrontal angle is difficult. It is best attempted with a sharp rasp reaching to the most cephalad portion of the bones. Removal of the thick forehead bone with an osteotome is difficult and serves to elongate the nose.

Caudal septum and nasal spine

If the tip of the nose requires elevation the caudal septum may be trimmed under direct vision with a No. 15 blade. A triangle is removed first from the anterior one third of the caudal septum. Then the columella may be raised if desired by trimming the more posterior part of the caudal septum. If the tip is elevated the anterior caudal angle of the upper lateral cartilages *may* require shortening. This should be done very judiciously, preserving all of the lining and removing only the smallest triangle of cartilage. If the anterior nasal spine is prominent, pushes the columella down, or is associated with a "short upper lip," it is trimmed judiciously.

Bony web

If a bony web is present at the base of the radix, satisfactory infracturing may be impossible. In such instances a V-shaped piece of bone may be removed from the web with a narrow osteotome or a narrow Converse forceps.

Lateral osteotomy

A double-guarded, straight 6 mm osteotome with a dorsal stabilizer is a satisfactory instrument for the lateral osteotomy. After each use it should be sharpened. The osteotome makes its own incision in the lining at the base of the piriform aperture. The assistant strikes the osteotome as it is directed as far as the level of the medial canthus. Some surgeons advocate starting the osteotomy low and curving it high on the lateral wall as the osteotome is advanced, the so-called *low-to-high osteotomy*. This results in a stepping that is unnatural; thus keeping it low on the plane of the maxilla is preferable.

Medial osteotomy

Although the medial osteotomy is not required for infracturing, it provides a smooth osteotomy and obviates against fragmentation of the bone or producing a spicule, both of which may mar the result. A 6 mm (nonguarded) osteotome is placed in the midsagittal plane, and the nasal bones are cut as far cephalad as the level of the medial canthus.

Outfracture/infracture

Through the medial osteotomy site the nasal bone is levered laterally, producing an outfracture. Then the bones are infractured. This sequence is preferred, because it assures that the bones are completely mobilized, and a green-stick fracture, which be definition retains its spring, is not produced. If a green-stick fracture is produced the bones later have a tendency to drift laterally. The outfracture lessens green-stick formation.

Final check

The dorsal profile is examined visually and tactilely. Then an Aufricht retractor is inserted, and the internal nose is inspected. Any small bone chips or cartilage irregularities are treated. Not infrequently the cartilage at the junction of the upper lateral cartilages and nasal bones needs trimming.

Closure

The mucosa of the transfixion incision (if one was made) is approximated with 5-0 chromic catgut sutures. Through-and-through ("orthopedic") sutures are not used. The intercartilaginous and piriform incisions are left open.

Dressing

Packs (see Chapter 27) are used if the inferior turbinates have been resected; otherwise no nasal pack is used. Then the nose should be degreased with freon and sprayed with Ace adherent. The nasal contour is maintained by Steri-strips, then plaster of Paris and an aluminum splint are applied.

Aphorisms

1. If it does not look right in the operating room, make it so.
2. Do only what has to be done, and do it conservatively.

REFERENCE

1. Courtiss, E.H.: Objectives of aesthetic surgery. In Courtiss, E.H., editor: Male aesthetic surgery, St. Louis, 1982, The C. V. Mosby Co.

19

Spreader Grafts for Reconstructing the Roof of the Upper Cartilaginous Vault

Jack Sheen

An overly narrow or collapsed middle nasal vault may occur after rhinoplasty when the roof of the upper cartilaginous vault has been resected, or an overly narrow middle vault may be naturally present in some patients who seek primary rhinoplasty. Therefore there are three instances when reconstruction of the middle vault is indicated: (1) primary rhinoplasty for patients with "narrow nose syndrome," (2) primary rhinoplasty for patients who are predisposed to middle vault collapse, and (3) secondary rhinoplasty for patients with collapse of the middle vault postoperatively. I believe the last instance to be the direct result of a failure to recognize the first two.

When I examine the preoperative photographs of patients who underwent secondary rhinoplasty, it is evident that certain aesthetic and functional problems might have been avoided by reconstruction of the middle vault during the primary operation. In a patient with narrow nose syndrome—an abnormally narrow nose with visible collapse of the lateral nasal walls and abnormal valving on inspiration—reconstruction of the middle vault is obviously necessary for a good functional and aesthetic result. Less obvious is the patient who is likely to have collapse of the middle vault after rhinoplasty. This is the person with short nasal bones, thin skin and soft tissue cover, weak cartilages, or any of these factors in combination. To understand how these factors affect and are affected by rhinoplasty, a brief review of normal anatomy is helpful.

The middle nasal vault is composed of the upper lateral cartilages, which are supported superiorly by the nasal bones and anteriorly by the dorsal edge of the septum. The shape of the septum may vary, but on cross-section the area of the middle vault usually corresponds to a T.[2] The medial edges of the upper lateral cartilages attach to the anterior lateral extension of the septum by end-to-end apposition. The wide anterior aspect of the septum (the top of the T), to which the upper lateral cartilages are attached, forms the dorsal roof.

Aesthetically the middle vault is the midsection of an integrated form composed of the three nasal vaults. These three vaults—bony, upper cartilaginous, and lower cartilaginous—are defined by smooth, slightly curved, divergent lines from the root of the nose to the tip.

With the normal confluence of these three vaults in mind, consider the effect of surgery on the middle vault, particulary resection of the dorsal roof. When the roof is resected several problems may result from cave-in of the lateral walls. Medial collapse of the middle vault produces a characteristic inverted V deformity caused by the visible borders of the bony pyramid (Figure 19-1). An oblique view of the structure may reveal the discontinuity of bony and cartilaginous vaults to be the result of an apparent bump at the caudal edge of the bone. This is very disturbing to patients, who are quick to point out that there was no "bump" preoperatively. Of course, what they are seeing is not a bump but a depression below the edge of the bone, an interruption of what should be a smooth lateral line.

Resection of the dorsal roof in certain patients may cause an even more disturbing problem: impaired breathing. The patient will have difficulty on inspiration because of collapsing internal valves. Without the spreading effect of the broad anterior septal edge, abnormal valving may occur. Patients with short nasal bones, narrow nose syndrome, or what Cottle describes as a *tension* nose frequently complain of difficulty on inspiration after operation. For these patients and for those predisposed to collapse of the lateral walls after resection, the middle vault should be reconstructed during the primary rhinoplasty.

THE SPREADER GRAFT

The following case demonstrates a technique for reconstructing the roof of the middle vault by placing strips of cartilage submucosally along the anterior edge of the septum. These grafts spread the walls of the middle vault laterally, aligning them with the bony vault, and well-functioning internal valves are maintained. I have placed over 500 spreader grafts to date and continue to be impressed by both the functional and the aesthetic results.

CASE REPORT

The patient was a 38-year-old anesthesiologist with a long history of obstructed airways. He had reported difficulty with nasal breathing and had to breathe through the mouth with any physical exertion. The nose had a high, convex dorsum and a narrow roof of the middle vault. Internally there was impaction of the airways at the internal valve bilaterally. Approximately 15% of the valve was open on each side (Figure 19-2, *A*). The septum was deformed, with most of the distortion near the floor of the nose. Both lateral walls were in intimate contact with the septum. Clear mucus covering the surfaces further obstructed the impaired airways.

With the base of the nose retracted and the septal angle exposed (Figure 19-3), the mucosa was infiltrated with 1% lidocaine with epinephrine. A small incision was made at the caudal reflection of the mucoperichondrium (Figure 19-4). *Incising into the caudal edge of the septum facilitates the placement*

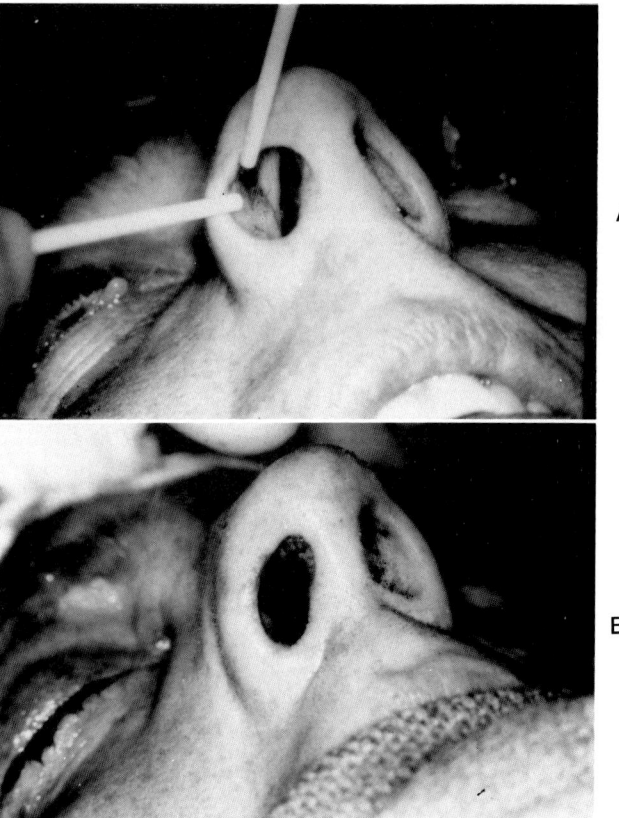

A

B

Figure 19-2. **A,** Preoperative view of obstructed airway caused by collapsed lateral walls. **B,** Postoperative view with spreader graft in place. Lateral wall is moved 2 to 3 mm away from septum.

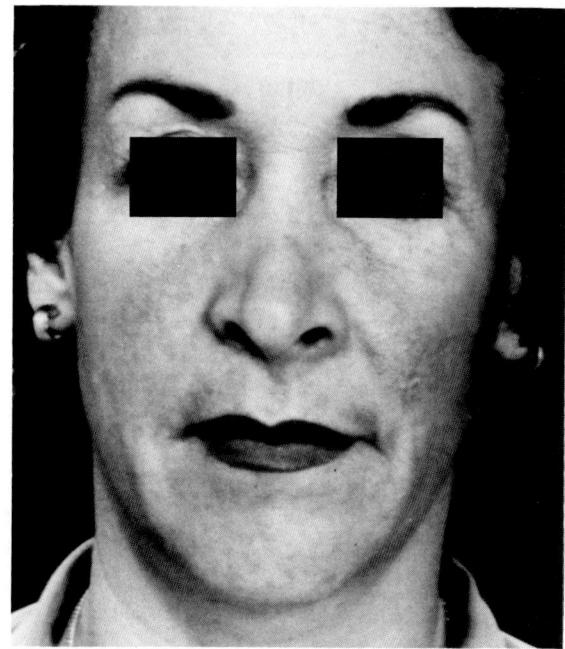

Figure 19-1. After surgery the middle cartilaginous vault collapses in patient with inverted V deformity.

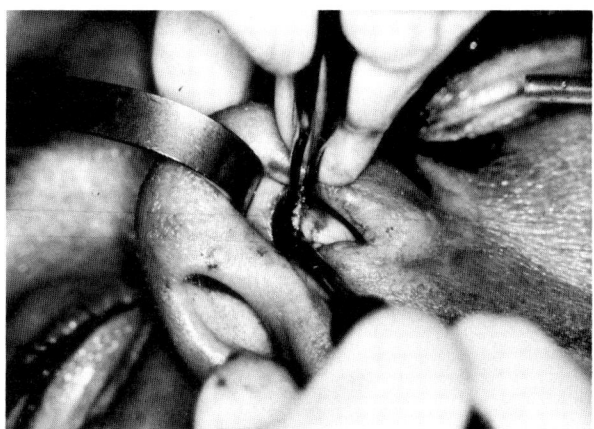

Figure 19-3. Incision at septal angle exposes anterior caudal septum.

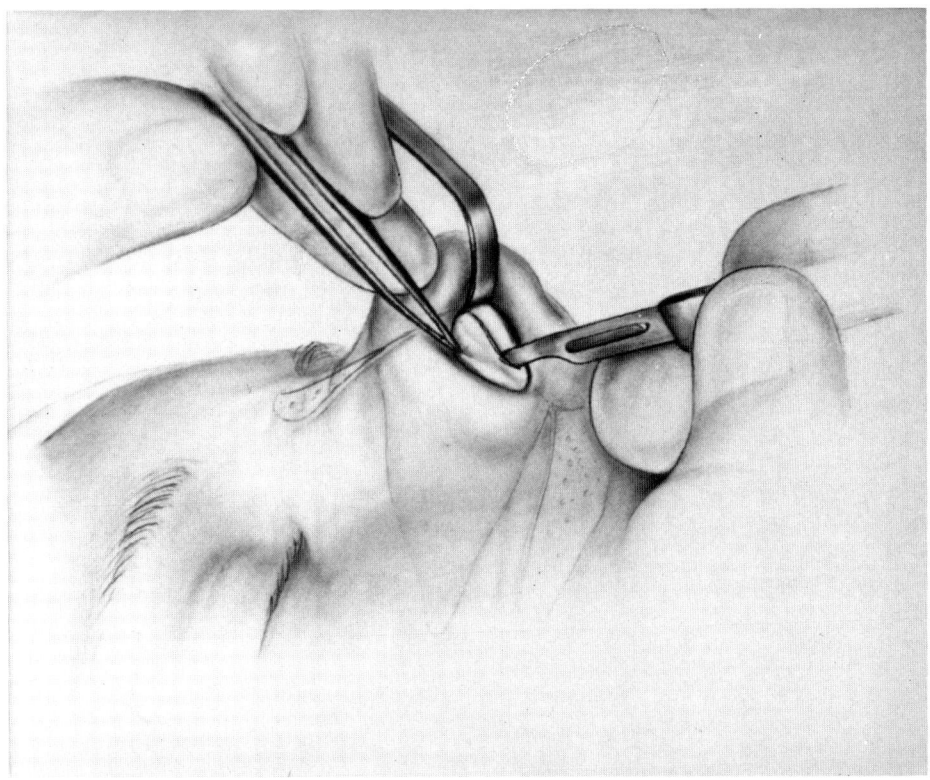

Figure 19-4. Incision into caudal edge of septum begins subperichondrial dissection. (From Sheen, J.H.: Spreader graft: a method of reconstructing the roof of the middle nasal vault following rhinoplasty, Plast. Reconstr. Surg. 73:230-239, 1984.)

of an elevator between the perichondrium and the cartilage. Dissection is simple and rapid, since the Cottle perichondrial elevator is inserted cephalad, past the arch of the bony pyramid (Figure 19-5).

A septoplasty was done to correct the airway obstruction and to obtain material for the grafts. Care was taken so the area of septal resection would not communicate with the pocket for the spreader graft. *If there is a communication the graft will slip posteriorly, losing its effectiveness.* Two strips of cartilage selected for the grafts were taken from the caudal end of the septum and part of the septum from the vomeral groove (Figure 19-6). *If more width is necessary small shims of ethmoid or cartilage can be placed medial to the grafts.*

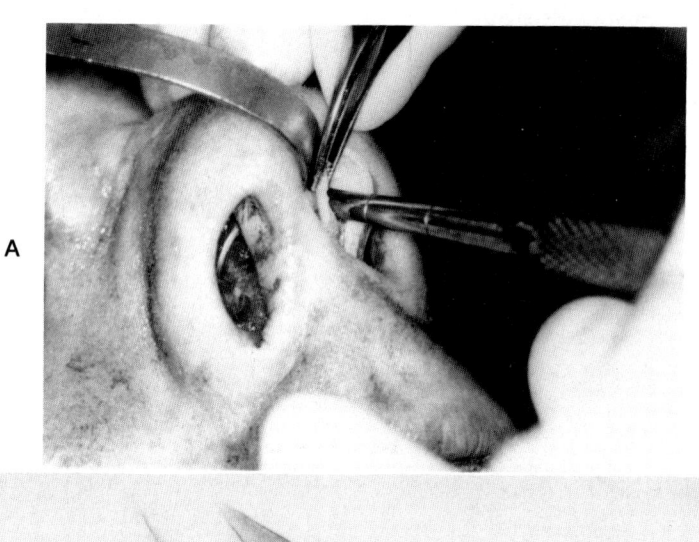

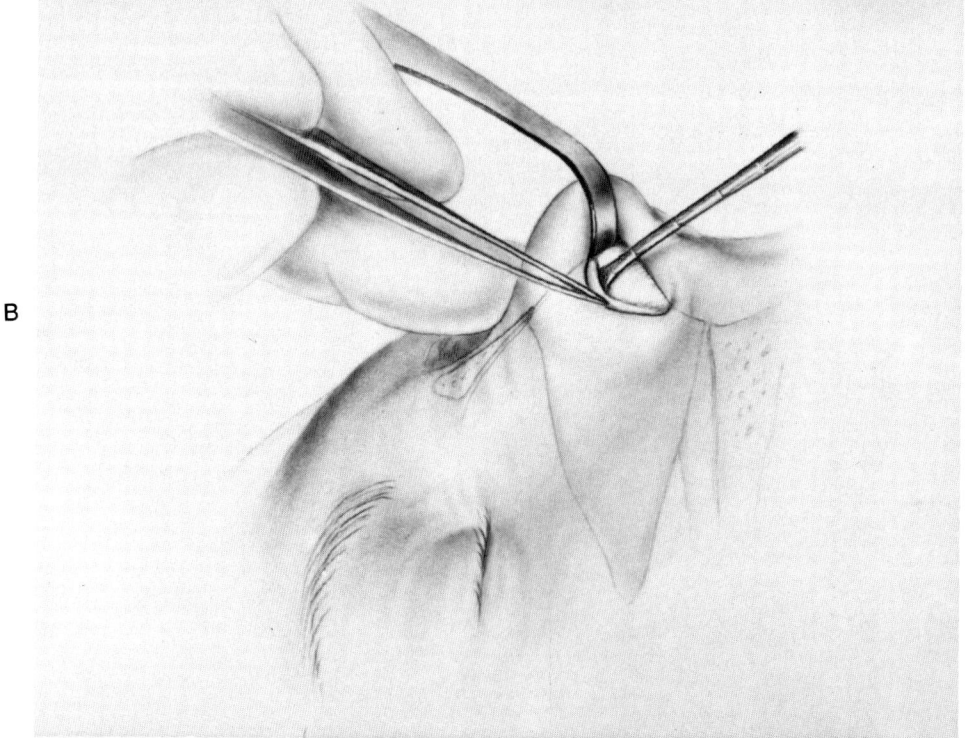

Figure 19-5. A, Subperichondrial dissection. **B,** Cottle perichondrial elevator is used to dissect pockets for spreader grafts. (From Sheen, J.H.: Spreader graft: a method of reconstructing the roof of the middle nasal vault following rhinoplasty, Plast. Reconstr. Surg. 73:230-239, 1984.)

The grafts were then placed into the prepared pockets (Figure 19-7), with the cephalic parts going under the arch of the bony pyramid and with the convex surface facing laterally (Figure 19-8). *The caudal part of the graft should be close to the at-* *tachment of the upper lateral cartilage* (Figure 19-9). After the spreader grafts were placed the walls of the middle vault were distracted laterally, effectively opening the internal valves (see Figure 19-2, B).

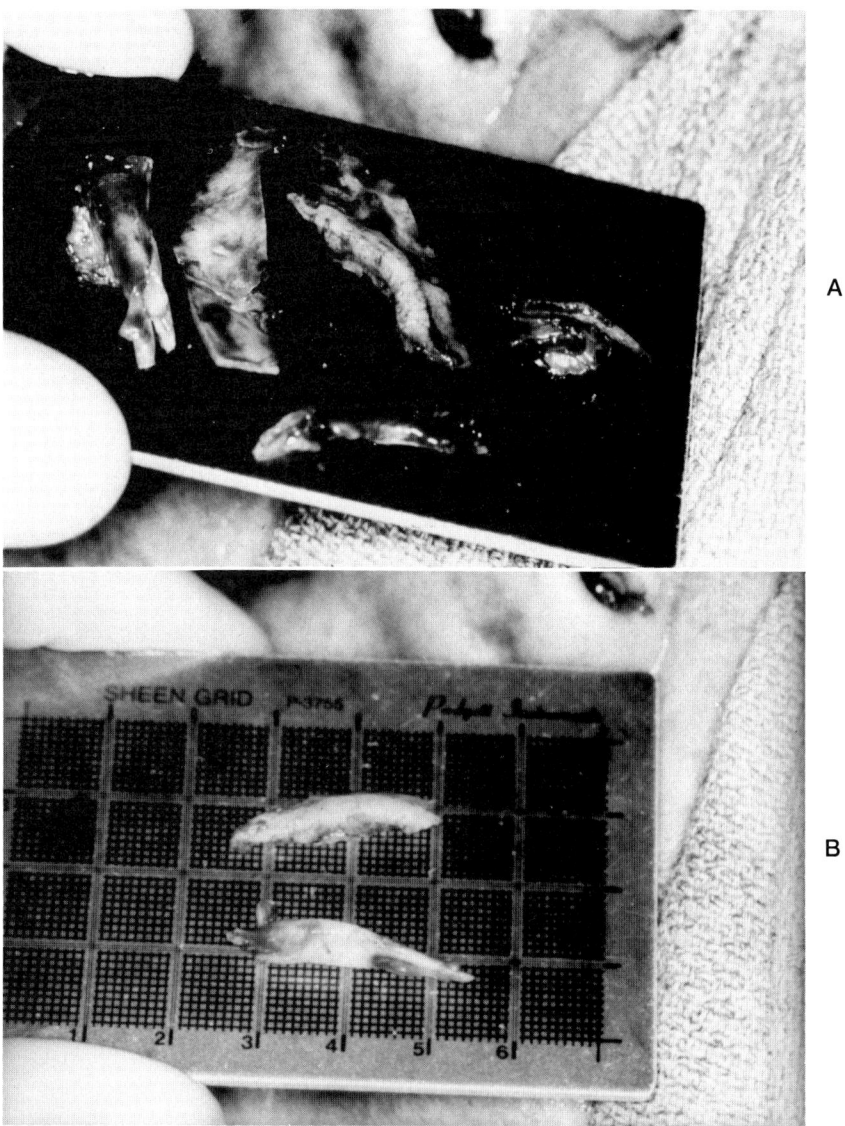

Figure 19-6. A, Specimen of distorted cartilage, vomer, and ethmoid obtained from submucous resection. **B,** Cartilage selected for spreader grafts.

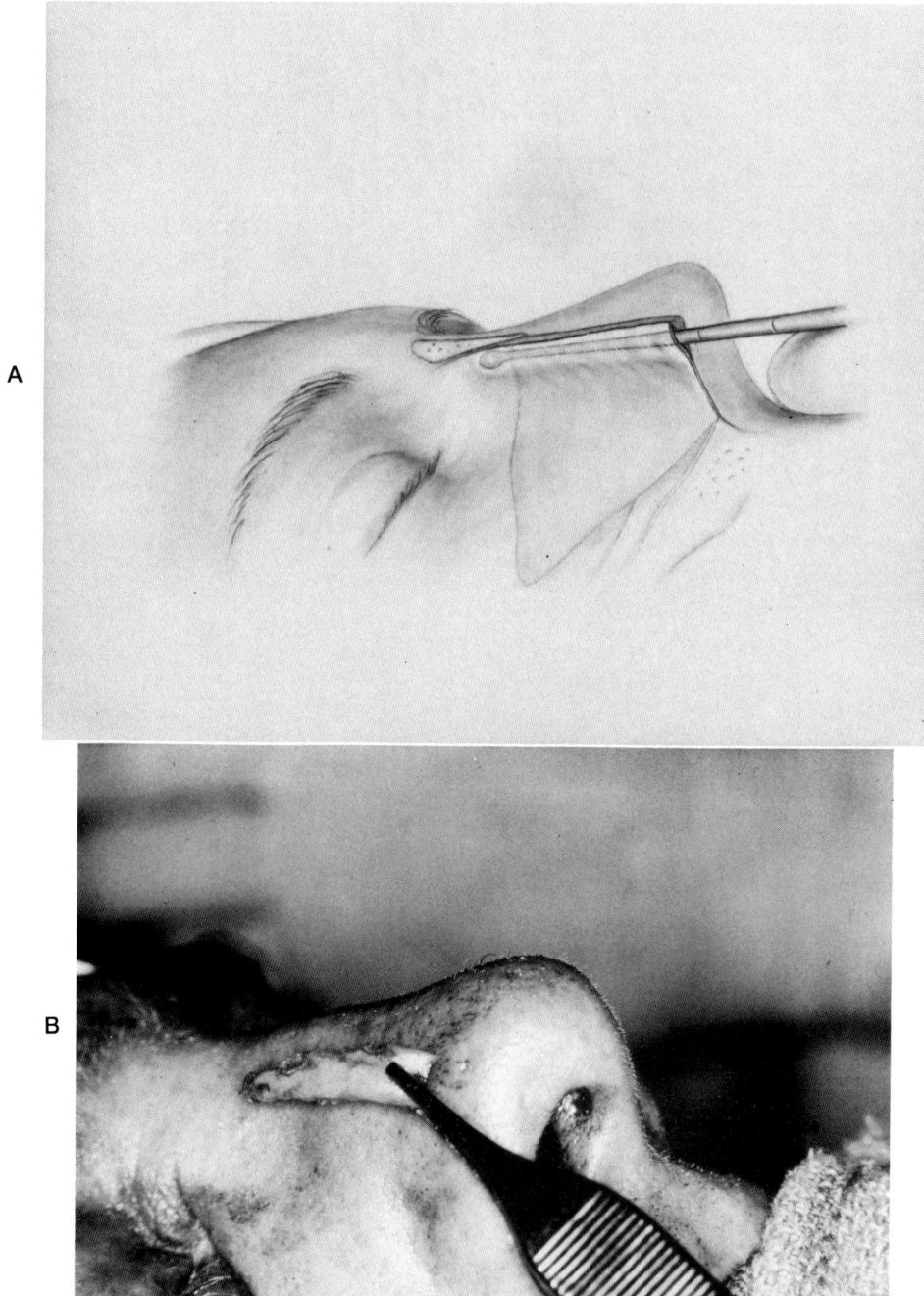

Figure 19-7. **A,** Correct position and extent of subperichondrial pocket. **B,** Graft shown externally in approximate position. (From Sheen, J.H.: Spreader graft: a method of reconstructing the roof of the middle nasal vault following rhinoplasty, Plast. Reconstr. Surg. 73:230-239, 1984.)

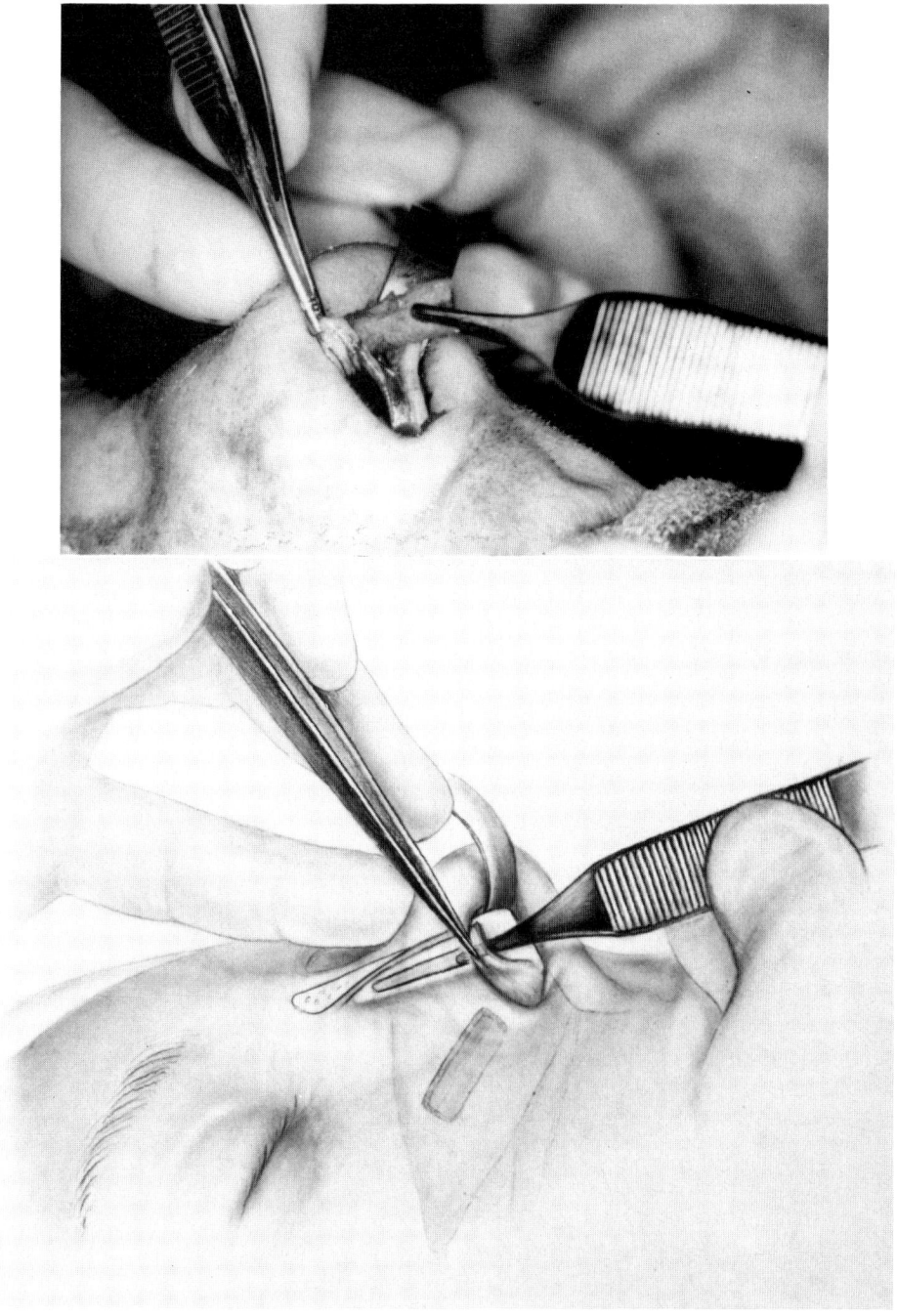

Figure 19-8. Spreader graft inserted into pocket. From Sheen, J.H.: Spreader graft: a method of reconstructing the roof of the middle nasal vault following rhinoplasty, Plast. Reconstr. Surg. 73:230-239, 1984.)

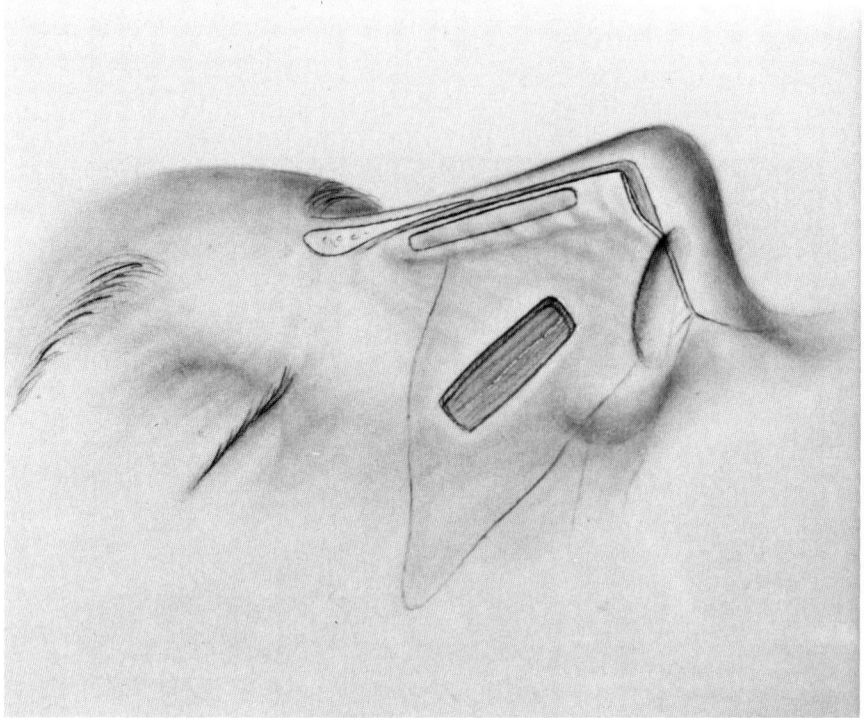

Figure 19-9. Spreader graft in place. Caudal end of graft is placed at caudal border of upper lateral cartilage. (From Sheen, J.H.: Spreader graft: a method of reconstructing the roof of the middle nasal vault following rhinoplasty, Plast. Reconstr. Surg. 73:230-239, 1984.)

DISCUSSION

This case shows the need for reconstruction of the middle vault during a primary rhinoplasty. The internal valves, which were collapsed because of the patient's high, thin nasal structure, were effectively opened by placement of spreader grafts. Although septoplasty alone would have relieved the obstructed airway, only by spreading the walls of the middle vault laterally would this patient enjoy optimal nasal function.

REFERENCE

1. Straatsma, B.R., and Straatsma, C.R.: The anatomical relationship of the lateral nasal cartilage to the nasal bone and the cartilaginous nasal septum, Plast. Reconstr. Surg. 8:443-445, 1951.

20

The Osseocartilaginous Vault

Thomas Rees

An interesting technique was developed by Tord Skoog[1] for dealing with large humps. The technique is described by Dr. Mühlbauer in Chapter 16. Skoog knew, like all rhinoplastic surgeons, that the removal of a large bony hump often led to an open-roof deformity, especially in the presence of a wide pyramid. The lateral bones simply cannot close the gap and obliterate the open space despite lateral and even superior osteotomies and even outfracturing. Neither does removal of a piece of bone from either side of the septum at the root of the nose always do the trick in such noses. To maintain the natural curvature of the dorsum of the nose, Skoog conceived the idea of removing the hump as a single and rather large unit, trimming it, and then replacing it in the dorsal pocket. The open roof was thereby closed, and a smooth naturally shaped dorsum resulted. The only problem is that in some patients the replaced hump can be somewhat mobile, and there is always the question of absorption, which in practical terms has not been a problem for those surgeons who elect to use this technique. I favor use of the technique in very large, wide humps and in some externally deviated noses also with large dorsal humps.

The patient in Figure 20-1 is, in my opinion, an ideal patient for a hump replacement procedure. He has a high dorsal profile, much of which is bone. He did not want a small nose and was fearful that the surgeon would overcorrect his profile. Of course the alternative to replacing the entire (but sculpted) hump in such a patient would be the addition of dorsal onlay grafts of cartilage. The hump was removed very generously with an osteotome, angled deeply into the nasion. Then the entire hump was refashioned by carefully stripping out the mucosa and using a file and an air drill to reduce and reshape it. It was then reinserted back into the nose. As does Dr. Mühlbauer, I favor an extramucosal dissection technique in such patients to isolate the replaced bony cartilaginous tissue from the internal nose, thereby reducing the possibility of contamination of the pocket and infection. This approach maintained the natural convexity and curvature of the dorsum as well as the attachment of the periosteum to the skin on the lateral sides of the bony vault.

This procedure is essentially a free graft into the dorsum of the nose, in which respect the nose is a very forgiving recipient site. The blood supply is excellent. Iliac bone grafts or autogenous cartilage grafts are rarely lost as a result of infection, as we all know. Sometimes these grafts can even survive infection. The Skoog technique is also applicable in patients with a marked deviation of the external nose in conjunction with a large hump (Figure 20-2). In such patients one can remove the hump, trim it, and replace it more in the midline. The approach is essentially a camouflage technique. I frequently camouflage a crooked nose with grafts of various shapes, rather than fruitlessly attempting to straighten a crooked septum, which can often be a most unrewarding procedure.

The heavy nose with a strong hump provides every possibility for an open-roof deformity, which is a nuisance to correct. Dr. Sheen's spreader grafts are most helpful in dealing with such problems, as they are in dealing with the very thin nose, as Sheen has described. I previously alluded to the closure of the open roof with cartilage grafts. For smaller degrees of open-roof deformity I often employ small strips of cartilage, which may or may not be soften by crushing.

163

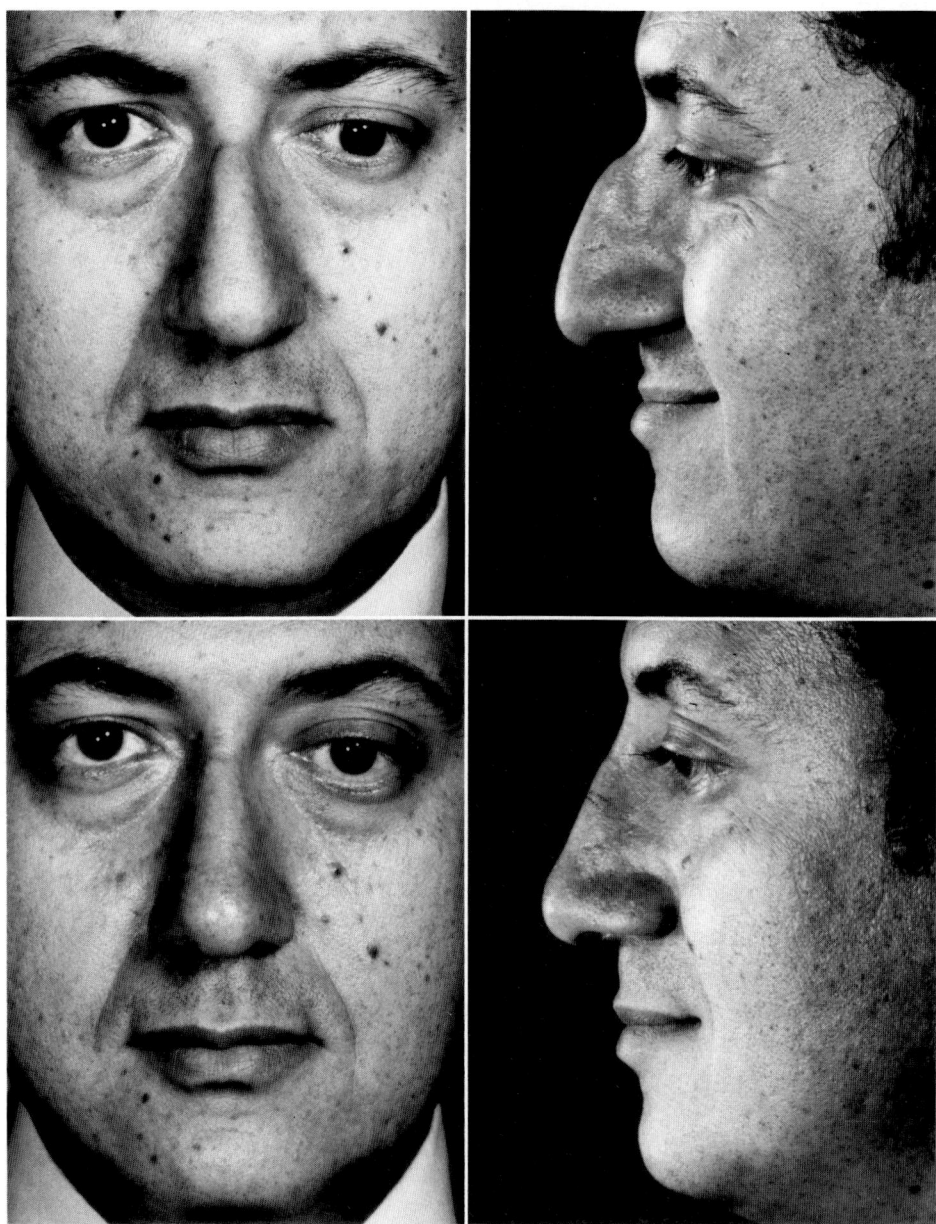

Figure 20-1. Hump replacement (Skoog) technique to maintain adequate size and proportion and to augment a small nasion. (From Rees, T.D.: Aesthetic plastic surgery, Philadelphia, 1983, W.B. Saunders Co.)

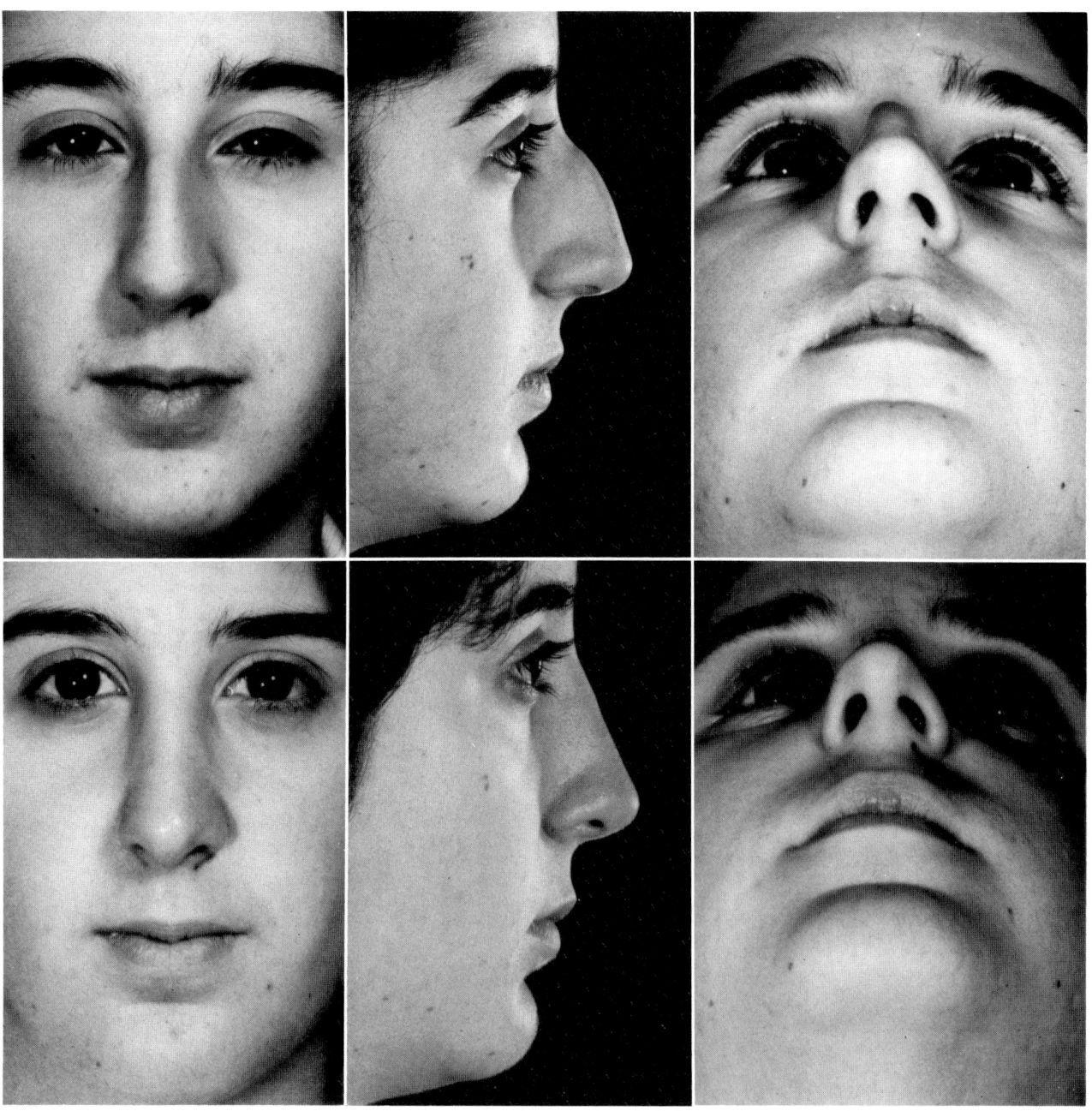

Figure 20-2. Hump replacement was used to reconstruct an open roof in this high, thin hump.

In reducing the nasal dorsum I often reduce the most offending portion first, especially if I am unsure how I am going to deal with the tip in a given patient. I most often separate the upper lateral cartilages from the septum cleanly and directly with a No. 11 blade (Figure 20-3). I take great care to preserve the upper lateral cartilages and the mucosa. I have had very little trouble with the internal valve over the years. If sufficient cartilage and mucosa are preserved, one should not have a problem with the internal valve. Synechiae will not occur in the absence of unsatisfied soft tissue coverage. Problems with the internal valve, in my opinion, result more often from collapse of the upper lateral cartilages against the septum. As I have repeatedly stated, I favor use of the extramucosal dissection technique for difficult septal problems and for the externally and internally twisted nose. I see no purpose for its use in the routine, uncomplicated rhinoplasty.

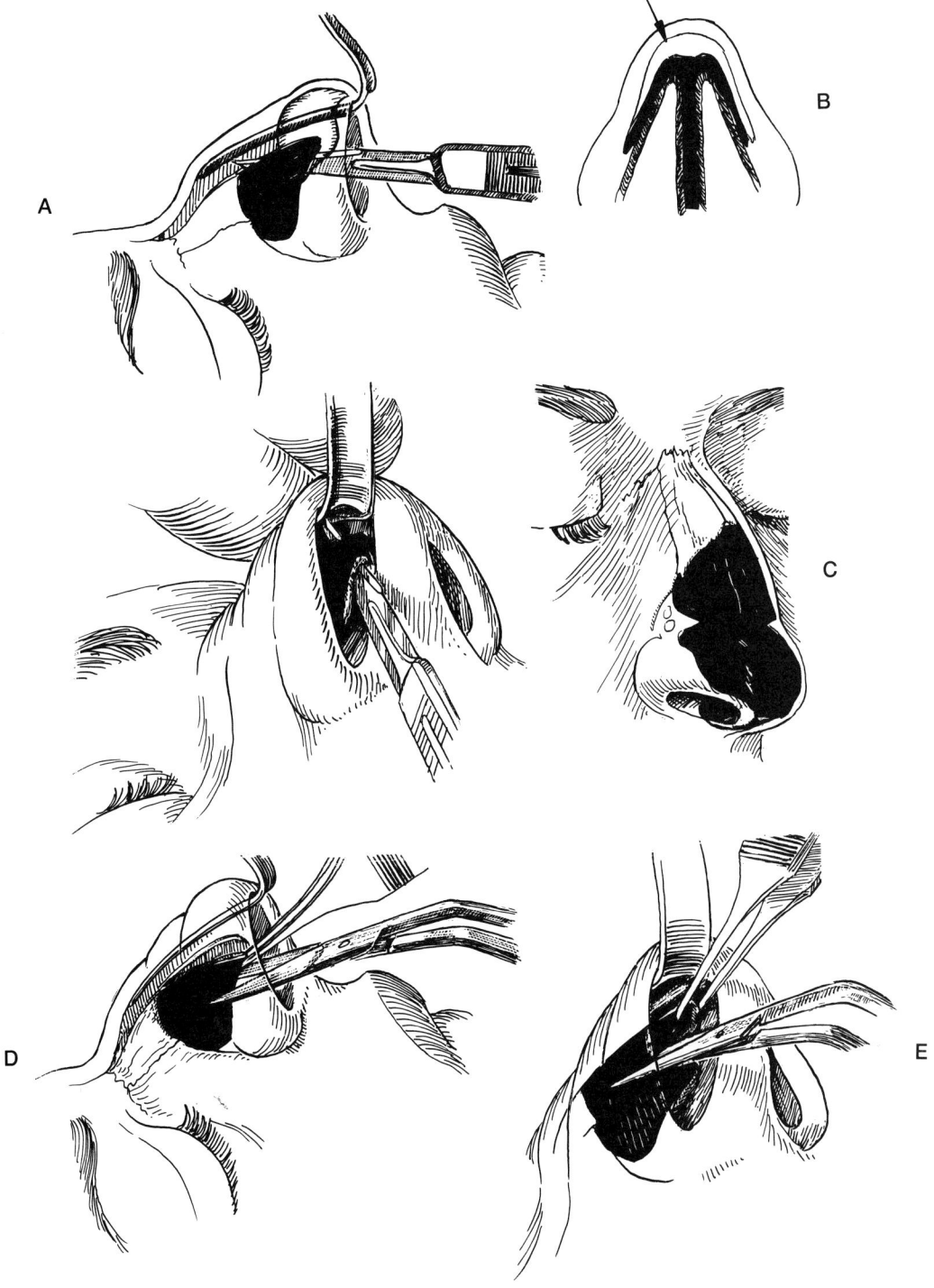

Figure 20-3. A, Protect dorsal skin with an Aufricht retractor and pass a No. 11 blade from upper lateral cartilage nasal bone junction inferiorly to sever attachment of upper lateral cartilage at cartilaginous septum. **B,** It is important that the knife hug the nasal septum as closely as possible so that a "shelf" of upper lateral cartilage does not remain attached to the septum. **C,** Detached upper lateral cartilages. **D,** Amount of dorsal border of upper lateral cartilage to be removed is estimated and excised by a single closure of the scissors. **E,** Cartilage is steadied by gentle inferior traction to produce a straight, single cut. (From Rees, T.D., and Wood-Smith, D.: Cosmetic facial surgery, Philadelphia, 1973, W.B. Saunders Co.)

I often lower the cartilaginous profile first, as shown in Figure 20-4. This approach leaves the bony dorsum in sharp relief so that it can be readily removed with a rasp or a very sharp osteotome (Figure 20-5). The osteotome must be precisely controlled. The rasp, however, can be used very safely and is controllable in these little spicules of bone.

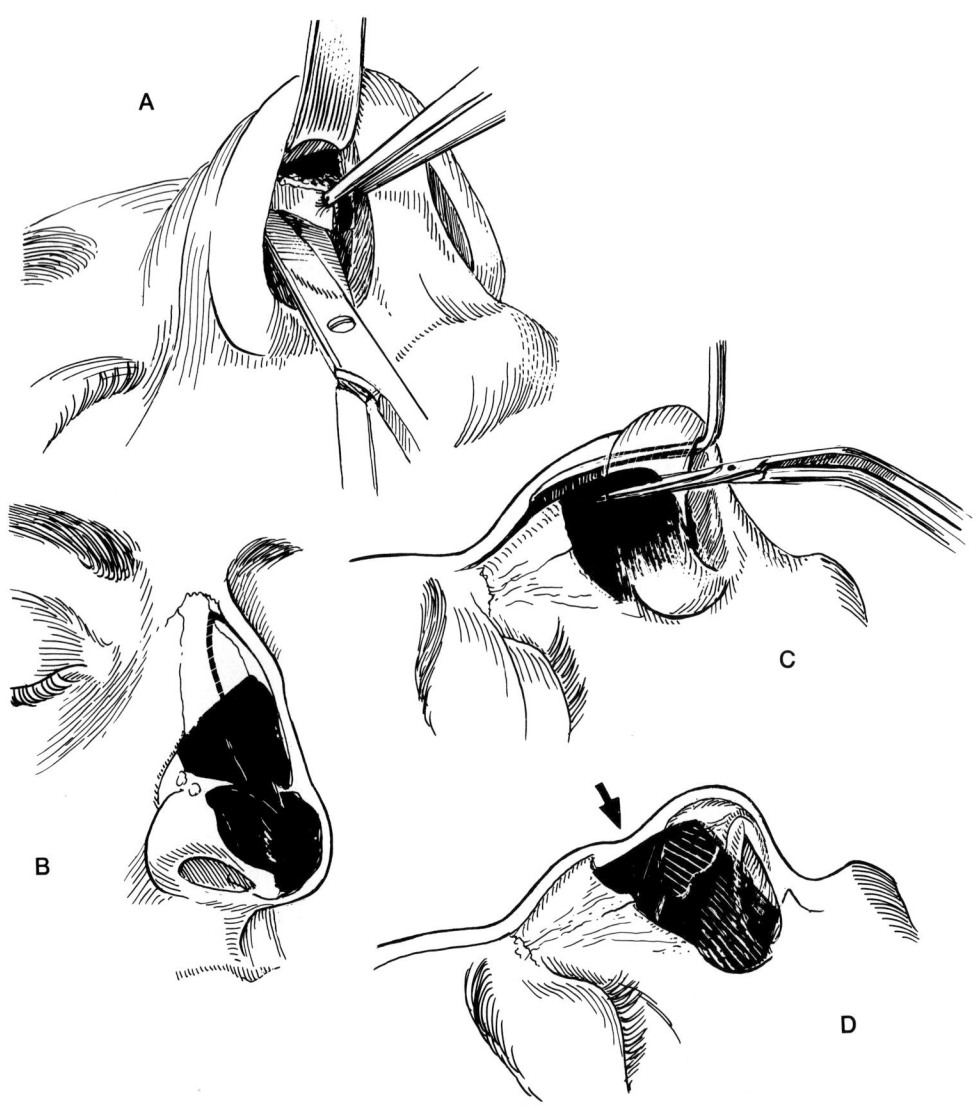

Figure 20-4. Method of preliminary lowering of nasal septum to bring both nasal tip and osseous hump to prominence. **A,** Dorsal cartilaginous septum is lowered by angled scissors to estimated new profile line. **B,** Dorsal borders of upper lateral cartilages are resected to a level slightly lower than that of the septum. **C,** Projected lines of the osteotomy, after cartilaginous resection. **D,** Nasal tip and osseous hump are brought to prominence; in many cases, this aids the operator's judgments in planning tip cartilage resections and contouring. (From Rees, T.D., and Wood-Smith, D.: Cosmetic facial surgery, Philadelphia, 1973, W.B. Saunders Co.)

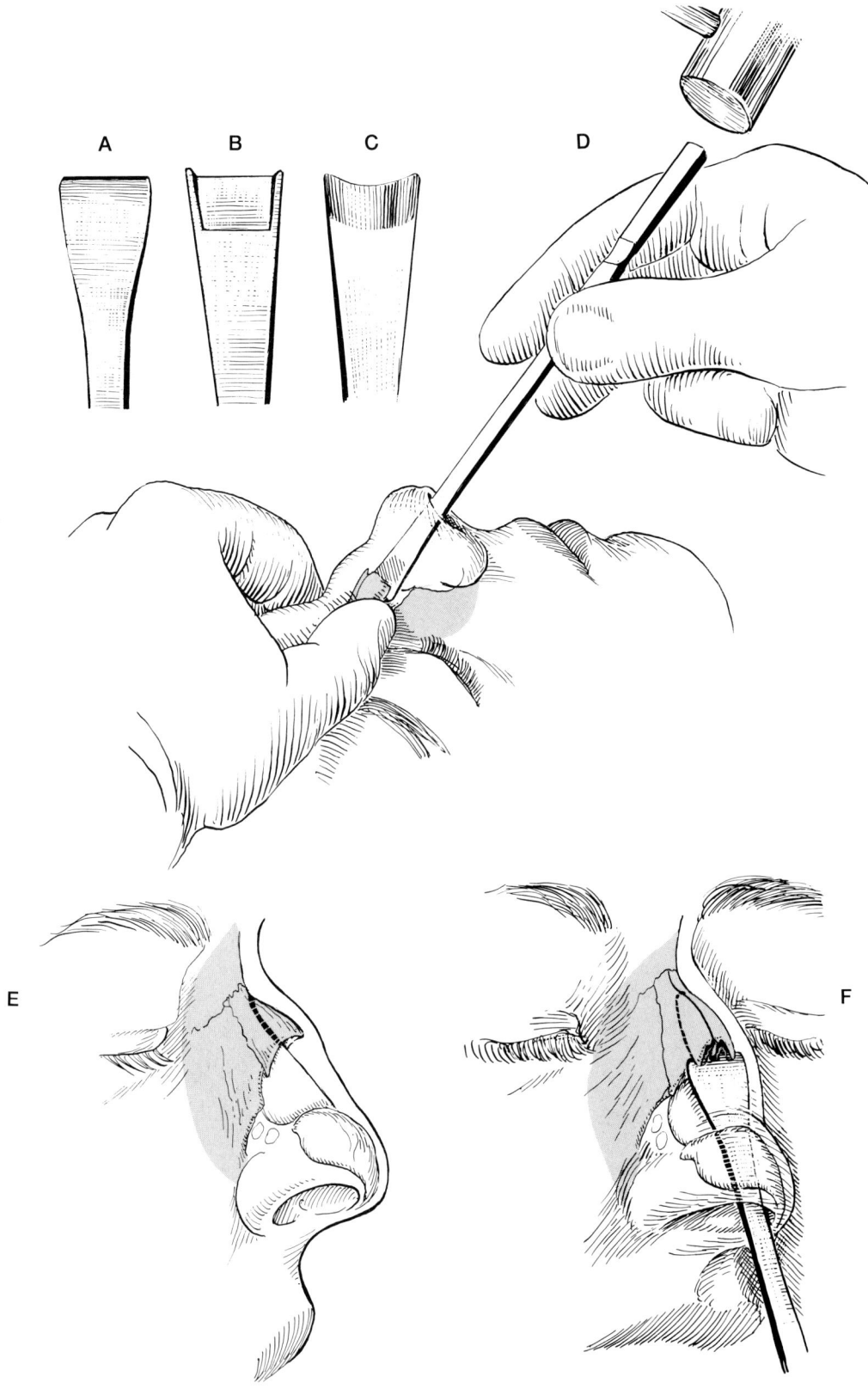

Figure 20-5. A, B, and **C,** Different types of chisels used. **D, E,** and **F,** Sharp removal of remaining small bony hump with chisel or osteotome.
(From Rees, T.D., and Wood-Smith, D.: Cosmetic facial surgery, Philadelphia, 1973, W.B. Saunders Co.)

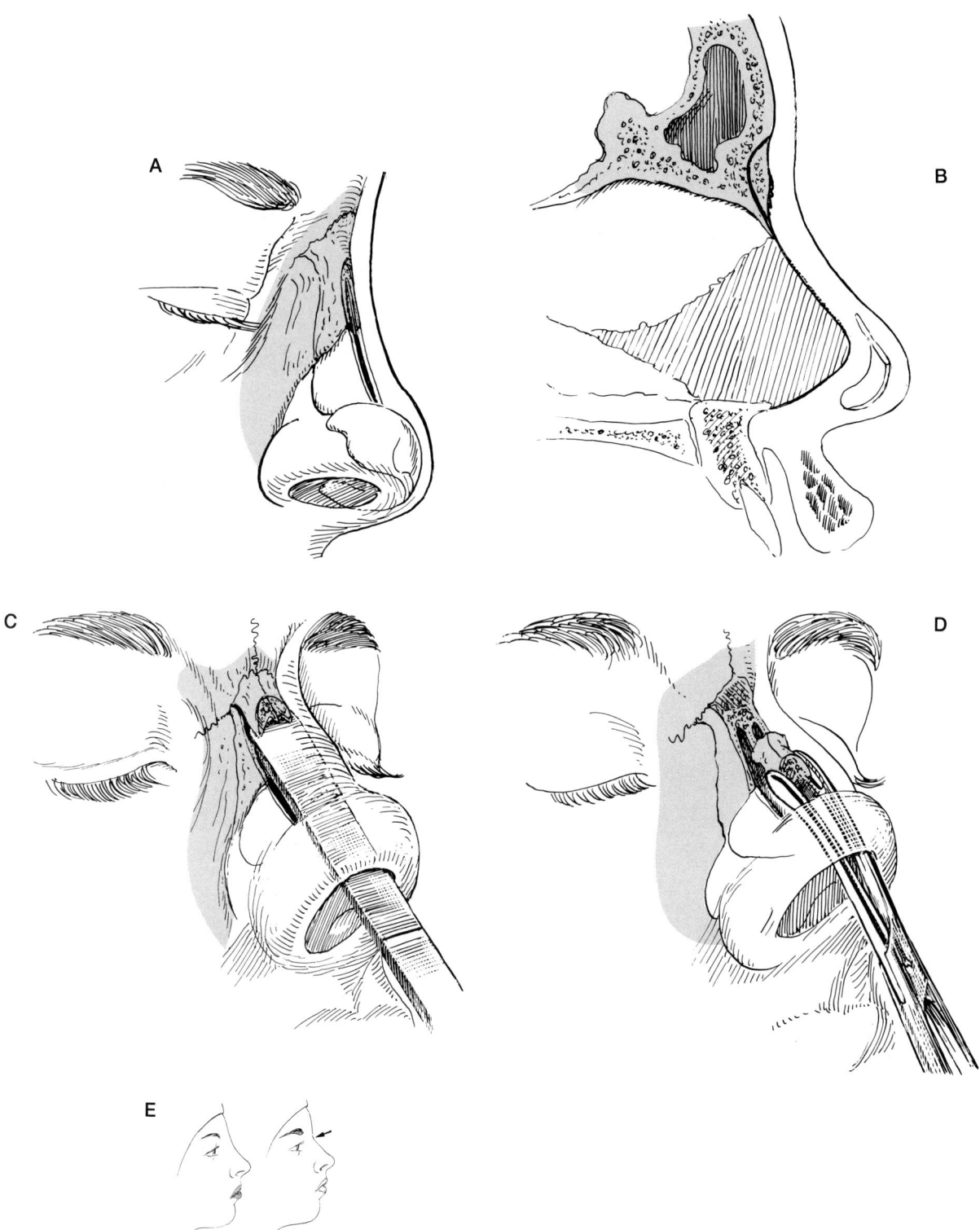

Figure 20-6. A, Excessive bone at nasofrontal angle after otherwise adequate removal of nasal dorsum. **B,** Area of nasofrontal bone considered excessive, preventing creation of desirable new nasal profile. **C,** A 10 or 12 mm osteotome or chisel is passed along new nasal dorsum and tapped into position. When adequate penetration of bone has been achieved, the instrument is levered slightly upward to produce a fracture at upper end of osteotomy. **D,** Nasal bone is removed with Converse forceps. **E,** Common form of profile, resulting from failure to remove nasofrontal angle bone, shown in "before" and "after" states. It must be emphasized that, in many patients, there is a practical limit to the amount of deepening that can be realistically achieved in this region. Attempting to take out too much bone will frequently result in a webbing of soft tissue across the depression, obviating the correction. (From Rees, T.D., and Wood-Smith, D.: Cosmetic facial surgery, Philadelphia, 1973, W.B. Saunders Co.)

Deepening the nasion below the glabella is a special problem and is not quite as simple to solve as we have frequently been led to believe. An osteotome or chisel can be used to knock out a piece of the thick bone at the root of the nose (Figure 20-6), but it is exceedingly difficult to narrow the bones at this level because of their thickness and because at this level we are operating above the nasal cavity. Figure 20-7 shows the kind of result one can achieve by removing a piece of bone. The improvement is minimal in my opinion, but notice the real problem with this patient, one that is very often the case in patients with no depression at the nasion. The fault is not with the nose but is related to the absence of frontal bossing and the presence of a flat, sloping forehead. The surgeon is hard pressed to create a nasion in such a patient unless the forehead bossing can be built up in some way.

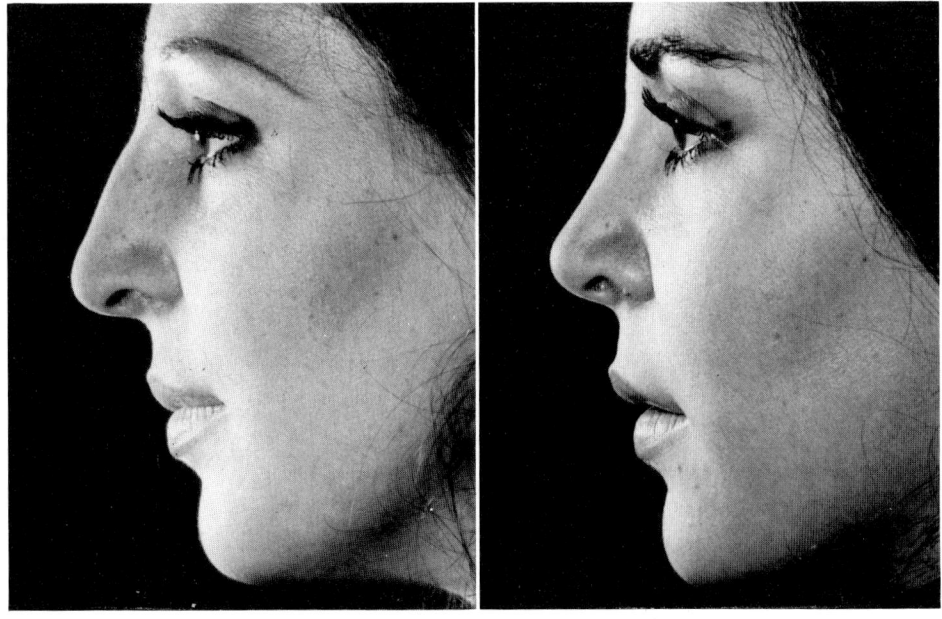

Figure 20-7. Result of chiselling away a portion of corlex of alabella. Note the flat slanting forehead. (From Rees, T.D.: Aesthetic plastic surgery, Philadelphia, 1983, W.B. Saunders Co.)

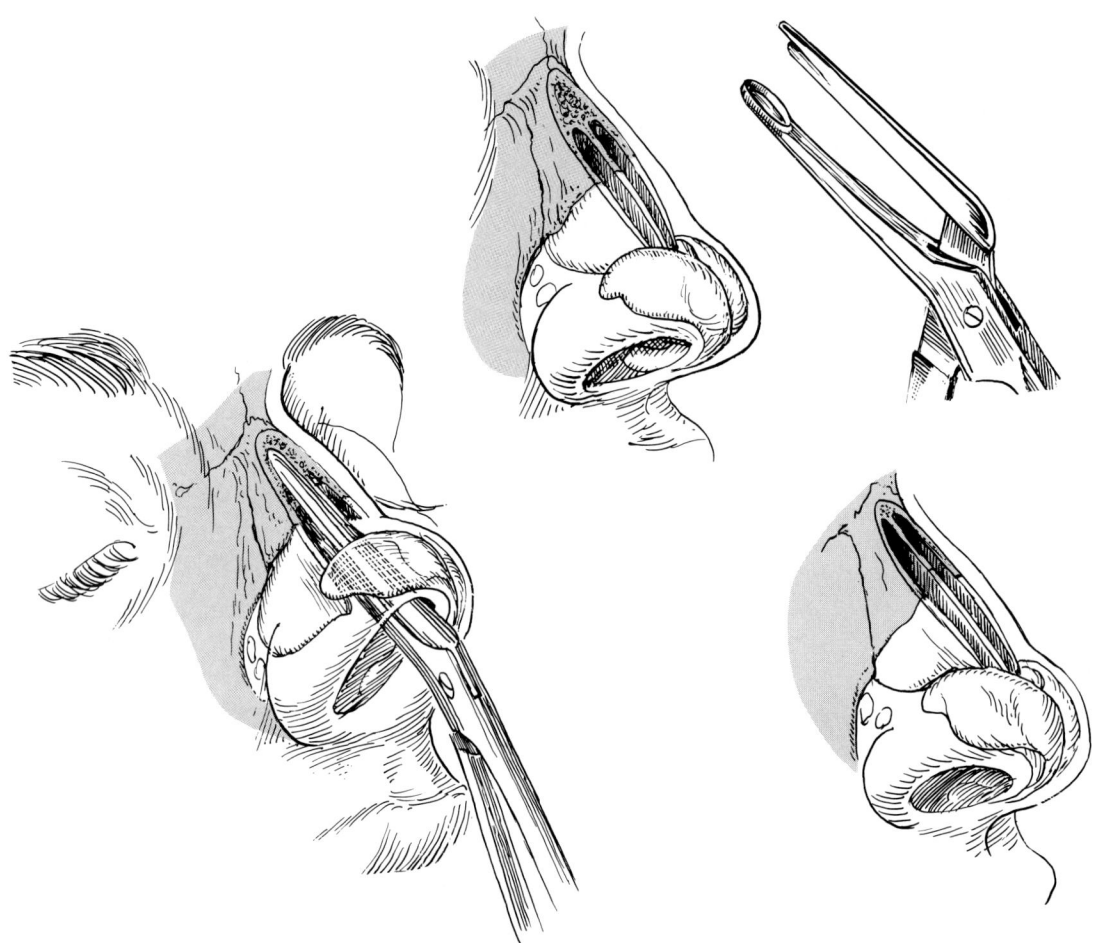

Figure 20-8. In many patients, a web of bone in the nasal root region remains after dorsum is modified. Left intact, this bone will prevent complete narrowing of nose in upper third. Web may be removed with osteotomes or, as illustrated, with nasal root forceps. A small sharp chisel can accomplish this same task with more precision. (From Rees, T.D.: Aesthetic plastic surgery, Philadelphia, 1983, W.B. Saunders Co.)

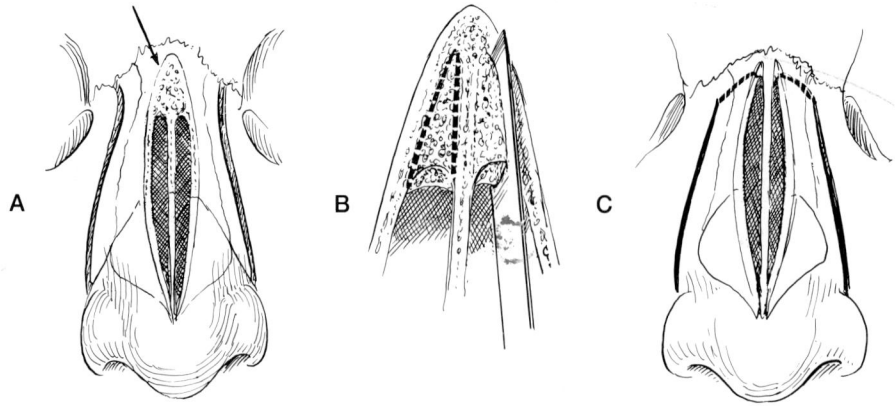

Figure 20-9. A, Sufficient narrowing of the bony nose requires complete fracture and room for fractured bones to move medially. **B,** Removal of a medial wedge of bone at root of nose may be necessary to achieve this medial movement. **C,** The complete lateral osteotomies and clean superior fracture necessary for success. (From Rees, T.D., and Wood-Smith, D.: Cosmetic facial surgery, Philadelphia, 1973, W.B. Saunders Co.)

If the nasal bones are not positioned correctly after a lateral osteotomy and infracture, then before I resort to a dorsal-onlay graft or even a Skoog maneuver, I frequently do a superior osteotomy or, as a last resort, an outfracture. As has been pointed out, it is sometimes necessary in patients with wide humps and wide nasal roots to remove a small sliver of bone from either side of the septum. This can be done with a small osteotome or a special Kazanjian forceps, provided in either case it is very sharp (Figures 20-8 and 20-9, *A* through *C*.

A superior osteotomy is often helpful in displacing the nasal bones medially. It is quite simple to perform and is done with a 2 mm osteotome inserted through the skin directly at the base of the nose, at the nasion (Figure 20-10). I used to puncture the skin through the hair-bearing brow, but this is quite unnecessary, since the skin wound is inconsequential. Also, I sometimes fracture the perpendicular plate of the ethmoid. The point I wish to make is that one must do whatever is necessary to place the bones in position at the primary rhinoplasty, and one should not have to count on special clamps, eyeglasses, or other gadgets to exert pressure on them postoperatively to move them medially. If one of the bones should be depressed or an open roof should result on one or both sides, a piece of cartilage can be used to camouflage the defect.

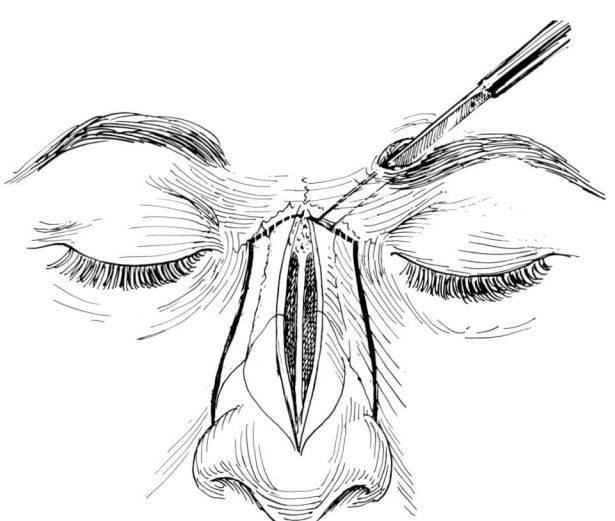

Figure 20-10. Percutaneous osteotomy to mobilize nasal bones. A 2 mm osteotome is used.
(From Rees, T.D.: Aesthetic plastic surgery, Philadelphia, 1983, W.B. Saunders Co.)

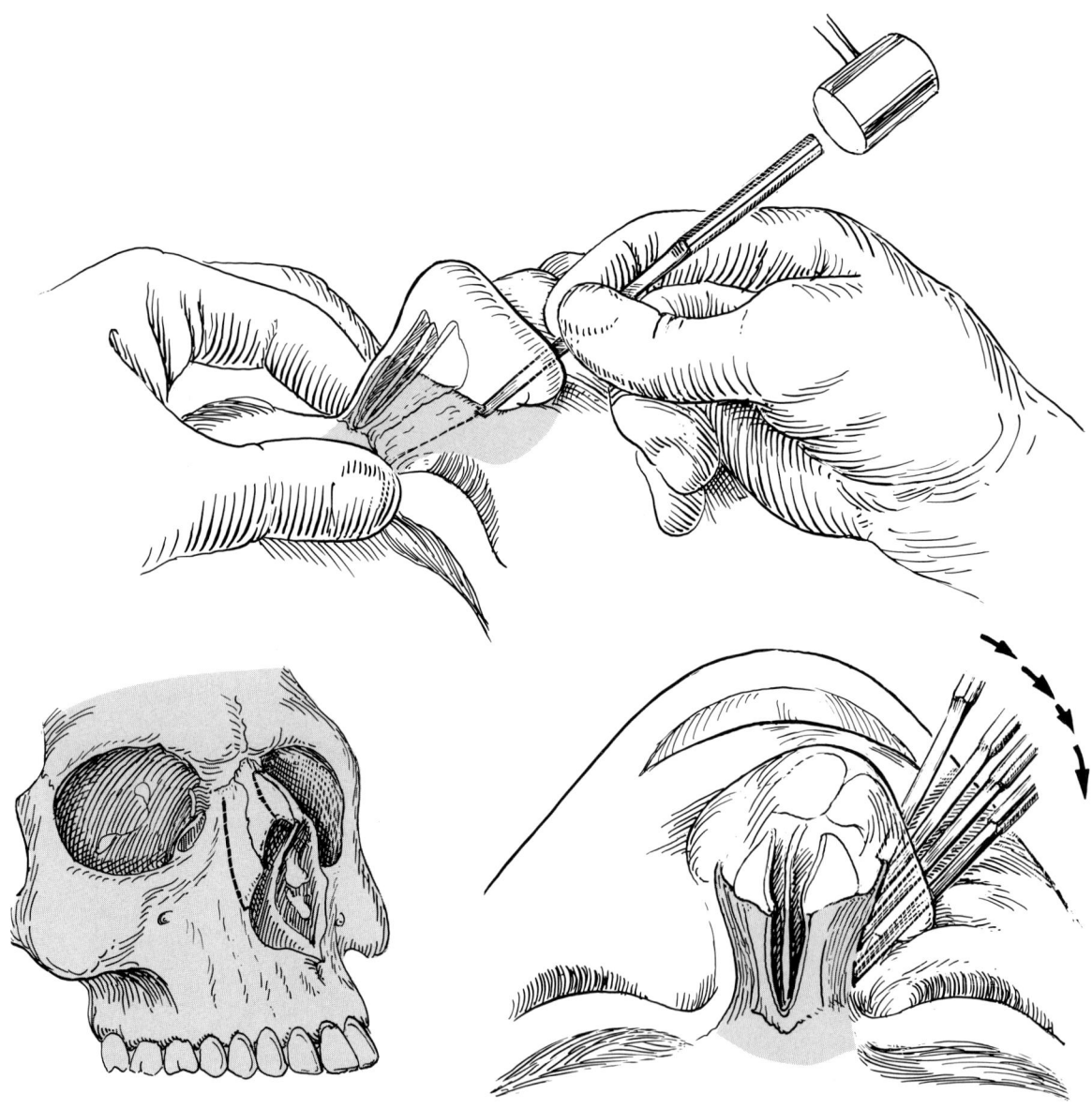

Figure 20-11. Lateral osteotomy by multiple puncture wounds from 2 or 3 mm osteotome. Control afforded by this technique is excellent. (From Rees, T.D.: Aesthetic plastic surgery, Philadelphia, 1983, W.B. Saunders Co.)

I have no pearls of wisdom about lateral oste-otomy. I am still unclear in my own mind what all of the terminology means: "high to low," "low to high," and so forth. I try to get the infracture as low as possible in the frontal process of the maxilla and to extend it as high as possible toward the level of the inner canthus. Thereafter what happens is often related to a bit of luck. If I feel the nasal bones are thick and unyielding, I will resort to a medial os-teotomy and outfracture. For lateral osteotomy I once again favor a small osteotome, usually 3 mm, inserted through the piriform sinus or directly through the skin of the cheek (Figure 20-11). The lateral osteotomy and infracture are at times the most important steps to be carried out in the pro-cedure and can yield the most significant improve-ment. This can be especially true in rhinoplasty for non-Caucasians (Figure 20-12).

REFERENCE

1. Skoog, T.: A method of hump reduction in rhinoplasty, Arch. Otolaryngol. 83:556, 1952.

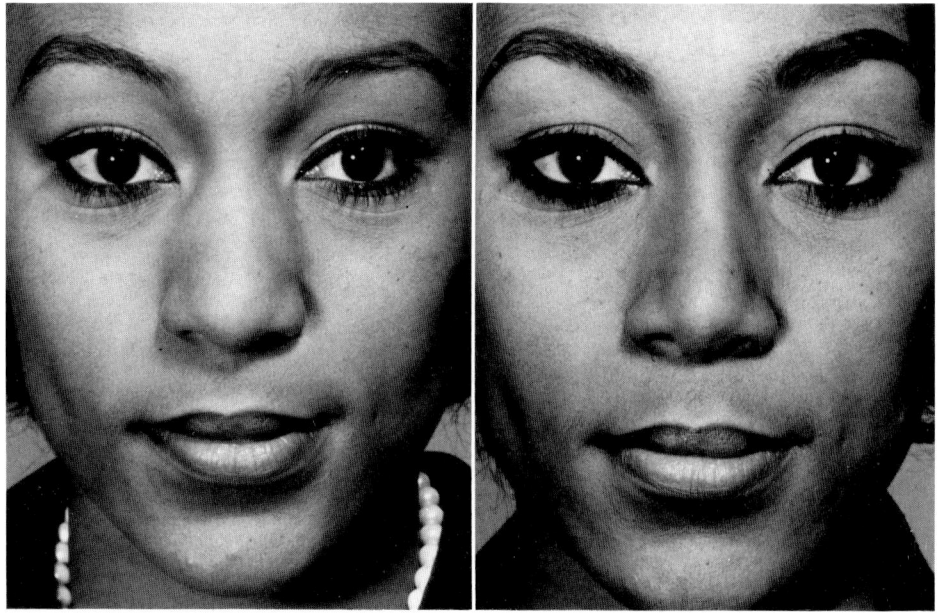

Figure 20-12. Lateral osteotomy and infracture may yield the most significant improvement in many patients.

Point & Counterpoint
Parts III & IV

Question: Is a lateral osteotomy always neccessary?
Comment (Eugene Courtiss): No, nothing is *always* necessary. However, a lateral osteotomy is *often* indicated, because the angular relationships of the bone often require change. The maneuver is done when the *individual patient* needs it.

Question: How often do you see lateral drift or spreading of nasal bones? Why does it occur, and how can it be avoided?
Comment (Jack Sheen): Very rarely do I see lateral drift of the nasal bones. I believe this is because I make a green-stick fracture whenever possible. When drifing does occur, however, I will do a secondary osteotomy. I must add that I firmly believe the root of the nose should not be too narrow. Many of the postoperative noses have an unnatural appearance, because they are overly narrow and the nasal walls are parallel. The nasal walls should diverge. Few noses need to be narrowed at the root; most noses need only a slight narrowing at the caudal portion of the bony pyramid. In some cases no osteotomy is required.

Question: Should the periosteum be elevated from the dorsum and lateral walls in all cases?
Comment (Gene Tardy): No. The area over the dorsum periosteum is routinely elevated only enough to gain access to and resect the bony hump.

Preserving all of the periosteum over the lateral bony walls reduces trauma and swelling and facilitates an "internal splinting" of the bony fragments during healing. Elevating a wide periosteal tunnel laterally before performing lateral osteotomies is totally unnecessary and simply increases surgical trauma and potential ecchymosis. Microosteotomes eliminate the need for lateral periosteal elevation, substantially reducing tissue trauma.

Comment (Eugene Courtiss): No, the periosteum need not be elevated.

However, I elevate enough periosteum to gain access to the bony hump if I am going to do anything to the bony hump. The only time that I elevate periosteum widely and nonconservatively is in the aging patient who may need redraping of skin and soft tissue or in the patient who has a huge nose and in whom the skeletal framework must be reduced enough to allow redraping. Otherwise the soft tissue granulation may result. Also, I think periosteal elevation ought to be minimal over the dorsum and not done at all laterally.

Question: Can you explain the advantages and disadvantages in using only the chisel for reducing the dorsum?
Comment (Walter Berman): The gouge chisel, I believe, has some advantage for reducing the dorsum. It can remove a little more from the essential segments or the perpendicular plate of the ethmoid so that you can proceed a little further up in the glabellar area while you are removing a little of the anterior or dorsal hump. Also, you can carry through superiorly if you want to decrease that glabellar groove. Other than that, certainly there are many ways of doing things, and of course, the largest of humps can be reduced with a rasp.

Question: Since you have had a great deal of experience with this trauma, how do you correct a nearly comminuted infracture?
Comment (Claus Walter): I use basically the same principle Dr. Sheen illustrates with his spreader graft. If the infracture is comminuted during the surgery, cartilage or bony onlay grafts can be used to create a smooth surface. Such an onlay is provided by the little bone always left in the perpendicular plate of the ethmoid. Because it does not move once it is put in place, this bone is a better material than cartilage.

For the past 15 years I have used a gouge chisel for osteotomies. The forces of mechanics work for me when I use this tool because of the way I turn the chisel. I turn it 180 degrees so that it will go outward, or inward, and am able to carve out the bone at the nasal frontal angle.

For lateral osteotomies I use only 2 to 3 mm chisels. They are small enough to fit any situation and are quite helpful. I do not elevate the periosteum on either side. I do elevate the periosteum only in the area of the hump when the hump must be reduced.

Question: Will the spreader graft improve the appearance of an upper lateral cartilage that has been traumatically avulsed from its attachment to the undersurface of the nasal bone? Is a spreader graft a better solution than an onlay graft for avulsed, depressed, upper lateral cartilages?

Comment (Jack Sheen): There are some cases where an onlay graft is indicated—total collapse of the lateral walls, for example. However, the spreader graft has three advantages. First, it does not create a stiff lateral wall, which is not normal in function or appearance; second, it actually spreads or opens the anterior portion of the airway, resulting in improved breathing for the patient; and third, it allows the surgeon better control over minor asymmetries.

Question: We have not brought up the "rocker." If you do both a medial osteotomy and a lateral osteotomy and you do them too thoroughly, a rocking sensation or rocking effect of the nasal dorsum will be the result when you make your infracture. Because of the rocker effect this approach has lost popularity. Have you had any rockers with medial osteotomies?

Comment (Gene Tardy): I am not sure I have ever seen a "rocker." The rocker phenomenon is described as resulting from a nasal bone that is relatively concave inward. It occurs, according to Dr. William Wright, when an osteotomy is done superiorly and high that frees the bone in the thick portion of the nasal bone and then when a lower osteotomy is done that creates an unstable bony segment that projects laterally when one pushes the caudal or cephalic part of the bony segment much in the fashion of a teeter-totter. If you make osteotomies medially and laterally on the thin portion of the ascending process and thin portion of the nasal bone, I don't see how you can create a rocker unless you encounter a major bony deformity or anatomic variant.

Question: No one has mentioned the separation of the upper lateral cartilages from the septum, either through a mucosal tunnel or otherwise. Are there any indications for trimming them, and can you elaborate on this point?

Comment (Eugene Courtiss): There are two techniques for managing the junction of the upper lateral cartilages and septum: One is to divide them with a scissor or knife, thus totally separating the upper lateral cartilages from the septal cartilage. This involves cutting through the lining, which I try to avoid. The second technique, and the one I prefer, is to shave the dorsal projection of the septum and upper lateral cartilages with a knife (or scissor), leaving the lining intact. Unless a very large reduction in the cartilages is needed, the latter technique does not cut through the lining. Although the first technique provides better exposure, it causes more scarring of the lining, which is why I prefer leaving the junction intact.

Question: What is your approach to saving mucosa or removing humps submucosally?

Comment (Eugene Courtiss): The underlying mucosa usually remains intact because so little bone is removed. The mucosa under the cartilages is removed *only* when considerable cartilage is trimmed. The point is to try to preserve the integrity of the lining. To preserve the lining some surgeons go so far as to elevate the mucoperichondrium submucosally, a maneuver that may be difficult technically and that also may be unnecessary.

Question: Please comment on the technique of extramucosal dissection.

Comment (Tom Rees): The technique of extramucosal dissection is quite popular in Europe and with some surgeons in North America as a routine part of all rhinoplasty procedures. The mucosa is dissected carefully from the roof of the internal nose. There are a couple of tricks to it: One is to start laterally on the upper lateral cartilage and work medially, then perform a submucosal dissection beneath the perichondrium of the septum and join the two over the apex of the junction of the septum and the upper lateral cartilages. As one gains the bony level superiorly the dissection is much simpler. I reserve it for very difficult septums and the twisted noses. I see no compelling reason to use it in every case, and I certainly do not accept the often-stated axiom that cutting through the mucosa and releasing the upper lateral cartilages from the septum results in damage to the internal valve, unless of course the surgeon excises too much upper lateral cartilage.

PART

V

ALAR BASE RESECTION

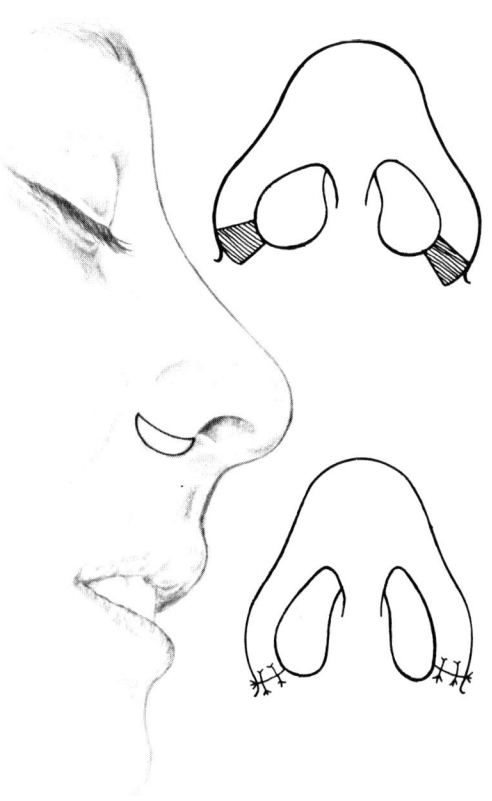

21

Approach to Alar Base Resection

Jack Sheen

The goal in alar base resection is narrowing of the nasal base while preserving or recreating normal contours. Although this basic concept seems obvious it is frequently overlooked by those who use an all-purpose approach to alar resection. An all-purpose approach, such as a standard wedge resection, does narrow the base but too often at the expense of natural-appearing nostrils (Figure 21-1). However, with careful preoperative evaluation and appropriate modifications in technique, the goal of a narrowed, natural-appearing nasal base can be obtained. To achieve this goal I rely on (1) the preservation of a medial flap whenever vestibular skin is removed and (2) a two-surface concept for operative planning.

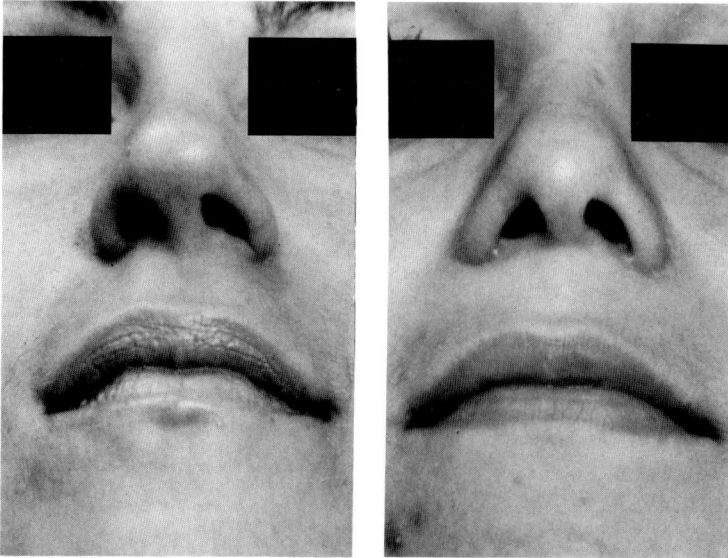

Figure 21-1. Two patients demonstrate unnatural appearance of nasal sill resulting from excision of alar wedge. (From Sheen, J.H., and Sheen, A.P.: Aesthetic rhinoplasty, St. Louis, 1978, The C.V. Mosby Co.)

180

THE MEDIAL FLAP TECHNIQUE

Standard alar base excision frequently leaves a notch in the floor of the vestibule, which interrupts the natural continuity of the sill (Figure 21-2, *A*). To prevent this notching I preserve a small, triangular medial flap in all cases where vestibular skin is excised (Figure 21-2, *B*).

An incision is made with an No. 11 blade along the alar base, progressing medially to within 3 mm of the rim. Then a back cut is made to create a small triangle of skin extending from the nasal sill (Figure 21-3, *A*). The excision is then completed by a superior cut (Figure 21-3, *B*). When the incision is closed the flap provides a small arc of tissue that ensures a smooth, natural curve to the nasal sill (Figure 21-3, *C*).

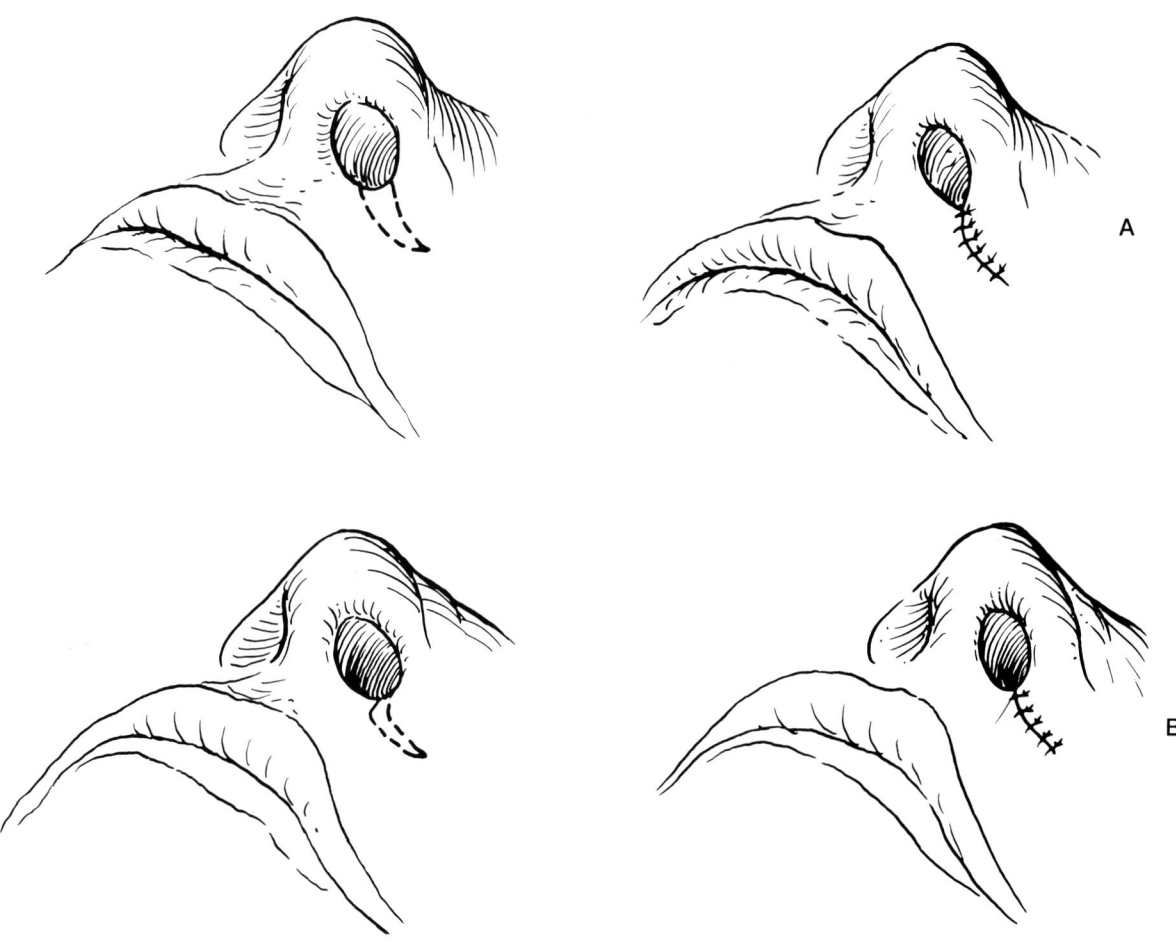

Figure 21-2. **A,** Standard alar sculpting incision. This type of alar wedge resection creates sharp notch at point of incision. **B,** Retaining medial flap creates smooth nasal sill. (From Sheen, J., and Sheen, A.P.: Aesthetic rhinoplasty, ed. 2, St. Louis, 1987, The C.V. Mosby Co.)

TWO-SURFACE CONCEPT

The alae have two surfaces: cutaneous and vestibular. Depending on the type of alar base, resection will involve either or both surfaces. For preoperative planning it is useful to categorize alar bases as types I, II, and III.

Type I includes heavy alar lobules with nostrils of proper size. With this type of patient only the cutaneous part of the lobule is reduced; the vestibular skin is left intact. Excision in the type I alar base should be conservative (rarely more than 3 mm), and the medial incision should not cross over the nasal sill (Figure 21-4, *A*). Because the sill is not

violated there is no need to plan a medial flap in this category. The skin is usually excised with a No. 15 blade, since the cut does not extend through the vestibular side (Figure 21-4, *B-C*).

Type II encompasses heavy alar lobules with slightly large nostrils. With type II alae the cutaneous portion is relatively larger than the vestibular portion. This type requires a proportionately large resection of alar lobule and a very small resection on the vestibular side (Figure 21-5, *A*).

The procedure proceeds as described in the section The Medial Flap Technique (Figure 21-5, *B*). For a natural contour it is important to preserve both

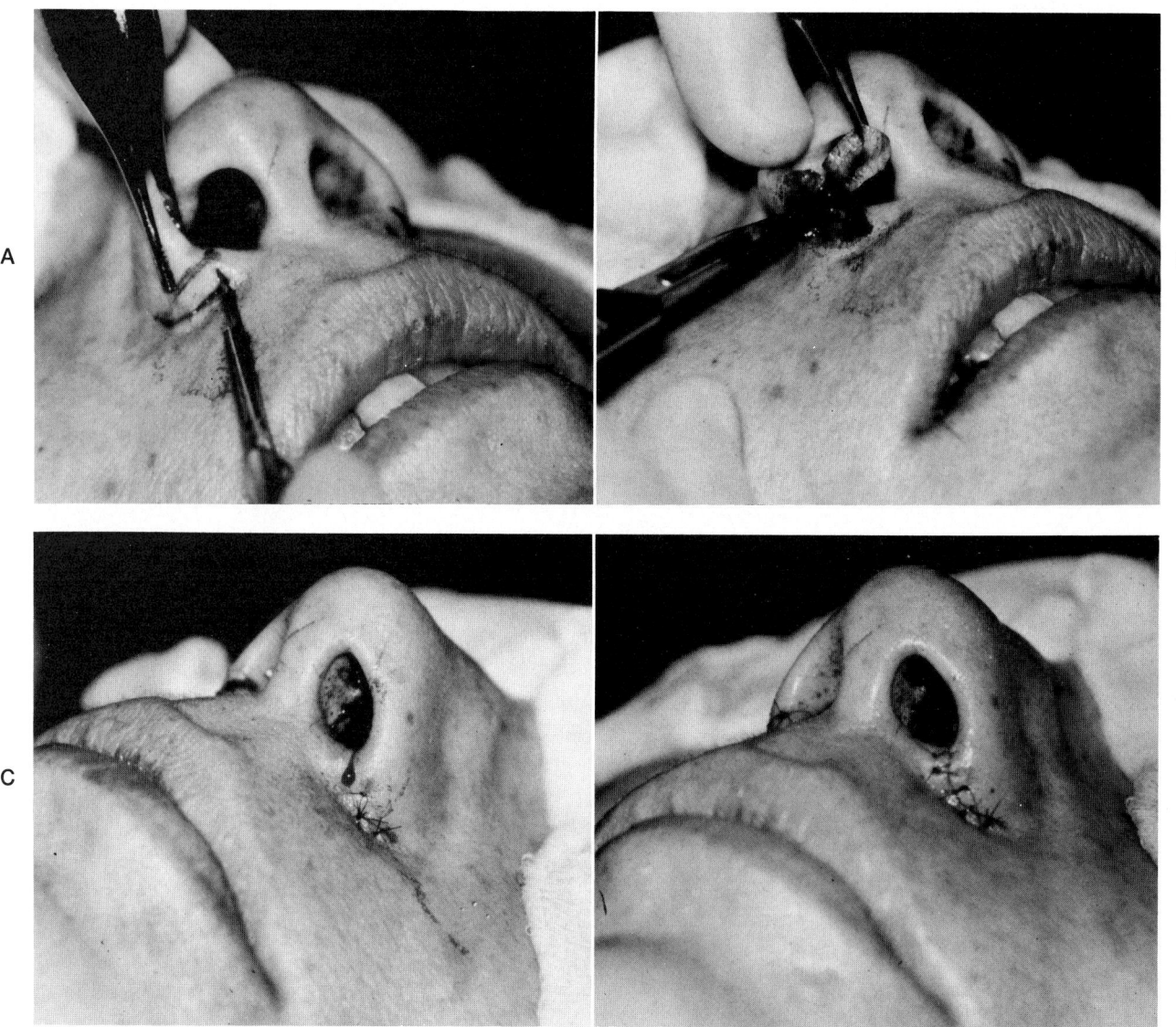

Figure 21-3. A, Back cutting to form the medial flap. **B** and **C,** Completed excision with medial flap retained. (From Sheen, J., and Sheen, A.P.: Aesthetic rhinoplasty, ed. 2, St. Louis, 1987, The C.V. Mosby Co.)

the medial flap and a margin of skin anterior to the alar-facial groove (Figure 21-5, C). The wound is closed with 6-0 nylon suture on the cutaneous side and interrupted 5-0 plain sutures on the vestibular side (Figure 21-5, D).

In the *Type III* alar base the curve of the lobule is parallel to that of the nostril. This type requires that equal amounts be resected from the vestibular and cutaneous sides. Distortion can easily occur if the balance of lobule and nostril is not carefully maintained (Figure 21-6). Resection must be conservative because these patients require surprisingly little reduction in nostril size, and the risk for postoperative nostril/lobule disproportion is great.

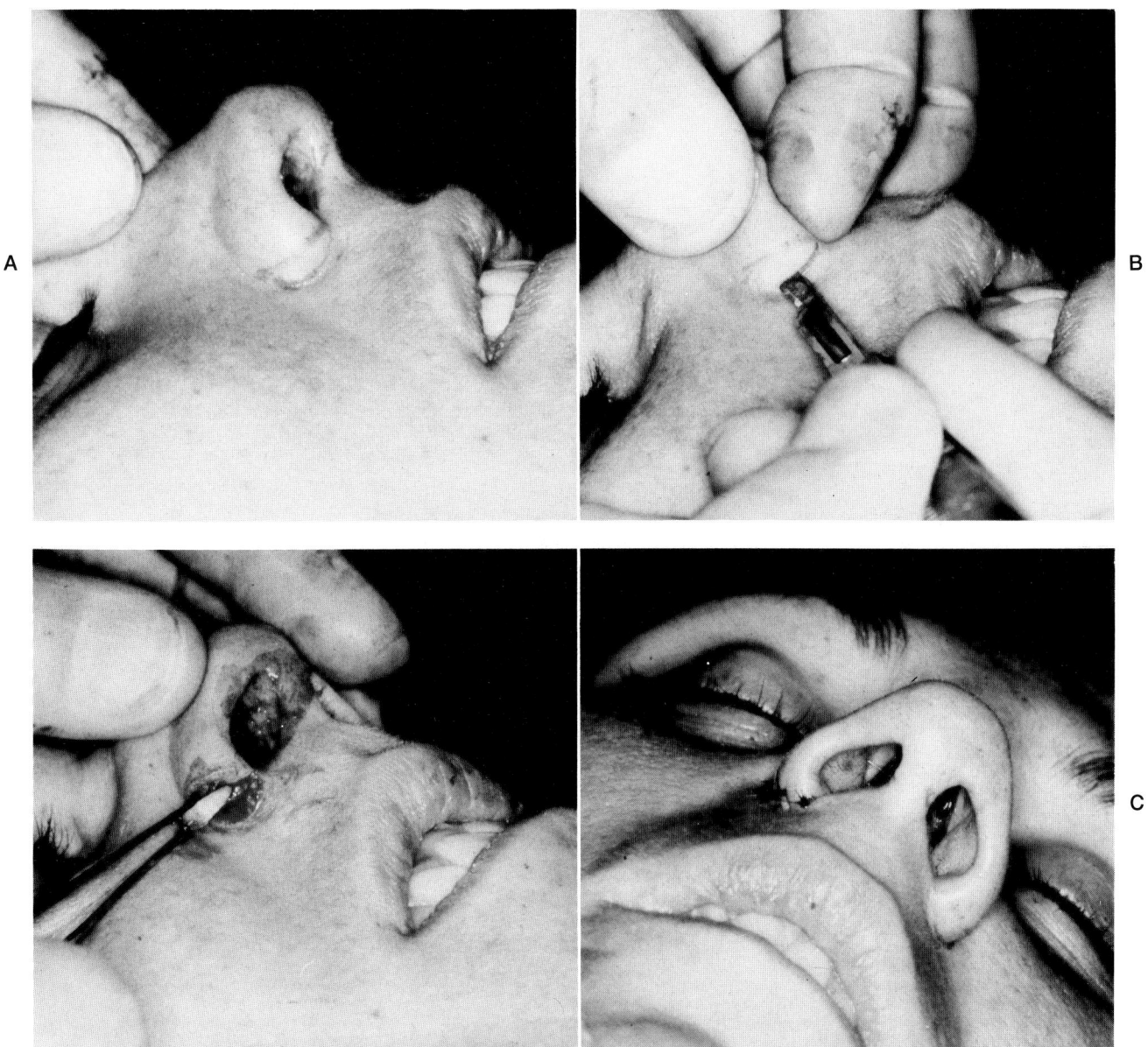

Figure 21-4. A, Type I alar base with planned excision outlined. **B,** Using No. 15 blade. **C,** Elliptic excision. Note small margin of skin preserved anterior to alar-facial groove. (From Sheen, J., and Sheen, A.P.: Aesthetic rhinoplasty, St. Louis, 1978, The C.V. Mosby Co.)

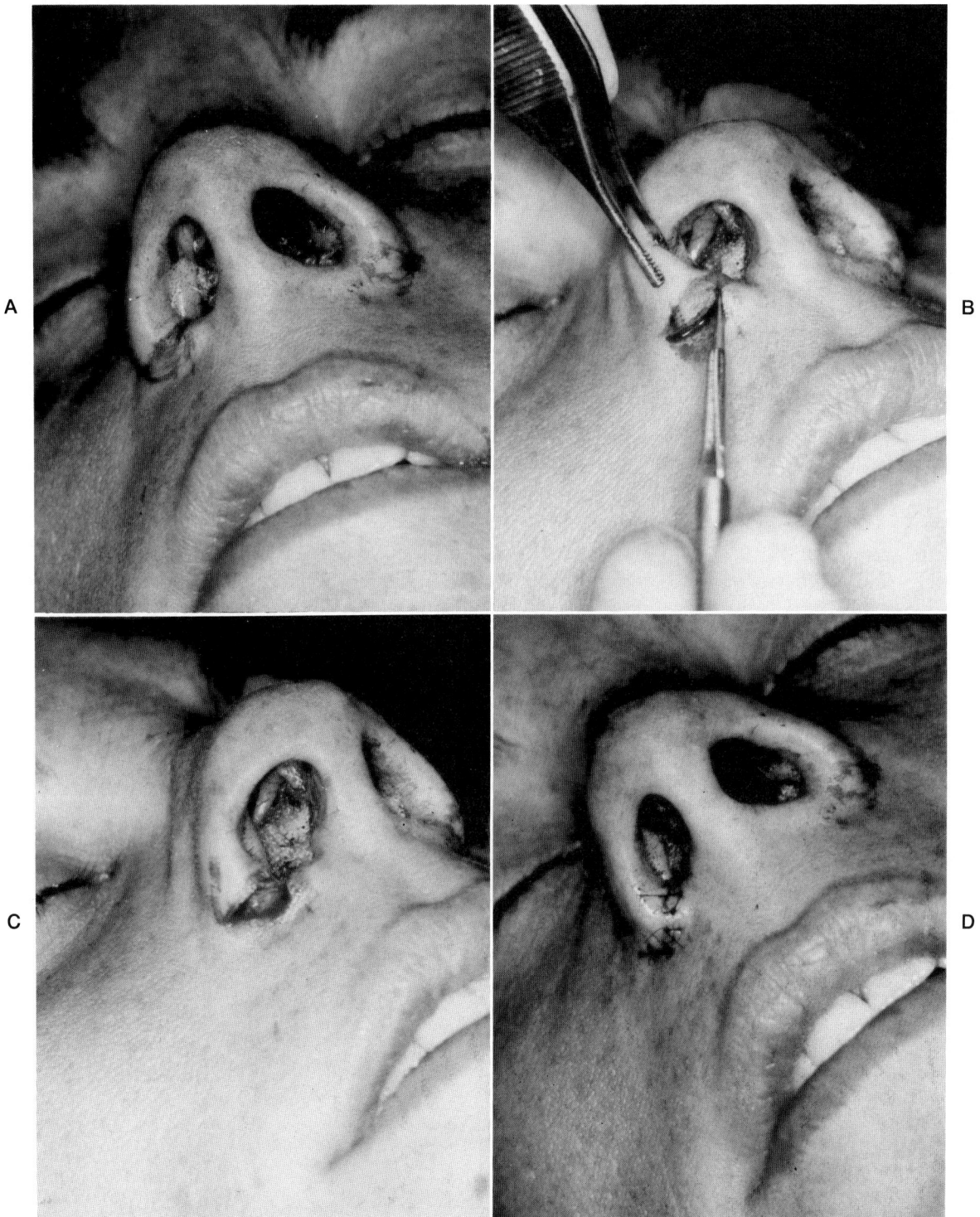

Figure 21-5. Type II alar base. **A,** Size of nostril is proportionately smaller than lobule. **B,** Cutting through nasal sill with No. 11 blade. Medial flap is retained with this type of base. **C,** Basal view of patient shows area of excision, medial flap, and small margin of remaining skin anterior to the alar-facial groove. **D,** Completed resection. Note improved size and position of nostril.
(**A,** From Sheen, J., and Sheen, A.P.: Aesthetic rhinoplasty, ed. 2, St. Louis, 1987, The C.V. Mosby Co.; **B, C,** and **D,** From Sheen, J., and Sheen, A.P.: Aesthetic rhinoplasty, St. Louis, 1978, The C.V. Mosby Co.)

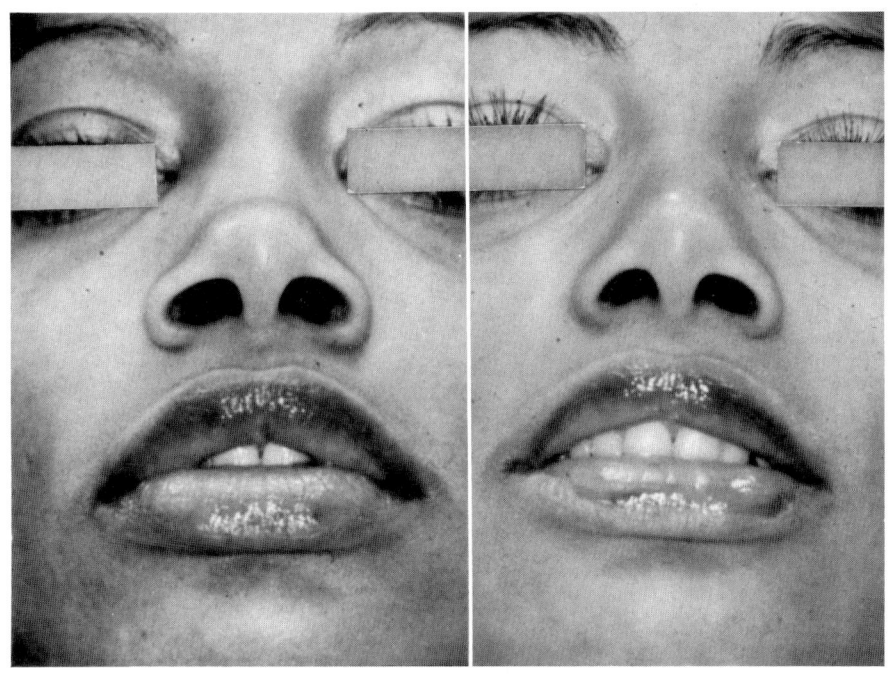

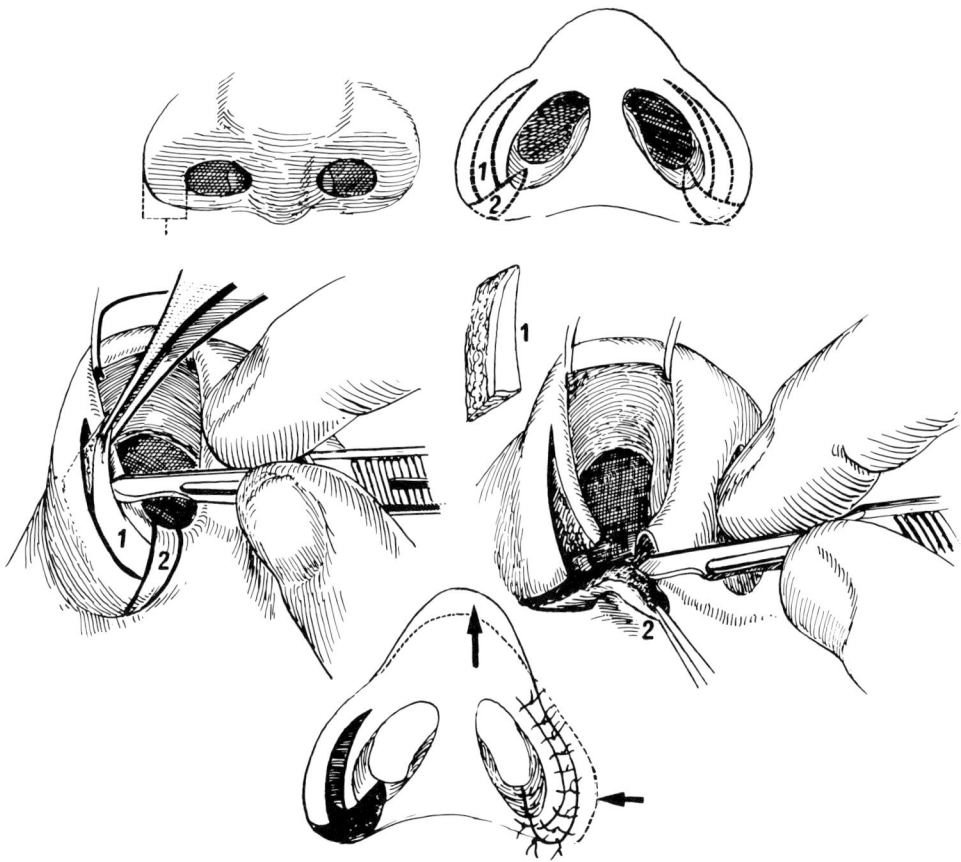

Figure 21-6. Preoperative and postoperative views of a type III alar base. Natural character of nose has been preserved. (From Sheen, J., and Sheen, A.P.: Aesthetic rhinoplasty, ed. 2, St. Louis, 1987, The C.V. Mosby Co.)

APPLICATIONS

I am often asked about the percentage of cases in which I do alar base resections. This is an important question, because the percentage of alar resections reveals something about the operation's effect on tip projection. When the height of the tip is decreased by lowering the dorsum and by resecting the angle of the septum, bowing of the nostrils will result.[1] If the surgeon is performing a high percentage of alar base resections, especially if many of them are unexpected (that is, unplanned preoperatively), I believe that surgeon is overresecting the dorsum. My experience indicates that about 10% of rhinoplasties require alar resection, and unless the surgeon has a special patient population with characteristically flared nostrils, I think only 10% to 15% of cases need alar narrowing; more than 15% of cases are probably due to iatrogenic loss of tip height.

REFERENCE

1. Sheen, J., and Sheen, A.P.: Aesthetic rhinoplasty, St. Louis, 1978, The C.V. Mosby Co., p. 571.

BIBLIOGRAPHY

Millard, R.D., Jr., editor: Symposium on corrective rhinoplasty, St. Louis, 1976, The C.V. Mosby Co., pp. 270-272.

Editor's Comments
Part V

Thomas Rees

Dr. Sheen has presented the technique and its intricacies very well. I find designing and executing the alar base resection to be one of the most difficult small procedures in plastic surgery. That is, it is challenging to get the design and symmetry exactly right, since the symmetry can often be distorted by a natural asymmetry of the face, which of course includes the nose, as well as any minor deflection of the nostrils or the septum or any imbalance formed by the maxilla in the skeletal floor.

I am often able to anticipate the need for an alar base resection and plan for it. If I suspect that the procedure will be required, I generally advise patients of the possibility before surgery, since they should know about the external scars in the nostril rim. Obviously, large alae, marked flaring, and a very prominent tip all require alar base resections to finish off the rhinoplasty. However, it is not always possible to anticipate the need for resection, and I am naturally conservative about performing alar base resection. In reducing and thereby relaxing the profile, "setting back the tent poles" so to speak, there is a relaxation of the soft tissues and a certain amount of sag. The nostrils are then apt to bow or collapse outward, and increased flaring is the end result. This flaring cannot always be anticipated and is not necessarily the result of excessive size of the nostril circumference but more a question of the shape after reduction. At the end of rhinoplasty, after the final minute trimming of the caudal ends of the upper lateral cartilages has been done, I assess the shape and size of the nostrils. If there is any doubt about whether an alar base resection is necessary, I postpone the procedure. It can always be done as a minor outpatient procedure a few weeks or months after the initial rhinoplasty, but it is quite interesting to know that I rarely do it after delaying the decision. One of the reasons for my change of

plan is that I would like to prevent alar base scars if possible, as well as avoid minor difficulties that can be encountered, such as asymmetry.

I perform alar base resections in approximately 15% of my primary cases. This percentage is certainly in sharp contrast to some; for instance, I believe Dr. Ralph Millard does them in more than 90% of his patients. I note that Dr. Sheen and I roughly agree on our percentages, which is gratifying, since we do not always agree on either procedure or statistics.

It is important to realize that one must tailor the alar base to accomplish what is required, to solve a specific problem. When a tip setback is required to overcome excessive projection, a full-thickness wedge must be removed from the entire curve of the alar bases where they attach along the cheek. This is the Weir method and should be used only in these specific cases, because the tradeoff involves scars along the alar crease. These scars can be quite noticeable and are prone to small stitch tracts and sebaceous accumulations. Reduction of flare or displacement of the nostrils in a more medial position requires resection of only variously designed wedges from the nostril sill; this is not difficult, but precision is required. A study of the contour of the nostril rim and sill is essential in placing the incision. Patients who have a natural groove will hardly notice a scar placed exactly in the groove, whereas those with a perfectly round sill do not appreciate a notch. Therefore, when the sill is round and smooth it is a good idea to place a small dart in the flap. We have all been taught to break up a straight-line incision; likewise, this small dart will break up an otherwise contracting scar across the sill.

One helpful technical hint is the technique of fracturing the nasal spine, and sometimes the anterior portion of the vomeris, in those patients with a minor septal deviation that will make it exceedingly difficult to achieve perfect symmetry in the alae. Even a slight deviation of the septum off the midline can cause enormous problems in designing these excisions. It is a simple matter to insert a 2 or 3 mm osteotome through the base of the transfixion incision and loosen the bone. Sometimes a 1 or 2 mm shift is all that is required.

Finally, in those patients with overhanging sidewalls where the nostril margins hang down like a curtain, obscuring the visibility of the columella from the profile, a direct excision of the overhang is required (see Figure 21-6). This procedure removes a long "piece of pie" from the entire length of the columella, frequently also in continuity with an alar base resection of the floor. The design can be varied to simultaneously elevate and defat the nostrils. Suturing must be exact, but the scars are remarkably benign if all the sutures are removed on the third or fourth day postoperatively. Elevation of the hanging nostril rim can of course be combined with a grafting of cartilage to the columella to make this structure more prominent.

PART

VI

IMPAIRED NASAL BREATHING: EVALUATION AND PHYSIOLOGY

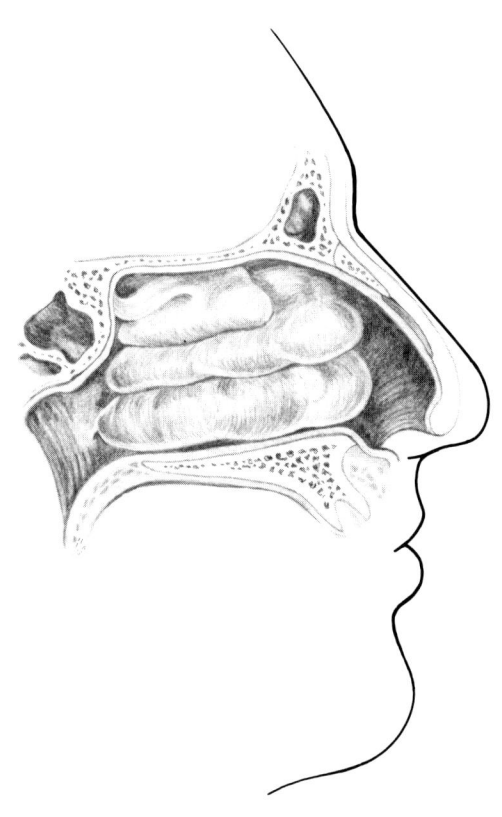

22

Nasal Physiology, Patient Evaluation, and Effects of Surgery

Eugene Courtiss

Because nasal form and function are interrelated it behooves surgeons performing nasal surgery to understand nasal physiology.

The nose has seven functions: as an airway; to condition the air; to clean the air; in olfaction; in phonation; with several nasal reflexes; and as a secondary sex organ. Only its main function as an airway will be discussed here; the reader is referred elsewhere for information on the other functions.

NASAL PHYSIOLOGY
Physical principles

When a difference exists between the pressure at the nasopharynx and that at the external nares, air flows through the nose. According to Ohm's law flow is directly proportional to the difference in pressure and is inversely proportional to the resistance. At low flows nasal airflow is laminar; that is, the air next to the nasal wall is almost motionless, whereas that in the center moves rapidly.

According to Bernoulli's principle, when a tube narrows the flow in the narrow area increases. On the other hand, the flow decreases in an area of dilation.

Of great importance is the radius of the channel (nose). According to Poiseuille's law, flow is directly proportional to the radius to the *fourth* power. Thus minor increases in the size of the nasal cavity result in major effects on airflow. In addition, the length of the channel (nose) inversely affects airflow.

Laminar flow applies to low flow rates, as in quiet nasal breathing. However, during most activity the flow rates are increased, and the flow is turbulent. In turbulent flow the air as a whole progresses at a constant velocity, but within the nose it follows random paths (eddy currents) and constantly changes velocity. To maintain the same flow turbulent flow requires a greater pressure gradient than does laminar flow (Figure 22-1).

The cross-sectional area of the airway is not constant: Through the internal valve it is small; through the turbinates it is larger; and through the posterior choana it is quite large. The nasal surgeon should preserve or enlarge the airway at the critical areas—the internal valve and turbinates—where airway obstructions usually occur.

Anatomic course

On inspiration most of the air passes through the middle meatus. A smaller amount travels through the inferior meatus, and a still lesser amount courses toward the olfactory area (Figure 22-1).

On expiration more air passes into the higher reaches of the nose, and the airflow is more turbulent, as verified by studies performed in 1941 that used cadaver halves, glass, and smoke.[2] However, the nose is a dynamic, changing structure. The course followed by the airstream needs further study.

When length is altered and the angle of the nares is changed, airflow is affected. When the nose is shortened air travels along the inferior meatus, and the flow is increased. Conversely, in patients with long, hanging noses, the airflow is less. In addition, the turbulence is greater, and the air travels higher on inspiration.

Because of the multiple factors that affect production of mucus, activity of the cilia, vasoconstriction, vasodilatation, and the nasal reflexes, the air flowing through the nose is constantly changing. These changes are associated with the *nasal cycle,* which is present in 80% of the population. (Those who have it are unaware of its presence.) During the nasal cycle the total airflow and total resistance remain constant; however, there is a reciprocal flow between the two nasal cavities. As the flow increases on one side it decreases on the other, and vice versa. The nasal cycle takes about 3 to 4 hours to complete.

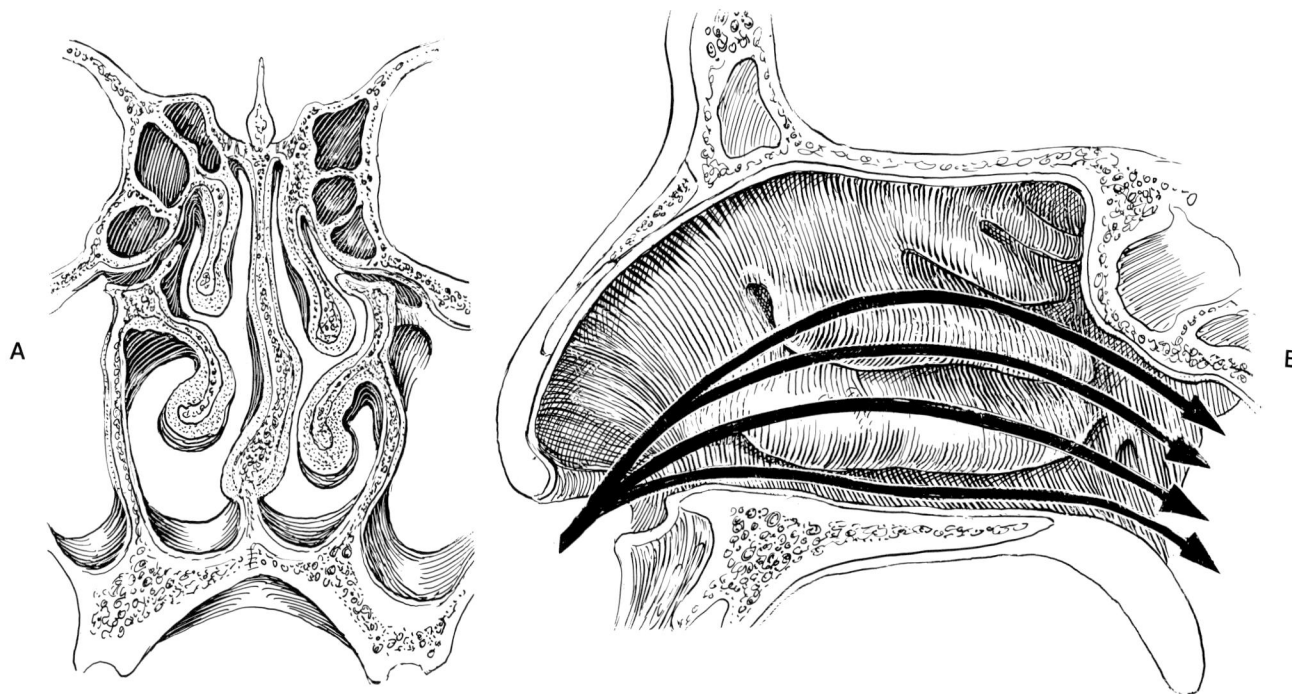

Figure 22-1. A, Coronal section through midnose shows available airspaces in "normal" nose. Slight septal deflections must be considered the norm. **B,** Passage of air through meatus in presence of normal mucosa. Main air current takes parabolic curve to pass through middle meatus over inferior turbinate. Lesser stream travels through inferior meatus and along nasal floor. Least airflow is through narrower superior aspect of nasal cavity. (From Rees, T.D.: *Aesthetic plastic surgery,* Philadelphia, 1983, W.B. Saunders Co.)

Valves

An important consideration is the nasal valves, which, like all valves, regulate flow. The nose has four valving mechanisms: the external valves, the internal valves, the inferior turbinates, and the nasal septum.

External valve. The paired external valves are formed by the alar cartilages, the columella, and the nasal floors. They are dynamic structures that on inspiration dilate actively and on expiration dilate passively. Because they are dynamic they may be adversely affected by trauma or surgery. Patients with Bell's palsy lack the motor function to dilate the ipsilateral external valve on inspiration.

NASAL VALVE PATHOLOGY

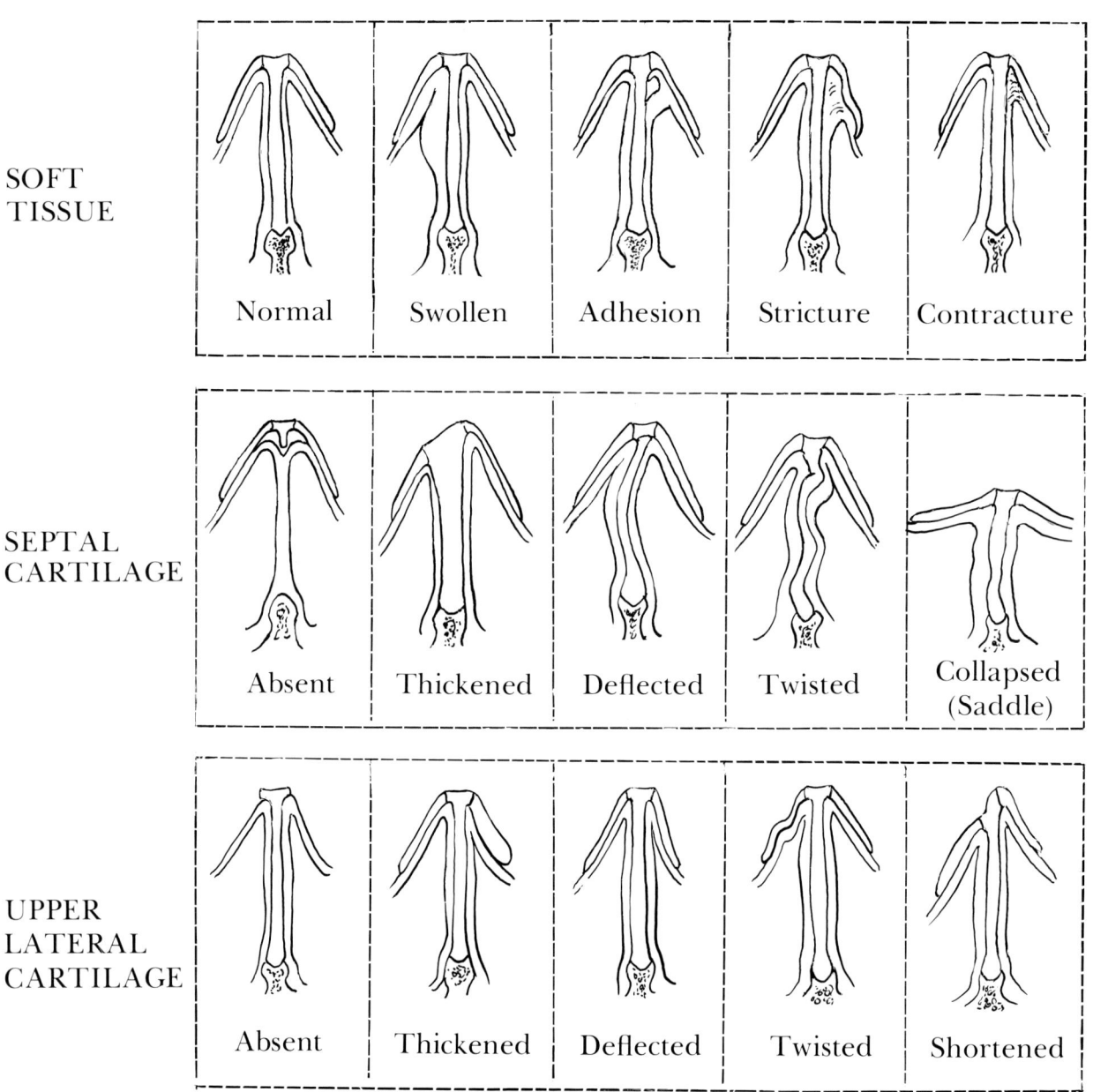

SOFT TISSUE

Normal   Swollen   Adhesion   Stricture   Contracture

SEPTAL CARTILAGE

Absent   Thickened   Deflected   Twisted   Collapsed (Saddle)

UPPER LATERAL CARTILAGE

Absent   Thickened   Deflected   Twisted   Shortened

Figure 22-2. Abnormalities of nasal valve may be caused by changes in mucocutaneous soft tissue that covers skeletal structures of nasal valve *(top row),* abnormalities or deficiencies of nasal septum *(middle row),* and deformities and injuries to upper lateral cartilages *(bottom row).* (From Rees, T.D.: Aesthetic plastic surgery, Philadelphia, 1983, W.B. Saunders Co.)

Internal valves (Figure 22-2). The paired internal valves (also known as the limen vestibuli, the limen nasi, the liminal valve, the os internum, the ostium internum, the liminal chink, the nasal valve, the valve area, the valve region, the flow-limiting segment, and area 2) are formed by the caudal ends of the upper lateral and septal cartilages, which join at a 10- to 15-degree angle. The caudal end of the upper lateral cartilages is not rigidly fused to the septal cartilage. Instead, a loose ligamentous tissue attaches the caudal end of the upper lateral cartilage to the septal cartilage. The angle is important: When the angle is increased airflow increases; when the angle is decreased airflow decreases.

The internal valves change the air from a column into a sheet. These valves are dynamic structures that function paradoxically: On inspiration the internal valves close, and then airflow is decreased; on expiration they open, and the airflow is increased.

The internal valves are the most important valves in Caucasians; the inferior turbinates are the most important valves in blacks. As with the external valves the internal valves may be damaged by surgery to the lining or cartilage. Damage to the internal valves may be avoided by the following three steps.

Location of incisions. Incisions made directly in the internal valves should be avoided, because they may produce scars that contract and thereby obstruct the airway. Instead, infracartilaginous, transcartilaginous, or intercartilaginous incisions should be made.

Excess lining. Excess lining should be trimmed judiciously, if at all. Excess mucosa will contract; a shortage may produce a contracture.

Cartilaginous resection. Resection of the caudal-dorsal angle of the upper lateral and septal cartilage should be conservative, if done at all. If too much is resected the angular relationships change, and rigid scar tissue forms.

Inferior turbinates. The paired inferior turbinates regulate airflow by vascular congestion and decongestion. They are the most important valves in blacks. Hypertrophy of the inferior turbinates is the most common cause of airway obstruction (Figure 22-3). Consequently treatment of the airway often requires treatment of the turbinate which is the subject of Chapter 29.

Nasal septum. In contrast to the internal and external valves and turbinates, all of which are dynamic, the nasal septum is a static valve. Deviation of the septum is normal; not all septal deviations adversely affect airflow. Furthermore deviations *parallel* to the airflow do not obstruct the airway; only deviations *perpendicular* to the airflow obstruct it. In the past the classic Killian submucous resection has been performed overly often.

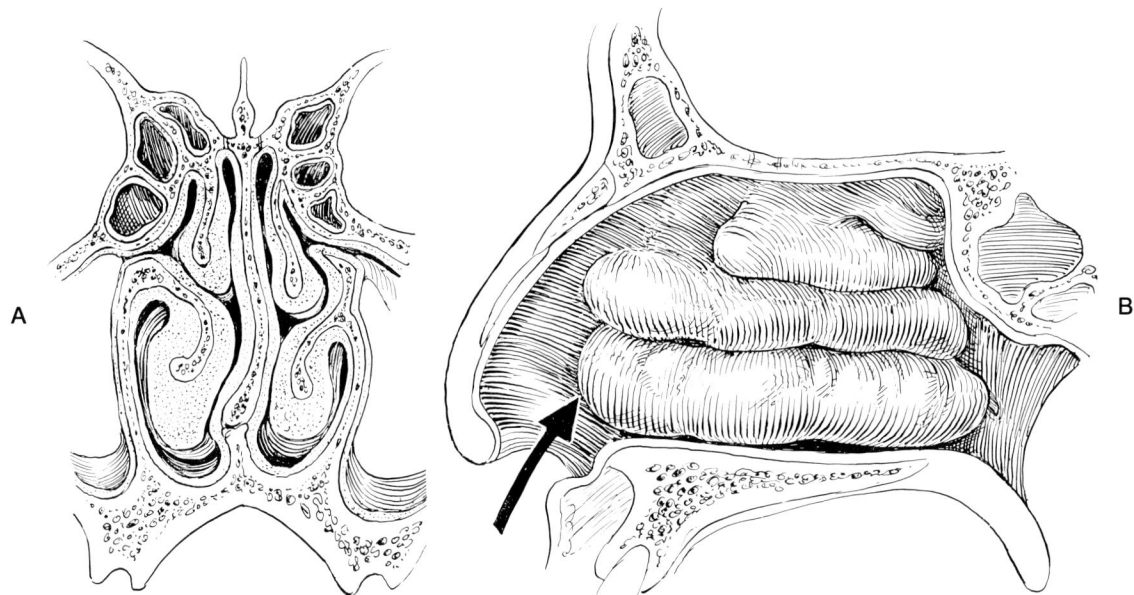

Figure 22-3. A, Severe crowding of the airways occurs in vasomotor states, with edema and swelling of the membranes. This is by far the most common cause of airway obstruction. **B,** Air current is blocked at anterior nose. (From Rees, T.D.: Aesthetic plastic surgery, Philadelphia, 1983, W.B. Saunders Co.)

PATIENT EVALUATION
Evaluation of the nasal airway

As pertains to all patients, an appropriate history is the first step in evaluating any patient's airway. However, patients often are unable to assess their nasal airway[1]; they have nothing with which to compare it. They do not know what is "normal" and may be influenced by other factors. Patients often do not know how long their airway has been impaired, and not infrequently they are unsure whether their breathing problem is congenital or seasonal. Some patients find it more difficult to breathe during the pollen season; however, evaluation by an allergist is indicated only if the patient has other allergic symptoms.

A history of trauma is difficult to evaluate. Nasal trauma occurs in almost everyone's past. Establishing a causal relationship between the past and trauma and current nasal obstruction is difficult unless the patient has been examined previously. Radiographs are of little value.

Physical examination

The nose should be examined externally and internally. The external examination includes a notation of nasal movements as the individual breathes.

Internal examination, rhinoscopy, should be performed with proper lighting, by means of either a headlight or head mirror. The nose should be examined carefully by looking into all of its reaches. Then the lining should be shrunk with 2% ephedrine and the nose reexamined. Any scars, obstructions, or changes in the turbinates should be noted.

Rhinomanometry, the measurement of nasal airflow, is helpful as a research tool but is rarely of value clinically.[1]

SELECTION OF OPERATIVE APPROACH

The choice of treatment of a given patient's nasal obstruction should be *individualized* according to the patient's *pathologic anatomy*. My philosophy of treatment is as follows: If the airway obstruction is due to hypertrophy of the inferior turbinates, then the inferior turbinates should be treated. (My preference is resection, the subject of Chapter 29.) If the airway obstruction is due to a septal deviation, then the septum should be treated, the subject of Chapter 32.

EFFECT OF AESTHETIC RHINOPLASTY ON AIRFLOW

As indicated by statistically significant studies,[1] which measured the airflow through the nose before and after surgery, an aesthetic rhinoplasty does *not* adversely affect the nasal airflow. However, preserving the integrity of the external and internal nasal valves is important.

Infracturing does not adversely affect the airway, because it does not change the angle between the caudal end of the upper lateral cartilages and the septal cartilage (the internal valve).

REFERENCES

1. Courtiss, E.H., and Goldwyn, R.M.: The effects of nasal surgery on airflow, Plast. Reconstr. Surg. (In press.)
2. Proetz, A.W.: Applied physiology of the nose, St. Louis, 1941, Annals Publishing Co.

23

Evaluation of Nasal Breathing:
An Objective Method

Eugene B. Kern

How much do you weigh? How do you know that? How well does your patient breathe? How do you know that? What the scale is to measuring a person's weight, the rhinomanometer is to measuring a person's breathing. The purpose of this chapter is to describe the technique and clinical value of an objective method for evaluating nasal breathing.

Rhinomanometry is a method of determining nasal airway resistance by the simultaneous measurement of nasal pressure and airflow.[4,9,10] This is an objective study. In order for rhinomanometry to be a clinically useful study of the functional nasal airways during breathing, it must meet several criteria: (1) Measurements of nasal airway resistance should be reproducible; (2) the quantitative measurement of nasal airway resistance should correlate with the clinical symptoms of the patient (usually nasal obstruction); (3) normal values and ranges of nasal resistance should be available for comparison; and (4) rhinomanometry measurements should provide information not available with other methods that assist in the diagnosis of nasal disorders and subsequent treatment. Rhinomanometry does meet these criteria and is an essential tool in the diagnosis of nasal obstructive disorders.

DETERMINATION OF NASAL RESISTANCE

Nasal airway resistance (R) is the relationship of transnasal pressure (P) to airflow ($\dot{V}$), the simplest formulation being:

$$R = P/\dot{V}$$

When airflow is laminar, resistance is independent of airflow rate. During laminar flow the pressure drop between two points in the system (P_1 and P_2) is proportional to airflow ($\dot{V}$). The formulation of this relationship is:

$$P_1 \, P_2 = K \, \dot{V}$$

Reynolds' number is a theoretic measure of the degree of turbulence. For laminar flow Reynolds' number is less than 2000. K is a constant.

When airflow is turbulent the relationship between pressure and flow is not simple, and there is not a unique value for resistance.[9] During turbulent flow the pressure drop between two points in the system (P_1 and P_2) is proportional to the airflow ($\dot{V}$) raised to the 1.75 power. The formulation of this relationship:

$$P_1 \, P_2 = K \, \dot{V}^{1.75}$$

Nasal airflow is turbulent, and the resistance calculated is dependent on flow rate. This is another way of saying the pressure-flow relationship is curvilinear. The nasal pressure-flow relationship is shown in Figure 23-1. If nasal resistance measurements are compared it is necessary to specify a specific point on the pressure-flow curve that is used to calculate resistance. Three systems have been used to specify a point for measurement. These are shown in Figure 23-1. A specific pressure point can be designated, such as 1.5 cm of water. Flow is measured at this pressure and the resistance calculated by dividing the pressure by the flow. It is also possible to specify a specific flow such as 0.25 L/sec. Pressure is measured at this flow, and the resistance is calculated by dividing the pressure by the flow. A third method has been proposed in which a circle of spe-

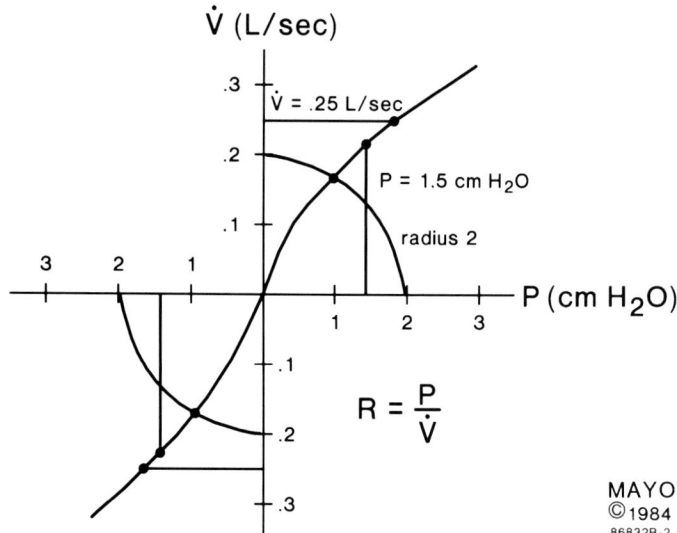

Figure 23-1. Three possible ways to select point on pressure-flow curve for determining nasal resistance *(R)*. Particular flow *(V̇)*, pressure *(P)*, or radius can be used to define point on the pressure-flow curve used to determine resistance. When radius is used ratio of pressure and flow axes must be 10:1.
(By permission of Mayo Foundation.)

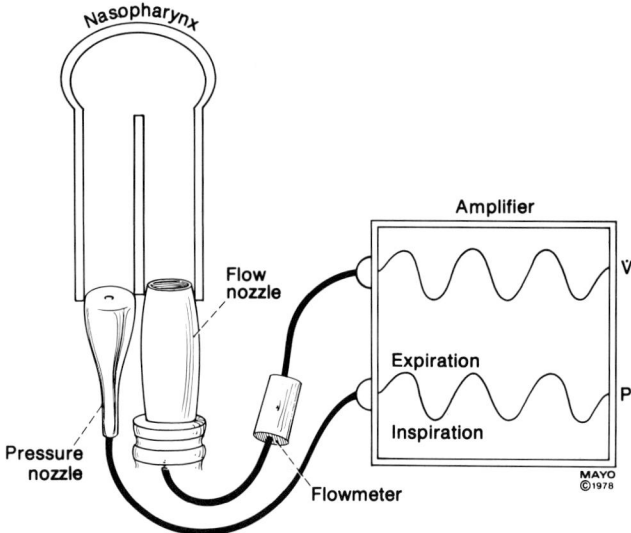

Figure 23-2. Anterior rhinomanometry. Transnasal pressure is measured by occluding pressure transducer in nostril of opposite nasal airway. This is measure of transnasal driving pressure. Flow through measured nostril is determined with pneumotachograph flowmeter.
(By permission of Mayo Foundation.)

cific radius is drawn at the origin.[10] The point at which this circle crosses the pressure-flow curve is used to calculate resistance in the same manner as the previous examples. In this case the pressure axis and the flow axis must have a 10:1 ratio. Any of these methods provide a consistent determination of nasal resistance; however, in all these cases nasal flow properties are specified only at a single value of pressure and flow. Different values for resistance would be obtained by alternative methods of specifying the point of measurement. For this reason all comparisons between individuals must be made at the same point.

METHOD OF RHINOMANOMETRY

To determine the resistance of the nose it is necessary to measure simultaneously pressure and flow through the nose. Practical methods of performing rhinomanometry can be characterized according to the method used to measure transnasal pressure and the method used to measure transnasal airflow. If the measurement of nasal pressure is performed at the nares, the technique is known as anterior rhinomanometry. If the measurement of transnasal pressure is made at the mouth, the method is known as posterior rhinomanometry.

Anterior rhinomanometry

Figure 23-2 schematically depicts the technique of anterior rhinomanometry. In this case one nostril is occluded with a pressure transducer. Since no airflow occurs through an occluded nostril, the pressure measured at the nostril will equal nasopharyngeal pressure (transnasal pressure). This is the driving pressure for nasal airflow through the nonobstructed (opposite) nostril. Airflow through the nonobstructed nostril is measured with a pneumotachograph. A mask is applied to the face so that all airflow through the nose is directed through the pneumotachograph. Simultaneous measurement of nasal pressure and flow will then permit calculation of nasal resistance. Only unilateral nasal resistance can be measured with this method. Total nasal resistance (R_T) can be calculated by the parallel resistance formula:

$$R_T = \frac{R_R \cdot R_L}{R_R + R_L}$$

Therefore the total nasal resistance is the product of the resistance on the right side of the nose (R_R) and the left side of the nose (R_L) divided by the sum of those resistances. The method of anterior rhinomanometry also cannot be used in cases of total

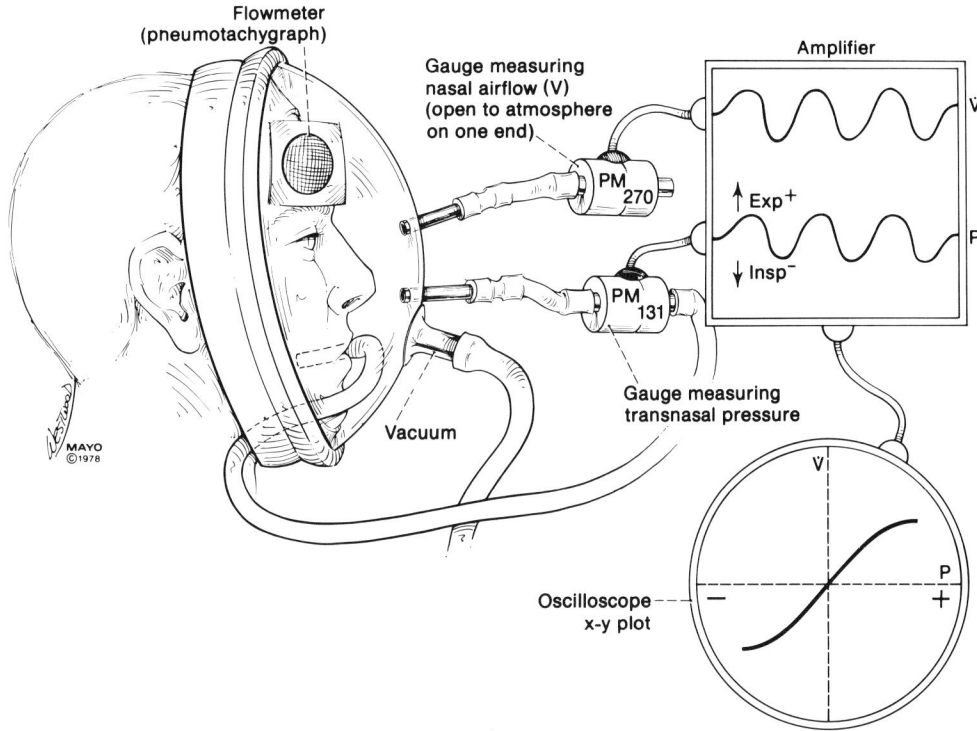

Figure 23-3. Posterior rhinomanometry. Transnasal pressure is measured by pressure catheter placed in mouth. If palate is relaxed pressure represents transnasal driving pressure. Nasal airflow is measured with a pneumotachograph flowmeter. (From McCaffrey, T.V., and Kern, E.B.: Rhinomanometry. In English, G.M., editor: Otolaryngology, vol. 2, Philadelphia, 1979, Harper & Row Publishers, Inc., pp. 1-18.)

unilateral nasal obstruction or in cases of septal perforation, since nasal pressure does not reflect nasopharyngeal pressure accurately in these cases.

Posterior rhinomanometry

To perform posterior rhinomanometry nasopharyngeal pressure or nasal driving pressure is measured by placing a catheter in the mouth rather than in one of the nostrils (Figure 23-3). In this way it is possible to measure the nasal resistance through both nasal passages in parallel or to measure nasal resistance in cases of nasal septal perforation in which the nasal chambers communicate. Nasal airflow is measured as in anterior rhinomanometry by a face mask and pneumotachograph. If unilateral nasal resistance is to be measured with posterior rhinomanometry, one of the nostrils is obstructed. Although posterior rhinomanometry can be applied to more situations than anterior rhinomanometry, it is not often used clinically because of the difficulty of obtaining reliable nasopharyngeal pressures through the mouth. Palatal muscles need to be re-

laxed, and this may be difficult for some individuals during nasal breathing. Whether anterior or posterior rhinomanometry is used, the pressure and flow recordings are displayed simultaneously on an XY recorder or oscilloscope. The resulting S-shaped curve depicts the resistance properties of the nose. These data can be used graphically, in which case increasing resistances are noted by clockwise rotation of the S-shaped curve, or nasal resistance ($\Delta P/\dot{V}$) can be calculated at a specific point on the curve by means of one of the three methods previously described, constant pressure, constant flow, or constant radius.

**CLINICAL EVALUATION
OF NASAL OBSTRUCTION**

Rhinomanometry provides only one aspect of the clinical evaluation of a patient with nasal obstruction. The measurement of nasal resistance must be interpreted along with the clinical history and physical examination. A recent study of a large number of patients with nasal obstruction has shown

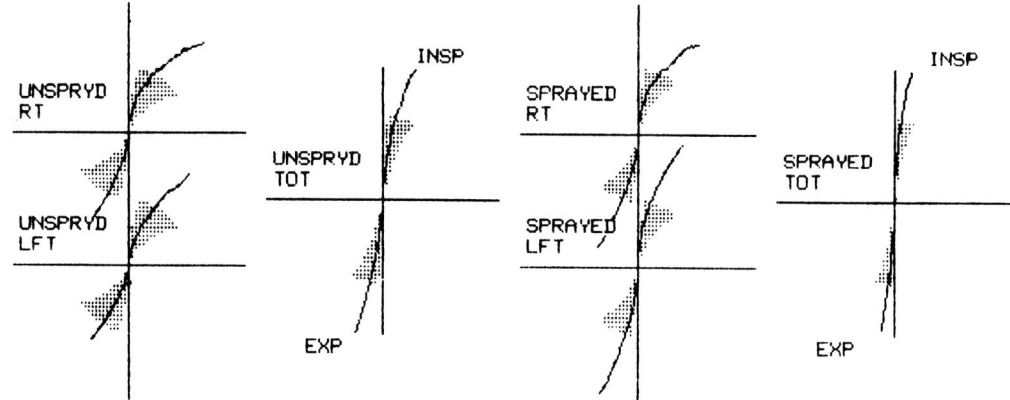

Figure 23-4. Normal nasal resistance. Nasal pressure-flow curves calculated before and after decongestion with phenylephrine. Shaded areas represent area bounded by 5th and 95th percentile limits of normal nasal resistance. Total nasal resistance curve is derived mathematically from unilateral nasal resistance measurements. Notice that after spray is used variability is less, as shown by a smaller range of normal. (By permission of Mayo Foundation.)

that in general the nasal resistance determined by rhinomanometry correlates with the subjective degree of nasal obstruction.[11] In addition, rhinomanometry provides information on the type and degree of nasal obstruction, which could not be assessed by rhinoscopic examination, because function cannot be determined by observation alone.

In general, there are two causes of nasal obstruction: (1) mucosal hypertrophy or congestion and (2) structural deformity of the nasal airway. By assessing nasal resistance before and after maximum nasal decongestion with topical phenylephrine, it is possible to determine the relative importance of mucosal versus structural nasal obstruction. For this reason rhinomanometry in a clinical setting is usually performed in the following sequence:

1. Right-sided nasal resistance (no decongestion)
2. Left-sided nasal resistance (no decongestion)
3. 1% Phenylephrine nasal spray—wait 10 minutes
4. Right-sided nasal resistance (after decongestion)
5. Left-sided nasal resistance (after decongestion)
6. Calculation of total nasal resistance from the measured unilateral resistances (equation 4)

The calculated resistance can then be compared to predetermined normal values (Figure 23-4). Mucosal obstruction usually could be expected to be corrected by decongestion, whereas in a structural

abnormality causing nasal obstruction, resistance would not come into the normal range after decongestion. Normal nasal resistance and ranges are given in Table 1. It is accepted that a nasal resistance greater than the 95th percentile is definitely abnormal.[3] However, the threshold of subjective obstruction will vary among individuals, and some individuals with apparently normal nasal resistance may at times experience obstructive symptoms.

INTERPRETATION OF NASAL RESISTANCE MEASUREMENTS

Nasal obstruction that is reversed by topical decongestion usually suggests a mucosal cause for the obstruction such as nasal hyperreactivity as a result of allergy, vasomotor rhinitis, or exaggerated nasal cycle. In general, with mucosal hyperreactivity the

TABLE 1. Normal nasal resistance during *inspiration,* at designated radii on pressure-flow curve before and after decongestion (based on 80 normal subjects)[13]

Radius	Before decongestion		After decongestion 1% phenylephrine	
	Mean	Range 5%-95%	Mean	Range 5%-95%
1	2.5	0.8-7.7	1.6	0.7-3.5
2	3.3	1.1-9.9	2.2	0.9-5.3

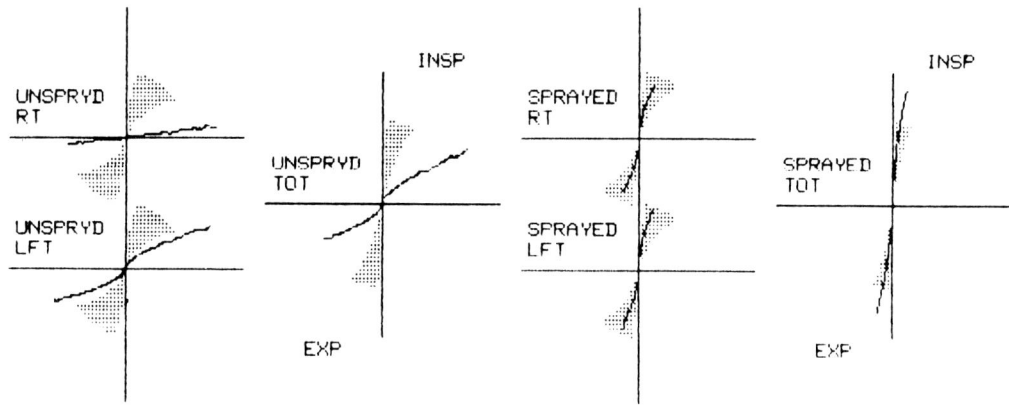

Figure 23-5. Mucosal nasal obstruction. Before decongestion there is markedly elevated nasal resistance bilaterally (all curves outside the normal range). After decongestion nasal resistance is within normal limits. This demonstrates reversibility of nasal mucosal obstruction. (By permission of Mayo Foundation.)

nose will have a greatly elevated resistance before decongestion and a normal resistance after decongestion with a topical vasoconstrictor (Figure 23-5). A slightly elevated nasal resistance on one side that returns to normal after decongestion and that does not produce an elevated total nasal resistance

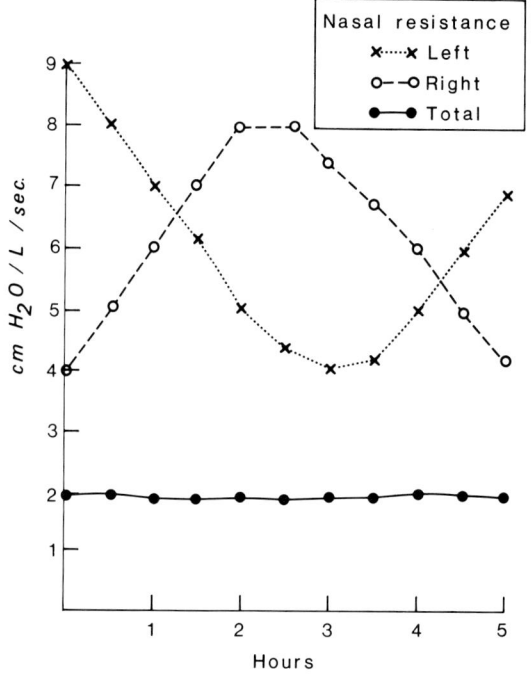

Figure 23-6. Fluctuation of nasal resistance with time. Alternating congestion of right and left nasal airways is nasal cycle. Note total nasal resistance remains constant. (By permission of Mayo Foundation.)

can be considered to be an exaggerated nasal cycle. The nose normally undergoes variations of nasal resistance with a pattern of alternating congestion and decongestion of the mucosa. In many individuals the right nasal chamber is congested while the left is decongested, with the pattern alternating over a period of 2 to 4 hours. This sequence of alternating congestion is termed the *nasal cycle.*[7] It is usually not of clinical significance, since total nasal resistance remains nearly constant (Figure 23-6). However, if a concomitant structural abnormality of the nasal airway exists, the cycle may produce a symptomatic obstruction during periods of congestion.

If nasal resistance remains elevated after topical decongestion, there is a structural abnormality of the nasal airway (Figure 23-7). This could be a septal deformity, scarring, synechiae, or irreversible mucosal abnormalities such as nasal polyps or hypertrophic mucosal changes on the septum or turbinates. The precise cause of the structural abnormality is usually apparent on rhinoscopic examination.[11]

Rhinomanometry is particularly useful in diagnosis of nasal obstruction that occurs as a result of dynamic changes in a nasal airway, since rhinoscopic examination may not detect these abnormalities. For example, nasal alar collapse (or nasal valve collapse) is a dynamic phenomenon in which the resilient cartilaginous structures of the nasal ala (or valve) collapse during inspiration. This phenomenon may be due to very localized obstruction in the area of the nasal valve or loss of structural cartilaginous support as a result of aging or nasal trauma or surgery. Rhin-

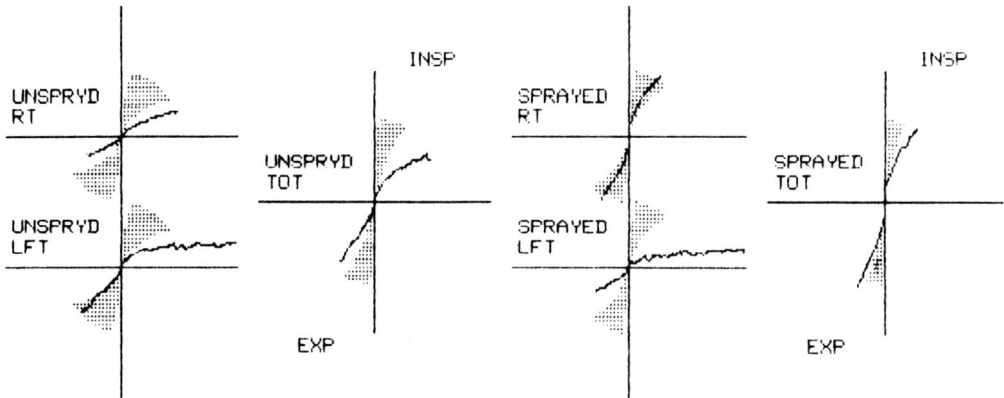

Figure 23-7. Structural nasal obstruction. Obstruction of left nasal airway is not reversed by decongestion, and total nasal resistance remains elevated. (By permission of Mayo Foundation.)

oplastic surgery with extensive resection of skin and cartilage in the nasal valve area can produce nasal valve collapse as a late complication. If the negative pressure of the nasal airway is sufficient to overcome the elasticity of the cartilage, the airway collapses and nasal resistance increases.[1] The typical rhinomanometric finding in such collapse is an asymmetric nasal pressure-flow curve. Since collapse occurs only during inspiration inspiratory resistance is higher than expiratory resistance. In addition, collapse produces a flow limitation that can be detected

as a plateau of the pressure-flow curve (Figure 23-8). Correction of nasal valve collapse may require grafting of cartilage to improve the support of the nasal airway and relieve the obstruction.

RHINOMANOMETRY FOR PRESURGICAL PLANNING

Rhinomanometric studies have indicated that the success of nasal septal surgery can be predicted by preoperative rhinomanometry.[12] If nasal airway resistance is high before surgery, there is a greater

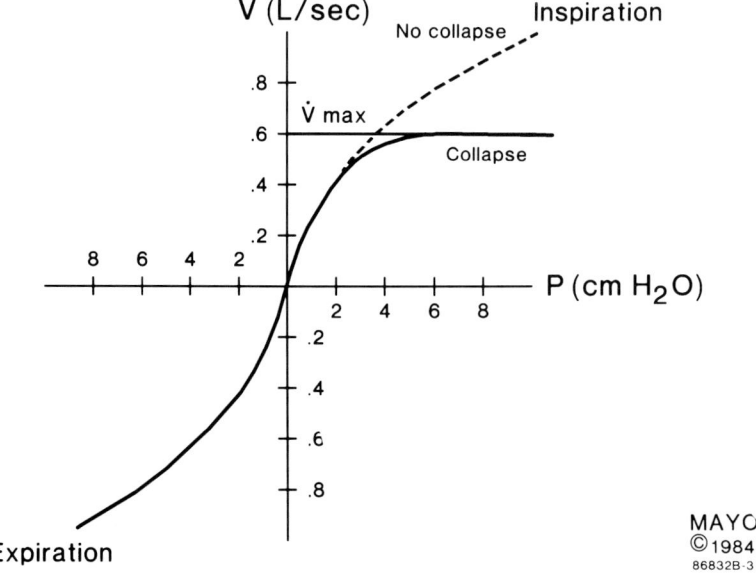

Figure 23-8. Dynamic collapse of nasal airway shown on pressure-flow curve. Collapse of nasal valve will produce limitation of inspiratory airflow ($\dot{V}_{max}$). In spite of increased efforts (pressure) inspiratory flow cannot exceed this value when collapse occurs. (By permission of Mayo Foundation.)

probability of symptomatic improvement than if nasal resistance is within the normal range before surgery. In those patients in whom the obstruction is corrected, as demonstrated by decrease in nasal airway resistance, the symptoms of nasal obstruction are generally eliminated. Rhinomanometry can also be helpful in the objective evaluation of nasal obstruction after rhinoplasty. In my 20 years of experience I have found that in patients who have had rhinoplasty and subsequent nasal breathing difficulties, the nasal obstruction was a result of an uncorrected septal deformity or was due to an obstruction of the nasal valve as a result of scarring or collapse. The physiology and surgery of the valve are covered in Chapter 25. Rhinomanometry is helpful in directing attention to these areas so that subsequent surgery can be planned to alleviate these most annoying symptoms.

REBUTTAL TO THE DISSENTING VIEW OF RHINOMANOMETRY

Courtiss and Goldwyn[5] recently presented an excellent summary of the theory of nasal airflow and its application to the diagnosis of nasal airway disturbances and the assessment of surgical results. The most significant observation they made was that there is an observable decrease in nasal airway resistance after successful surgery for nasal obstruction. This observation has been made by others[12] investigating nasal resistance, so it is unquestionably accurate. Therefore it is safe to assume that the physiologic change responsible for the subjective improvement in these patients was a reduction in nasal airway resistance.

Despite that finding, those authors remain skeptical about the clinical utility of measuring nasal resistance by rhinomanometry.[5] They cited three reasons for this opinion: (1) Nasal resistance may not correlate with the subjective feeling of obstruction; (2) nasal resistance may not correlate with rhinoscopic evaluation; and (3) there is a high degree of variability in nasal resistance measurements. These points will be discussed.

Although Courtiss and Goldwyn stated there was no consistent correlation between subjective symptoms and absolute nasal resistance, no numeric data were presented to support that point. However, an earlier review of 1,000 patients demonstrates a consistent relation between subjective symptoms and absolute nasal resistance.[11] Although most individuals can detect a change in nasal resistance more accurately than an absolute level, the evidence does support the concept that nasal resistance is the basis for the perception of subjective nasal obstruction. It is not surprising that the measurement of nasal resistance does not always clearly distinguish between the normal and the abnormal nasal airway. The human nose has been shaped by multiple evolutionary demands. On the one hand, the nasal airway must function as a low-resistance passage for respiratory air, but on the other, it also must provide sufficient turbulence to adequately humidify the air reaching the lower airways and olfactory nerve endings. As in most biologic systems, these opposing demands are met by compromise. Since the nasal airway is not a low-resistance passage, a certain degree of resistance must be and is tolerated. Symptoms may therefore appear at various levels of resistance, but in general the higher the resistance, the more likely symptoms will occur. The lack of absolute correlation, therefore, is not an indication of the imprecision of the technique but rather of a variability in the ability to perceive the obstruction.

Courtiss and Goldwyn[5] were also concerned about the lack of correlation between nasal resistance measurement and rhinoscopic findings. This has been noted previously.[11] However, this does not represent a defect in the method but rather demonstrates the difficulty in predicting the functional importance of an internal nasal deformity. A large posterior deformity often will produce little change in nasal resistance, whereas a slight narrowing of the nasal valve area will produce a large increase in nasal resistance. The ability of nasal resistance measurements to identify functionally significant deformities is probably the most valuable asset of the technique. Again, you cannot determine function by observation alone.

Those authors have commented on the great variability in the resistance data between individuals and even in the same individual at different times. This is the result of the dynamic nature of the nasal airway and is not due to imprecision in the technique.[8] The nasal cycle has been observed for many years.[10] Decongestion of the mucosa with phenylephrine reduces variability by eliminating the mucosal factors responsible for obstruction and allows the importance of structural deformities to be assessed. Comparison of measurements before and after decongestion also provides an indication of the reversible component of the obstruction.[2]

SUMMARY

Rhinomanometry is an objective method for the evaluation of nasal breathing. It provides useful information that has important clinical value in the diagnosis of nasal obstructive disorders and the treatment of patients:

1. Nasal resistance is determined (normal versus elevated).
2. Reversible (mucosal) versus irreversible (structural) obstruction *can* be differentiated.
3. Dynamic changes of the nasal airway (such as alar or valve collapse) can be detected.

The information derived from nasal resistance measurements can be used to determine which therapy would be most beneficial in a particular patient. In addition, nasal resistance measurements are useful after therapy, since they provide a comparison of pretreatment and posttreatment nasal resistance. Thus the effectiveness of the treatment and the possible need to modify a therapeutic program can be assessed objectively.

The question of whether nasal resistance measurements are a clinically useful tool must be answered with a qualified "yes," because these data must be intergrated with the clinical history and physical examination. The information thereby provided on the functional status of the nasal airway cannot be obtained by any other method.

ACKNOWLEDGMENT

I am deeply indebted to and wish to thank my colleagues Thomas V. McCaffrey, M.D., and John F. Pallanch, M.D., and my secretary Mrs. Barbara Chapman for their assistance in this work.

REFERENCES

1. Bridger, G.P.: Physiology of the nasal valve, Arch. Otolaryngol. **92**:543-553, 1970.
2. Broms, P.: Rhinomanometry: III. Procedures and criteria for distinction between skeletal stenosis and mucosal swelling, Acta Otolaryngol. [Stockh.] **94**:361, 1982.
3. Broms, P., Jonson, B., and Lamm, C.J.: Rhinomanometry: II. A numerical description of nasal airway resistance, Acta Otolaryngol. [Stockh.] **94**:157-168, 1982.
4. Clement, P.A.R.: Committee report on standardization of rhinomanometry, Rhinology **22**:151-155, 1984.
5. Courtiss, E.H., and Goldwyn, R.M.: The effects of nasal surgery on airflow, Plast. Reconstr. Surg. **72**:9-19, 1983.
6. Hamilton, L.H.: Nasal airway resistance: Its measurement and regulation, Physiologist **22**:43-49, 1979.
7. Hasegawa, M., and Kern, E.B.: The human nasal cycle, Mayo Clin. Proc. 53:28-34, 1977.
8. Hasagawa, M., Kern, E.B., and O'Brien, P.C.: Dynamic changes of nasal resistance, Ann. Otol. Rhinol. Laryngol. **88**:66, 1979.
9. Kern, E.B.: Rhinomanometry, Otolaryngol. Clin. North Am. 6:863–874, 1973.
10. Kern, E.B.: Rhinomanometry. In English, G.M., editor: Otolaryngology, Hagerstown, Md., 1979, Harper & Row Publishers, Inc., vol. 2, pp. 1-18.
11. McCaffrey, T.V., and Kern, E.B.: Clinical evaluation of nasal obstruction: A study of 1,000 patients, Arch. Otolaryngol. **105**:542-545, 1979.
12. Mertz, J.S., McCaffrey, T.V., and Kern, E.B.: Objective evaluation of anterior septal surgical reconstruction, Otolaryngol. Head Neck Surg. **92**:302-307, 1984.
13. Pallanch, J.F., McCaffrey, T.V., and Kern, E.B.: Normal nasal resistance, Otolaryngol. Head Neck Surg. **93**:778-785, 1985.

THE NASAL VALVE

Extramucosal Rhinoplasty and Reconstruction of the Nasal Valve

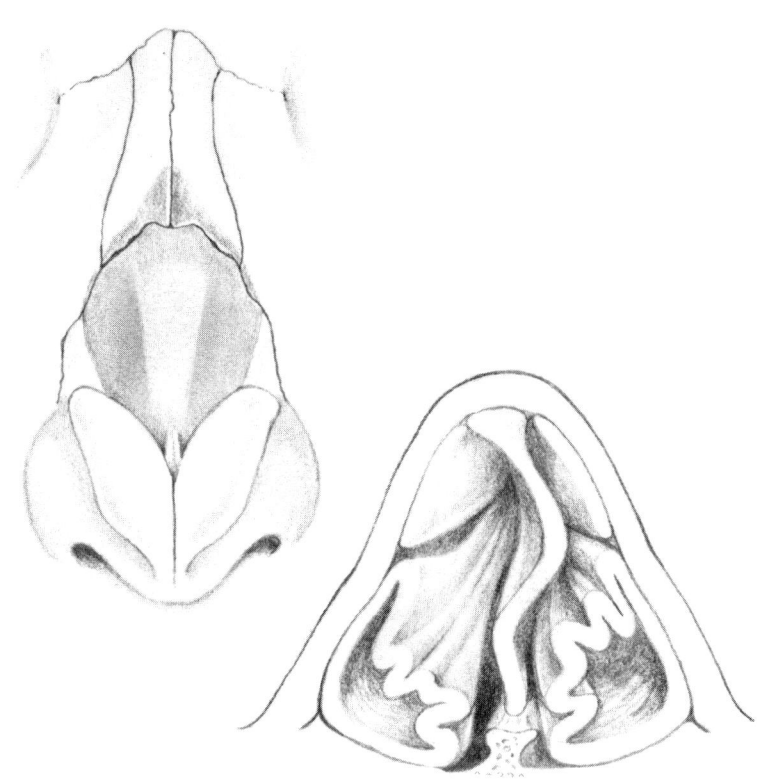

24

Surgical Approaches to Problems of the Nasal Valve Area and the Extramucosal Rhinoplasty

Claus Walter

When dealing with nasal airway problems one should be aware of an often overlooked fact: There are cases in which the piriform aperture is somewhat too small or has become smaller after extensive surgery or after several rhinoplasties. There may be a thickening of the periosteum and bone, resulting in a narrowing of the nasal vestibule. Such a condition justifies removal of a piece of bone at the edge of the piriform aperture. Only the injudicious removal of bone can cause injury to the lacrimal system.

Other procedures to consider are the double, triple, and quadruple osteotomies to widen the bony vault. These can be done with very small chisels to mobilize the bones without injuring the periosteum and while keeping the wall intact. After operation it is mandatory to use obturators to keep the structures dilated for 3 weeks.

EXTRAMUCOSAL RHINOPLASTY

Extramucosal rhinoplasty is helpful in treating airway problems. Through this approach the underlying mucous membrane is better visualized, since it can be dissected away in the area of the nasal valve. The central portion of the hump, which consists of the dorsal septum and a part of the nasal bones, is then removed. If a patient has breathing problems the free end of the upper lateral cartilage is not removed but only severed from the septum so as to widen the nasal valve area (Figure 24-1).

Other approaches in treating impairment of the nasal valve are possible. For instance, a piece of cartilage can be used to stabilize the nasal entrance.

It is inserted through an incision in the alalabial junction, under tension to spread the base of the nostril. When, however, the cartilage is large and malpositioned, one can remove the entire upper lateral cartilage, turn it over 180 degrees, and insert it in a new position (Figure 24-2). Fixation with mattress sutures is mandatory. Another approach to this problem is use of an island flap of skin to enlarge the nasal vestibule after excision of scar. It is possible to obtain a piece of tissue from the nasolabial junction for relining of the base of the vestibule.

In cases of destruction of the nasal valve, one can overlap the triangular cartilage with the lower lateral cartilages to advantage. A medially based mucochondral flap, cut from the lower lateral cartilage,

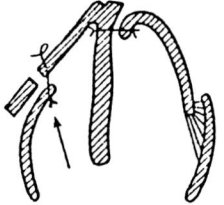 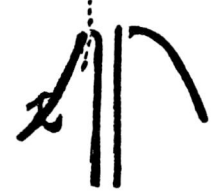

Figure 24-1   Figure 24-2

Figure 24-1. Upper lateral cartilages are divided from septum and sutured into another position in relation to septum.

Figure 24-2. Excision of entire lower lateral cartilage in a case of alar collapse. Cartilage is turned 180 degrees and reinserted.

is turned into the ensuing defect after the upper lateral cartilages are divided from the septum. This widens the internal valve with a local tissue (Figures 24-3 and 24-4).

Long ago, before Sheen introduced his spreader grafts (Figure 24-5), I described a method of dividing the upper lateral cartilages from the septum and inserting a composite graft, taken from the auricle, into the defect for reconstruction of the inner valve. This is another method for enlarging the nasal passageway.

One can also reverse the position of the upper and lower lateral cartilages to open up the nasal airway, or one can enlarge the base of the nasal entrance with a composite graft (Figure 24-6).

In certain cases cartilage is needed only for stabilization and is inserted as a saddle graft on top of the septum. Sutures are used to connect the graft with the upper lateral cartilages for better healing. A composite graft containing cartilage and skin is used instead, to enlarge the nasal entrance after all scar tissue has been removed. I like to cover any transplant for a week to protect it from drying out. Transplanted cartilage examined months and years later has remained quite viable.

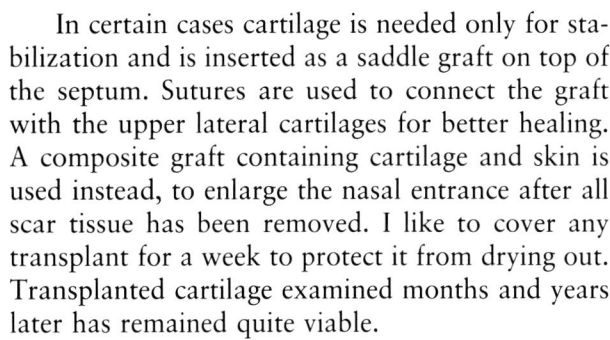

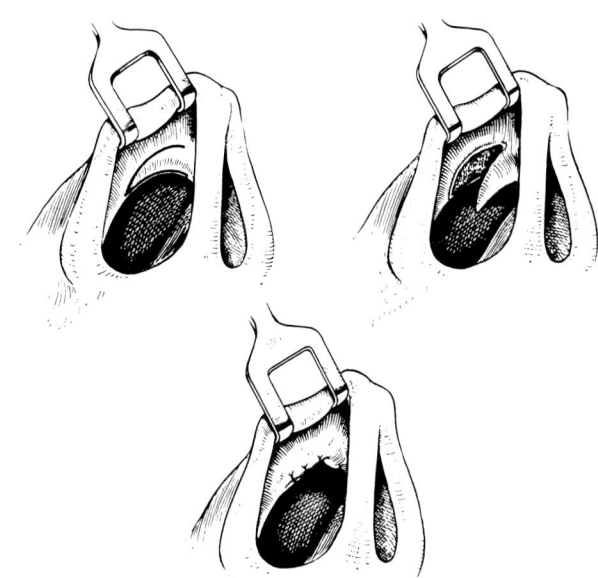

Figure 24-4. Nasal diagram of folds of cartilage of larynx and its envelope going inward cranially.

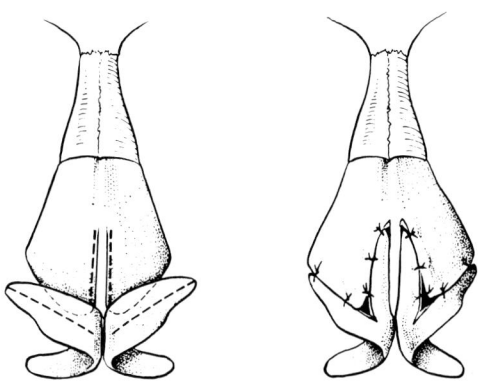

Figure 24-3. A, Anatomic view of cartilages of larynx and epiglottis with marked guide for sectioning. **B,** After mobilization membranous cartilage folds of vestibulum are pushed into septal suture defect.

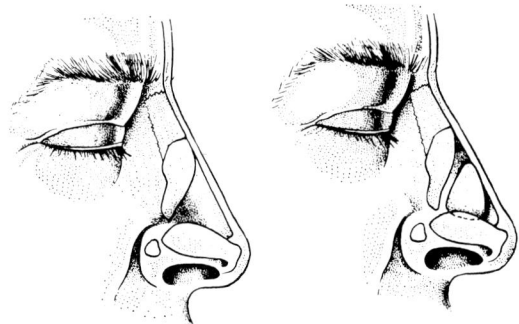

Figure 24-5. Correction of so-called *pinched nose* caused by extensive removal of cartilage in region of upper lateral cartilages or lateral portion of lower lateral cartilages. Either auricular cartilage or auricular composite grafts are used if inner lining of nose is missing also. (From Walter, C.D.: Secondary nasal revisions after rhinoplasties, ORL J. Otorhinolaryngol. Relat. Spec. 80:519-526, 1975.)

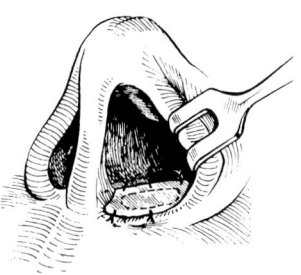

Figure 24-6. Treatment of postoperative atresia of nasal entrance by insertion of composite graft from inner aspect of helix rim or concha after scar is excised in nasal vestibule. (From Walter, C.D.: Secondary nasal revisions after rhinoplasties, ORL J. Otorhinolaryngol. Relat. Spec. 80:519-526, 1975.)

SUPRATIP DEFORMITIES

The typical supratip deformity is characterized by a flat or nonexisting tip with a thickened supratip area. These deformities arise because of excessive resection of the lower lateral cartilage. The skin of the tip and the leftover alar cartilage only hang on the nasal dorsum. After the skin is retracted the nose becomes even smaller, and the same deformity appears. The solution is adding cartilage! For the correction of such tips I favor the Goldman technique, and I augment those medial crura with additional cartilage. Sometimes the excess cartilage left in the lateral portion of the the tip can be used to advantage (Figure 24-7).

The preferred method includes augmentation with that taken from the existing nasal cartilage or from the ears. If the nose has been foreshortened the scar tissue can be excised, regardless of skin and fibrous cartilage. Then a small piece of cartilage and mucosa on the cranial portion of the septum is excised to allow placement of a composite graft from the auricle on top of the septum. The skin portion of this graft is divided to facilitate suturing the skin parts of the graft to the surrounding mucosal parts of the nose (see Figure 24-7). The composite graft is taken from the anterior portion of the concha. The nose can then be lengthened and occasionally widened. The defect at the donor site is closed from behind by an island flap or by a full-thickness free skin graft. A cartilaginous strut is inserted into the columella for additional support.

A retracted columella can be corrected at the same time by excising the inferior crus of the ear or the part where the helix begins. There is a perfectly matched cartilage that resembles the medial crura. After the skin is divided one has a perfectly suited graft to duplicate the area of columella. Such a composite graft is then inserted after a caudal transfixion incision is made.

A composite graft for inner lining should always come from the front of the concha, because the skin is attached very tightly, and such a graft resembles the internal nasal structure. An incision is made from the mastoid area through the skin and subcutaneous tissue. After the postauricular skin is incised this piece of skin is rotated on its subcutaneous pedicle forward into the conchal defect. Color match is perfect, and there is no danger of necrosis. The postauricular skin is closed directly.

The composite graft can then be trimmed as necessary. Sometimes small strips of skin and larger pieces of cartilage are left, or vice versa. The patient should be instructed to pack the nose with a little foam rubber for 4 weeks after operation.

Figure 24-7. A, Replantation of cartilage after extensive excision of septal cartilage with retraction of columella, producing hanging tip. Cartilage is specially shaped to compensate for missing anterior nasal spine. **B,** Postoperative parrot-beak deformity. After resection of residual cartilaginous hump molded piece of resected cartilage or some septal cartilage secured in same operation is placed on top of lower lateral cartilages from rim incision. **C,** Cranial portion of lower lateral cartilages are inserted into nasal septum to counterbalance postoperative tendency of contraction in region of nasal spine. Additional cartilage is important to keep nasolabial angle well stabilized. **D,** Additional implantation of cartilaginous strut into columella is mandatory. In case epithelium is lacking composite graft is used instead of plain cartilage. **E,** Donor sites for composite grafts to be used in nasal reconstruction. **F,** Postoperative short-nose deformities are best corrected by insertion of composite graft taken from anterior aspect of concha. **G,** Short columella is best treated by horizontal incision and implantation of composite graft from postauricular site, with skin and cartilage incorporated in reconstruction of columella. **H,** Correction of high nasal rim is best carried out by wide undermining of skin and alae and insertion of composite graft into resulting vestibular defect. (From Walter, C.D.: Secondary nasal revisions after rhinoplasties, ORL J. Otorhinolaryngol. Relat. Spec. 80:519-526, 1975.)

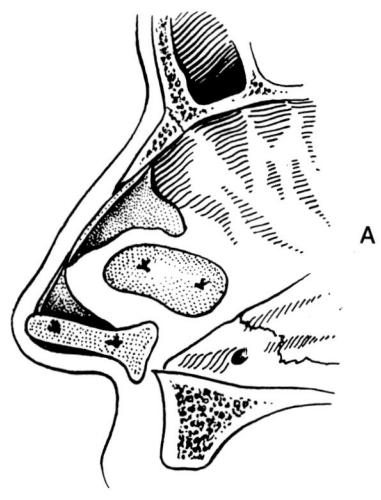

A

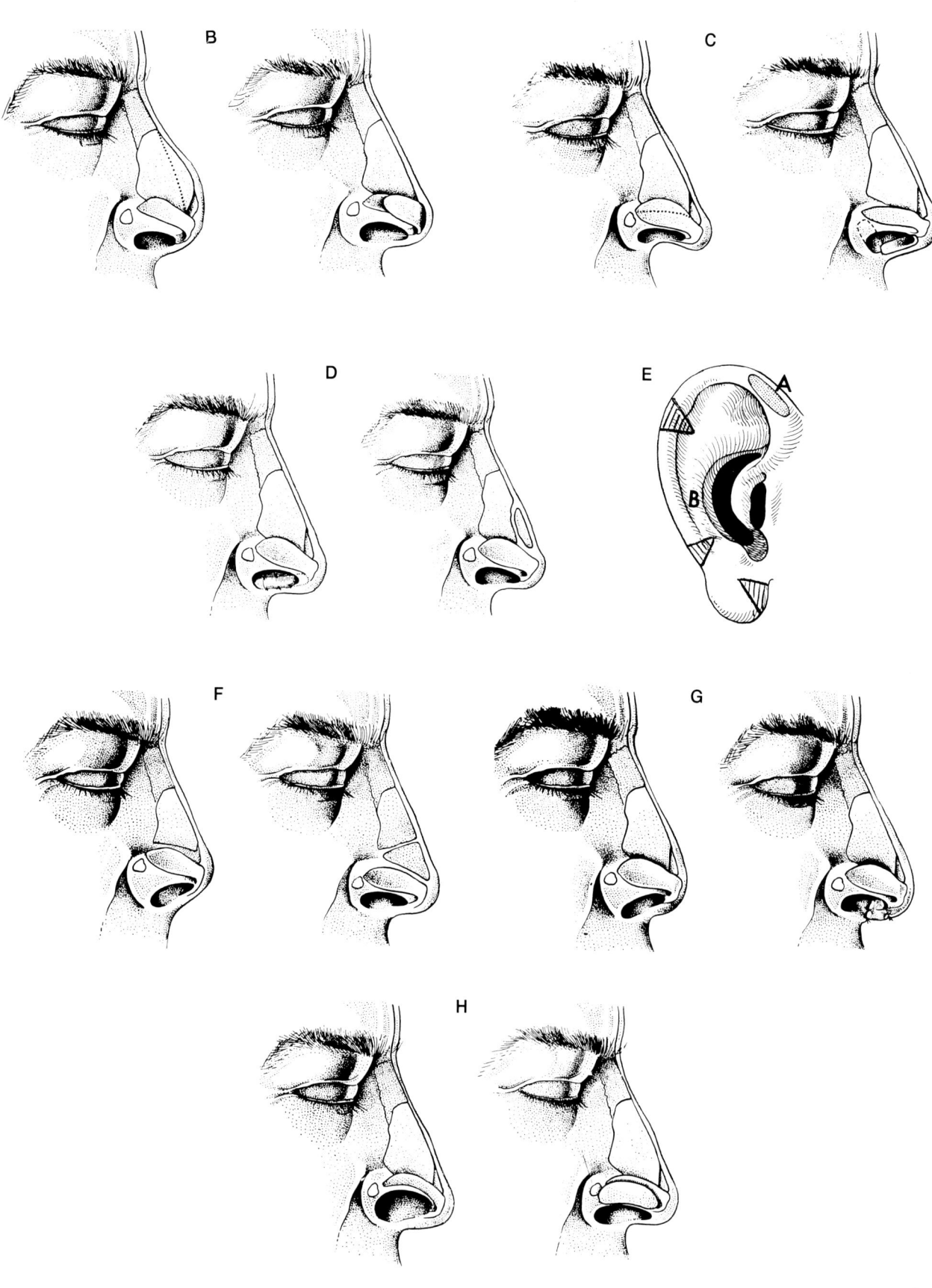

BIBLIOGRAPHY

Converse, J.M.: Reconstructive plastic surgery, ed. 2, Philadelphia, 1977, W.B. Saunders Co.

Rees, T., and Wood-Smith, D.: Cosmetic facial surgery, Philadelphia, 1973, W.B. Saunders Co.

Rogers, B.O.: Rhinoplasty. In Goldwyn, R., editor: The unfavorable result in plastic surgery. Avoidance and treatment, Boston, 1972, Little, Brown & Co.

Sheen, J.: Achieving more nasal tip projection by the use of a small autogenous bone or cartilage graft, Plast. Reconstr. Surg. 56:35, 1975.

Sheen, J.: Finesse in rhinoplasty. In Millard, D.R., editor: Symposium on corrective rhinoplasty, St. Louis, 1976, The C.V. Mosby Co.

Sheen, J.: Secondary rhinoplasty, Plast. Reconstr. Surg. 57:137, 1975.

Walter, C.: Beitrag zu korrektiven Operationen am Nasensteg und am vorderen Septum, HNO Wegw. 13:104-105, 1965.

Walter, C.: Composite grafts in nasal surgery, Arch. Otolaryngol. 90:622-630, 1969.

Walter, C.: Nasenbehinderung durch Nasenflügelkollaps und seine Korrektur. HNO Wegw. 7. Bd. S. 338-340, 1959.

Walter, C.: Secondary nasal revisions after rhinoplasties, Aesth. Plast. Surg. 2:317-329, 1978.

Walter, C.: Secondary revisions after rhinoplasties, ORL 80:520-525, 1975.

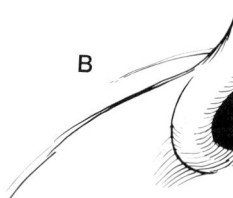

A

B

25

Surgery of the Nasal Valve

Eugene B. Kern

determined that altho
sistance was due to the
two thirds of the nasa
vicinity of the piriforn
part to the congestive
(head) of the inferio
that the entire nasal
whereas Masing,[17] in
64 mm[2]. The narrowe
is this opening of the
that specific triangula
caudal end of the up
nasal septum. The na
degrees and represent
lateral cartilage and tl
valve angle ranges bet
leptorrhine nose. The
the primary inflow r
of the inspiratory resi
the head of the inferic
valve area plays an ir
inant role as an inflo
casian (leptorrhine nc
tyrrhine nose). The na
unit that includes the
piriform aperture (floc
tissue, and frontal pr
terior head of the inf

FUNCTION OF THE

The complete fur
known. Williams[26] ha
as an inflow device (
of respiration. Hinder
sal valve controls ins
them from a column t
shape, velocity, direc
rents. Gray* has also
inferior turbinate is a
valve area, because i
tance to breathing du
Among the functi
spiratory regulation,
nasal valve area is a
tance, because the val
the narrowest portic
pointed out by Bridge
sidered to function ir
fluenced by Bernoulli
resistor consist of a s
lapsible segment (the

to see the valve
the upper lateral
10 to 15 degrees
angle is consister
the nasal valve.
and is normal in
associated with
nose because of
terations in nasa
nasal resistance.
A useful clir
of an abnormali
nasal valve is tl
breathes quietly
from the midlin
and the patient
airflow through
maneuver relieve
sidered a positiv

*Gray, V.D.: Personal comm

The nasal valve region plays a key role in nasal breathing. Physiologic studies demonstrate that this complex yet compact region significantly regulates both nasal airflow and nasal resistance. Surgical incisions in tissues adjacent to the nasal valve can produce abnormalities of the valve with the postoperative symptom of difficulty in breathing. A patient who cannot breathe through the nose after a rhinoplasty can be a most dissatisfied patient. Knowledge of the structure and function of the nasal valve region is required by all those who operate on the nose. The goals of this chapter are to present (1) definitions and a classification of abnormalities of the nasal valve region, (2) the principles, goals, and details of surgery of the nasal valve region, and (3) strategies used to avoid or minimize complications in this region, especially when cosmetic rhinoplasty is performed.

DEFINITIONS

A valve is defined as a movable structure that regulates the flow of a gas or fluid. The human nose has a number of valves. The erectile tissues of the turbinates (turbinal valve) and of the nasal septum (septal valve) can regulate the flow of air in the nose; therefore, these two tissues are nasal valves. However, specifically, the nasal valve, which was first described by Mink[21] in 1903, is usually referred to as the slitlike opening between the caudal end of the upper lateral cartilage and the nasal septum. The nasal valve is only a portion of the nasal valve area and should not be confused with the entire nasal valve area, which includes the distal end of the upper lateral cartilage, the head of the inferior turbinate, the caudal septum, and the remaining tissues surrounding the piriform aperture. The *nasal valve area*

is the narrowest portion of the nasal passage and has many synonyms: os internum, ostium internum, limen vestibuli, valve area, valve region, and area 2. The *nasal valve* itself also has several synonyms, including the liminal valve, flow-limiting segment, and liminal chink.

PERTINENT ANATOMY OF THE NASAL VALVE AREA

The external portion of the nose can be divided into three parts (Figure 25-1): the upper bony portion; a middle third, which is the roof cartilage (upper lateral cartilage) and which is in fact connected as one cartilage to the nasal septum; and the lower third of the nose, which is composed of the paired lower lateral or lobular cartilages (or also called the *alar* or *great alar cartilages*). This skeletal structure is covered by skin, muscles, neurovascular tissues, connective tissues, and mucocutaneous tissues intranasally. The upper lateral cartilage is attached proximally beneath the nasal bones by fibrous tissue. It is also supported caudally and laterally by fibrous tissue, and it extends beneath the lower lateral cartilages and out laterally to the maxilla. The upper lateral cartilage is usually separated caudally and medially by a narrow cleft from the nasal septum.

The entire *nasal valve area* extends from the region of the caudal end of the upper lateral cartilage in its relationship to the nasal septum medially, laterally to the bony point of the piriform aperture and the soft fibrofatty tissue in this region, and it is bounded below by the floor of the nose and posteriorly by the head of the inferior turbinate (Figure 25-2). Haight and Cole[11] recently investigated the nasal valve and determined the site by using "head-out" body plethysmography in 10 subjects. They

TECHNIQUE (Figure 26-1)

Dissection of the septal mucosa region is technically simple. The dissection could be performed with a view to septoplasty. The flap is detached with pointed scissors 0.5 to 1.0 cm above the columellar edge of the septum and then with an elevator along the dorsal edge. When the bony hump is reached the sharp end of the elevator is turned outward; in this way the hump is divested of its mucosal covering.

A beginner may find dissection of the lateral face of the mucosal vault a more difficult procedure to perform. The mucosa is drawn downward with dissecting forceps and dissected in situ by opening the blades of the pointed scissors. Rapid dissection upward is avoided. The upper lateral cartilage is exposed, and in a certain manner it is exteriorized (the dorsal portions of the lateral crura and of the sesamoids are involved). This edge of the cartilaginous zone is resected in continuity with the adjacent soft tissue, leading to exposure of the lower border of the superior lateral cartilage. It is then a simple matter to dissect the mucosa a length of 2 to 3 mm, maintaining the mucosa under constant tension with dissecting forceps. Pointed scissors are used, the points often being visible through the very thin cartilage.

All that remains is to free the mucosal flaps by pushing them downward with the elevator. Continuity with the dissection conducted previously is maintained at a higher level on the deep surface of the bony hump.

Fi
pa
ca
(a
re
an
m
Ke
re

ment (Figu
main colla
expiration
influence tl
cles preven
inspiratory
flaccidity o
sues would
ing. The n
in concert
to provide
the wide r

CLINICAL
VALVE

The na
tion in eve
airway obs
an anatom
dysfunctio
valve in th
need trimr
without a
relationshi
cartilage to
nose can b
or four-pro

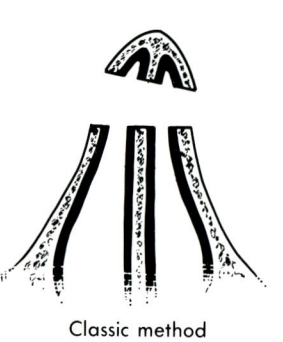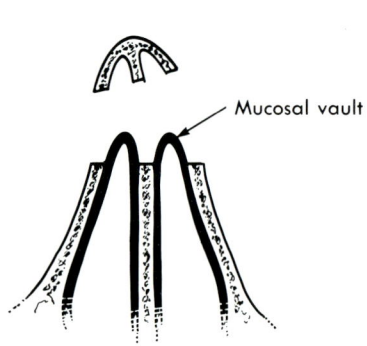

Classic method   Extramucosal method

Mucosal vault

Figure 26-1

ADVANTAGES

What are the advantages of the extramucosal method? First, it prevents the parrot-beak deformity. Several causes exist for this convex deformity of the supratip area. Cartilaginous excess is one cause that is easily corrected. The accumulation of scar tissue is also a cause; this should disappear with time and massage (the idea of a pseudokeloid" is an excuse rather than a true explanation). Finally, the most difficult type of parrot-beak deformity arises from excessive sacrifice of the mucosa behind the supratip area. This leads to retraction of the deep surface of the skin, creating a fearful deformity in the form of a watchglass. Conservation of two intact mucosal flaps constitutes a double layer, which prevents development of this formidable complication.

A second advantage of this extramucosal method is that it protects the deep surface of the skin from contact with packing (Figure 26-2). If after an accidental splinter fracture occurs the lateral wall should collapse, packing becomes necessary to provide support. If the mucosa has been resected the packing will be in contact with the deep surface of the skin and may draw the skin inward when it is removed. Conversely, if the mucosa is preserved the deep skin surface is protected against direct contact with the packing.

The third and most important advantage of the extramucosal method is that grafts can be reinserted in the dorsum with a minimum of risk. The two mucosal flaps constitute a floor that prevents the graft from falling into the nasal fossae and provides a barrier against infection.

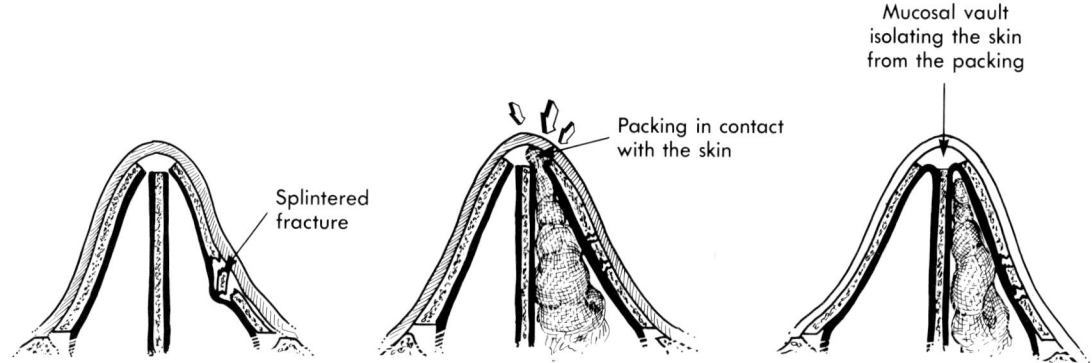

Figure 26-2. Advantages of the extramucosal technique.

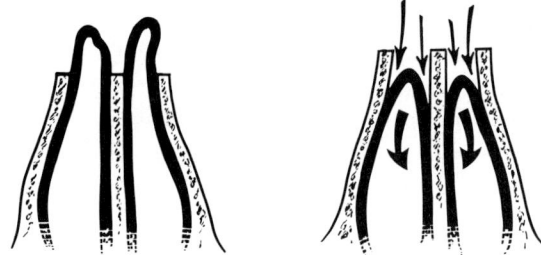

Figure 26-3. The danger of an excess of mucous membrane is avoided by the undermining.

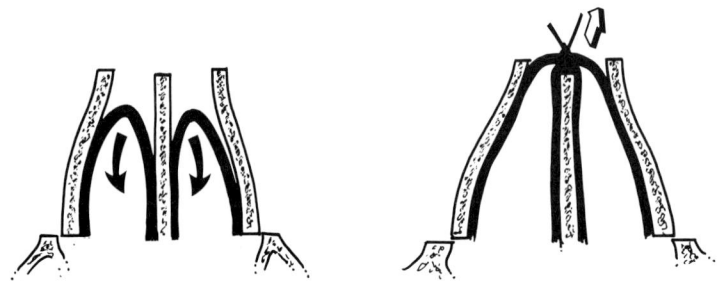

Figure 26-4. The creation of a web retraction is avoided by a U-stitch uniting the two mucosal vaults at the edge of the septum.

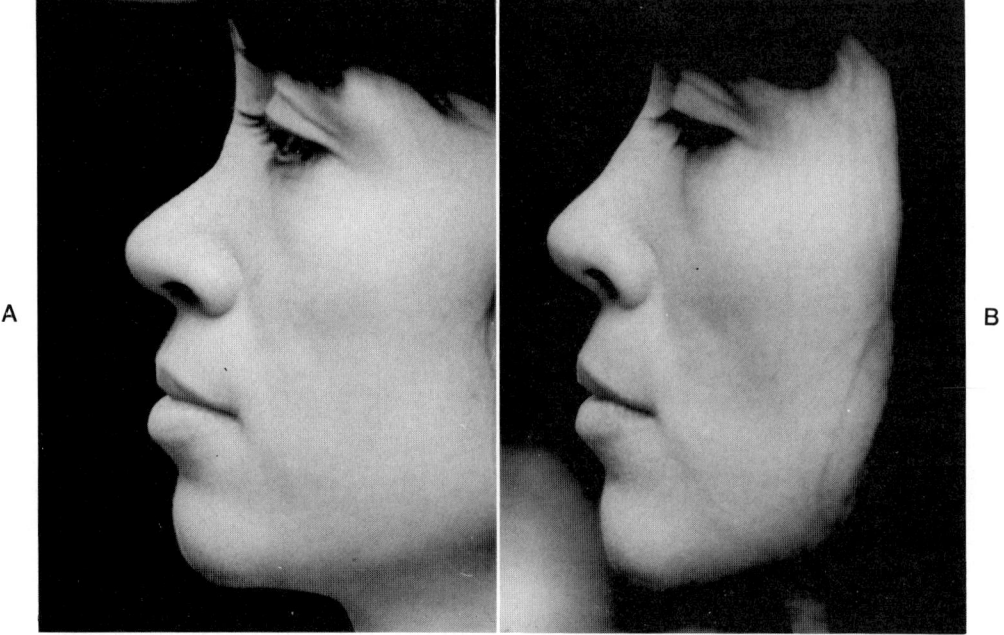

Figure 26-5. A, "Bird-beak" deformity following loss of dorsal graft at primary rhinoplasty caused by loss of mucosa. **B,** Secondary correction with a bone graft.

DISADVANTAGES

The most frequent criticism of the extramucosal method is that it creates an excess of mucosa (Figure 26-3). This could be the case in extensive resection of the hump. However, one should keep in mind that the mucosa retracts in a manner similar to skin. Retraction is facilitated by detaching the septal mucosae. To avoid creating a web at the anterior angle, the two mucosal vaults above the dorsal edge of the septum are united by submucosal stitching with catgut. The anterior angle of the vestibule than regains its normal acute character (Figure 26-4).

This suture point has never given rise to problems and has never contributed to a supratip deformity. On the contrary, the extramucosal method is one of the most effective means of avoiding the parrot-beak deformity.

The young girl in Figure 26-5, A, has a birdlike profile; such a profile can be the result when the extramucosal technique is not used. This accidental collapse could have been avoided if the surgeon had used the extramucosal procedure. Realizing, during the operation, that he had accidentally resected too much of the dorsum, the surgeon reintroduced the hump in the form of a graft. Unfortunately, since the graft was unprotected because of extensive sacrifice of mucosa, it was extruded. Two weeks later an attempt was made to introduce an auricular cartilage graft, but this also was extruded, creating a birdlike deformity. Grafting of bone was necessary to correct this deformity. An accident of this type will not occur if the mucosa is left intact. Happily, this is a rare accident.

Whenever I resect a relatively large hump I routinely reinsert it to ensure more natural contours of the dorsum and improved definition. In fact, when a large hump has been resected lateral osteotomies do not suffice to bring the edges of the hump into contact—a gap persists because of the shape of the lateral walls, which are not flat like a sheet of plywood but are convex, facing outward.

Infracture of the nose after operation produces a nicely rounded dorsum, but this is only an *illusion.* The dorsum is flat, and two lateral "rails" exist that correspond to the dorsal borders of the lateral walls (a third "rail" can appear medially if the septum is a little higher than the lateral walls) (Figure 26-6).

Fortunately for the surgeon, in most cases the subcutaneous pouch created by resection of the hump is filled with a "providential" scar tissue that masks the projecting "rail." If, however, this tissue is absorbed the dorsum is poorly defined and marked by the projection of the "rails." This anomaly of the upper part of the dorsum constitutes a veritable "signature" of the operation. It occurs frequently.

The object of reinserting the hump is to assist formation of this "providential" scar tissue, and it can be considered a "scar inducer" rather than a true graft.

The technique used by me and my colleagues differs greatly from that described by Skoog,[2] who resected the hump in a rather extensive manner, creating a slight hypercorrection. This hypercorrection was then "corrected" by reinsertion of a relatively large fragment of the osteocartilaginous hump. Without the graft the nose was slightly overcorrected, whereas insertion of the graft caused the profile to change, with improved definition but also more projection of the dorsum.

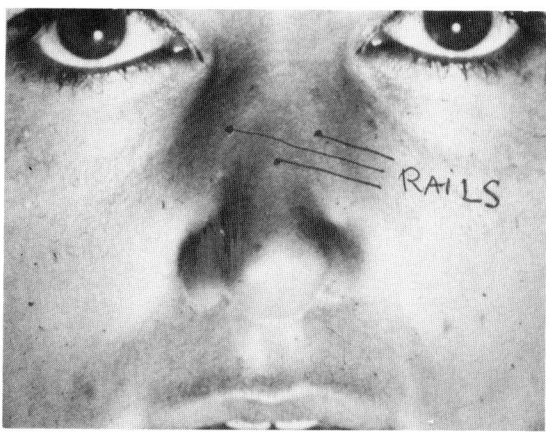

Figure 26-6. "Rails" formed by the dorsal borders of the lateral walls of the nose and the dorsal border of the septum. An inevitability in most rhinoplasties.

Our approach is quite different. We do not use an onlay graft but an inlay (Figure 26-7). When inserted, this inlay graft should fill the gap between the lateral walls; this requires that the dorsal border of the septum be further lowered slightly to provide a space. To be more precise, the profile shape remains the same with or without the inlay grafts. Remember that the role of this implantation is to guide cicatrization to allow better definition of the shape of the dorsum as *seen from the front*.

Reinsertion can be performed in three ways. First, the lateral osseocartilaginous part of the hump can be used—an excellent method but one requiring the availability of a flat, thin bone (thin as a nail), which is a rare finding. Second, the two lateral cartilages taken from the hump can be presented head to tail and fused by pressure between the jaws of crushing forceps (Figure 26-8). Finally, the septal cartilage can be used when the lateral cartilages are unsatisfactory. Since the former is too thick it has

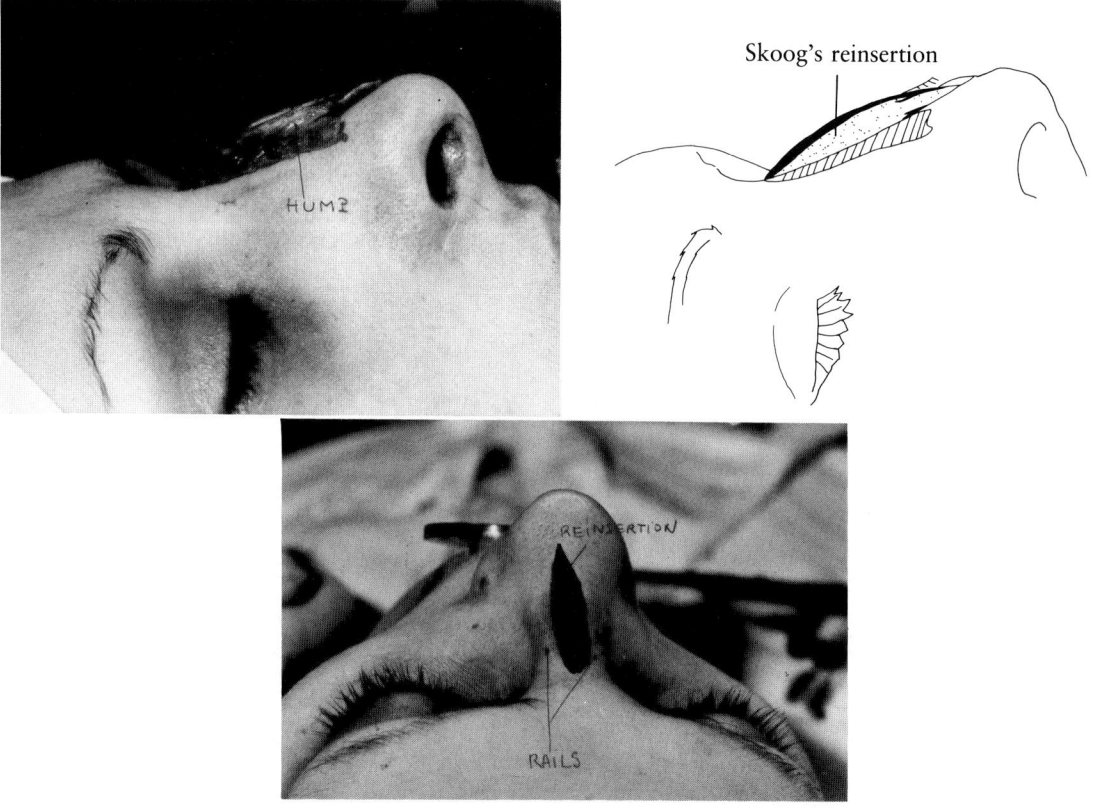

Figure 26-7. The use of an inlay graft to provide contour to the dorsal "open roof."

to be crushed with a "screw-crusher," which has one flat surface and one surface lined with horizontal bands. In this way the fragment is not only thinned but has a tendency to curl on itself, a particularly favorable feature for creating a nicely rounded dorsum.

It is obvious that when an *onlay* graft is necessary, the two mucosal flaps provide perfect protection for the graft against infection and *secondary resorption*. Moreover, insertion of the fragment contributes toward improved correction of the deviation. To use the extramucosal method is, above all, to respect anatomic structures. This procedure contributes more than any other to obtaining at the end of operation an anatomically normal and anatomically complete nose.

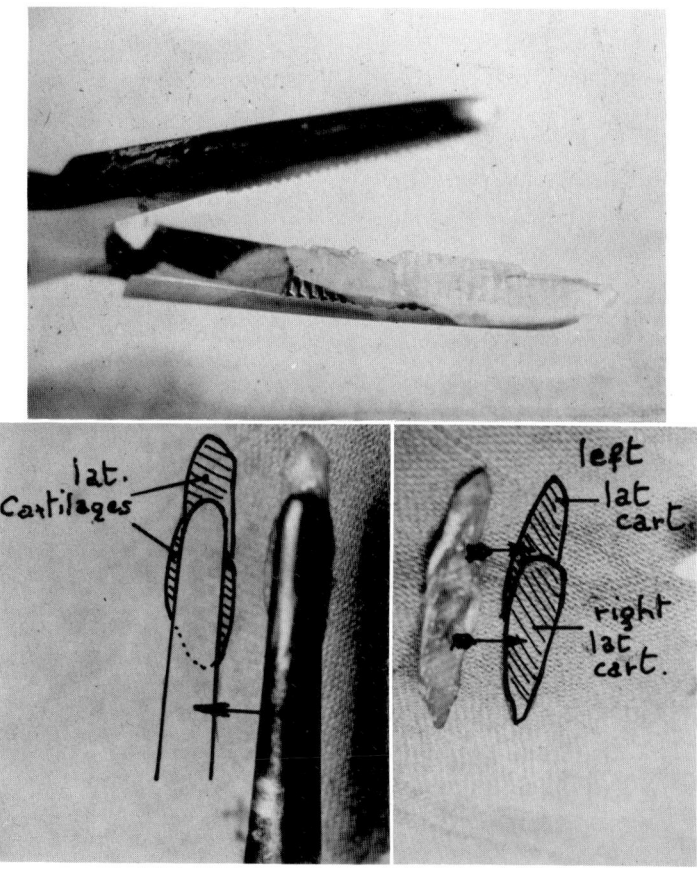

Figure 26-8. The cartilage inlays are crushed with a "screw-crusher." They are then more useable as inlays for the dorsum.

Uses of the extramucosal technique
Rodolphe Meyer

Eitner's diagram of the extramucosal technique showed the dissection of the mucoperichondrium and section of the upper lateral cartilages.[1]

The extramucosal technique can be extremely useful in elongating the nose. It may be used in noses with a pig-snout appearance and in other similar problems of nasal shortness. The dissection of the mucoperichondrial vault and section of the upper lateral cartilages at their attachment to the septal cartilage permit a sliding downward and forward of the tip-columella complex.

Another use of the extramucosal technique is found in the repair of harelip noses. We began using this approach to repair harelip noses as well as for extremely difficult septoplasties and crooked noses in the early 1960s.

We also use it in some perforations of the septum. In perforations with a diameter up to 3 cm, we achieve the closure with an extramucosal technique. For a perforation more than 3 cm in diameter, we have a three-stage procedure at our disposal; it involves a three-layered buccal mucosa flap reinforced with ear cartilage, which is transferred into the nasal cavity to fill the septal defect. We first described this technique in 1970. We can close practically every type of septal perforation with one of these two techniques.

Another important use of the extramucosal approach is the surgical treatment of the collapsed ala at the level of the valve. After one accomplishes the extramucosal dissection and section of the upper lateral cartilages, one has only to perform a transalar fixation of the upper lateral cartilages. The alae are now in a newly detached and lateralized position. The mattress sutures include the ala and the medial third of the nose.

The extramucosal technique is useful in removing the hump of the nose in two maneuvers. In the first the caudal cartilaginous part of the hump is resected with a scissor. The next step is removal of the bone with the Rowland forceps. In both steps there is no cut through the mucoperichondrium, since it has been dissected and pushed toward the lumen of the cavity. The procedure of Skoog is applied sometimes in correcting a huge hump. One removes it, reduces it in size, and reinserts it to obtain an appropriate, slightly undulated dorsum.

Hump reduction with reinsertion of the cartilaginous part of the dorsum can also be done. The remnant of the cartilaginous hump when reinserted can act as a spreader in cases of narrow medial nasal segment (Chapter 19). We occasionally move a part of the bone from the upper nasal dorsum to the lower dorsum in order to model its profile.

Extramucosal dissection

Tom Rees

Since first introduced by Eitner the technique of extramucosal dissection has been widely adopted by rhinoplastic surgeons in preference to through-and-through separation of the upper lateral cartilages from their attachment to the nasal septum. I by no means favor this technique in most of my operations; rather, I usually transect the upper lateral cartilages flush with the nasal septum with a No. 11 blade. However, in specific instances the extramucosal technique is highly advantageous, as has been pointed out by Drs. Jost, Meyer, Mühlbauer, and others.

I reserve the technique for severely twisted noses and obstructed septums, since it provides wide access to the entire osseocartilaginous structure of the nose, including the septum and the nasal bones, permitting exact sculpting of these structures. Also, in such twisted noses I usually find it necessary to replace one or more grafts of cartilage or bone or, indeed, sometimes the entire hump to restore the natural contours of the dorsum and to camouflage any deviation that might remain. In such cases, where grafts are required, it is only logical to preserve a pocket for reception of the graft that does not directly communicate with the internal nose, thereby decreasing the possibility of contamination of the biologic implant from the bacterial contents of the nose and lessening the chances of infection and extrusion. Likewise, in a very large hump with a wide base to the bony pyramid, I prefer the extramucosal technique even if the septum is straight, since I usually plan to replace part or all of the hump or skin grafts of septal cartilage to restore the dorsal con-

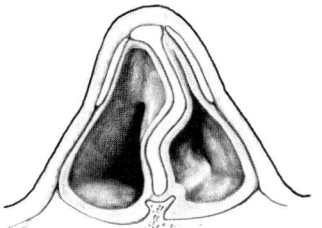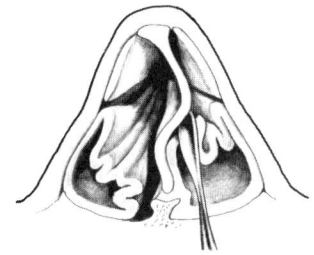

Figure 26-9. In the extramucosal technique the mucosa is dissected free and dropped like a "curtain" to permit access to the osteocartilaginous skeleton.

tours and obviate an open-roof deformity of sufficient width to be noticeable in the postoperative result. The technique has been well described by Drs. Jost and Meyer, and I can only add my recommendation of copious subperichondrial injection of local solution to provide a "hydrolic dissection" effect, which greatly facilitates the dissection. Figure 26-9 illustrates what happens to the lining. It is dropped like a curtain into the nose. After repair on the osseocartilaginous framework is completed, the flaps are elevated to their normal position and fixed in place with mattress sutures of fine, plain catgut threaded back and forth through the full thickness of septum. I have not found it necessary to suture them above the level of the septum as recommended by Dr. Jost.

REFERENCES

1. Eitner, E. (Cited by Jost, 1975): Jost, G., and Legent, F.: Atlas de chirurgie ésthetique plastique, Masson et cie, pp. 30-46, Paris, 1934.
2. Skoog, T: A method of hump reduction in rhinoplasty, Arch. Otolaryngol. 83:556, 1952.

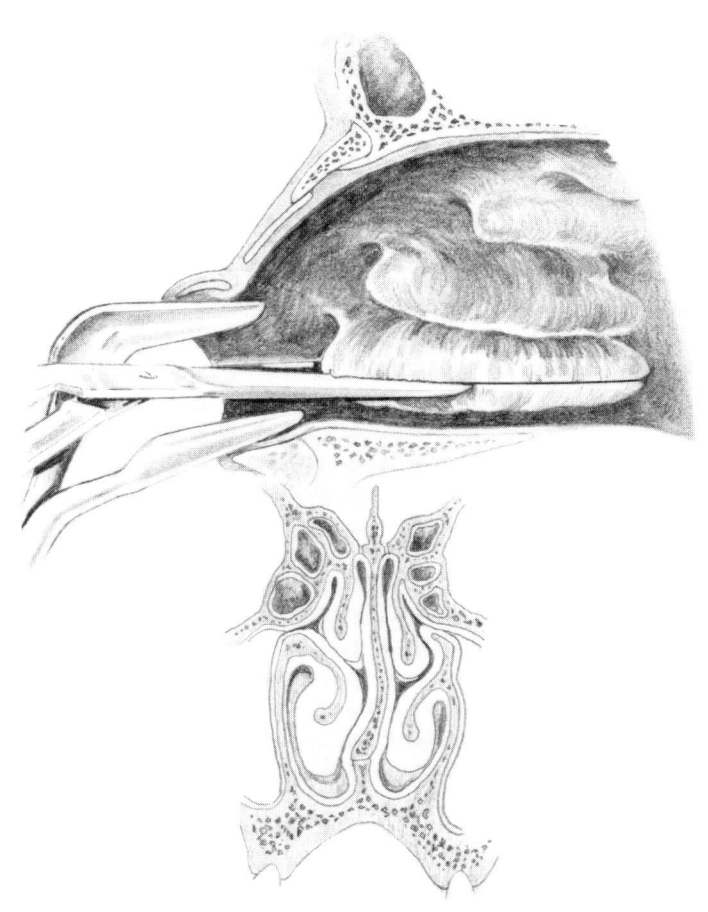

27

Turbinate Obstruction: Causes and Surgical Techniques in Resection

Eugene Courtiss

Historically, various techniques have been used to manage hypertrophied turbinates. Various caustics have been injected; sodium morrhuate has been injected into the inferior turbinate. The inferior turbinate has been scarified by various techniques. Some surgeons have crushed it, others have outfractured it. Electrocoagulation has been espoused by many, and cryosurgery is suggested by some authors; other authors have published their results with the use of steroids. One author recommended treatment by resection.

One of three things allegedly happens if one resects an inferior turbinate. One may encounter ozena. Ozena is an obliterating endarteritis. I do not believe that this occurs after resection of the turbinate. Another alleged sequela is rhinitis sicca, characterized by drying, crusting, a loss of cilia, and hypertrophy of the turbinate. Another is atophic rhinitis, a condition that follows a suppurating sinus infection, that destroys turbinate bone, and that is accompanied by a *round cell infiltrate*.

Normal turbinate mucosa has pseudostratified columnar epithelium with goblet cells, a thin basement membrane, and serous and mucous glands. There is a very thin lining underneath the mucosa. The mucosa is rich in vascular channels, a very vascular organ.

If you biopsy an obstructing turbinate you find pseudostratified columnar epithelium, the serous and mucous glands remain, and round cells are seen. These are plasma cells. The plasma cells were not known in 1934 when Roskin described atrophic rhinitis. he mistook the plasma cells for lymphocytes.

The vascularity of the organ remains after resection of the turbinate.

CAUSES OF TURBINATE OBSTRUCTION

What are the causes of turbinate obstruction? One cause is compensatory turbinate hypertrophy caused by deviation of the septum. Turbinate hypertrophy may also be caused by allergies, medications, vasomotor disturbances, dust, tobacco, hyperthyroidism, pregnancy, or emotional problems, or it may have nasogenital origins, where the turbinates enlarge as a result of excessive sexual stimulation.

RESECTION—SURGICAL TECHNIQUES

Before the turbinates are resected the nose is packed with epinephrine solution to shrink the lining. The turbinates are injected with local anesthetic. The turbinate is fractured in a cephalad direction with a Joseph elevator so that the scissor blade can be placed underneath it (Figure 27-1). A double-action turbinate scissor is used. One blade is placed beneath the turbinate and the other blade on top. The scissor is closed and the specimen produced. The specimen is about 3 cm long and contains mostly soft tissue. It may have bone. The scissor sometimes does not cut the tissue cleanly; in that case a pituitary forceps works reasonably well.

Turbinate resection need not be radical. The lateral nasal wall and the middle turbinate need not be removed. Since the middle turbinate provides the mucus to the nose, I do not recommend its removal (Figure 27-2).

The turbinates are highly vascular, and bleeding must be controlled by packing. The pack I prefer is compressed Gelfoam.

It can be cut into small strips; five or six of these may be gripped in bayonet forceps and used in tandem. One of my patients needed a transfuion. However, since I began using the Gelfoam pack no others have required a transfusion.

Results of turbinate resections have been good in a series of 88 patients who were suffering from turbinate problems. Many of these patients had allergies and had previously undergone surgery of the

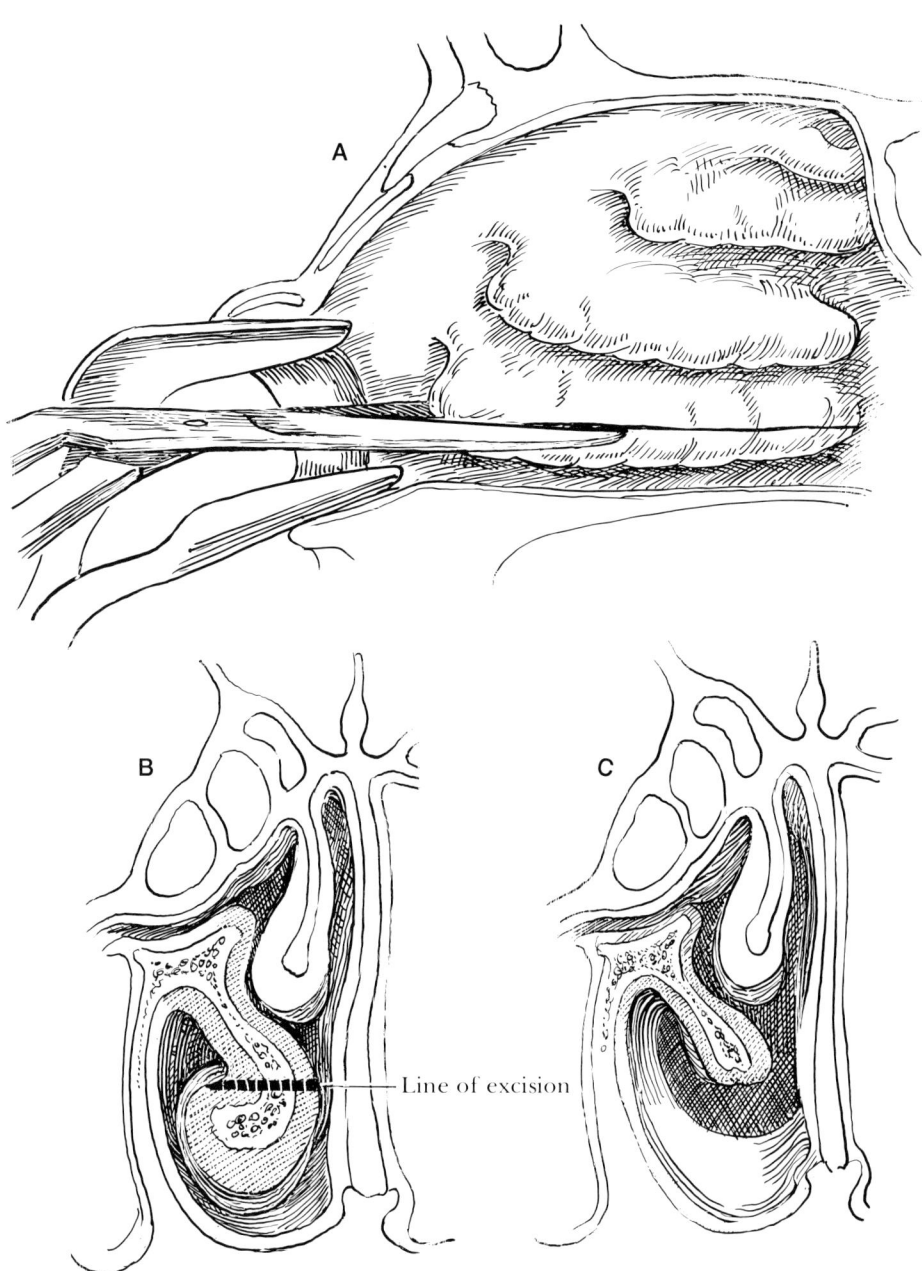

Figure 27-1. Resection of inferior turbinate. **A,** Angled scissors placed with vertical orientation to resect portion of hypertrophied mucosa and bone. **B,** Gelfoam or Avitene should be used to cover raw edge of turbinate to help prevent hemorrhage. **C,** Final result after healing. Remaining soft tissue of turbinate may hypertrophy again, causing obstruction. (From Rees, T.D.: Aesthetic plastic surgery, vol. 1, Philadelphia, 1980, W.B. Saunders Co.)

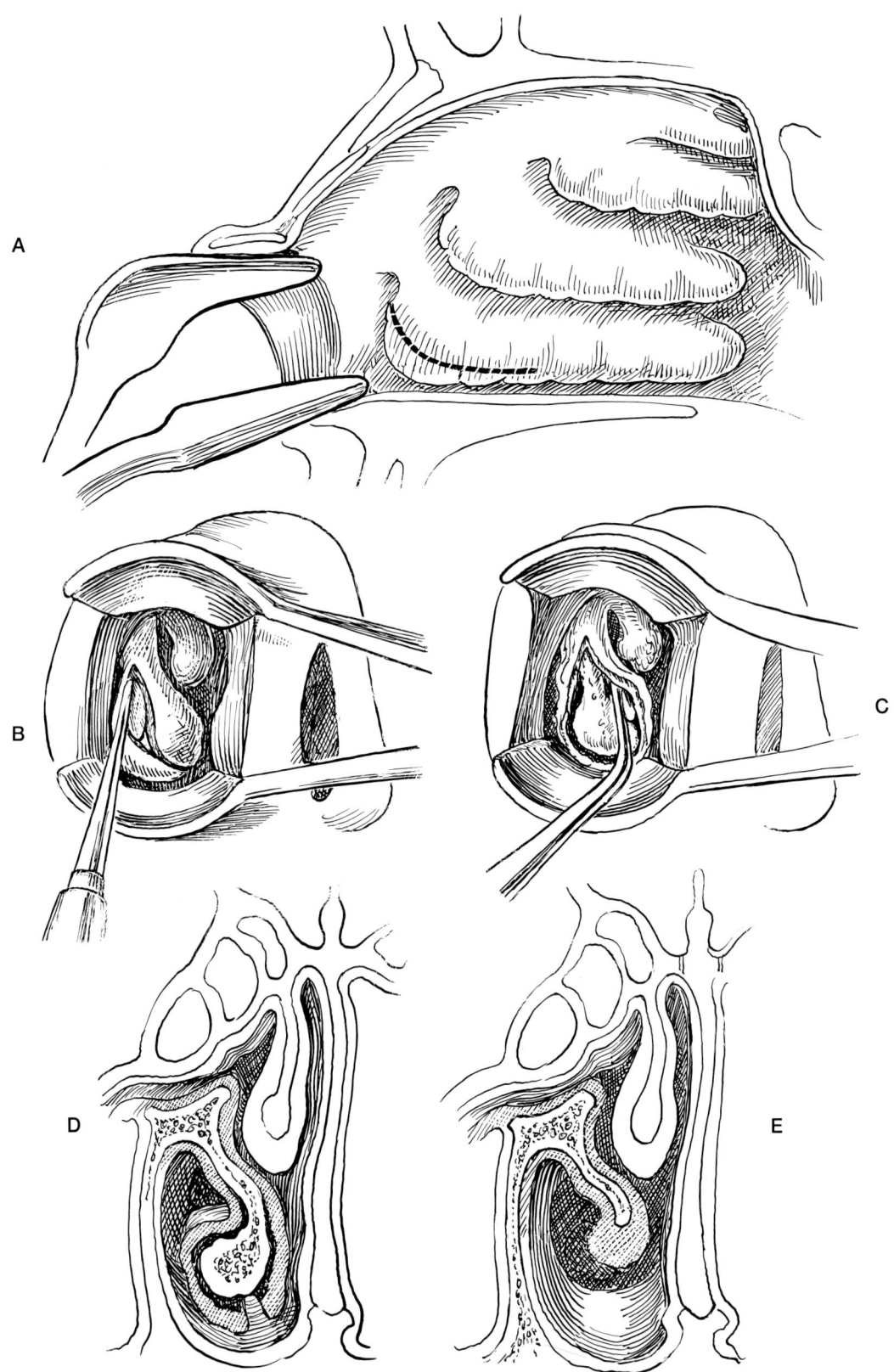

Figure 27-2. Submucous resection of turbinate bone. **A,** Curved incision down to bone over anterior inferior edge of turbinate. **B,** Mucoperiosteum and submucosa elevated off medial and lateral surfaces of conchal bone up to its attachment with lateral wall. **C,** Hypertrophied bone excised with angled scissors. (From Rees, T.D.: Aesthetic plastic surgery, vol. 1, Philadelphia, 1980, W.B. Saunders Co.)

septum or were dependent on nasal spray to improve their breathing. Many of these patients also had aesthetic rhinoplasty performed simultaneously. Follow-up in this series was 2 to 37 months. Six or seven years have now elapsed. All of the patients except two reported feeling better, as supported by objective evidence, after turbinectomy. The patients were asked the following question after surgery: "Do you breathe better, worse, or the same after your operation?" The response given most frequently was "I don't know what you did, Doctor, but I now breathe better." Thus the patients appeared to be satisfied with the results of this surgery.

I have yet to see a single intranasal problem caused by removal of the turbinate. Yet, I was taught, as many others were also, that atrophic rhinitis, rhinitis sicca, or ozena would appear if the turbinates were removed. I believe this attitude about turbinate surgery dates back to the 1930s when the lateral nasal wall was removed in the treatment of chronic sinus disease.

In a rhinomanometric study Dr. Robert Goldwyn and I evaluated patients by means of a technique not too dissimilar to the one described by Dr. Kern. We found that evaluation by individuals of their own airway was questionable. Many patients believed that their airways were quite satisfactory. Yet, on examination we found the airway to be decreased and obstructed. Many others said "I can't breathe through my nose," but examination revealed normal flow rates and no evidence of intranasal pathosis. Patients were unable to correctly identify their own airway problems because they lacked a standard of comparison. A patient's ability to identify his or her problem may also be linked to insurance coverage. Patients want the cost of their operations covered by insurance, so they will often state they are having trouble through their noses or that they have a septal deviation in the belief that their insurance will cover the cost of the operation.

Several problems are associated with turbinate resection. First, if the resection is done with a local anesthetic, obtaining satisfactory anesthesia may be a concern. I have not used a sphenopalatine block. Instead, I ensure that the patient is adequately sedated and that the topical anesthetic has had time to take effect.

A second problem is bleeding. I have not used electrocoagulation. It is very difficult to fit an electrocautery device inside the nose through a nasal speculum. The blood pressure obviously must be controlled. A patient with a systolic blood pressure at 200 mm Hg and a diastolic pressure of 150 mm Hg is going to bleed freely. I pack with epinephrine during the operation; postoperatively I have used Avatine, Surgicel, or Gelfoam.

A third problem is the occurrence of synechiae. They are best prevented by avoiding a raw area between the septum and turbinate. The nose should be cleaned often and early with peroxide and an applicator stick. If a synechia occurs anesthesia should be induced, the adhesion divided, and the raw surface splintered apart with silicone plates until healing occurs.

Turbinate resection does have a place in rhinoplasty. If the airway obstruction is due to septal deviation, the septum should be the focus of treatment, but if the airway obstruction is caused by turbinate hypertrophy, then the turbinate hypertrophy is the focus. In my experience resection of obstructing inferior turbinates is a safe procedure that will help patients.

Point & Counterpoint
Parts VI, VII & VIII

Question: How much of the turbinate do you resect, and what do you identify as specific indications for turbinectomy?

Comment (Eugene Courtiss): Resect as much turbinate as is required to relieve the obstruction, usually about 75%; however, quantitating the resection is difficult. What is resected is not important; what is left is important.

Resection of the turbinate is indicated when the patient's airway is obstructed because of hypertrophy of the inferior turbinate, and I emphasize the word *inferior*. I have never resected a *middle* turbinate whose function is production of mucus.

Question: Dr. Kern mentioned atrophy in his study. Atrophy of what and after what? What is the incidence of atrophy for turbinectomy?

Comment (Eugene Kern): I have seen atrophy of the mucosa in patients who have had turbinectomies (done elsewhere), patients who had submucous resection, and patients with septal perforations. If you were to biopsy the mucosa and look at the submucosa, you would find thin atrophic changes. Vascularity is decreased when compared to that in normal subjects. So when we speak about atrophy we are talking about histopathologic changes in the mucosa and submucosa. I cannot give you an exact number of patients who had resections of the submucosa and then developed atrophy. It seems, however, that the literature cites evidence of nasal trauma, surgical or nonsurgical, that produced changes in the mucosa and submucosa accompanied by decreases in functioning of cilia and decreases in the glandular population; these decreases then produced the symtoms of dryness and crusting. The nasal chambers seem more patent, and concomitant to that is the patient's complaint of difficulty in breathing.

I believe I have performed turbinate surgery on no more than 20 patients, and perhaps this small number is the result of my concern about what might occur. I have been taught that atrophy develops slowly; it will not be seen immediately. The age of the patient at the time of total turbinectomy may also influence the development of atrophy. Certainly I don't know all the physiologic factors in the development of atrophy.

Question: What percentage of patients undergo turbinectomies in your rhinoplasty practice?

Comment (Eugene Courtiss): At least 75%.

Question: If there is a strong allergic history do you advocate a more conservative treatment first, before turbinectomy? Do you try treatment with antihistamines or any other type of treatment?

Comment (Eugene Courtiss): If the patient has a *strong* history of allergy, I refer the patient to a doctor who specializes in allergies. However, I do not refer the "average patient". I do a turbinate resection instead. In my experience medical treatment does not provide permanent relief of airway obstruction caused by hypertrophy of the turbinate. I don't administer steroids or antihistamines either systemically or in sprays; they have too many side effects, and surgery is more direct, is more permanent, and has fewer side effects.

My patients with turbinate resections now number more than 500. I have never seen an adverse sequela. In addition, I am unaware of a single case in the literature where a partial resection of the inferior turbinate was followed by the development of atrophic rhinitis. Incidentally, atrophic rhinitis is seen in patients who have not had surgery of any type.

Dr. Robert Goldwyn and I have reviewed our original 88 patients, at this point between 6½ to 9½ years after operation. None of them has developed dry nose. That fact dispels the argument of "it takes time to develop," for which there is no evidence.

One last comment, the teaching that turbinate resection causes atrophic rhinitis has an almost religious fervor. This fervor dates back to the preantibiotic 1930s when chronic sinus disease was endemic in this country and otolaryngologists were resecting the inferior *and* middle turbinates *plus* the lateral nasal wall to provide drainage from the maxillary sinus. I suspect that the problems those patients had were due to the *radical* nature of the surgery.

Question: Do you resect the compensatory turbinate caused by deviation of the septum, or does it, in reality, shrink to normal after the septal problem is corrected?

Comment (Eugene Courtiss): I resect it because a better airway is provided. Furthermore, if the hypertrophy is due to bone enlargement, no shrinking will occur.

I am not sure anyone has proved that correction of the septal problem is, a priori, followed by "shrinkage" of the turbinate.

Comment (Eugene Kern): I would have to evaluate the situation, of course. If the turbinate responds to decongestion, then I would probably consider that physiologic compensation. If, on the other hand, it does not respond to decongestion because of hyperplastic mucosa obstructing the airway, then I would consider limited removal of that tissue. Some patients have problems after turbinate surgery, and I do not think it is necessarily important to remove those turbinates and then to follow the course of that patient to see whether or not atrophy occurs. In fact, if functioning cilia and glandular tissue are lost, atrophy can and does occur. The unifying point here is that you need to be cautious and you need to make an accurate diagnosis. If the turbinate is hyperplastic and swollen and will not decongest, then turbinate surgery is something you want to consider. On the other hand, if the turbinate is swollen because of a physiologic change, then you have to be careful in operating on such a patient, because atrophy can and does occur.

Another point should be made about physiology. Turbinectomy decreases resistance needed to expand the lung tissue. One function of the nose is to provide resistance and, I believe and have demonstrated that, without sufficient resistance the patient will complain of difficulty in breathing, a problem that may cause changes in the pulmonary system. Also, it has been noted that resistance is necessary to expand the chest.

Question: Do any of you decompress the middle turbinate as described by Dr. Cottle? Has anyone had experience with resecting the middle turbinate? (It certainly is done in tumor surgery.) And do you think this may or may not have an adverse effect?

Comment (Eugene Kern): In polypoid degeneration of the turbinate and inflammatory diseases, the middle turbinate on occasion has been removed or destroyed by the disease process itself. At other times it has been inadvertently removed during ethmoidectomy because of the extent of the disease process. In general, in my opinion, the middle turbinate should be preserved. I don't know much about the function of the middle turbinate, whether it is involved in reflexes or whether or not it has a cybernetic function, so I try to preserve it if I can.

Concerning the middle turbinate compression syndrome described by Dr. Cottle, I have seen patients who complain of headaches because of impaction of middle turbinate against the septum in that region. You may want to treat that region with cocaine, and if you are able to relieve the symptoms of headache or pressure, then a judicious outfracture in that area may be of benefit. I don't have hard data on this approach, but I know that some patients have been relieved of these symptoms by this limited procedure.

Question: Turbinates are dynamic (i.e., one swells and the other shrinks). Which one should be resected, or should both be resected?

Comment (Eugene Courtiss): In *most* patients both have to be resected. However, in the presence of a septal deviation the one on the side to which the septum is deviated may not need resection.

PART

IX

CORRECTION OF THE DEVIATED NOSE

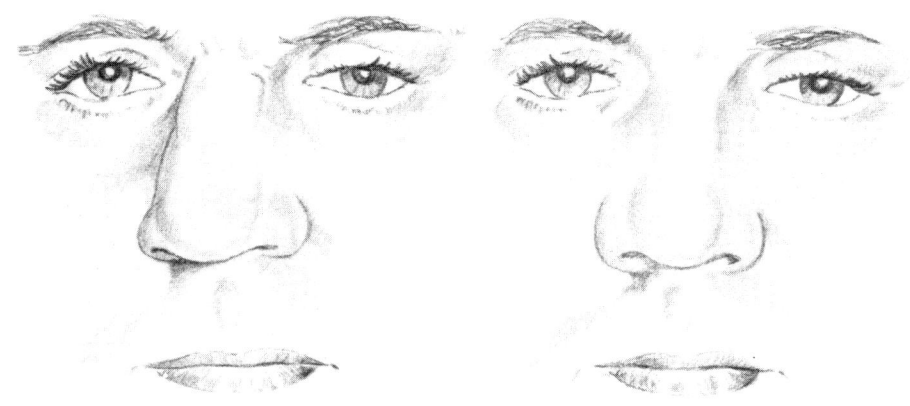

28

Nasal Septal Reconstruction

Eugene B. Kern

Do you perform submucous resections? If so, why? Have you had postoperative problems with this procedure? Are patients still complaining of nasal breathing difficulties? The causes of nasal breathing difficultes are legion. Most can be classified as either mucosal, structural, or a combination of these. The main thrust of this chapter is to discuss the concept of reconstruction of the nasal septum to treat structural abnormalities that produce problems in nasal breathing. I assert that this reconstruction is a surgical evolutionary step beyond the submucous resection that allows correction of numerous septal deformities that are not amenable to submucous resection. Pearson and Goodman[16] have stated that "an open mind is just as important to the production of an open nose as it was at the turn of the century."

Mine is an ambitious communication, because it was spawned of a desire to change ideas. Consequently it is offered in the hope that it will be read with an open mind. Consider therefore that the classic submucous resection is but a limited surgical procedure, because it deals with only a portion of the septal skeleton that is capable of producing nasal airway obstruction. Before this subject is discussed an exact definition of terms should be introduced.

What is a submucous resection? The *submucous window resection*, as Killian[9] called it, classically involves removal of cartilaginous or bony septum (or both) that obstructs the nasal airway. In the submucous resection an adequate caudal and dorsal strut of quadrangular cartilage is left intact (Figure 28-1). Theoretically this remaining caudal and dorsal strut of cartilage prevents changes in the cartilaginous dorsum and averts a saddle-nose deformity. Thus, in the submucous resection only the central portion of the nasal septum (Cartilaginous or bony) is removed, and a caudal or dorsal portion remains.

What is a nasal septal reconstruction? It also involves resection or removal of cartilaginous or bony septum (or both), but it also includes *access* to and *reconstruction* of all parts of the septum (including its extension, the upper lateral cartilage) that are capable of obstructing the nasal airway (Figure 28-2).

Both operations are primarily designed to bring about improved nasal respiratory function.

The pioneer work of E. Fletcher Ingals[7] and Otto T. Freer[5] both of Chicago, and Gustav Killian[9] of Freiburg, Germany, led to modern, nonmutilating, mucosa-preserving surgical techniques for the nasal septum that culminated in the submucous resection. This was a giant stride in relieving nasal airway obstruction but just the first step in this field. Unfortunately the dictum of preserving the caudal end of the septum and the dorsal septum as a strut (submucous resection) is a limited concept in the total surgical approach for relief of nasal airway obstruction caused by abnormalities of the septum. The idea that these structures are not to be removed has filtered down through the decades as a basic tenet and a philosophic concept to be followed assiduously, lest serious and potentially disfiguring cosmetic and nasal respiratory sequelae should become clearly apparent, even to the casual observer, not to mention to the patient. "Beyond Killian thou shall not go" lurked in the collective subconscious of many rhinologic surgeons as evidenced by the fact that the submucous resection is still being widely advocated and practiced today.

It was patient dissatisfaction that prompted scientific investigation of the reasons for the failure of some operations on the septum. The imperfect results in patients with nasal obstruction rallied the curious. Thus the question was asked "Why were

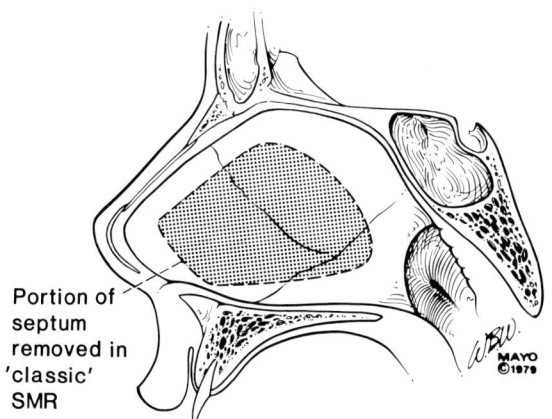

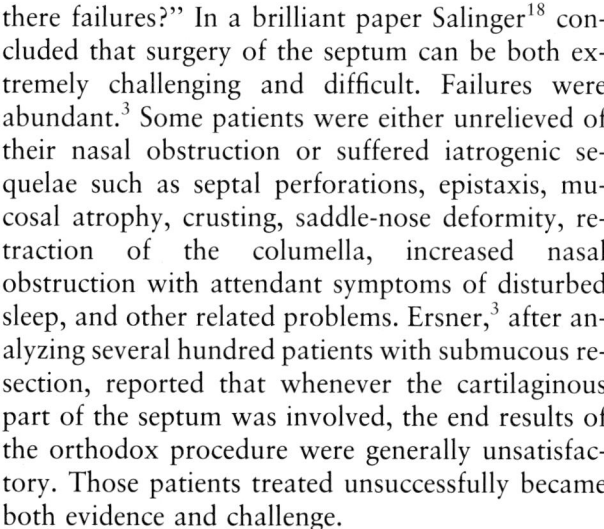

Figure 28-1. Shaded area represents portions of nasal septum that can be approached by submucous resection *(SMR)*. (By permission of Mayo Foundation.)

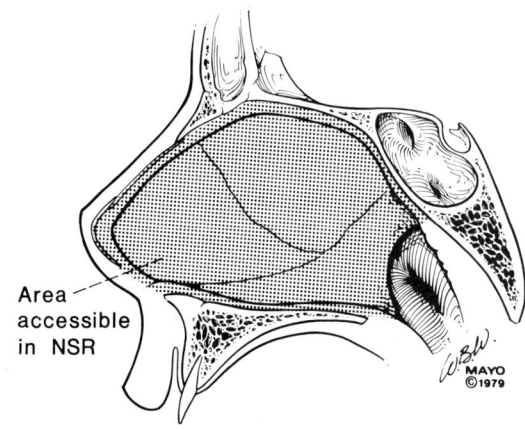

Figure 28-2. Structures of nasal septum *(shaded area)* and upper lateral cartilage that can be approached by nasal septal reconstruction. (By permission of Mayo Foundation.)

there failures?" In a brilliant paper Salinger[18] concluded that surgery of the septum can be both extremely challenging and difficult. Failures were abundant.[3] Some patients were either unrelieved of their nasal obstruction or suffered iatrogenic sequelae such as septal perforations, epistaxis, mucosal atrophy, crusting, saddle-nose deformity, retraction of the columella, increased nasal obstruction with attendant symptoms of disturbed sleep, and other related problems. Ersner,[3] after analyzing several hundred patients with submucous resection, reported that whenever the cartilaginous part of the septum was involved, the end results of the orthodox procedure were generally unsatisfactory. Those patients treated unsuccessfully became both evidence and challenge.

Even earlier, Metzenbaum[13] realized and wrote that the submucous resection falls short of dealing with all abnormalities producing obstruction of the nasal airway. Obstruction obviously may be produced by abnormalities at the caudal end of the septum, the anterior nasal spine, the premaxilla, the dorsal portion of the septum, and the upper lateral cartilage, which are extensions of the septum and are not amenable to submucous resection. These deformities of the caudal end can produce severe obstruction of the nasal airway with symptoms of insufficiency in nasal breathing. This clinically supported observation prompted the surgical attempts by Metzenbaum[13], Peer[17], Seltzer[19], Fomon and colleagues,[4] and others to deal with the problem of the caudal-end deformity that produced both cosmetic and functional (breathing) disturbances. In ad-

dition, an abnormality of the nasal valve (the slitlike opening between the caudal end of the upper lateral cartilage and the nasal septum) is also capable of producing nasal airway obstruction. Surgery for nasal airway obstruction must therefore include treatment of the caudal end of the septum and of the valve. The function and surgery of the nasal valve are covered in Chapter 25. To operate on the entire nasal septum for nasal airway obstruction, the surgeon must go beyond the concept of submucous resection (which by definition leaves the caudal and dorsal septum intact) to nasal septal reconstruction (which by definition approaches and reconstructs the entire septum and its extension, the upper lateral cartilage) when indicated by the extent of the deformity.

Careful thinkers recognized that a posterior septal deformity alone did not constitute the major or predominant cause of nasal airway obstruction; the clinician realized that it was the caudal end of the septum, where significant airway obstruction could be produced by minimal skeletal deformities. Thus reflective surgeons transcended tradition, and valiant attempts were made to mobilize the caudal end of the septum to relieve nasal airway obstruction. Other procedures were explored in attempts to deal with nasal septal and external nasal deformities that were intimately associated with nasal airway obstruction. The rigid thesis that anatomic deformities deep within the nose were exclusively responsible for all cases of nasal airway obstruction was rejected overwhelmingly by the observations of astute people.

The Freer[5] and Killian[9] concept of submucous window resection that initiated an era comes to rest in the rhinologic "hall of fame" as the forerunner of the more encompassing idea of nasal septal reconstruction. The submucous resection properly replaced the previous traumatic, mucosa-sacrificing, septum-crushing procedures advocated by sincere, dedicated physicians who attempted to relieve the suffering of those with nasal airway obstruction. Submucous resection was directed toward resection of septal abnormalities that were neither at the caudal nor at the dorsal edge of the septal cartilage. Nasal septal reconstruction is directed toward of all parts of the septum—including its extension, the upper lateral cartilage—for relief of nasal breathing insufficiency.

ABNORMALITIES AND AREAS OF THE NOSE

Maurice H. Cottle of Chicago, according to Hinderer[6], suggested delineating five areas of the nose so that localization of abnormalities might be more specific. Each area is identified by a specific number, which is a convenience both for keeping records and for conveying information about given regions of the nasal cavities (Figure 28-3, *A*).

Septal deformities of area 1 (the caudal end of the quadrangular cartilage) and area 2 (the dorsal portion of the quadrangular cartilage and upper lateral cartilage) plus the anterior nasal spine and premaxillary crest are not approachable by submucous resection and therefore are not treatable by this method. All deformities of the septum in these regions are capable of producing nasal breathing insufficiency. In reviewing patients who had symptoms of upper airway obstruction but who had not undergone rhinoplasty, Bridger[1] noted that the most common deformity was in the caudal end of the septum (area 1) (Figure 28-3 *B*). He recognized that deformities of the caudal end of the septum were aggravated by changes in the columella caused by retraction, local scars, and spurs and deviations in the maxillary crest (premaxilla) and anterior nasal spine, all of which produced asymmetries of the nostrils. Bridger substantiated his observations by hard rhinomanometric data in 10 patients. He used a technique of maximum inspiratory flow and plotted the resultant flow-pressure data to prove the point.

Although the nasal valve and the pertinent surgery of that region is covered in Chapter 25, some introductory concepts concerning the nasal valve and its role in understanding the concept of nasal septal reconstruction will be offered here. The upper lateral cartilage is an extension of the nasal septal cartilage

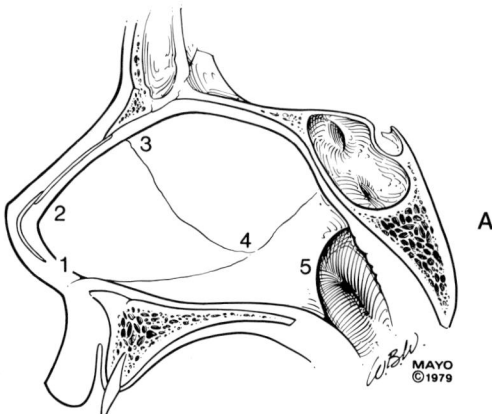

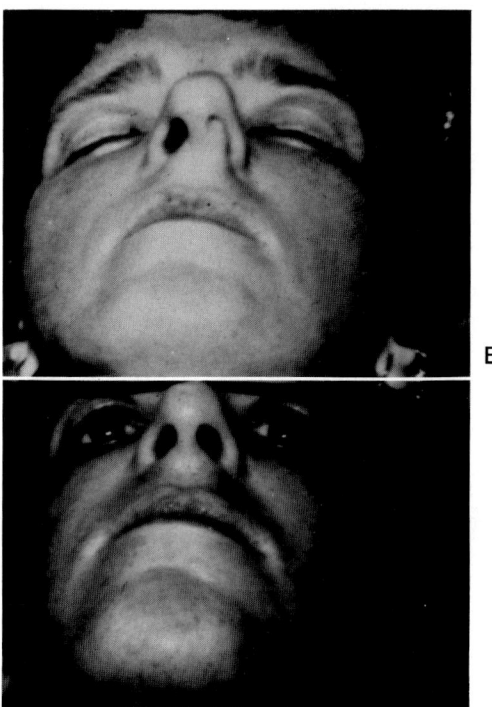

Figure 28-3. A, Areas of the nose. *Area 1,* vestibular area, is region of caudal end of septum in its relationship to anterior nares. *Area 2,* liminal valve area or nasal valve is the region where caudal end of upper lateral cartilage joins nasal septum. *Area 3,* attic area, is the area of nasal septum beneath bony vault of nasal bones. *Area 4* is anterior turbinate area. *Area 5* is posterior turbinate area in region of choana. **B,** *Above:* caudal septal deformity in area 1 obstructs left nasal chamber; *below:* postoperative photograph after caudal end of septum was repaired by nasal septal reconstruction with use of maxilla-premaxilla approach. (A by permission of Mayo Foundation.)

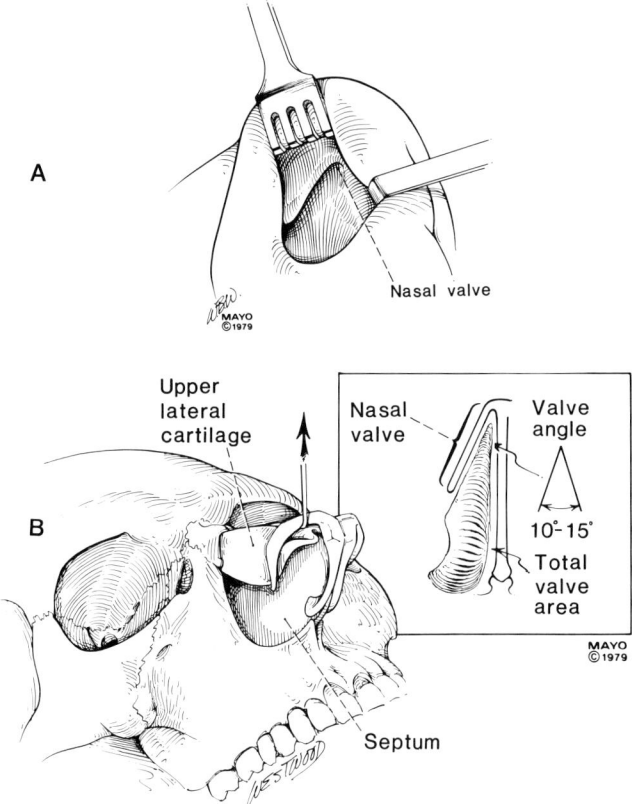

Figure 28-4. **A,** Clinical view of nasal valve *(area 2)*. Region is between caudal end of upper lateral cartilage and nasal septum. Note use of retractor to expose nasal valve. When nasal speculum is used, care must be taken not to obscure nasal valve. **B,** Nasal valve area is bounded by nasal septum, caudal end of upper lateral cartilage, and soft fibrofatty tissue overlying piriform aperture and floor of nose and posteriorly by head of inferior turbinate. Area is shaped like inverted cone or teardrop, slitlike apex of which is nasal valve angle, which normally subtends angle of 10 to 15 degrees. (By permission of Mayo Foundation.)

and an important component of the nasal valve.

The nasal valve is usually referred to (as mentioned earlier) as that slitlike opening between the caudal end of the upper lateral cartilage and the nasal septum, and it was first described by Mink[14] (Figure 28-4, *A*). The nasal valve is only a portion of the nasal valve area and should not be confused with the entire circumference of the nasal valve area, which includes the upper lateral cartilage, the septal cartilage, floor of the nose and piriform aperture, head of the inferior turbinate, and the mucocutaneous covering of these structures (Figure 28-4, *B*). Although the human nose contains a number of valves (direction and flow regulators of air), including the erectile tissues of the turbinates (turbinal valve) and of the nasal septum (septal valve), the nasal valve is the narrowest portion of the nasal passage. It has many synonyms for example, os internum, ostium internum, flow-limiting segment, liminal valve, liminal chink, limen vestibulum, valve area, valve region, and area 2. Anatomically, the upper lateral cartilage, which is an extension of the septal cartilage (Figure 28-5), is attached firmly at its proximal end beneath the nasal bones. It extends distally beneath the lower lateral cartilages and is supported caudally and laterally by fibrous tissue. Bridger[1] believed that the entire nasal valve area averaged 55 mm^2, whereas Masing[10] calculated the same area to be 64 mm^2. It is the narrowest portion of the nasal airway. The opening of the nasal valve angle is measured in degrees and represents the angle between the upper lateral cartilage and the nasal septum; it normally ranges between 10 and 15 degrees.

Figure 28-5. Histologic section demonstrates that upper lateral cartilage is extension of septal cartilage. This section of upper lateral cartilages and septum was taken just distal to nasal bones. (Original magnification X10.) (By permission of Mayo Foundation.)

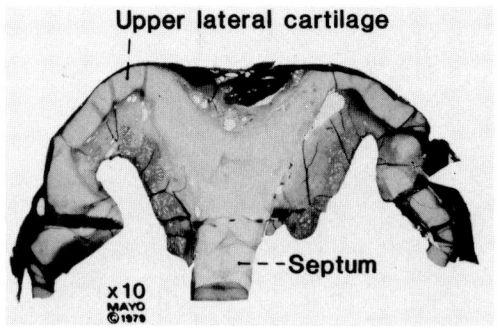

All of this is important, because the nasal valve is probably the crucial inflow regulator, accounting for most of the inspiratory resistance to airflow, and because disturbances of the nasal valve can produce symptoms of nasal airway obstruction. Bridger[1] offered two important concepts concerning the dysfunction of the nasal valve. First, the pathologic anatomy produces dysfunction of the nasal valve by causing this valve to collapse too early during inspiration rather than by changing the total nasal resistance. Second, increased nasal resistance is not always a consequence of nasal valve dysfunction. Early collapse of an already narrowed nasal valve seems to be important, although an increase in nasal resistance can be found in persons who have obstruction of the nasal valve. Bidger[1] arrived at these conclusions after studying the nasal valve with rhinomanometric techniques. He considered the nose as having a collapsible, flow-limiting segment (nasal valve) similar to a Starling resistor. His model involved a rigid tube (internal nose) with a short collapsible segment (the flexible external nose). The transmural pressure is the difference between the pressure outside the tube (atmosphere) and the intraluminal (nasal) pressure. The flexible external nose tends to resist collapse, apparently because of the way the cartilages are sprung open. Thus a critical transmural pressure can be reached in which a collapsible segment closes. This occurs when the inside or intraluminal intranasal pressure becomes negative from the effect of inspiration.

Bridger[1] pointed out that the maximum inspiratory effort can increase the flow-pressure curve to a point at which the airflow will no longer be increased by a further increase in negative pressure

(Figure 28-6). This finding was compatible with the concept of the nose having a flow-limiting segment or nasal valve. A simple experiment to demonstrate this is to try to prolong your own inspiratory sniff. You can recognize that a point is reached when an increase in negative pressure (inspiration) no longer increases airflow. Bridger[1] considered the mechanical deformities in areas 1 and 2 as upstream resistances; this concept is important clinically and functionally because an upstream obstruction (areas 1 and 2) usually produces an elevated nasal resistance or early collapse of the valve during inspiration, whereas a downstream obstruction (areas 3, 4, and 5) usually does not produce a pronounced elevation in nasal resistance unless the obstruction is quite large. In other words, abnormalities in areas 1 and 2 (upstream) are more likely to produce the symptom of nasal airway obstruction than are septal abnormalities in area 3, 4, or 5 (downstream).

Bridger[1] noted that the sagging and depression or twisting and buckling of the upper lateral cartilage also disturbed the relationship of this cartilage and the nasal septum and thereby narrowed the nasal valve. He demonstrated that individuals with these deformities had altered flow-pressure curves in comparison with curves in a normal population. This author concluded that these disturbances were attributable to small changes in the size and shape of the nasal valve, which had a pronounced influence on collapsibility. Therefore any abnormality in the nasal valve area could cause early collapse of the nasal valve and produce symptoms of nasal airway obstruction.

A basic approach to nasal airway obstruction requires something more in the surgical armamentarium than submucous resection; it requires the surgical ability to uncover totally and reconstruct deformities of the nasal septum that are capable of producing nasal airway obstruction, including deformities at the caudal end and the dorsal portion of the quadrangular cartilage, the upper lateral cartilage, the anterior nasal spine, and the maxillary crest (premaxilla), all of which are unapproachable and consequently untreatable by the submucous resection (Figure 28-7).

Nasal septal reconstruction is a surgical concept that allows all parts of the nasal septum to be approached and reconstructed when necessary for physiologic (breathing) and cosmetic reasons. Any sophisticated surgical handling of the entire septum and upper lateral cartilage therefore requires knowledge of the maxilla-premaxilla approach to extensive septal surgery as enunciated by Cottle and oth-

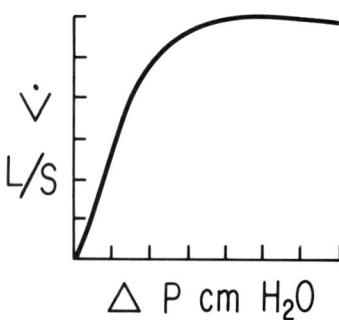

Figure 28-6. Representative nasal airflow $(\dot{V})$ and nasal air pressure curve (ΔP) demonstrates that point can be reached when increase in pressure (negative during inspiration) can no longer produce increase in transnasal airflow.

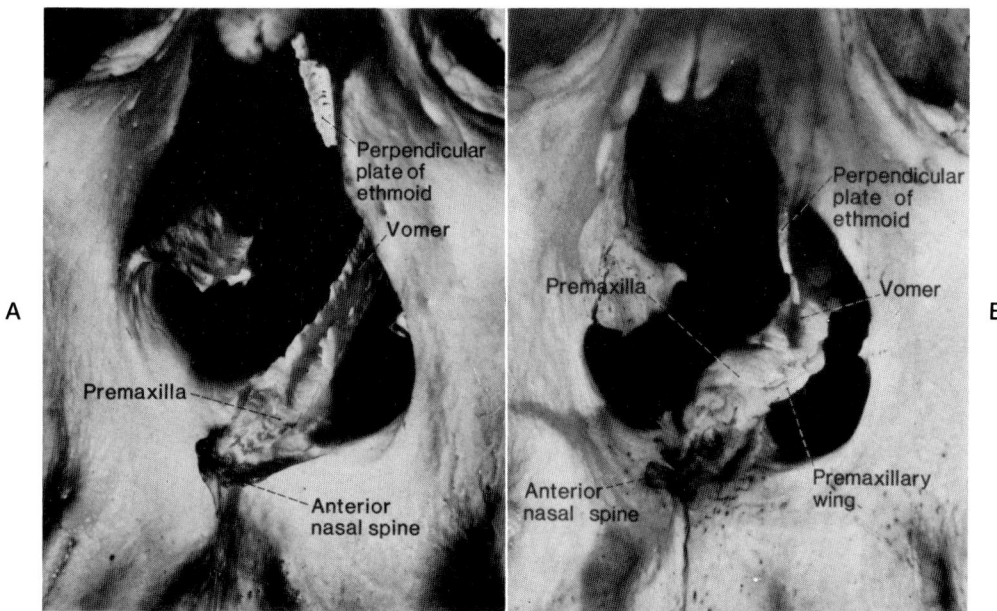

Figure 28-7. A, Normal bony anatomy in region of anterior nasal spine, premaxilla, and vomer. **B,** Example of abnormal bony anatomy in region of anterior nasal spine, premaxilla, and vomer, which is approachable by maxilla-premaxilla method of Cottle with development of inferior tunnels.

ers.[2] Although the technique must be tailored to each individual pathologic variation, the general principles and the sequence most frequently employed can be described.

APPROACH TO THE MAXILLA AND PREMAXILLA
Technique

The approach to extensive septal surgery requires understanding of the pertinent anatomic structures (Figure 28-8), as found in the work of Mosher.[15]

For the right-handed surgeon a right hemitransfixion incision is the most useful way of beginning almost all intranasal septal surgery (Figure 28-9, *A*). A left anterior tunnel is begun by sharp dissection, whether this is the concave or the convex side of the deformity (Figure 28-9, *B*). This mucosal elevation should be on the cartilage and beneath the perichondrium to avoid bleeding and to preserve the elevated perichondrium if a portion of the septum is resected (Figure 28-10). As the dissection continues this left anterior tunnel becomes a left anteroposterior tunnel, with elevation of the mucoperiosteum of the perpendicular plate of the ethmoid bone and the vomer in the posterior portion of the nose

(Figure 28-11). The lip is undermined with a Knapp scissors, the anterior nasal spine is exposed, and a right inferior tunnel is created along the floor of the nose (Figure 28-12). Remember, not every patient needs exposure of the anterior nasal spine or creation of inferior tunnels. Inferior tunnels are useful as an approach to septal impactions or anterior spurs. A left inferior tunnel is then developed (Figure 28-13). The left inferior tunnel is joined with the left anteroposterior tunnel by careful, sharp dissection (Figure 28-14). This completely isolates the caudal end of the septum, anterior nasal spine, premaxilla, and floor of the piriform aperture.

A vertical incision can then be made in the septal cartilage (Figure 28-15) 2 to 3 cm behind the caudal end of the septum, and a right posterior tunnel can be fashioned. This is done to eliminate any problems in the posterior septum that may be present (Figure 28-16). The excision may include the posterior aspect of the quadrangular cartilage, perpendicular plate of the ethmoid, and vomer, which may be removed when indicated.

The caudal end of the septum can then be dislocated from its attachments to the anterior nasal spine and the crest of the premaxilla and vomer by sharp dissection. This caudal end of the septum with

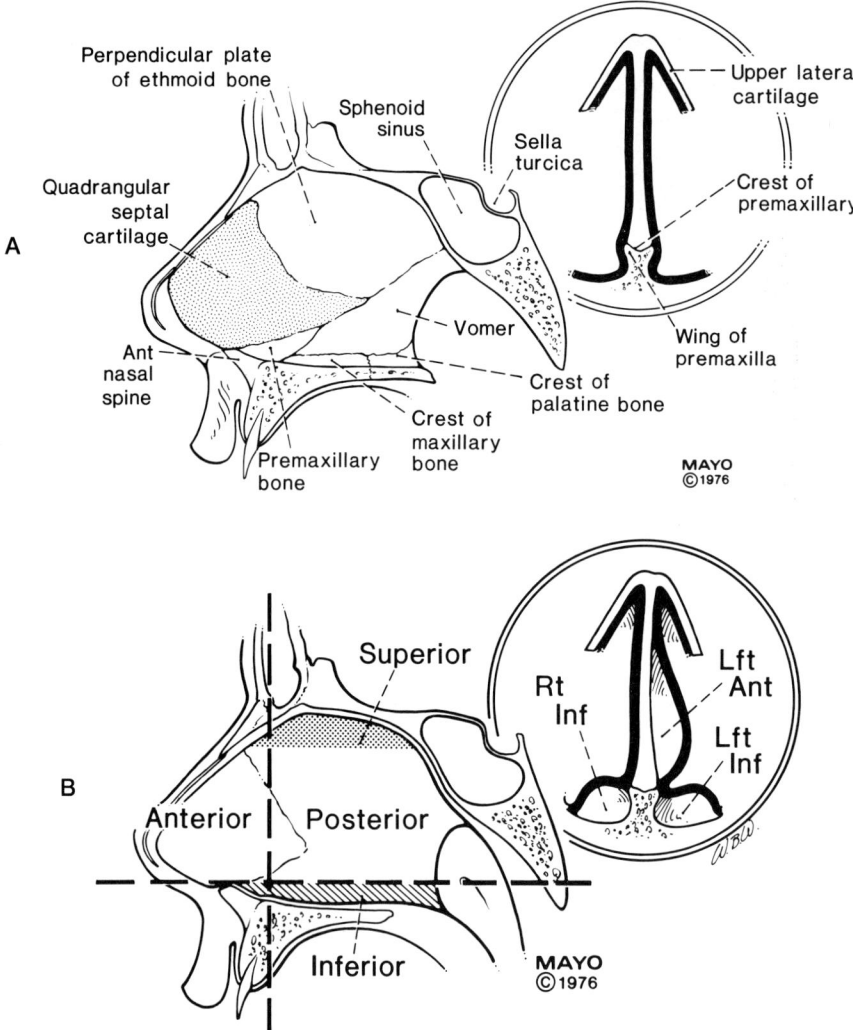

Figure 28-8. A, Pertinent anatomic terms and structures. **B,** Division of nose and nasal septum into anterior, posterior, superior, and inferior portions. Anterior portion of septum is that part of nose anterior to imaginary vertical line drawn from proximal end of nasal bones to hard palate. Inferior portion is that area of septum and floor of nose that lies below articulation of quadrangular septal cartilage with anterior nasal (maxillary) spine and crest and wings of premaxilla. "Superior" refers to portion of septum nearest cribriform area. Left anterior tunnel would be mucosal flap elevated from left side of septum back to imaginary line dividing anterior portion from posterior portion. Beyond that imaginary line mucosal elevation on same side would be left posterior tunnel. Mucosal elevation from floor of nose up to region of articulation of quadrangular septal cartilage with anterior nasal spine and premaxillary wings would be inferior tunnel. (By permission of Mayo Foundation.)

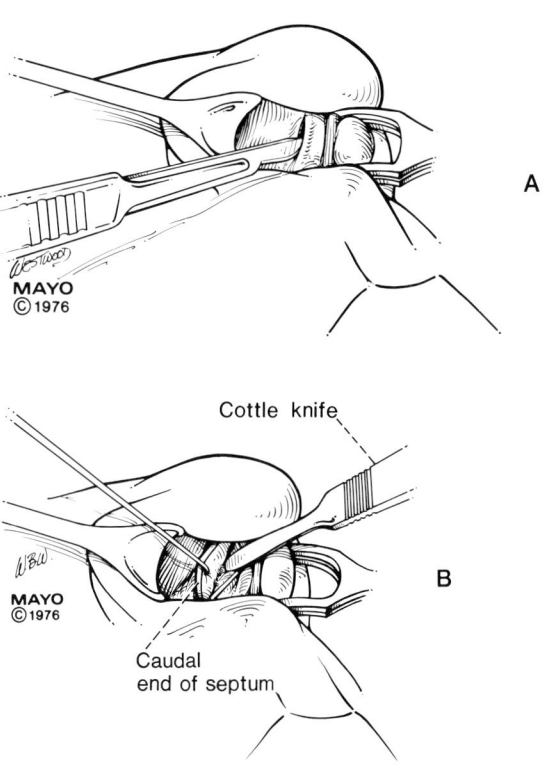

Figure 28-9. **A,** Right-handed surgeon holds Cottle columellar clamp in left hand, and assistant holds alar protector. After columellar clamp is applied to identify caudal end of septum, right hemitransfixion incision is made with No. 15 blade about 1 to 2 mm behind caudal end of nasal septum. **B,** Quadrangular septal cartilage is retracted, through right hemitransfixion incision, to right with hook, and Cottle knife is used to begin left anterior tunnel by sharp dissection beneath mucoperichondrium of septal cartilage. (By permission of Mayo Foundation.)

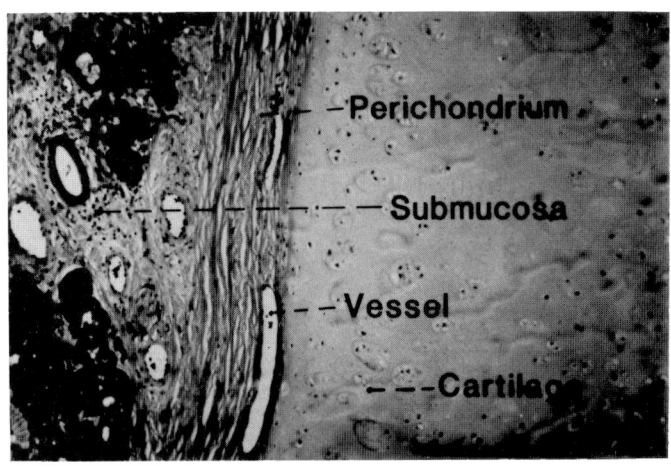

Figure 28-10. Histologic section of human nasal septal cartilage and overlying perichondrium and submucosa. Note presence of vessels in perichondrium and their relationship to septal cartilage. (Original magnification X100.)

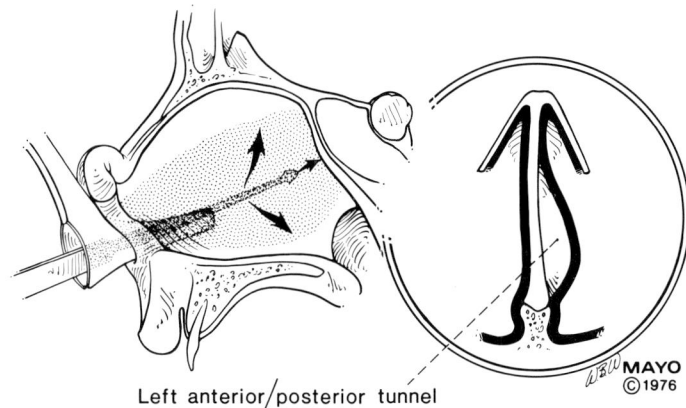

Figure 28-11. As dissection continues left anterior tunnel becomes left anteroposterior tunnel, with elevation of mucoperiosteum of perpendicular plate of ethmoid bone and vomer in posterior portion of nose. With nasal speculum placed through hemitransfixion incision into left anterior tunnel, Cottle elevator is used to continue mucoperichondrial and mucoperiosteal elevation back to face of sphenoid. (By permission of Mayo Foundation.)

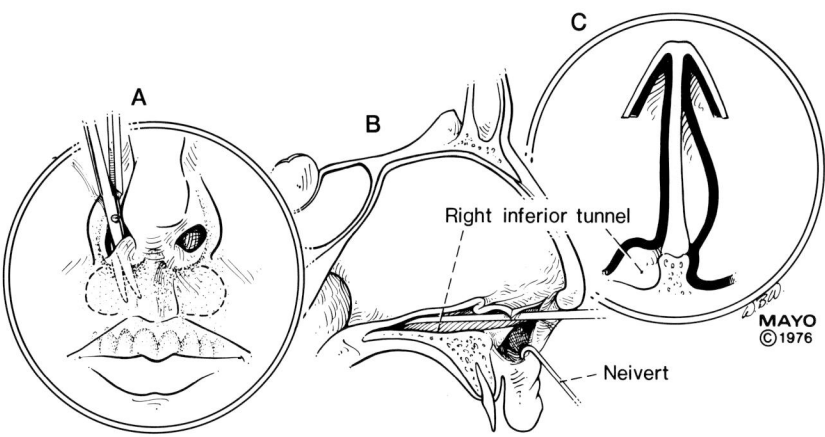

Right inferior tunnel

Neivert

MAYO
©1976

Figure 28-12. A, Lip is undermined by elevating tip of nose with left hand and placing a Knapp scissors into hemitransfixion incision between oral mucosa and orbicular muscle anterior to nasal spine. Nasal spine and floor of nose are exposed (within limits of broken lines) so that right inferior tunnel can be created. **B,** Narrow Neivert retractor, inserted into hemitransfixion incision, is used to retract soft tissues to expose anterior nasal spine, piriform aperture, and floor of nose on right. **C,** Curved Cottle elevator is used to elevate mucosa along floor of nose and to develop inferior tunnel. (By permission of Mayo Foundation.)

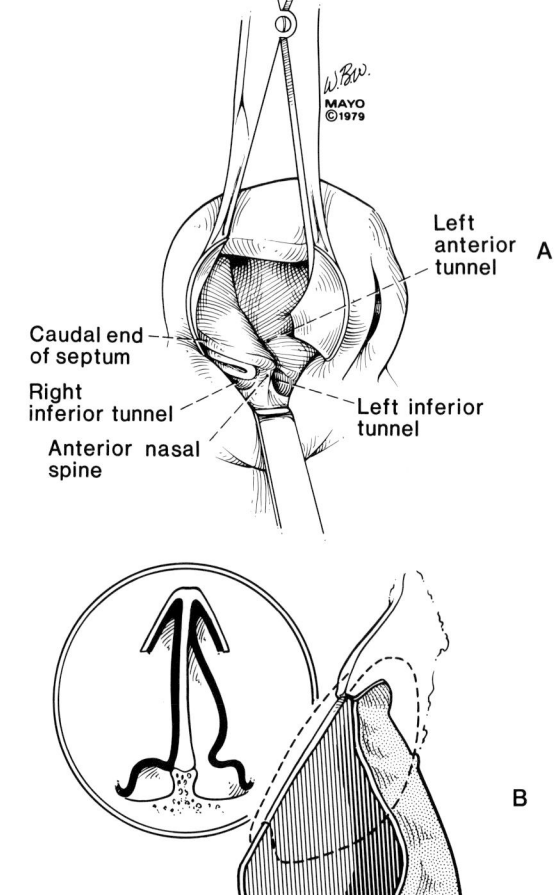

Left anterior tunnel **A**

Caudal end of septum

Right inferior tunnel

Left inferior tunnel

Anterior nasal spine

MAYO
©1979

B

MAYO
©1976

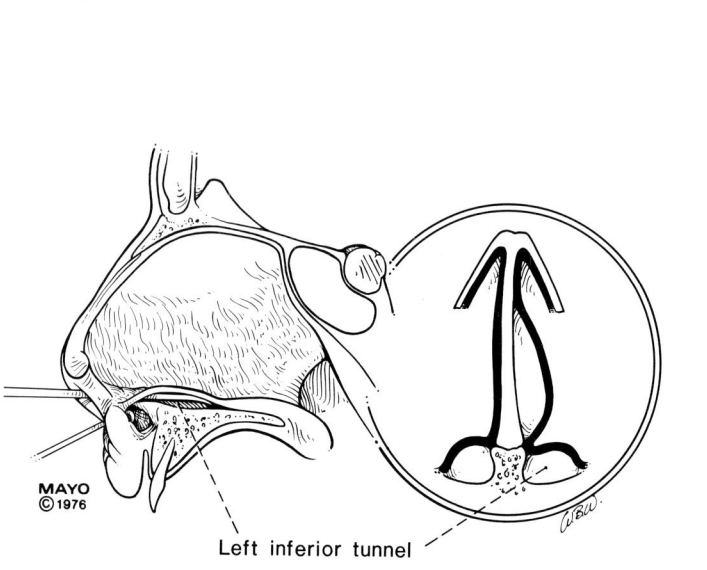

Left inferior tunnel

MAYO
©1976

Figure 28-13. Development of left inferior tunnel. Crest of piriform aperture is identified, and curved Cottle elevator is used to elevate mucosa along floor of nose on left. Three tunnels have now been developed—left anteroposterior, right inferior, and left inferior. (By permission of Mayo Foundation.)

Figure 28-14. A, Left-sided tunnels are not connected because tissue is firmly adherent to region of osseous and cartilaginous joint between quadrangular septal cartilage and crest of premaxilla. **B,** Joining of left anterior and left inferior tunnels by sharp dissection of fibrous tissue that binds mucosa in this area to crest of premaxilla. Care is taken not to perforate mucosa. (By permission of Mayo Foundation.)

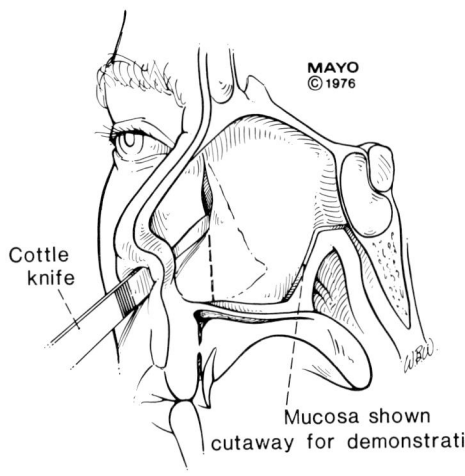

Figure 28-15. With Cottle knife in left anterior tunnel, vertical incision is made in quadrangular septal cartilage caudal to perpendicular plate of ethmoid bone at point 2 to 3 cm behind caudal end of septum. Care is taken not to perforate mucosa. This incision allows access to right side of septum so that right posterior tunnel can be elevated before posterior portion of septum is removed, when desired. (By permission of Mayo Foundation.)

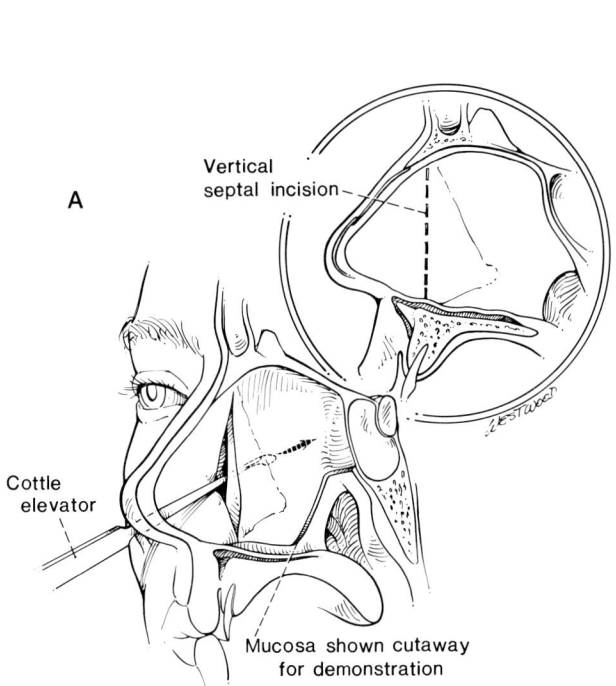

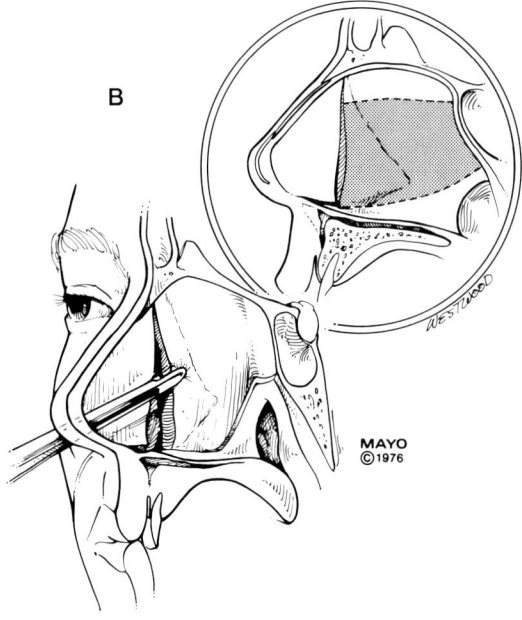

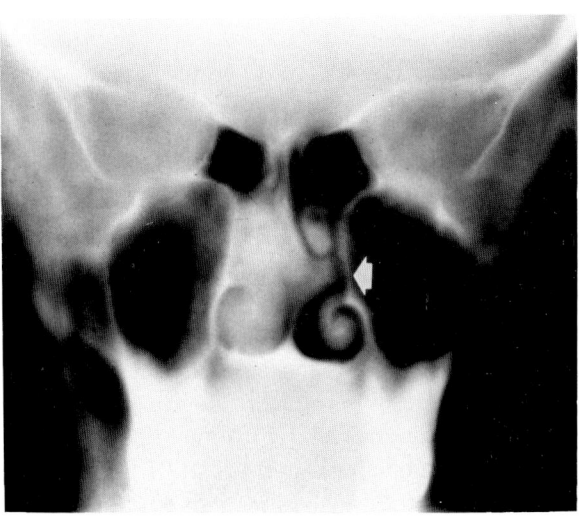

Figure 28-16. A, Development of right posterior tunnel. With Cottle elevator placed through vertical incision in cartilage, elevation begins on right side to create tunnel beneath mucoperichondrium and mucoperiosteum. **B,** Posterior septum (including posterior aspect of quadrangular septal cartilage), bony perpendicular plate of ethmoid bone, and vomer may be removed back to facce of sphenoid (shaded area) with a Koffler-Lillie bone forceps, when deformity is present in posterior areas 4 and 5. **C,** Roentgenogram of septal deformity in posterior area 4 on patient's left side in region of middle meatus. (By permission of Mayo Foundation.)

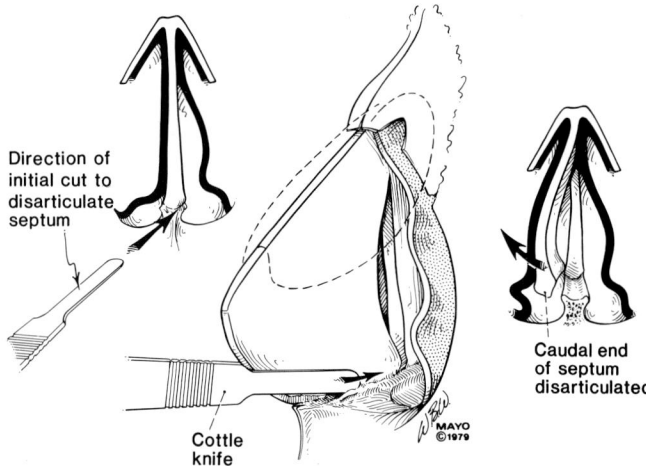

Figure 28-17. Caudal end of septum is disarticulated by sharp dissection from attachment to anterior nasal spine and crest of premaxilla and vomer. This allows caudal end of septum, with mucosa attached on right side anteriorly, to be swung into right nasal chamber. Caudal end of septum may be modified according to deformity present. If caudal end of septum is still deformed, it may be necessary to raise right anterior tunnel and totally free septal cartilage from its attachments to anterior spine and premaxilla. (By permission of Mayo Foundation.)

mucosa attached on the right side can be swung into the right nasal chamber (Figure 28-17) and modified as necessary. In some instances uncovering alone is all that is required for reconstruction and straightening of the caudal septum. If the caudal end of the septum is still deformed and abnormal, it may be necessary to raise a right anterior tunnel and totally free the septal cartilage from its firm fibrous attachments to the anterior nasal spine and premaxilla, separate it from the upper lateral cartilage, and replace it with, preferably, autogenous bone from the perpendicular plate of the ethmoid bone or vomer or from the cortex of the mastoid. Thus by the use of the maxilla-premaxilla approach, the caudal end of the septum may be exposed, examined, and reconstructed. The anterior nasal spine, premaxillary wings, and piriform aperture may also be exposed, removed, and reconstructed as indicated by the individual problem.

What are the indications for the maxilla-premaxilla approach to extensive nasal septal surgery? Remember, certainly not every patient with a septal abnormality requires the entire maxilla-premaxilla approach for structural correction. It is important to understand the cause of airway obstruction and

have the technical knowledge and skill to use inferior tunnels when needed to facilitate exposure of the abnormality and reconstruction. What are the advantages of the maxilla-premaxilla approach (as part of the concept of nasal septal reconstruction for nasal respiratory insufficiency) over the submucous resection? The answers to these questions have been addressed by Cottle and associates[2] but are repeated as part of this discussion.

Indications

Indications for the maxilla-premaxilla procedure are as follows:

1. Approach to and mobilization or removal and replacement of a severely deformed caudal end of the nasal septum
2. Approach to modify the length of the septum (this may include rotation of the tip)
3. Approach to and correction of deformities of the wings or bodies of the premaxilla (especially low, anteriorly located impactions)
4. Approach to and correction of the anterior maxillary spine
5. Approach to and correction of the floor of the piriform aperture
6. Approach to and transseptal exposure of abnormal skeletal structures in noses previously traumatized (surgically or nonsurgically)
7. Approach to and repair of nasal septal perforations [The maxilla-premaxilla approach allows adequate mobilization of tissues so that some small perforations (less than 1 cm) may be repaired when indicated.]
8. Approach to and management of septal abscesses and hematomas (The evacuation is accomplished by an incision placed not in the mucosa but in the skin of the vestibule; that is, a right hemitransfixion incision.)
9. Approach to and exposure for total removal of the septum and total replacement when indicated.
10. Approach to inferiorly placed impactions (especially after previous nasal septal surgery)
11. Accomplishment of intraseptal separation of nasal bones (because the septal space has been widely opened)
12. Implantation of tissues for patients with atrophic rhinitis (endonasal microplasty)
13. Intraseptal inspection and correction of recent septal fractures and dislocations

14. Approach to the wide or retracted columella
15. Approach to the sphenoid sinus, sella tur-
cica, and parasellar regions when indicated

Advantages

The advantages of the maxilla-premaxilla approach as part of the nasal septal reconstruction
concept, as contrasted with the submucous resection, include the following:

1. Since the maxilla-premaxilla approach de-
rives its access through a skin incision at the
caudal end of the septum (right hemitransfixion), it leaves undisturbed the mucosal
coverings for intranasal implantations and
averts mucosal scarring, atrophy, and disturbances in ciliary function.
2. It allows easy suturing of the original, anteriorly placed, right hemitransfixion incision
and thereby allows healing by primary inten-
tion.
3. It allows access to the chondro-osseous joint
fascia for cutting, scraping fibers, or freeing
septal mucosal flaps and thus joining anterior
and inferior tunnels.
4. It provides the opportunity for reconstruction of the entire bony septum.
5. It averts the inadequate operation that results
from the imposed limitations of the surgical
field, because now the entire bony and cartilaginous septum can be uncovered and exposed.
6. It makes feasible the performance of secondary septal operations, because it allows wide
exposure and the opportunity of elevating
mucosa from the bony floor of the nose. The
mucosa along the floor of the nose is usually
not scarred by previous surgery (unless inferior tunneling has already been preformed).

The technique and indications for along with the
advantages of the maxilla-premaxilla approach have
been presented as part of the basic knowledge required for nasal septal reconstruction to eliminate
airway obstruction. What is the role of surgery of
the valve in nasal septal reconstruction? As mentioned previously, please consider reading Chapter
25 for a more comprehensive discussion of valve
surgery breathing disturbances, if you have not done
so already.

Septal portion of nasal valve surgery

The surgeon must realize that nasal septal reconstruction is aimed at reconstruction of the nasal
septum (including its extension, the upper lateral

cartilage) for relief of nasal breathing insufficiency.
The septum and upper lateral cartilage are part of
the nasal valve. The surgeon must diagnose the patient's problem and modify the surgical technique
for each individual pathologic variation. The surgeon should have the technical ability to explore the
entire septum and the upper lateral cartilage and to
treat any mucocutaneous disturbance that may be
present in these regions. This systematic approach
to nasal septal reconstruction involves three types of
surgery (1) septal, (2) upper lateral cartilage, and (3)
mucocutaneous scar.

I will discuss in detail some technical aspects of
septal reconstruction that pertain to valve surgery
in this chapter. I have covered the other aspects of
the upper lateral cartilage that pertain to valve surgery in Chapter 25. Septal abnormalities that contribute to nasal valve problems may be due to an
absent, thickened, deflected, twisted, or scarred septum or to some combination of these problems. Surgery is carried out in a field as bloodless as possible
and is facilitated by local and topical (cocaine flakes)
anesthesia in a relaxed, well-premedicated patient.
Two-power optical loops are extremely useful for
the meticulous handling required of these tissues and
are recommended for all nasal surgery. The anterior
tunnels or flaps must be elevated on one side or both
sides so that the caudal end of the septum can be
exposed and the abnormalities can be revealed and
corrected as suggested by the maxilla-premaxilla approach previously discussed and summarized in Figure 28-18. For example, thinning of a thickened septal cartilage in this valve region may be all that is
required, and the valve surgery in this instance may
therefore be quickly terminated. If the septum is
more than just thickened, or presents other problems, the caudal end of the septum may have to be
freed and mobilized from the maxillary spine and
premaxillary wings. Mobilization can be achieved
by making a vertical incision in the quadrangular
cartilage anterior to the perpendicular plate of the
ethmoid bone, freeing the caudal end of the septum
from its crest and resecting the dislocated or deflected portions of the septum. The surgery can be
terminated if by uncovering the septum and freeing
it from its posterior and inferior attachments, the
deflection is reduced and the septum swings to the
midline, relieving the nasal valve obstruction. However, if a twisted piece of cartilage still obstructs the
nasal valve, it can be selectively removed, perhaps
by excising an almond-shaped portion of septal cartilage. If a large piece of cartilage must be removed,
the septum should be reconstructed by crushing, re-

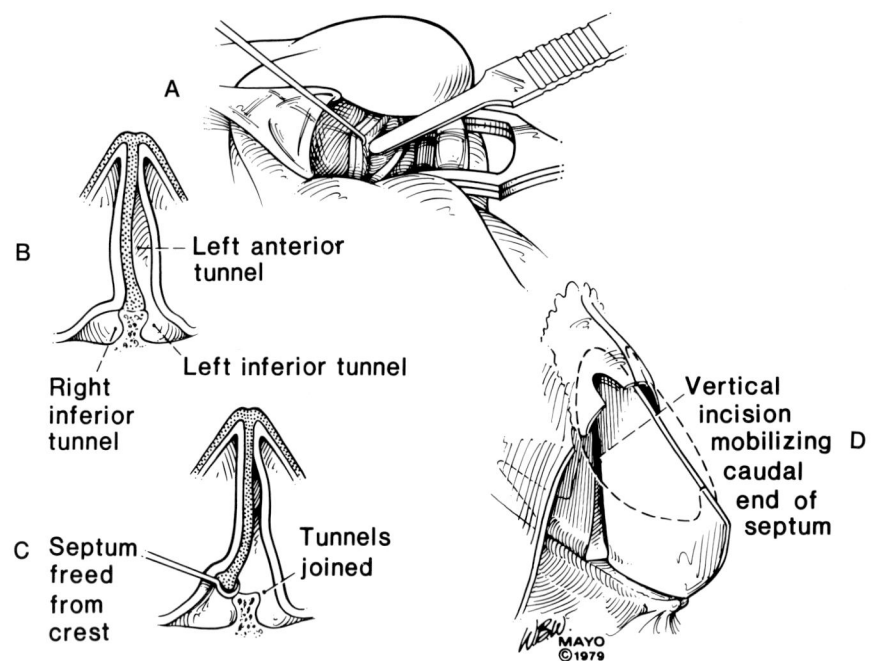

Figure 28-18. **A,** Right hemitransfixion incision and approach to nasal septum by creation of anterior and inferior tunnels, with joining of left anterior and left inferior tunnels (**B** and **C**) to free septum from the crest of maxilla and premaxilla. **D,** Mobilization of septum is completed by freeing, by vertical incision, caudal end of septum from perpendicular plate of ethmoid bone. (By permission of Mayo Foundation.)

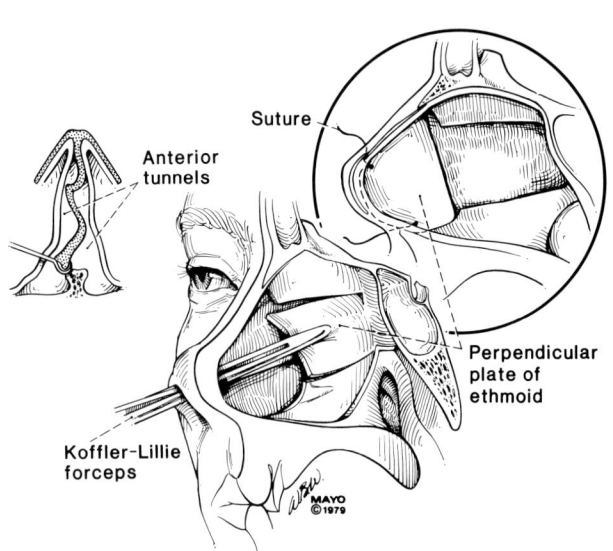

Figure 28-19. Bilateral anterior tunnels have been created to allow removal and replacement of deformed caudal end of septum with autogenous bone graft from perpendicular plate of ethmoid bone. (By permission of Mayo Foundation.)

placing, and fixing the cartilage between the septal flaps. Theoretically this will avert the problem of flaccidity and early collapse of the nasal valve caused by septal abnormality.

Surgery should attempt to reconstruct normal anatomy and avoid increased rigidity and collapsibility. At times the only way to correct a severe abnormality is to remove and replace completely the caudal end of the septum. Although other surgeons have already illustrated this procedure, the details are shown in Figure 28-19. In planning treatment for the nasal valve region, septal surgery should be considered first, since septal abnormalities are probably the most frequent causes of nasal valve obstruction. If surgery on the septum does not solve the nasal valve obstruction, the upper lateral cartilage should be explored next (Chapter 25).

DISCUSSION

The submucous window resection is a limited procedure in the total treatment of nasal airway obstruction. Evolutionary surgical principles that must now be considered include partial or total reconstruction of the nose for improvement of respiration

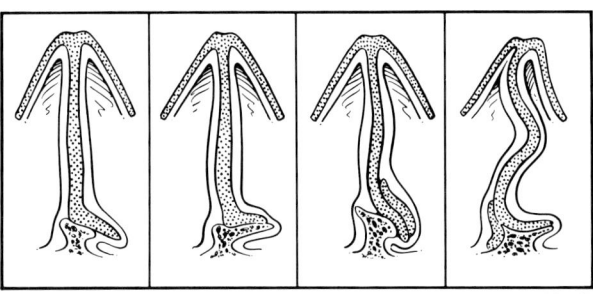

Figure 28-20. Various types of anterior septal deformities that are not amenable to submucous resection. Drawings represent merely a few of many examples seen in (surgically and nonsurgically) traumatized noses. Note that defect is along floor of nose and frequently involves joint region between septal cartilage and premaxilla, as represented in this series. See Figure 29-7, *B*, for abnormal bony anatomy in this region and Figure 29-21 for roentgenographic evidence of defect in this region. (By permission of Mayo Foundation.)

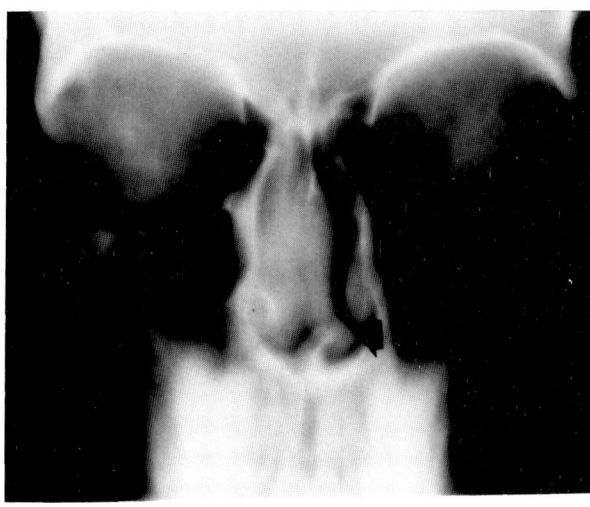

Figure 28-21. Roentgenogram demonstrates existence of anterior septal defect not amenable to submucous resection. Note that defect along floor of nose on left also involves joint area between septal cartilage and premaxilla.

and avoidance of surgical manipulations that may produce nasal respiratory insufficiency. An obstructing infracture of the frontal process of the maxilla should be avoided when lateral osteotomies are performed. Incisions in the valve region should be avoided whenever possible. The removal of excessive lobular cartilage, the removal of excessive soft tissues, and the sacrifice of functioning mucosal lining tissues should also be avoided if nasal breathing difficulties are to be prevented postoperatively.

The submucous resection is an operation. Nasal septal reconstruction is a concept, with the maxilla-premaxilla approach providing access for extensive septal surgery when required to correct nasal breathing problems caused by structural abnormalities. Abnormalities of the anterior nasal septum that are not amenable to submucous resection require newer methods of nasal septal reconstruction that reach beyond the pathologic anatomy originally designated to be within the operative field of the submucous resection. Some of the various types of anterior septal abnormalities near the floor of the nose that are encountered in the traumatized patient are seen in Figures 28-20 and 28-21.

An understanding of the interrelationship between nasal architecture and the dynamic physiologic principles of breathing is essential for improved reconstructive surgery. The submucous resection is performed within the septal borders by preservation of a caudal end and the dorsal strut, whereas nasal

septal reconstruction conceptually allows an option for a surgical approach at the borders of the septum. This includes the caudal end of the septum and the region of the valve where pathology may produce nasal airway obstruction.

The maxilla-premaxilla approach provides a conceptual framework for dealing with abnormalities of the caudal and dorsal portions of the septal cartilage. The surgical attack can now be taken to the floor of the nose, the nasal spine, the premaxilla, the piriform aperture, and the valve area—essentially all parts of the septum can be exposed. New vistas for solving problems of nasal airway obstruction have therefore been opened. The idea that nasal airway obstruction can be caused by upstream resistance, although known intuitively, was substantiated in the work of Bridger[1]. It is important to think aerodynamically, despite the fact that our knowledge is insufficient. Thus deformities of areas 1 and 2 produce the abnormalities most significant for disturbing nasal airflow. These are upstream resistances, and small deformities here (upstream areas 1 and 2) are capable of producing significant airway disturbances.

In patients with intranasal deformities this information should help to direct surgical intervention toward restoration of normal relationships between the cartilaginous and the bony skeletal structures of the nose and not merely toward enlarging the nasal airway. The maintenance of streamlined aerodynamic contours seems of paramount importance, as does the preservation of functioning turbinal tissue, so that excessive turbulent airflow (probably a significant contributor to abnormal increases in nasal airway resistance) does not result. All of these considerations are intended to help the patient breathe easily through the nose.

Conservative functional surgery means preserving mucosa and anatomy, yet being courageous enough to remove and reconstruct the caudal end of the septum, to replace tissue and to reconstruct, not just resect. Surgery for nasal airway obstruction should mean more than just operating on the posterior septum. It requires knowledge and ability brought to bear on the entire septum in order to preserve or restore nasal breathing.

The debate is not whether submucous resection is superior to nasal septal reconstruction. Nasal reconstruction is an evolutionary step toward solving problems that submucous resection could not solve, namely, nasal airway obstruction caused by deformities of caudal or dorsal septal cartilage. The concept of nasal septal reconstruction, with the maxilla-premaxilla approach, not only permits the exposure of septal deformities that are approachable by submucous resection but provides an approach to the caudal end of the septum, upper lateral cartilage, dorsal septum (involving the nasal valve), anterior nasal spine, premaxilla, and piriform aperture. Bridger[1] and others showed conclusively with rhinomanometry that abnormalities of these areas may produce nasal respiratory insufficiency. In one study of 1,000 patients McCaffrey and Kern[11], using rhinomanometry, clearly showed that as the patients' symptoms of nasal obstruction increase, an increase in nasal airway resistance can be documented. In another study by Mertz and colleagues[12] 50 patients who underwent nasal septal reconstruction for anterior septal deformities were examined preoperatively and postoperatively with anterior mask rhinomanometry. A high degree of correlation was found between the reduction in nasal resistance after operation and the patient's subjective assessment of improvement of breathing. This type of substantial physiologic data (rhinomanometry) facilitates our evaluation of our clinical observations and surgical techniques.

The submucous resection approach is inadequate for wide exposure of the septal structures. An abnormality that requires optimal exposure frequently benefits from the maxilla-premaxilla approach. Examples of instances in which optimal exposure is required include previous trauma or previous submucous resection with intraseptal scar-

ring, atrophy of mucosa, endonasal microplasty, septal hematoma, septal abscess, subtotal septal reconstruction, and total septal reconstruction with implantation or transplantation of the caudal end of the septum. Optimal exposure of the intraseptal space as an avenue to the sphenoid sinus and pituitary gland can be obtained by the maxilla-premaxilla approach (Kern and others[8]). This approach can be used to enlarge the endonasal space to facilitate repair of choanal atresia. It can also be used for exposure in intraseptal bony surgery not requiring removal of cartilage to correct abnormalities of the inferior portion of the septum of the joint fascia of the maxillary crest, since these situations are not amenable to submucous resection. Difficult cases in which the patient has persistent septal impactions and requires revision surgery are not amenable to submucous resection but are suited to the maxilla-premaxilla approach, which allows inferior tunneling. Intraseptal separations of the upper lateral cartilage from the nasal septum are possible, thus avoiding intranasal mucosal cuts with attendant bleeding and scarring. Intraseptal separation of the nasal bones is possible. Through the hemitransfixion incision it is possible to place cartilage or other graft materials over the dorsum. Surgery in persons who have small nostrils, such as children, surgery involving scarring at the base of the nose, and surgery involving the maxillary spine and premaxillary wings are amenable to exposure and reconstruction through the maxilla-premaxilla approach, when indicated, but are not usually amenable to the submucous resection approach.

When extension of the septal surgery to the pyramid is required, the submucous resection incision is often inappropriately placed. The hemitransfixion incision not only allows extensive septal surgery but also facilitates surgery of the upper lateral cartilage. A combined septal-rhinoplasty procedure can be accomplished by this approach, which makes feasible exposure and repair of cosmetic deformities and structural abnormalities that impair nasal breathing. Approach and access must always be given consideration.

Moreover, submucous resection does not address the question of the nasal valve. Bridger[1], using valid modern rhinomanometric techniques, examined 44 patients by the maximum inspiratory method. Of these, 17 suffered from nasal insufficiency; seven of these 17 experienced their problems or had their symptoms worsen after rhinoplastic surgery! Thus Bridger[1] clearly demonstrated that consideration of the function of the nasal valve is essential in all nasal surgery: "In seven of the people in the symptom group, the symptoms commenced or were aggravated after a rhinoplastic procedure, showing that consideration of the function of the nasal valve is important in nasal surgery." Bridger's objective breathing studies (rhinomanometric data) substantiated his point, which has been confirmed in another laboratory.[11]

Nasal septal reconstruction is a concept, an idea. The maxilla-premaxilla approach is a tool that allows the surgeon access to all parts of the septum and pyramid. The surgeon may use the entire maxilla-premaxilla approach or modify it as needed. Today the best functional results are achieved when the entire deformity is corrected, without sacrificing the resilience and stability of a cartilaginous septum. This may require the reintroduction or reconstruction of the cartilaginous and bony structures that were removed during the procedure. In the classic Killian operation the surgeon exchanges a semirigid medial wall for a flaccid membrane with limited stability. During inspiration even slight differences in pressure between the nostrils may amount to a transseptal pressure difference sufficient to produce collapse of the septum into one nostril. The importance of replacing cartilaginous and bony tissues in the intraseptal space cannot be overstated. If the skeptic does not accept the work of Bridger[1], the experienced rhinologic surgeon knows how difficult it is to separate two mucosal flaps in a patient who has had a submucosal resection. When bone and cartilage have been replaced in the intraseptal space, the required sharp dissection goes more smoothly, especially if the perichondrium has been saved. In other words, it is easier to reexplore a nose that has had bone and cartilage replaced in the septal space than one in which this space has been left vacant. Not only does replacement of skeletal tissue allow support and preserve the septal space, it also prevents or minimizes the inevitable scar tissue contracture.

The case rests with the words of Arbour* who has stated that the submucous operation *resects* within the borders of the septum, whereas nasal septal reconstruction *reconstructs* not only within the borders of the septum but also *at* the borders of the septum. Using the maxilla-premaxilla approach the surgeon has access to any part of the septum that may require removal and reconstruction to correct nasal breathing dysfunction. Nasal septal reconstruction allows an approach to and correction of the numerous septal deformities, including nasal valve abnormalities, that are not amenable to sub-

mucosal resection. This is no longer a dispute but an evolutionary surgical fact.

ACKNOWLEDGMENT

I owe a debt of gratitude for the diligent efforts of my secretary Barbara Chapman. I am also grateful to William B. Westwood, M.S., and John Hagen, from the Department of Medical Graphics, for their exceptional illustrative material.

REFERENCES

1. Bridger, G.P.: Physiology of the nasal valve, Arch. Otolaryngol. 92:543, 1970.
2. Cottle, M.H., and others: The "maxilla-premaxilla" approach to extensive nasal septum surgery, Arch. Otolaryngol. 68:301, 1958.
3. Ersner, M.S.: Rhinoplastic procedures to establish normal physiologic nasal function, Pa. Med. J. 1:749, 1948.
4. Fomon, S. and others: New approach to ventral deflections of the nasal septum, Arch. Otolaryngol. 54:356, 1951.
5. Freer, O.T.: The correction of deflections of the nasal septum with a minimum of traumatism, J.A.M.A. 38:636, 1902.
6. Hinderer, K.H.: Fundamentals of anatomy and surgery of the nose, Ed. 2, Birmingham, 1978, Aesculapius Publishing Co.
7. Ingals, E.F.: Diseases of the chest, throat, and nasal cavities, Ed. 4, New York, 1900, William Wood & Co.
8. Kern, E.B., and others: A transseptal, transsphenoidal approach to the pituitary: an old approach—a new technique in the management of pituitary tumors and related disorders, Trans. Am. Acad. Ophthalmol. Otolaryngol. 84:997, 1977.
9. Killian, G.: the submucous window resection of the nasal septum, Ann. Otol. Rhinol. Laryngol. 14:363, 1905.
10. Masing, H.: Experimentelle Untersuchungen über die Strömung in Nasenmodell, Arch. Otorhinolaryngol. 189:59, 1967.
11. McCaffrey, T.V., and Kern, E.B.: Clinical evaluation of nasal obstruction: A study of 1,000 patients, Arch. Otolaryngol. 105:542, 1979.
12. Mertz, J.M. McCaffrey, T.V., and Kern, E.B.: Objective evolution of anterior septal surgical reconstruction, Otolaryngology 92:308-311, 1984.
13. Metzenbaum, M.: Replacement of the lower end of the dislocated septal cartilage versus submucous resection of the dislocated end of the septal cartilage, Arch. Otolaryngol. 9:282, 1929.
14. Mink, P.-J.: Le Nez comme voie respiratoire, Presse Otolaryngol. (Belge.) 2:421-481, 1903.
15. Mosher, H.P.: The premaxillary wings and deviations of the septum, Laryngoscope 17:840, 1907.
16. Pearson, B.W., and Goodman, W.S.: S.M.R., septoplasty, and the surgical relief of nasal obstruction, Can. J. Otolaryngol. 2:238, 1973.
17. Peer, L.A.: An operation to repair lateral displacement of the lower border of the septal cartilage, Arch. Otolaryngol. 25:475, 1937.
18. Salinger, S.: Deviation of the septum in relation to the twisted nose, Arch. Otolaryngol. 29:520, 1939.
19. Seltzer, A.P.: The nasal septum: Plastic repair of the deviated septum associated with a deflected tip, Arch. Otolaryngol. 40:443, 1944.

---

*Arbour, P.G.: Personal Communication, 1978.

29

A Method of Submucous Resection

Jack Sheen

Since I long ago abandoned septoplasty techniques that transect, score, morcel, or otherwise manipulate septal cartilage without resecting it, my discussion will be limited to a technique of submucous resection that I routinely perform and the results of which I routinely evaluate in patients after operation. Because of my own failures in septoplasty and because of the many patients whose secondary rhinoplasties have resulted in inadequately treated airway problems, I now feel that a bold but well-controlled submucous resection ensures the most effective and complete correction of septal deviations. This technique also provides usable pieces of cartilage and bone for reconstructive purposes. Use of a swivel knife, a punch, or a button knife often proves to be a halfway measure that leaves the patient with persistant airway obstruction and the surgeon with a handful of useless fragments.

Whether the submucous resection is done to harvest cartilage for grafting, for septal deviations, or for both, the most important consideration is structural support. To maintain this support one must preserve substantial dorsal and caudal segments of septal cartilage. At least 1.5 Cm of unmolested cartilage should remain at the dorsal and caudal edges.

Having utmost respect for the integrity of the septum, I resect just what is necessary and no more. When the submucous resection is completed and the airways are clear, remnants of bone and cartilage are replaced into the septal pocket. As Cottle suggested, these remnants are often crushed to create larger, more manageable pieces that will not become displaced. Leftover pieces of cartilage and bone that are simply put back will frequently shift, resulting in postoperative airway obstructions. The Cottle cartilage crusher is most effective for splaying irregular pieces, which, when replaced, will add substance to the septal partition.

CASE REPORT

This 45-year-old man had a long history of airway problems. He did not recall specific injury to his nose. Approximately 3 years before he was seen by me, a septoplasty and partial inferior turbinate resection were done to relieve the obstruction but with very little improvement. At that time he was told by the operating surgeon that nothing further could be done without the possibility of worsening the problem.

On examination there was a caudal deflection of the septum that caused a narrowing of the nostril on the patient's left side. There was a septal convexity on his right that caused impaction of the internal valve on that side Figures 29-1, A and 29-1, B. Thus the patient had a compromised airway on both sides. The central part of the septum and the anterior third of the inferior margins of both inferior turbinates had been resected.

Surgical approach

To obtain a satisfactory airway on both sides, first, the caudal end of the septum must be placed in the midline and, second, the internal valve on the patient's right side must be opened to a functional angle. It has been my clinical experience that the methods of intrinsic modification of the cartilage (i.e., repositioning, morcellation, or scoring), do not provide a predictable or lasting result. On the other hand, resection of deformed cartilage from the caudal portion of the septum, including its removal from the vomer and reimplantation as a free graft, well seated and fixed in the columella, as first described by Galloway and cited by Fromon,[1] does provide a predictable and most satisfactory solution to the problem.

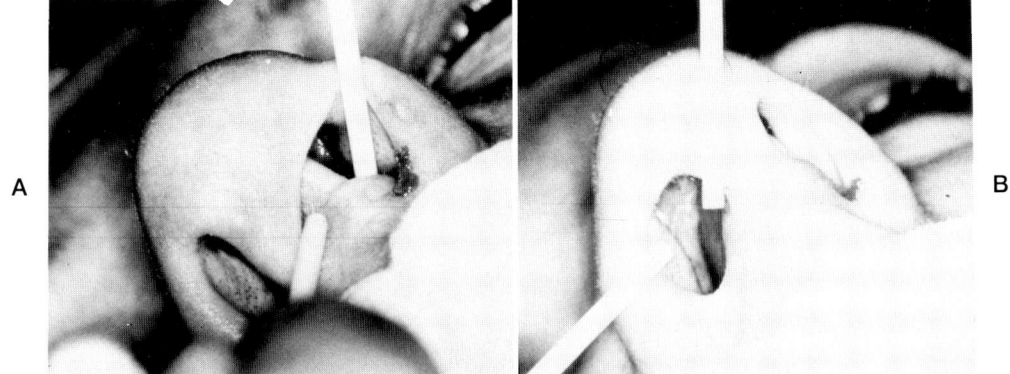

Figure 29-1. A, Columella retracted to show deflected caudal edge of septum. **B,** Caudal angulation is also responsible for obstruction in patient's right nostril.

Surgical procedure

A hemitransfixion incision is made from the angle of the septum to the base of the columella, exposing the caudal edge of the deformed cartilage (Figure 29-2). The mucoperichondrial flaps are dissected from both surfaces of the remaining cartilage. The flaps that do not contain septal cartilage are not separated. Inferiorly, the dissection extends over the vomer, exposing the remaining cartilage in the groove.

After the mucoperichondrial flaps are elevated, a Jackson turbinate scissors is used to transect the cartilage beginning at the caudal edge and continuing posteriorly past the bony junction. The specimen is removed, and the remaining dissection of all obstructing parts is completed, Figures 29-3, *A* and 29-3, *B*. The specimen is trimmed of all irregularities, leaving a straight, usable graft.

The columella is split to facilitate the seating of the caudal portion of the free cartilage graft. Occasionally a mattress suture is placed through the columella and the caudal edge of the graft to maintain its position (Figures 29-4, *A-C*). Mattress sutures are then placed through the mucosa and the columella to ensure a stable graft. At the completion of the suture placement, there is a normal external valve with good support. The resection of the septal convexity on the patient's right and placement of a spreader graft (Figure 29-5) have opened up the internal valve on that side.

Results

One year after surgery there has been no shift in the position of the caudal septum. There are good support to the base of the nose and an adequate airway on both sides of the septum.

REFERENCE

1. Foman, S., and others: Plastic repair of the deflected nasal septum, Arch. Otolaryngol. 44:155-156, 1946.

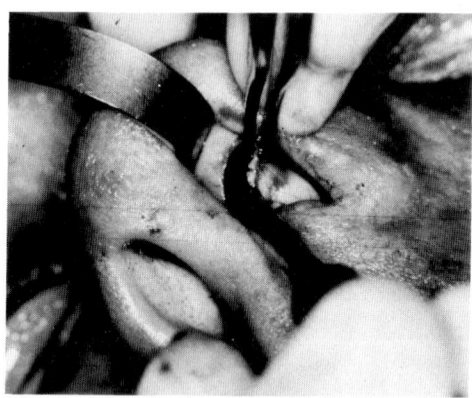

Figure 29-2. Intercartilaginous incision extending over angle of septum along caudal reflection of septum.

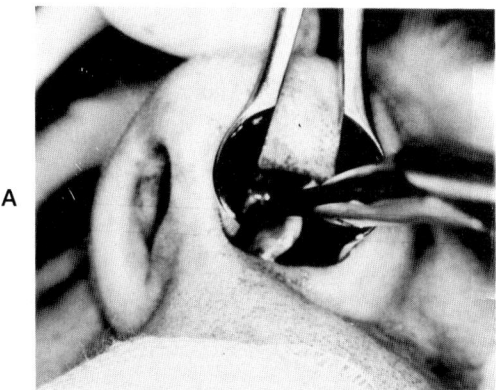
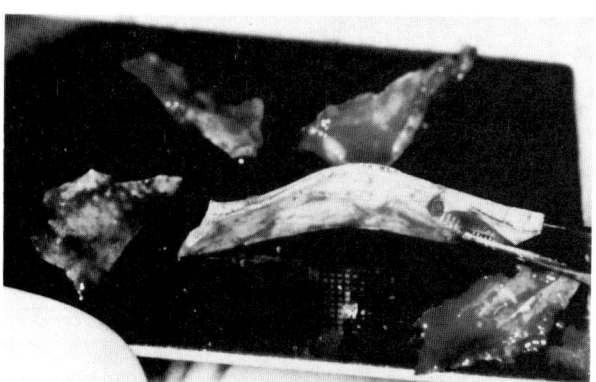

Figure 29-3. A, Septal scissors placed across caudal edge are directed cephalad. **B,** Specimen showing the angulation at the caudal third.

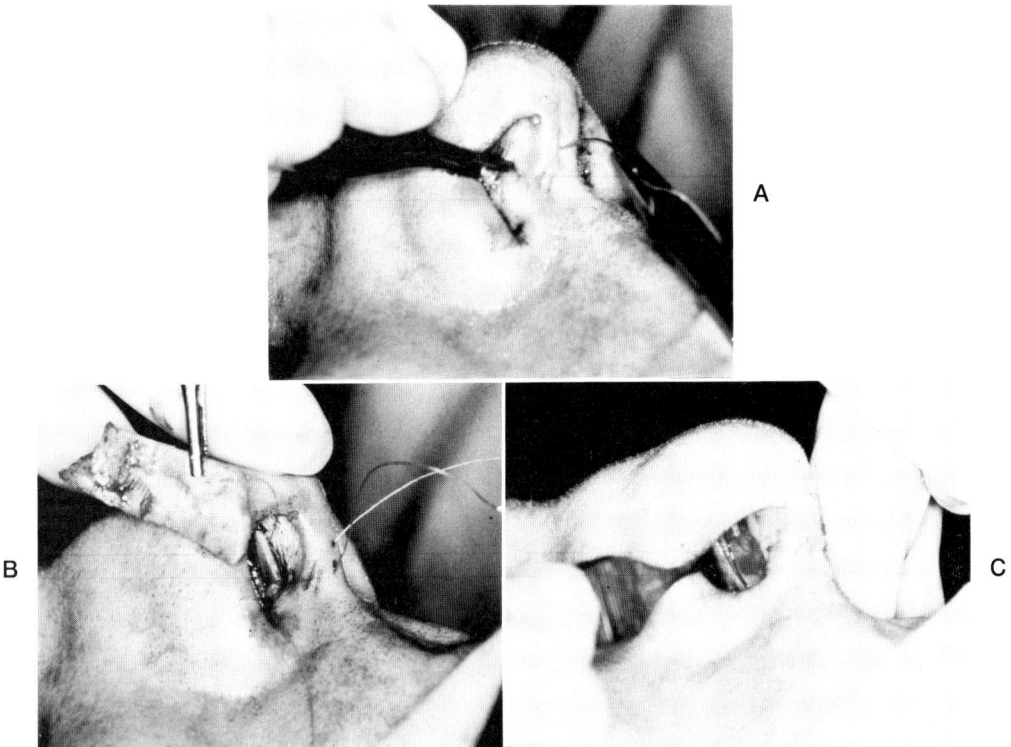

Figure 29-4. **A,** 4-0 Plain catgut suture being placed through columella, which has been cut with Joseph scissors. **B,** Mattress suture through columella and through caudal edge of graft to be placed. **C,** Graft being seated in split columella by placing traction on sutures.

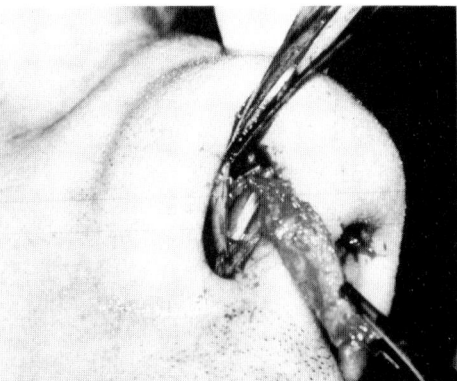

Figure 29-5. Spreader graft being placed on patient's right side to open up valve and to move anterior septal strut closer to midline.

30

Nonsurgical Closure of Nasal Septal Perforations

Eugene B. Kern

Closure of nasal septal perforations with silicone rubber prostheses has provided an effective alternative to surgical closure in treatment of patients symptoms associated with nasal septal perforations. At the Mayo Clinic many patients have been treated by prosthetic closure of septal perforations. I will present the data on 171 patients (97 female and 72 male patients, ranging in age from 6 to 87 years) with nasal septal perforations who were treated by insertion of silicone rubber septal buttons. Only patients with symptoms were fitted with buttons (Table 3). Investigations were done to rule out systemic disease as an etiologic factor. Previous nasal surgery was the most frequent cause of the perforations (Table 4).

The method of sizing the perforations by the use of a paper template and merthiolate has been described previously[4,5,8]. During the years 1972 to 1975 all of the buttons were hand-carved from medical-grade silicone rubber. In 1975 a septal button made of softer silicone rubber became commercially available. This proved to be smoother, more conforming prosthesis that alleviated the necessity of carving each button as it was needed. Some very large perforations have still warranted the use of custom-carved buttons.

In 145 cases the silicone rubber septal buttons were introduced in an office procedure with 5% cocaine used for topical anesthesia. The other proceudres were done in the operating room in association with other nasal surgery.

TABLE 3. Most frequent symptoms in 171 patients treated with septal buttons for nasal septal perforations*

Symptoms	No. of patients
Crusting	117
Epistaxis	104
Difficulty in breathing	67
Pain	47

*Less frequent symptoms included whistling sound, postnasal drainage, rhinorrhea, hyposmia, voice change, snoring, recurrent infection, and malodor.

TABLE 4. Reported causes of nasal septal perforations in patients with silastic septal buttons

Cause	No. of Patients
Nasal surgery	49
Other physical intranasal trauma	26
External trauma	14
Cautery	12
Chemical	4
Cocaine abuse	2
Infection	3
Lupus erythematosus	6
Wegener's granulomatosis	3
Nasal sarcoidosis	2
Rendu-Osler-Weber disease	3
Undetermined	47
Total	171

DATA AND RESULTS

Data were collected from questionnaires, follow-up examination, and patient records. Follow-up data were available on 136 of the 171 patients. Follow-up periods ranged from 1 month to 8 years. Buttons were in place at the end of the follow-up period in 100 of the 136 patients (73.5%). In 32 of these patients the button had come out or been removed at some point in time but had been replaced at the patient's request. In 36 of the patients (26.5%) the button came out or was removed and was not replaced. In these cases treatment was considered a failure.

Most frequent causes for loss of buttons included spontaneous extrusion, sneezing, blowing, sniffing, trauma, or patient manipulation. Some patients lost more than one button. Persistent discomfort and poor fit were most frequent causes for removal of a button in the 34 that were removed. Buttons were later replaced in several of these patients at their request.

When patients requested removal of a septal button, they tended to do so soon after placement. One third of the patients who had buttons removed requested removal within 1 week after placement. Two thirds of these patients had the buttons removed within the first 6 months. Some patients documented an early period of discomfort lasting 1 day to several weeks. Typical symptoms during this period were irritation, soreness, dryness, and persistent sneezing. In some cases this led to early removal of the button. Those who chose to keep the buttons seldom had further trouble after the initial period of adaptation.

Benefits reported by the patients most commonly included reduced epistaxis, reduced crusting, and improved breathing. Some patients commented that their nasal discomfort had decreased or that the whistling noise had ceased. Several patients mentioned that they could now blow their noses again. Others stated that they had noted improvement in olfaction, exercise tolerance, sleep, or voice quality.

Size of the perforations had been recorded in 125 cases. The perforations varied in size from 0.9 to 11 cm^2. Thirty-eight patients had perforations smaller than 5 cm^2. Perforations larger than 5 cm^2 were found in eight patients.

Since placement of prefabricated prostheses was begun, nine patients have needed replacements with a custom-made prosthesis because of poor fit of the original button. Nine other patients had custom buttons placed initially, because the perforation was obviously too large for a commercial button (3 cm in diameter) (Figure 30-1).

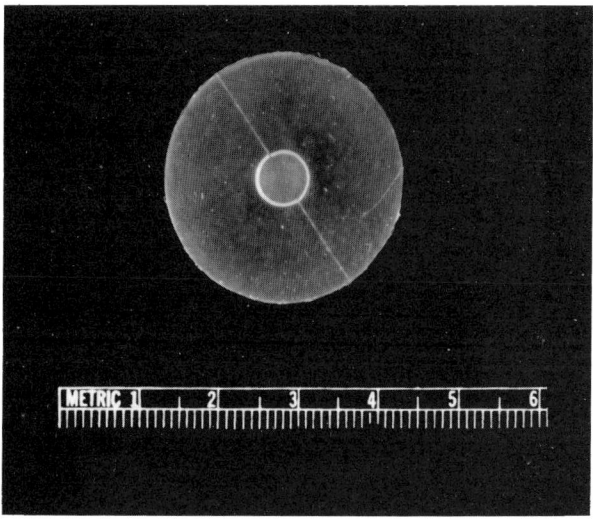

Figure 30-1. Commercially available silicone rubber nasal septal prosthesis (button), 3 cm in diameter, can be trimmed or modified and introduced into most septal perforations. Most nasal septal perforations are less than 3 cm in diameter.

Four patients with unusually large septal perforations were recently treated with custom-made silicone rubber septal prostheses. The most difficult problem in these cases was how to properly size the perforations. In these four patients the perforations were sized by means of computerized axial tomographic scanning with 1.5 mm cuts through the nasal region (Figure 30-2). This yielded the dimensions of the perforation and adjacent tissues within a tolerance of 1 to 2 mm. An accurate template was then made from the scaled dimensions of the successive axial cuts. A medical artist experienced in the fashioning of these buttons then made a button that fit exactly the perforation in each of these four cases (Figure 30-3). In one case the scan revealed that adhesions had impeded rhinologic assessment of the actual margins of the perforation. These were lysed at the time of placement of the prosthesis, and the button was fitted precisely within the true margins of the perforation.

Two of the patients had nasal septal perforations after submucous resection was done elsewhere. A cause was not found in the third and fourth patients despite thorough investigation. The second patient had had previous nasal biopsy that produced negative results and that had enlarged the perforation considerably.

All four patients had symptoms and complained of crusting, epistaxis, and headache. In addition, the

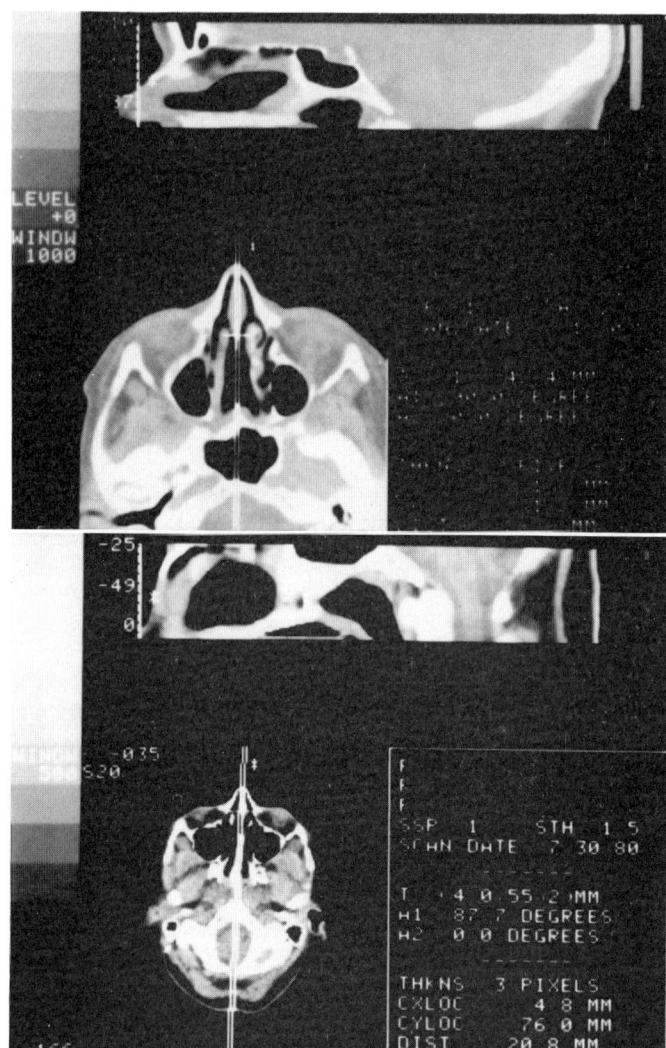

Figure 30-2. Examples of large nasal septal perforations in two patients. Both are larger than 3 cm in diameter. It was necessary to first determine exact size and configuration of perforation by means of computerized axial tomographic scanning with 1.5 mm cuts through nasal region. By obtaining actual dimensions of the septal perforation, it was possible to carve silicone rubber nasal septal prosthesis to exactly fit into irregular septal perforation.

first patient complained of facial pain, cough, and purulent nasal discharge. The second patient additionally complained of feeling more fatigued since the perforation had been present. The third patient had additional symptoms of nasal congestion, lethargy, and drainage. The fourth patient also complained of difficulty in breathing and nasal dryness.

In the first two cases physicians had attempted to close the perforations by sewing together two commercial septal buttons and then fitting them into the perforations. In both cases the attempts failed because of poor fit and cursting. In the second case silicone rubber sheeting glued together to cover the perforation had failed. A single prefabricated button in the fourth patient had fallen out, because its 3 cm diameter was smaller than the septal perforation.

The perforations varied in size and shape. The first perforation was trapezoidal in shape with a height of 2.8 cm and diagonal length of 5.2 cm.

The prosthesis was 6.5 cm long. In the second patient the perforation formed a large oval with no visible superior margin of tissue. At examination 2 years earlier it had been noted that there was nothing to offer the patient because the perforation was too large to outline well enough to fit a button. The third perforation measured 2.5 × 4 cm. The fourth perforation was quite similar in shape to the first, although slightly smaller in size.

In the first patient it was necessary to perform a lateral rhinotomy and remove a small portion of the frontal process of the maxilla to place the prosthesis (Figure 30-4). The second button was just small enough that placement was accomplished without an incision. In the third case a limited lateral rhinotomy was needed for placement, and in the fourth case a simple alar incision was sufficient (Figure 30-5). Button placement was aided by suturing the flanges of the button together on one side and

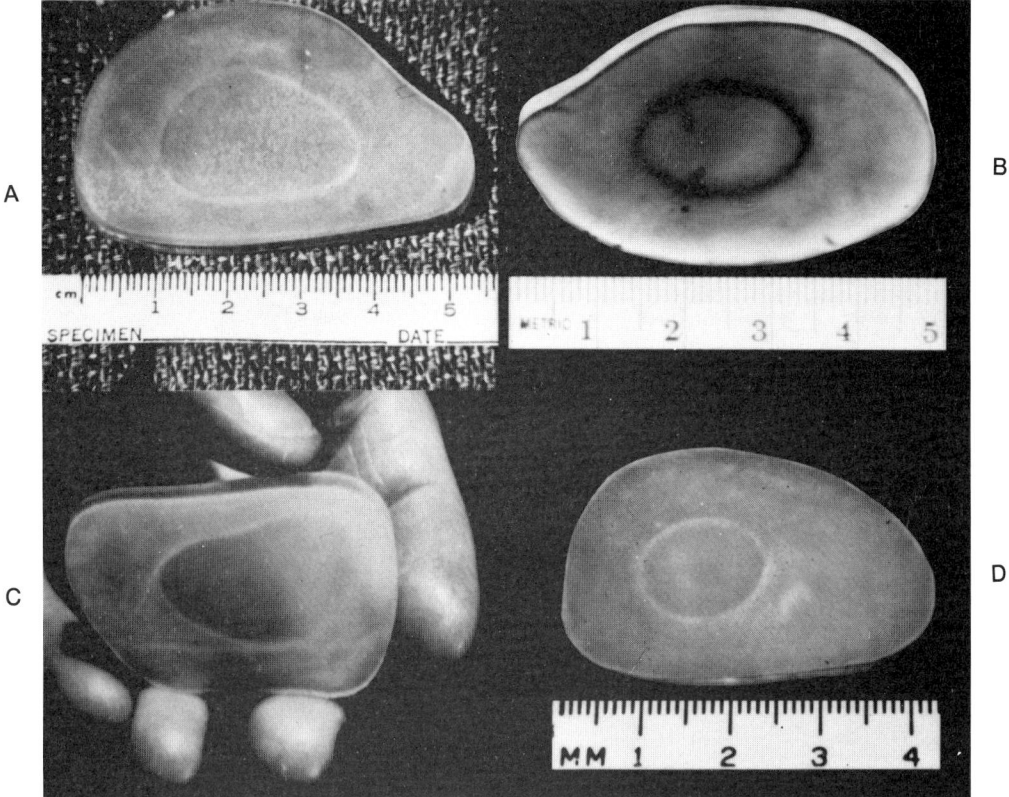

Figure 30-3. Four silicone rubber nasal septal prostheses prepared to fit into large nasal septal perforations.

Figure 30-4. A, Prosthesis before its placement. Since this was giant nasal septal perforation, large rhinotomy approach was needed to introduce the silicone rubber prosthesis into septal defect. **B,** Introduction of button into perforation. **C,** Closure of lateral rhinotomy incision. **D,** One year after operation.

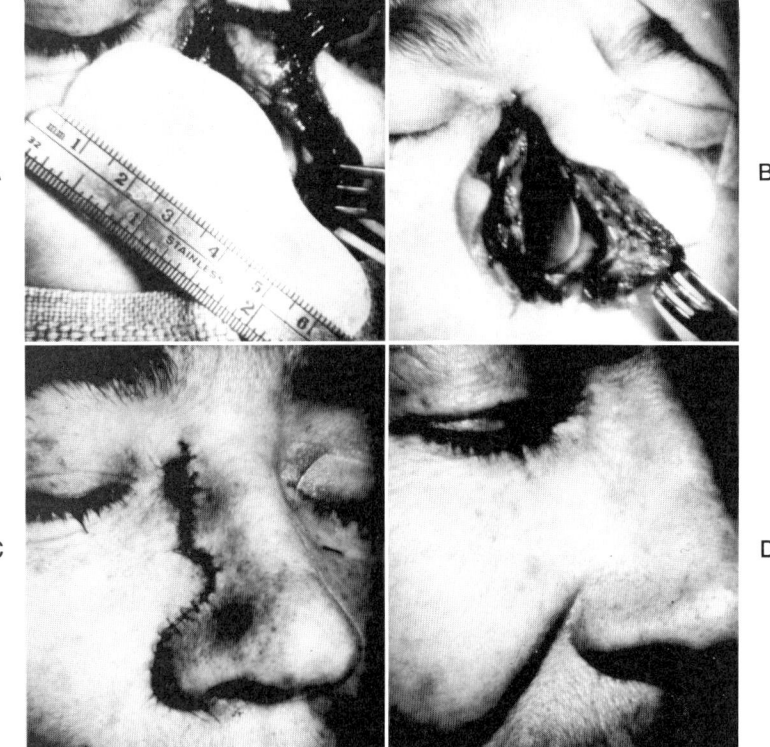

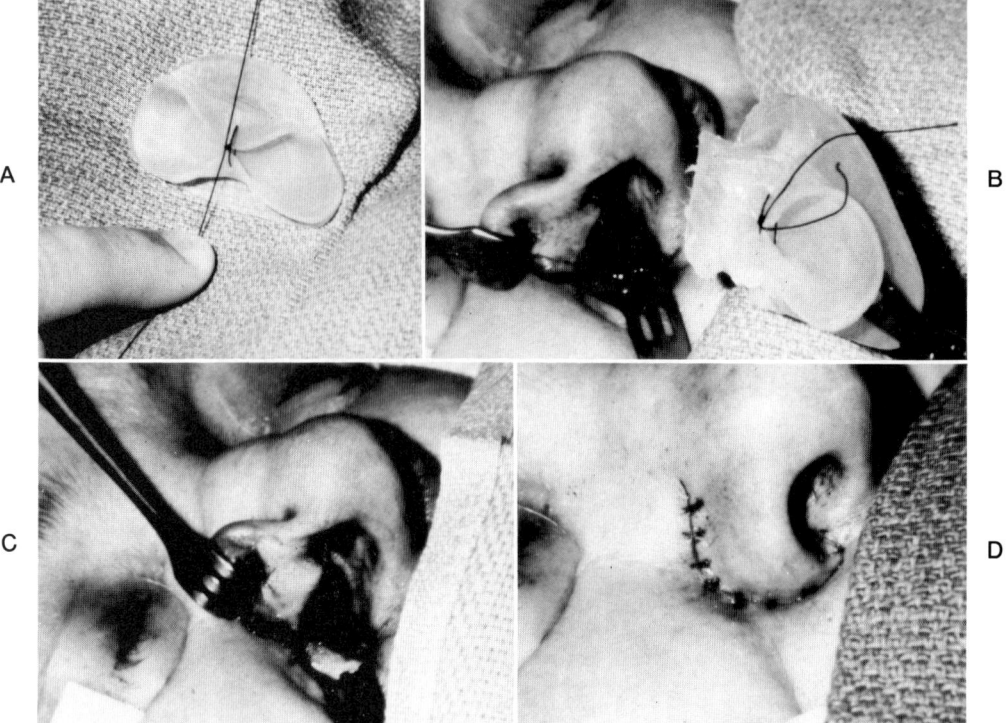

Figure 30-5. Alar incision is used to gain exposure required to introduce nasal septal prosthesis (**A, B,** and **C**). Closure of alar incision is seen in **D.**

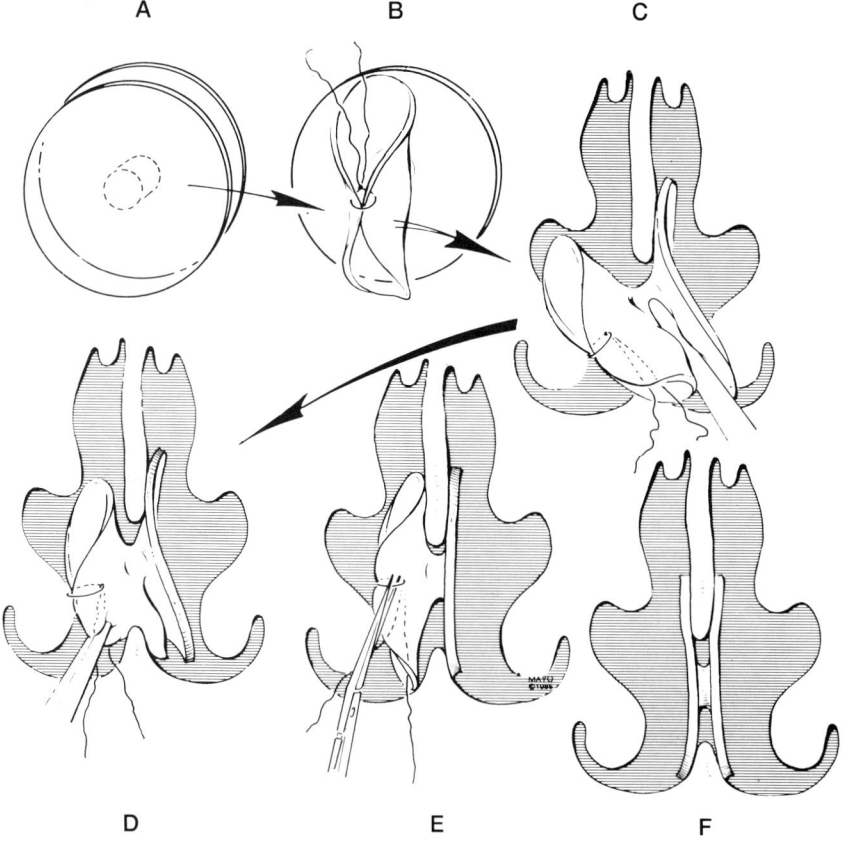

Figure 30-6. Schematic summary of technique by which nasal septal prosthesis is introduced. **A,** Septal prosthesis. Note that suture is placed through one of silicone rubber flanges of septal prosthesis (**B**). Silicone rubber prosthesis is introduced into perforation (**C**) and then pulled through (**D**), and after suture is snipped (**E**) prosthesis pops into place (**F**).

releasing the suture once the button was in place, as suggested by Arbour[1] (Figure 30-6).

Follow-up took place after 1 year in the first two patients, and the other two patients were contacted at 10 and 11 months after placement. All patients reported no further problem with epistaxis. In addition, each stated that their breathing had improved. Three noted disappearance of their pain, and one described improvement in her voice. One patient still had some problems with crusting.

DISCUSSION

Meyer,[9] in 1951, described the use of an obturator to close septal perforations. He reported a method of sizing the perforation by means of a template made from wax. The template was then used to create a nylon button. In his original article Meyer reported success with five patients, with follow-up periods ranging from 1 to 4 months. Link is reported to have used a superpolyamide septal obturator in the same year.[3]

Van Dishoeck and Lashley,[11] in 1975, reported a method of sizing obturators by injecting material into the perforation space after the rest of the nose had been walled off with cotton wool and discs of X-ray film. A soft plastic obturator was then cast in a mold of plaster of Paris.

Janeke,[7] in 1976, described a method of sizing anterior inferior perforations with blotting paper. The outline of the perforation appeared on the paper where the mucus had soaked into it. A disc of silicone rubber was then cut 3 to 4 mm wider than the paper outline. The circumference was then grooved and the prosthesis placed.

Zaki[12] described a method for making an impression of the defect with impression material on a cotton swab or tongue depressor. The material was placed in the perforation, and pressure was applied on each side to fill out the area of the defect. After the material had set it was removed and used to make a mold, from which a button was created out of heat-cured acrylic resin. The button was finished by polishing. Zaki believed it was mandatory to use an impression so that the stem of the button would be the right size. In that way one could avoid spreading by the button flanges of any adjacent open area near the flanges that might contribute to crusting. He also stated that a highly polished acrylic button would induce less crusting and bleeding and not be dislodged as easily as one of silicone rubber.

Brain[2] reported a technique in which an impression was taken with "silicone rubber." From this a silicone rubber obturator was constructed. He reported good results in 19 of 20 patients but mentioned that with larger perforations the results were not as favorable. Gray introduced the technique our group at Mayo had described[4,5,8] in which medical-grade silicone rubber is used.

The foremost problem in closing the four large perforations in the present series was finding an adequate method for sizing the perforations. It was important that the button fit exactly, since the margins of these perforations were so small. The center portion of the prosthesis must be of the proper size to avoid slippage of the button while allowing the flanges to conform to adjacent tissues so as not to obstruct the airway. All tissue margins of the perforations must be adequately covered so that crusting and bleeding will be minimized.

In all four of the cases of unusually large septal perforations in this series, it was impossible to size the defect with paper and merthiolate, since the paper could not be held against the slim margins well enough to get an accurate outline. Making a wax or synthetic impression was not feasible in such large defects, since it would have been difficult to fill all the areas of the defect and still remove the impression material. The use of computerized tomographic scanning proved quite effective for obtaining accurate sizing of the septal perforations. These cases were unusual, however, and the need for such measure is certainly an exception.

It is apparent that the nasal septal prosthesis is a useful alternative to surgical treatment for symptomatic nasal septal perforations. In 15 patients in this series it was the only treatment option remaining after attempts at surgical closure failed. It should also be noted that two of the patients who had buttons removed had subsequent successful surgical closure. Fairbanks,[6] in discussing surgical closure of septal perforations, commented that prostheses are an important treatment mode for patients with symptoms who are poor operative risks or who have perforations caused by active granulomatous or vascular disease. Reiter and Meyers[10] commented that closure of septal perforations in patients with diseases such as lupus erythematosus would probably best be accomplished with silicone rubber buttons.

There were no harmful complications in our series. The two buttons that dislodged posteriorly remained in the nasopharynx before they were retrieved. An external incision was necessary to introduce a septal button in only the three cases mentioned. This is not without precedent. Denecke and Meyer[3] stated that in very large perforations, when the nostril is too small to admit the obturator, the approach could be enlarged by incising the columella and extending the incision as far as the perforation.

Further review of the courses of patients with symptoms associated with nasal septal perforations has verified the success of treatment by septal prosthesis in 73% of patients. Use of prefabricated buttons has proved to be an efficacious, safe, and cost-effective means of treating patients with smaller perforations. In some patients with larger perforations use of a custom button has been necessary for successful treatment. Four patients for whom no previous satisfactory treatment had been available were successfully treated by introducing a carefully sized, custom-made nasal septal prosthesis.

ACKNOWLEDGMENT

I thank my colleagues George W. Facer, M.D., and John F. Pallanch, M.D., for their contributions to this work and William B. Westwood and Peter M. McDonahey, of the Department of Medical Graphics, who created these large septal obturators.

REFERENCES

1. Arbour, P.G.: Practical suggestion in cases of septal perforations: an easy way to insert the Kern's septal obturator, Laryngoscope **89**:1170-1171, 1979.
2. Brain, D.J.: Septorhinoplasty: the closure of septal perforations, J. Laryngol. Otol. **94**:495-505, 1980.
3. Denecke, H.J., and Meyer, R.: Corrective and reconstructive rhinoplasty. In Plastic surgery of the head and neck, vol. 1, New York, 1967, Springer-Verlag, pp. 137-140.
4. Facer, G.W., and Kern, E.B.: Nasal septal perforations: use of silastic button in 108 patients, Rhinology **17**:115-120, 1979.
5. Facer, G.W., and Kern, E.B.: Nonsurgical closure of nasal septal perforations, Arch. Otolaryngol. **105**:6-8, 1979.
6. Fairbanks, D.N.F.: Closure of nasal septal perforations, Arch. Otolaryngol. **106**:509-513, 1980.
7. Janeke, J.B.: Nasal perforations closed with a Silastic button, S. Afr. Med. J. **50**:2146, 1976.
8. Kern, E.B., and others: Closure of nasal septal perforations with a Silastic button: results in 45 patients, ORL Dig. **39**:9-17, 1977.
9. Meyer, R.: Neurungen in der Nasenplastik, Practica Otolaryngol. **13**:373-376, 1951.
10. Reiter, D., and Meyers, A.R.: Asymptomatic nasal septal perforations in systemic lupus erythematosus, Ann. Otol. Rhinol. Laryngol. **89**:78-80, 1980.
11. Van Dishoeck, E.A., and Lashley, F.O.N.: Closure of a septal perforation by means of an obturator, Rhinology **13**:33-37, 1975.
12. Zaki, H.S.: A new approach in construction of nasal septal obturators, J. Prosthet. Dent. **43**:654-657, 1980.

31

The Septum in Rhinoplasty

A few practical hints and technical suggestions

Mark Gorney

Form follows function.
FRANK LLOYD WRIGHT

In contrast to Frank Lloyd Wright's classic architectural dictum, quite the opposite applies in septorhinoplasty: Function is almost wholly dependent on form.

No septum is really straight. Heredity, birth, and repetitive trauma all combine to give most of us some degree of septal irregularity.[7] As long as the nasal vault is adequate, minor septal deviation is of little concern. However, it is self-evident that any narrowing or lowering of that vault without simultaneous correction of the septum will lead to some limitation of airflow. The externally deviated nose calls for aesthetic as well as functional correction. What we are concerned with is the essentially straight or slightly deviated nose inside of which there is a potential for both functional and aesthetic failure. A crooked nose cannot be straightened without correcting the septum; a simple rhinoplasty can create a crooked nose if the septum is not corrected.

A structurally sound and straight septum is the foundation of a satisfactory rhinoplasty result. As obvious as this may seem there is still substantial disagreement among surgeons as to appropriate corrective techniques. Among plastic surgeons there is also some misunderstanding of nasal physiology, particularly of the valve area, and sometimes there is a cavalier disregard for the integrity of the nasal airway. I suspect that the rate of obstructive complications is much higher than rates officially reported in the literature. In other words, it is nice to make them (the patients) beautiful, but can they breathe?

Volumes have been written on the functional aspects of nasal surgery. Neither this material nor the internal anatomy or function of the nose will be belabored here. Rather we should limit our attention to one facet of a broad field: an overview of the structural aspects of septoplasty as it relates to cosmetic rhinoplasty.

INFORMED CONSENT

In an "informed consent" session with the patient who has a potential nasal obstruction, one can draw the following metaphor: "Your nose is like an A-frame cottage. The front half of the cottage is made of canvas, and the back is made of wood. Down the middle, from front to back, there is a main bearing wall that supports the spine of the roof. If a giant tree were to fall on the house, the spine of the roof would cave in, and the central bearing wall would probably bend to a much greater degree on the weak front than on the hard rear. The bearing wall will buckle to varying degrees, thereby obstructing the rooms on either side. Imagine further that this wall at its bottom is set into a trough that also runs from the front to the back of the house. Both sides of the central bearing wall and the sides of the trough are covered with thick, red velvet wallpaper. On the slanting side walls of the roof there are some broad shelves that protrude into the room.

If the center wall is bulging into the space on either side, it will be difficult to pass from one end to the other. If the wall is crooked enough that the shelves on each side touch it, there is no passage at all. If the wall is only partly crooked and I wish to make the house narrower by moving the side walls in, I will achieve the same obstructive effect (no passage) unless I straighten out the main bearing wall first. To do this I must raise the wallpaper, get under it, and remove or straighten the crooked portion of the dividing wall. However, I cannot remove all of it, because then the roof might collapse. I must leave at least an L-shaped support at the front and under the roof. If this portion is also crooked I must then straighten it out. The wallpaper on both sides then rejoined, back to back, and there will be better passage on either side."

Although this may seem an oversimplified version, it has served me well over the past 25 years, even in cases where results have been less than optimal.

NASAL PHYSIOLOGY

For the purpose of this discussion we should focus on several limited but important facets of internal nasal physiology of significance to the plastic surgeon.[2,8]

1. The way in which air currents traverse the nasal conduits, the direction, their shape, and the speed of the stream are determined as much by nasal configuration as by the natural anatomic constriction found approximately 2 cm inside the nostrils. This area, commonly referred to as the *internal valve,* is the confluence of the caudal edge of the upper lateral cartilages and the septum (under the overlap of the upper border of the alar cartilages). This valve converts a round column of air into a flat stream, as the nozzle of a garden hose shapes the stream of water. The length and capacity of the hose mean nothing; the stream it throws and its direction are characterized by the shape of the nozzle (Figure 31-1, *A*).

2. On normal inspiration in the intact nose the air is directed upward and backward, arching up between the septum and turbinates to the face of the sphenoid, down through the choana, and into the pharynx. Relatively little air passes along the floor. The choana has essentially no effect on the stream.

3. Over the turbinates air becomes humidified to approximately 90% relative humidity before it reaches the larynx.

4. On expiration air passes through the lower choana and is thrown into the eddies by the baffle effect of the posterior aspect of the burbinates and the nozzle effect of the nostrils.

5. As the air currents are moved over the ciliated surfaces, particulate matter is deposited, probably by electrostatic principles. The mucous glands deposit a lubricating blanket, which is moved by the cilia and carries off debris. Tear flow assists this mechanism.

6. The function of the nasal cilia has been detailed by Proetz.[8] Cilia line the inner surface of the nose except for the olfactory areas. Going back to the metaphor, one can visualize a house through the center of which run two corridors covered with thick, velvet-pile, self-cleaning, wallpaper. The dust entering the house is passed along the wall, ceiling and floor, down the corridor, through the back door, and into the ashcan; it makes a complete trip in 20

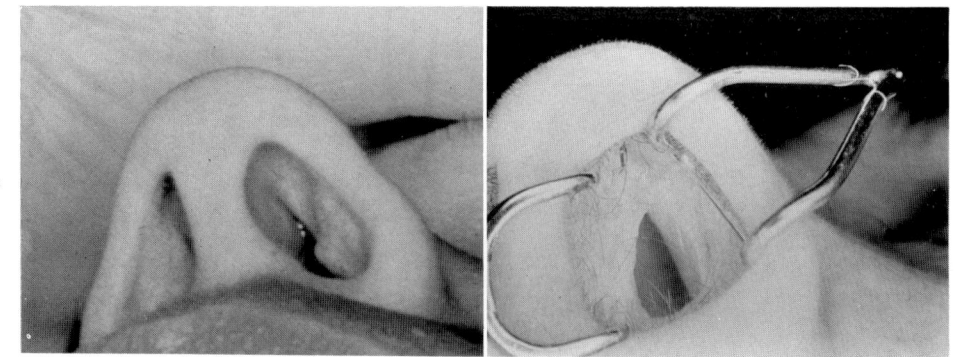

Figure 31-1. A, Normal configuration of internal valve on deep inspiration. **B,** Constriction of internal valve as result of surgery. Excessive loss of mucosa or upper lateral cartilage results in cicatricial webb and direct volumetric reduction of airflow.

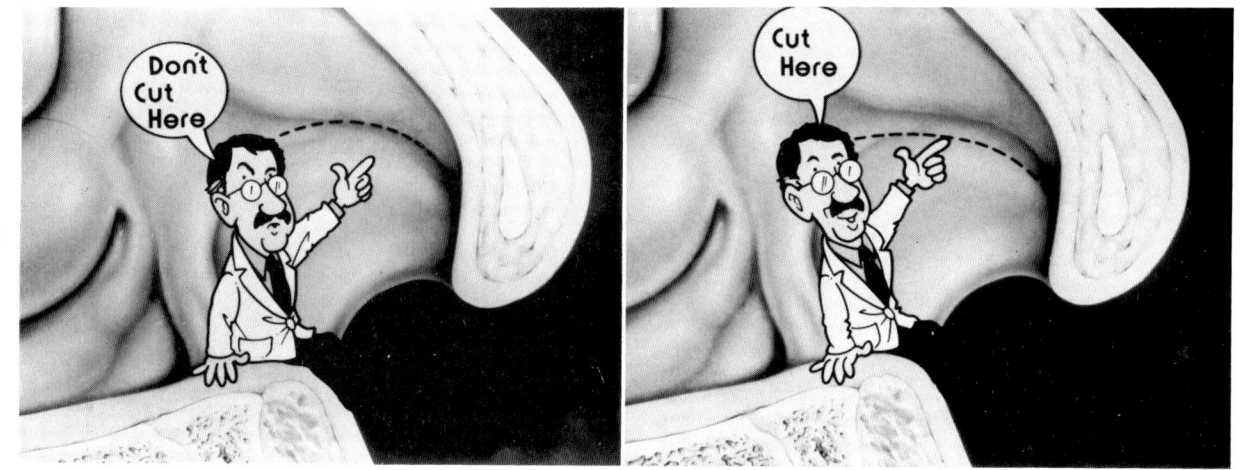

Figure 31-2. A, Preserve margin of upper lateral cartilage during rhinoplasty. **B,** Intercartilaginous incisions are acceptable but should be located at least 2 mm caudal to valve.

minutes. This self-cleaning wallpaper works 24 hours a day unless something happens. Cilia are tough and have only one natural enemy: drying. This eliminates their ability to function and move mucus.

7. The principal iatrogenic enemy of cilia is scar tissue, which makes hurdles over which cilia cannot move the mucous blanket. Annular scars not only bar the flow but further narrow the nozzle, thus creating not only a mechanical but also a physiologic barrier (Figures 31-1, *B* and 31-2).

8. The valves must be of sufficient size to allow free flow of air, and they should be nearly identical. If disproportionate amounts of air are allowed to enter one side only, that side will tend to dry and undergo metasplasia. This may be reported by the patient as a feeling of nasal obstruction. Underventilation will lead to constant accumulation of mucus.

ARCHITECTURAL SIGNIFICANCE OF THE SEPTUM

Converse[1] and others have thoroughly detailed the role of the septum in nasal architecture. I would like to reemphasize a few vital points.

1. It is generally agreed that if one drops an imaginary line from the nasion to the nasal spine, anything posterior to that line can be resected from floor to ceiling without fear of collapse. Anything anterior to it must be resected with descretion and forethought, lest insufficient support and subsequent functional (and aesthetic) distortion occur. Even if there seems to be an adequate dorsal cartilaginous support remaining, beware of the effect of contracture of the mucosal leaves and the plane of the scar

between them. If there have been perforations, this contracture will be more significant.

2. If one considers the upper lateral cartilages as the wings sprouting from the upper edge of the septum (an embryologically correct concept), then if the upper edge of the septum is deviated, it must be freed from the wings that tether it. If one fails to do this their guidewire effect will eventually deviate the dorsum again. This separation should be done at a submucoperichondrial level. If one keeps the mucoperichondrial flap attached to the underside of the upper lateral cartilages, except where they join the septum, then the mucoperichondrial flaps will not sag. In this way one can avoid cutting away the upper lateral cartilages, mucosa and all. In my opinion this maneuver creates scar and synechiae, which later may restrict inspiratory airflow.

3. High septal deflection, often undetected, can frustrate a perfect rhinoplasty. The hump, which is in the normal midsagittal plane, may be covering a crooked septum just below it, a configuration easy to miss in cursory preoperative examination. Operative edema may deceive the surgeon. After infracture is finished the nasal bones and upper lateral cartilages are then brought together against an undiscovered deviation of the new upper border of the septum. Two weeks later, when the edema recedes, the beautiful result at the end of the operation may appear distinctly off center.

4. The sequence of the septal correction at surgery is important. Figure 31-3 shows a typical subluxation and override of the septum-vomer junction at the anterior inferior corner of the quadrilateral

cartilage. What happens here can have a profound effect on the new profile line. If the dislocated lower edge of the cartilage is freed up and replaced within the vomer, this will tend to lift the lower end of the nose (Figure 31-4). On the other hand, if the extremely deviated lower edge of the septum must be cut off, or the vomer groove must be chiseled out to replace the septum in the center, or both, the surgeon may end up lowering the end of the nose, whose support depends on the remaining cartilaginous strut. Thus the surgeon must know what he or she intends to do ahead of time. It is poor planning to make a beautiful profile and then correct the septum only to find the profile lowered in the tip area. It is wiser to do the septal correction first, leaving more than adequate dorsal buttress so that the profile line can still be corrected or the nose shortened at the end of the rhinoplasty without weakening the remaining support. If in doubt, the hump resection and dorsal correction must be done first and then the septoplasty so that enough cartilage is left behind to guarantee integrity of the profile line. Correcting the septum first, particularly if it is badly bent, is much easier from the standpoint of visibility, neatness, and safety.

5. The hump may be a relative or absolute one. A large Arabic or a Romanesque hump can be characterized as an absolute one. If the profile line suddenly dips below the end of the nasal bones, this is a relative hump, which is almost invariably caused by septal abnormality. If the septum has been distorted severely enough to be noticeable externally, oftentimes almost total removal of the septum will barely affect the profile line. In this nose it is wise to consider using the resected septum to bridge the sag between the self-supporting tip and the end of the nasal bone.

6. In severe internal deviations the remaining L-shaped strut may remain deviated or subluxated. If the surgeon fails to straighten it out, he or she is guaranteed a deviated nose. Until recent years most authors advised various maneuvers to score, cut, crosshatch, or remove strips vertically from the convex side of the deformity, with the idea of allowing the remaining septum to swing back into the midline (Figure 31-5). There are also a number of maneuvers described to keep it in the original position, but generally speaking, this has been at the best chancy. At least as many noses have redeviated as have maintained the improvement. Gibson[6] and, more re-

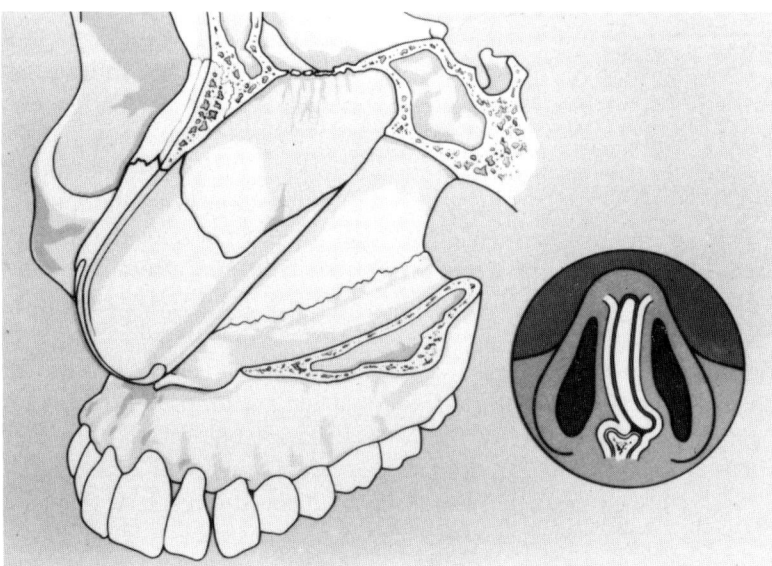

Figure 31-3. Typical subluxation-override of cartilaginous septum on vomer. This presents as "shelf" (see *inset*). Note that cartilage is invested in its own perichondrial envelope and vomer in its own periosteal sheath.

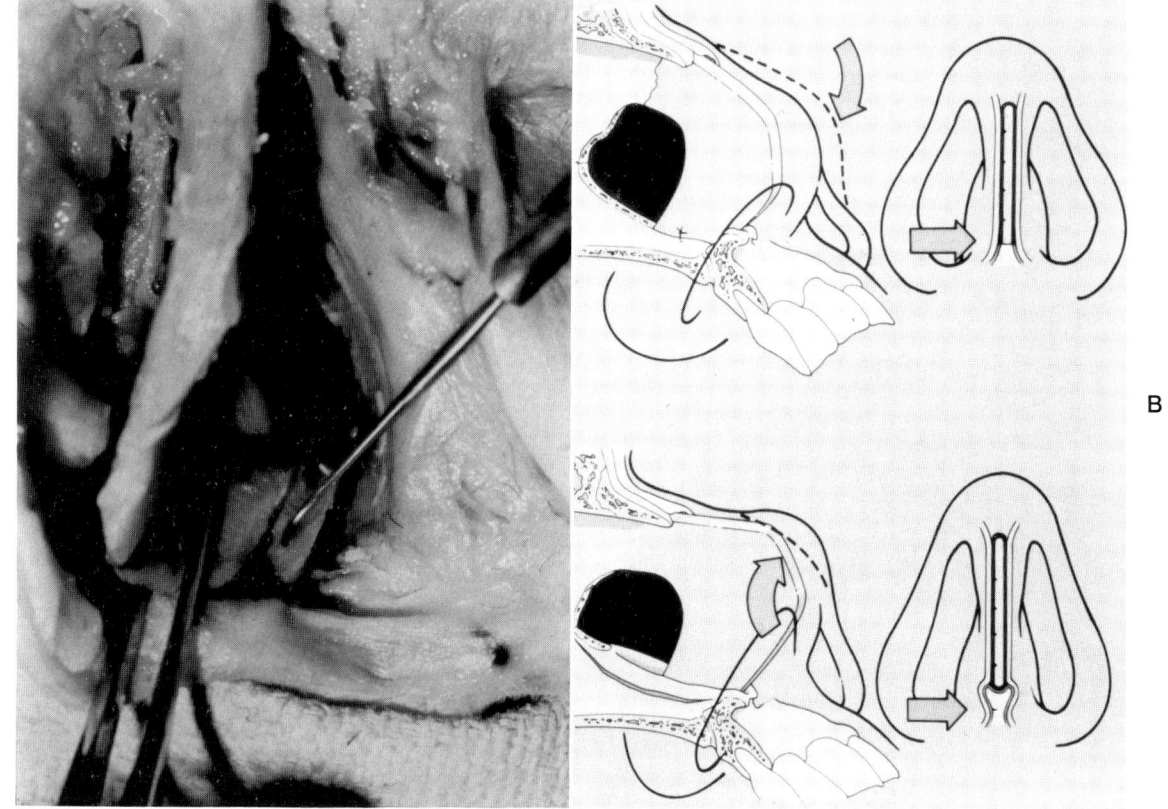

Figure 31-4. A, Intraoperative perspective as viewed by surgeon. Elevator is in vomer groove, which is shifted to left in this case. **B,** Resection of vomer (top) in such a case would likely result in sagging of remaining framework of nose and depression of nasal tip. Maintenance of vomer and replacement of the remaining cartilaginous stut into vomer (below) would more likely preserve forward thrust of nose, especially at tip region.

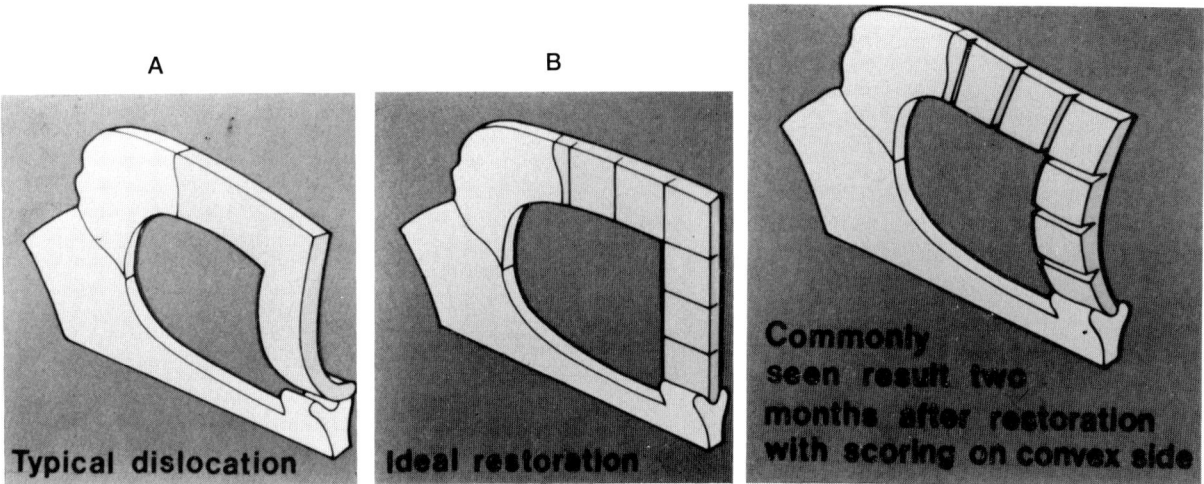

Figure 31-5. A, Typical dislocation of septal cartilage remnant out of vomer groove. **B,** Restoration of cartilage strut into groove after weakening of cartilage by crosscutting. It is important to maintain mucosal connection to cartilage on at least one side during such reconstruction. **C,** Postoperative bowing of vertical strut, even though it was weakened by crosscutting, is not unusual.

cently, Fry[3-5] have effectively demonstrated the existence of interlocking stresses within cartilage. Most significantly, Fry has dramatically illustrated the tendency of cartilage to curl to the opposite side from which it is scored. Thus the septum should be scored on the concave side (Figure 31-6, *A* and *B*). If the deviation is a complex one both sides should be scored but always on the concave portion (Figure 31-6, *C*).

7. In a particularly badly deviated septum it helps to reinforce the scoring by placing a small batten of surplus septal cartilage or vomerine bone on the unscored side to act as a reinforcement. If possible redeviation is feared this batten can be placed diagonally across the remaining septum. This maneuver is illustrated in Figure 31-7, *A*.

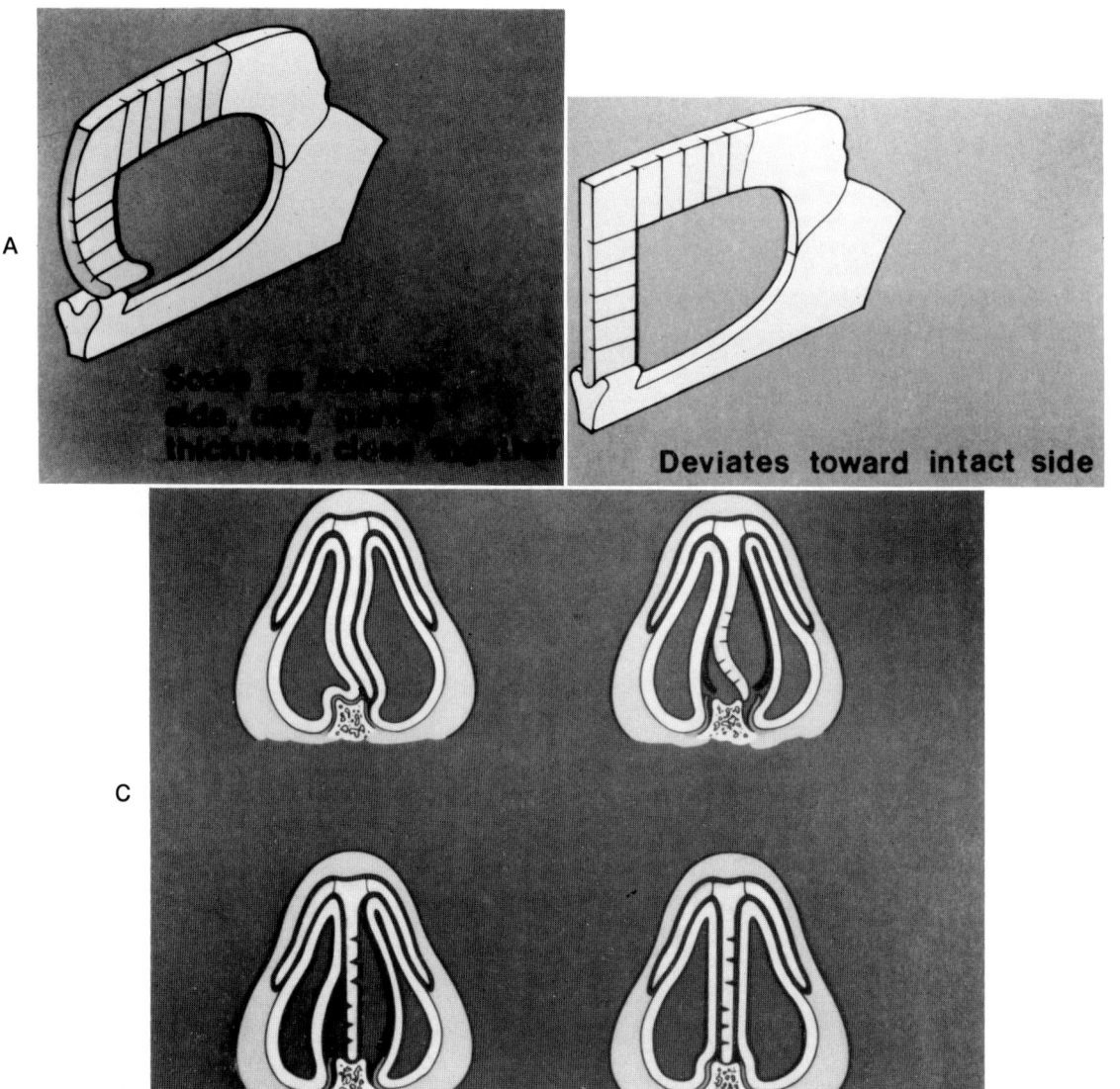

Figure 31-6. A, Septum should be crosscut on concave side and only part way through thickness of cartilage. Redundant lips of cartilage that are dislocated from vomer can be conservatively trimmed. **B,** Cartilage crosscut in such a manner will tend to deviate toward intact side, with forces of healing. **C,** Wherever concave surface exists crosscutting can be done. These cartilaginous incisions should be placed as close together as feasible. Theoretically at least, such weakening of concave side results in straightening force in septum, as shown; however, such is not always the result.

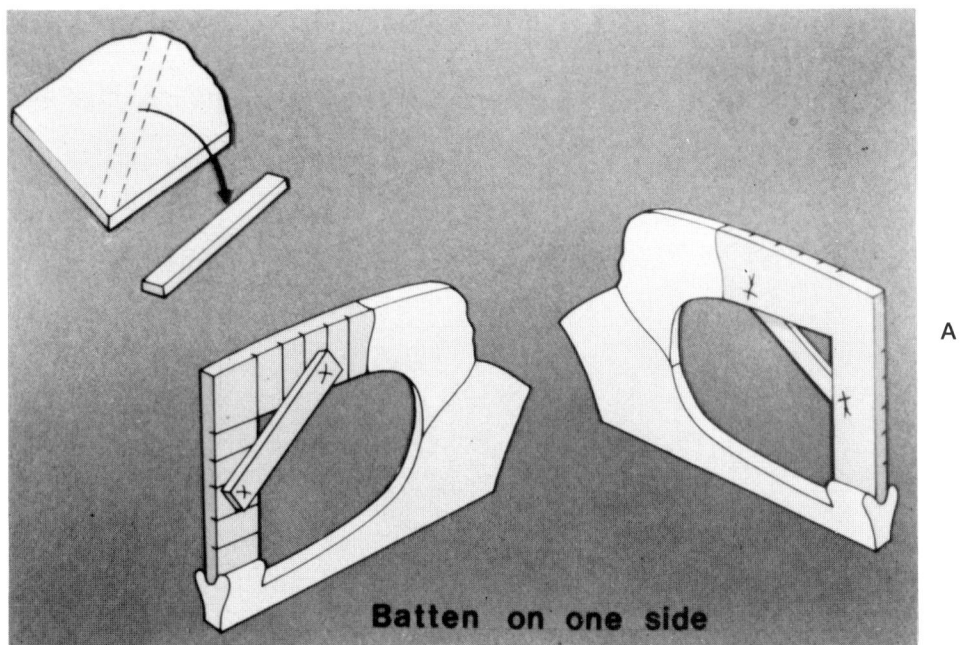

Batten on one side

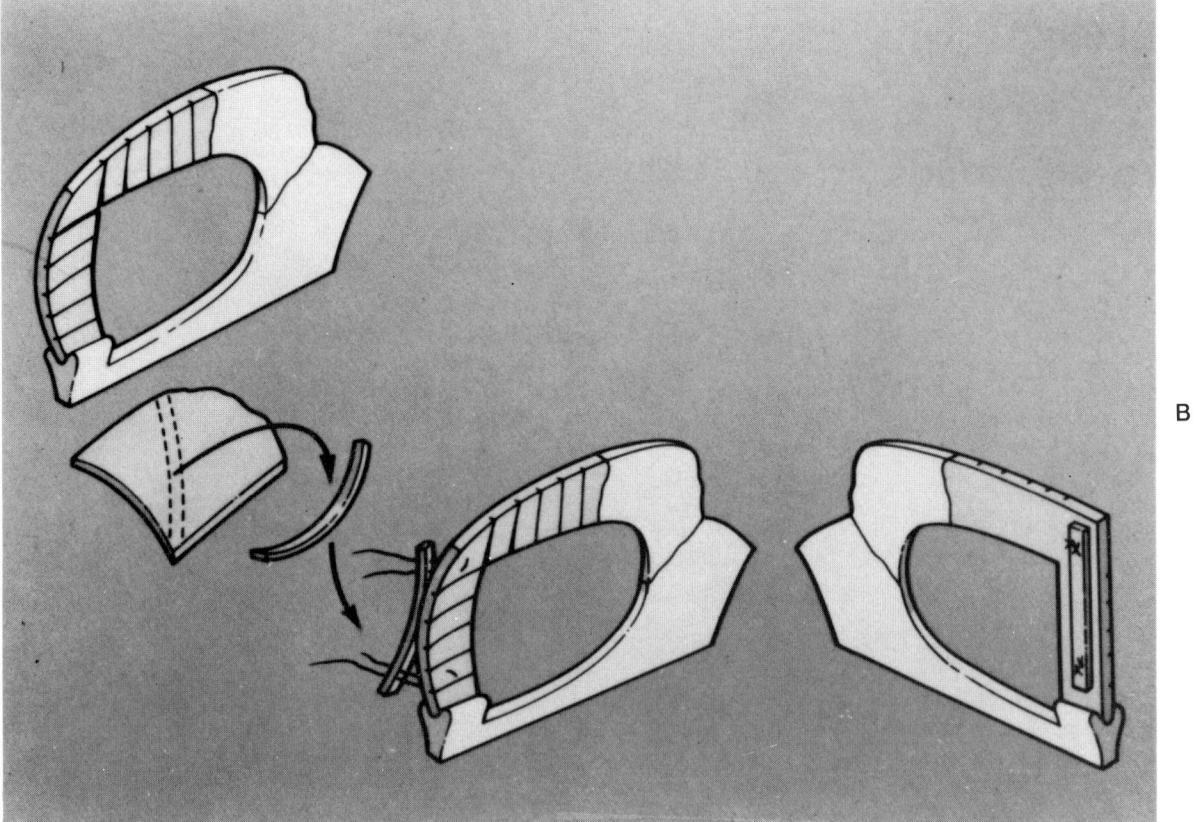

Figure 31-7. **A,** Straight, thick portion of septal specimen can be used as cross brace or batten to keep septum straight (either one or both sides). **B,** Curved cartilage spear can be used as countersplint on opposite side to prevent recurvature.

Alternatively, one can cut a curved batten out of a segment of curved cartilage that has been resected and can suture it on the "convex" side of the remaining septum. This strong curve will then act as a "counterspring" and prevent redeviation (Figure 31-7, *B*).

TECHNICAL SUGGESTIONS

No one operation can correct a deformity so infinite in its variables. What must be done is an operation that will (1) restore function, (2) correct deviation, and (3) prevent saddling, columella retraction, and tip droop. The principle of the operation is to divide every attachment of the cartilaginous septum except for a mucosal flap on one side, to release the interlocking stresses in the twisted cartilage, or to resect what cannot be straightened. The goal should be maximum mobility with the least removal of tissue possible (Figure 31-8).

A few caveats may be in order.

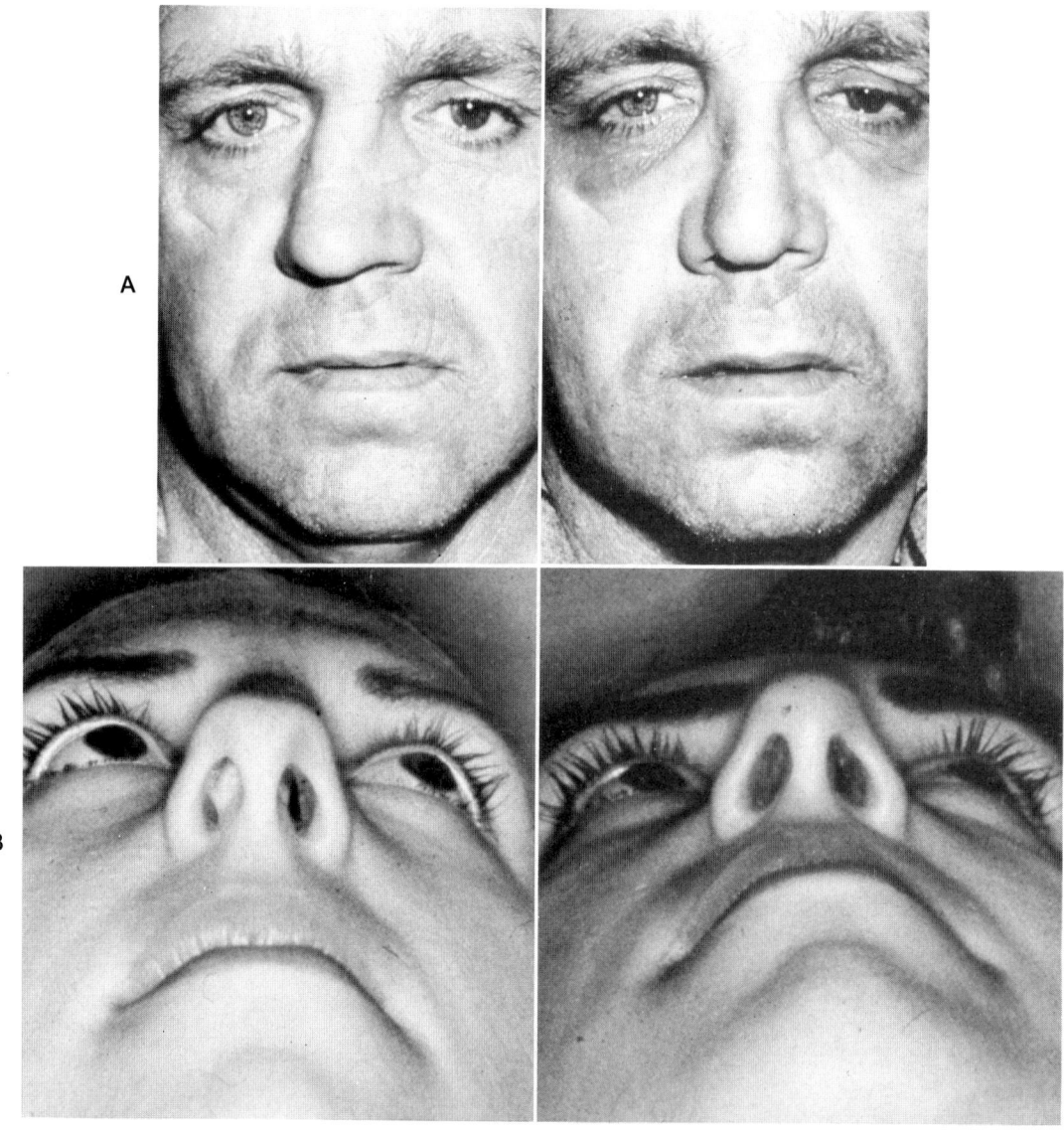

Figure 31-8. **A,** Severely twisted nose corrected by partial resection and scoring. Replacement of morceled cartilage and cross-bracing on right with batten (see Figure 31-7). **B,** *Left:* severely deviated caudal septum after attempted correction; *right:* permanent midline position after scoring on concave side and bracing of convex side with counterspring of curved cartilage (see Figure 31-7, *B*).

1. The secret to avoiding perforation is to elevate the flap at the right level—subperichondrially. In the distal 1 or 2 cm of cartilaginous septum, the mucosa is intimately attached to the cartilage. After an incision is made along the protrusive leading edge, a pair of Converse scissors or a sharp elevator is useful in finding the correct plane. It is easy to start down the wrong one, and this virtually guarantees perforations and tears, particularly along the spurs, crests, and ridges where the mucosa is as thin as wet tissue paper. There is a characteristic gray-blue reflex visible on entering the right plane. There is also a clean, smooth feel on the instrument, which will glide along easily. When the instrument passes from the cartilage to the vertical plate of the ethmoid, there is a characteristic change in the feel to one of scraping. It is best to proceed in semicircular, upward motions rather than to push straight ahead, then back. Do not try to go past the angle of deviation or around ridges, since this will also produce perforations. (Small perforations are of no consequence unless they are on both mucosal leaves; in this case permanent perforation will result.)

2. Along the inferior anterior aspect of the cartilaginous septum, where it fits in the vomerine ridge, it is difficult to pass the instrument down from the subperiosteal space of the vomer. The quadrilateral septal cartilage is invested completely by perichondrium, even along its lower edge, which may or may not sit in the vomerine groove (see Figure 31-3, A). The vomerine ridge, in turn, has periosteum tightly adherent over it. Therefore undermining from the roof of the nose to the septum-vomer ridge should not be continued inferiorly, but a new tunnel should be started under the periosteum of the vomer. It is much easier to joint these two spaces without tearing once they have been independently developed (see Figure 31-3, B-E).

3. Remove only what is necessary: Sometimes simple correction of the subluxation override will allow the septum to swing back into midline after scoring. If a substantial section must be removed or there are perforations, morcel what was removed, and put it back between the mucosal flaps (see Figures 31-3, F, and 31-6).

4. If the vertical element of the remaining L-shaped cartilage support is still crooked, do not depend on columellar pockets or transfixion devices to straighten it. It not only will not work, but it will carry the tip of the nose with it when it redeviates. Score it on its concave side, and if need be, stiffen it on the intact (convex) side with a thin cartilage batten as previously described (see Figure 31-7).

5. Totally intact, accurately closed mucoperichondrial flaps, if inadequately splinted, may be dangerous. Septal hematomas are not uncommon, and if they are not evacuated properly they can give a thick, obstructive septum. There is no harm in making a couple of stab wounds with a No. 11 blade at separate sites on either side at the base of the mucopericondrial flaps to drain the hematomas.

6. The turbinates are often part of the problem. Time and space do not permit a detailed account of this aspect; however, if may be appropriate to deal with troublesome turbinates at the time of surgery by several simple maneuvers. They can be outfractured by forceful pressure with a long speculum, cauterized along their edge, or trimmed away. Beware of overly enthusiastic treatment. Intraoperatively and postoperatively they also respond nicely to intranasal injection of corticoids directly into the submucosa. Injection of 0.5 ml of methylprednisolone acetate into the bulging portion of the middle turbinate will help.

REFERENCES

1. Converse, J.M.: Corrective surgery of nasal deviations, Arch. Otolaryngol. **52**:671, 1950.
2. Fomon, S., and others: Physiological principles in rhinoplasty, Arch. Otolaryngol. **53**:256, 1951.
3. Fry, H.J.H.: Nasal skeletal trauma and the interlocked stresses of the nasal septal cartilages, Br. J. Plast. Surg. **20**:146, 1967.
4. Fry, H.J.H.: The importance of the septal cartilage in nasal trauma Br. J. Plast. Surg. **20**:392, 1967.
5. Fry, H.J.H.: Interlocked stresses in human nasal septal cartilage, Br. J. Plast. Surg. **19**:276, 1966.
6. Gibson, T., and David, W.B.: The distortion of autogenous cartilage grafts: its cause and prevention, Br. J. Plast. Surg. **10**:257, 1958.
7. Gray, L.: The deviated nasal septum, J. Laryngol. Otolaryngol. **79**:567, 1956.
8. Proetz, A.W.: Physiology of nose from the standpoint of plastic surgeon, Arch. Otolaryngol. **39**:514, 1944.

BIBLIOGRAPHY

Becker, O.J.: Problems of septum in rhinoplastic surgery, Arch. Otolaryngol. **53**:622, 1951.
Dingman, R.: Correction of nasal deformities due to defects of the septum, Plast. Reconstr. Surg. **18**:291, 1956.
Fomon, S., and others: New approach to ventral deflections of nasal septum. Arch. Otolaryngol. **54**:356, 1951.
Fomon, S., and others: Plastic repair of obstructing nasal septum, Arch. Otolaryngol. **47**:7, 1948.
Goldman, I.B.: Rhinoplastic sequelae causing nasal obstruction, Arch. Otolaryngol. **83**:151, 1966.
Goldman, I.B.: New techniques in surgery of deviated nasal septum, Arch. Otolaryngol. **64**:183, 1956.
Horton, C.E.: Combined septoplasty and rhinoplasty. In Masters, F.W. and Lewis, J.R., Jr., editors: Symposium on aesthetic surgery of the nose, ears and chin, St. Louis, 1973, The C.V. Mosby Co.
Kazanjian, V.H., and Converse, J.M.: Surgical treatment of facial injuries, Baltimore, 1974, Williams & Wilkins Co.
Killian, G.: Die submucose Fensterresektion der Nasenscheidewand, Arch. Laryngol. Rhinol. (Berlin) **16**:362, 1904; The submucous window resection of the nasal septum, Ann. Otol. Rhinol. Laryngol. **14**:363, 1905.
Metzenbaum, M.: Replacement of lower end of dislocated septal cartilage versus submucous resection of dislocated end of septal cartilage, Otolaryngol. **9**:282, 1929.
Peer, L.A.: Operation to repair lateral displacement of lower border of septal cartilage, Arch. Otolaryngol. **25**:475, 1937.
Seltzer, A.P.: Nasal septum: plastic repair of deviated septum associated with deflected tip, Arch. Otolaryngol. **40**:433, 1944.
Steffensen, W.H.: Reconstruction of the nasal septum, Plast. Reconstr. Surg. **2**:66, 1947.

Point & Counterpoint
Part IX

Question: Is there ever an indication for total septectomy?

Comment (Mark Gorney): Very, very rarely. This approach should be used only in the traumatically injured nose, the one that is completely smashed, that is, in the old boxer or old wrestler. I have occasionally had to remove the septum, because the problem could be corrected only in two stages. First, I removed the obstruction, then I reconstructed the septum. Nowadays I would more often complete the correction in one procedure.

Comment (Jack Sheen): No, I have never had any reason to totally remove the septum.

Comment (Gene Tardy): I have removed the entire septum only for malignant disorders. I will consider a partial or complete removal if there is trauma, as Dr. Gorney mentioned, but then obviously I must provide total replacement with fixation and stabilization.

Question: You seem to have some very strong feelings about minimal trauma to the cartilage and gently tissue handling. Could you elaborate on that topic?

Comment (Gene Tardy): I do have strong feelings about the handling of cartilage, because finally we, as a group of doctors interested in doing reasonable work, understand that currently cartilage is the best replacement substance to use in the nose. This realization has taken some time to develop. I am pleased to learn the group assembled here have general agreement on the importance of cartilage.

Anecdotal experience is helpful and should be a part of any common input to continuing education. However, based on laboratory studies and biopsies of crushed and uncrushed cartilage. I am convinced that you run less risk of eventually losing the work you have put in to the restored anatomy if you do not crush or fragment cartilage severely. Cartilage grafts provide a slender, delicate support with shape, form, and contour. We exploit those properties in all kinds of reconstruction of the lovely curved lines of the nose; after all, there are no straight lines anywhere in the nose. The evidence of resorption after chondroitin sulfate has been liberated through the crushing of cartilage remains unclear. The work in Europe and Sweden on cartilage and its long-term fate is compelling. I urge you to read the literature on cartilage and then employ the most conservative technique possible. By simply shaving the cartilage you can make a delicate, thin wafer that looks like a piece of Gelfoam; it is not crushed, it possesses structural integrity, it is live cartilage, and it will persist.

Question: Do you have any feeling about use of crushed cartilage?

Comment (Jack Sheen): I can speak only from a clinical point of view, but I feel quite the opposite. I have in the last 10 years placed more than 1,000 crushed-cartilage grafts; I use crushed cartilage to modify the thickness or the shape, and I do this with lateral walls. For the last 3 to 4 years I have been placing crushed cartilage over the dorsum to close the roof or to make an absolutely normal palpating dorsum with no ridges. In recent years I have been crushing cartilage to place in the tip, and I have not seen any degree of absorption in any of these patients over the long term. I cannot give you any hard data that would support my position; I can only tell you as a clinician that crushed cartilage does work and it has worked well for me for the last 12 years.

Question: Why do you like splints for your septal work?

Answer (Mark Gorney): I like the splints, but I don't leave them in long, just about 4 to 5 days, or 2 weeks maximum in a severly injured nose. I feel more comfortable with splints; whereas a lot of people still pack noses. I have not packed a nose in 10 years. I have tried some of the magnetic splints that Dr. Tardy described, but I never feel secure that those magnets are working across two layers of mucosa. Maybe I am wrong. But I do believe in using the splints, and I find the Xomed ones to be very satisfactory.

Question: Over what period of time does the cartilage reshape itself in the healing process? We know the cartilage has a memory, but does this memory cause redeviation after 6 months? Is it advisable to leave some type of splint in place for 6 months or a year?

Comment (Mark Gorney): First, the splint would be messy and cause an odor. Second, I am not convinced that the splint will keep the nose straight. I agree with Gene Tardy that the forces and the memory within cartilage are extremely strong; I have seen septa stay straight about 3 months, then suddenly at about 6 months, redeviate.

Comment (Gene Tardy): It seems to me that the inherent interlocked stresses in cartilage cannot be easily overcome by some kind of semirigid, semipermanent splint. No one really believes that a favorable rhinoplasty result can be substantially influenced long term by an external splint. Why can't the same be true internally? I believe if the cartilage is not properly repositioned without tension and force at the time of surgery, then a high probability exists that the septum will redeviate.

A great deal of controversy exists about scoring the concave side of the cartilage. In our studies scoring the cartilage on the concave side has resulted in a little release and a little improvement. It is only, however, when partial-thickness wedges are taken out on the *convex* side (the opposite side) that the cartilage straightens sufficiently to be stabilized with sutures. Therefore what you are treating in essence is like a crescentic scar; there is one long side and one short side. The surgeon must lengthen the short (concave) side and shorten the long (convex) side, functionally equalizing the two sides.

Question: Do you perform the septal work initially at the time of septorhinoplasty or after the dorsum has been changed? Do you do a submucous resection at the time of rhinoplasty? Do you ever separate the two—work on the septum and then do an external correction several months later?

Comment (Jack Sheen): I do a large percentage of septorhinoplasties in one step, and I don't see any reason not to, as long as the integrity of the dorsal and caudal struts is maintained.

Comment (Mark Gorney): I rarely separate the two, and I always do the septum first.

Comment (Gene Tardy): I usually attack the septum first, because I find that part of the procedure the hardest to do. Also, while I am doing that the rest of the nose is usually undergoing vasoconstriction. There are times, however, when this order is reversed, particularly when one wants to ensure adequate residual support. I try to complete the work in one stage. The nose is made up of variety of components that need to be rearranged and fitted together like pieces of a puzzle.

Comment (Mark Gorney): Before we abandon this topic I would like to point out that the ear is a superb source of extra cartilage. Jack Sheen has demonstrated, better than anyone, how beautifully you can use almost the entire concha. You need never be afraid that cartilage is lacking inside the nose.

Question: Is there a minimal age limit for the patient when operating on the deviated septum?

Comment (Gene Tardy): I don't believe there is an age limit. If the child has a bilateral blockage that child needs to breathe for general health reasons as well as for normal facial growth. I will do a conservative although complete dissection of the tissues, then do a reconstruction. If I can construct at least one very good airway and another that is at least passable, I am happy and satisfied. I then tell the child that at 15 or 16 years something more will need to be done. Many children in this country smash their noses on the basketball court or in a bicycle accident, and suprisingly few of those noses fail to develop properly. I think surgical dissection can be safely done without disturbing growth centers.

Question: Would any one of you ever do a submucous resection on a child?

Comment (Eugene Kern): I agree with Gene Tardy; I operate on a septum if and when it is indicated for improvement of the airway in a child. It has been demonstrated convincingly that you can do these procedures safely in children, in a controlled setting, with minimal trauma. Of course in a certain number of cases you will have to do a secondary procedure, but the goal is to improve the airway and thereby breathing.

Comment (Eugene Courtiss): The real problem we have is not in the young child, but it is in the child of 11 or 12 years, the young girl who is pretty and just beginning to develop. The orthodontist is now ready to go to work, and he says "Fellas, she can't breath through her nose. Would you take care of it right now?" She wants her rhinoplasty at that stage, and at that point you have to hold a lot of hands, for about 3 years.

Question: Are there any specific guidelines or indications as to when to do a septoplasty or when a submucous resection is specifically indicated? Do you ever run into problems with the so-called *flapping flap* where medial support of the septal wall is lost and mucosal flaps vibrate on inspiration or expiration?

Comment (Jack Sheen): As Dr. Tardy has pointed out, the decision of whether to do a septoplasty or a submucous resection depends on the abnormality. It also depends on whether or not septal cartilage is needed to reconstruct the nose. This is one of the indications I have used over the years for doing a submucous resection. I have not found any problems clinically with the so-called *flapping septum,* and I have certainly removed my share of vomer and cartilage. I have seen patients who have had the entire septal partition removed except for the anterior and dorsal caudal supports, without flapping mucosa.

Comment (Mark Gorney): The only reason for doing a resection would be for extrusion of an isolated, small knuckle of cartilage or spur. In any other case I would attempt a septoplasty.

Comment (Eugene Kern): I believe it is important to replace the cartilage and bone in the interseptal space to provide support. Also, as mentioned, if and when it is necessary to enter the septal space at a later date, it is much easier to perform dissection. Aside from any physiologic consideration, I believe it is important to replace tissue in the interseptal space.

Comment (Gene Tardy): I always try to put something back between the flaps, because that cartilage or bone may be needed later on in that patient. I would rather put it there than in the bottle. Alternatively, that cartilage or bone can be stored behind the ear up in the hairline. It won't bother the patient very much if you explain that you will be able to use it years later if you need it, perhaps for some of these very difficult reconstructions.

Question: The next question is a rather practical one. Unfortunately, I suppose, about 75% of the normal population has a deviated septum. In a standard rhinoplasty without submucous resection, how do you address the problem of insurance coverage in terms of the diagnosis? Is this a relevant factor; do you just put down "straight rhinoplasty," or do you always do some work on the septum?

Comment (Jack Sheen): I do in fact indicate "septoplasty/rhinoplasty." However, when absolutely nothing is done on the septum, this information is indicated on the operative note. About half of these notes are picked up by the insurance company, and payment is denied. I do all I can to ensure that the insurance company pays for the part for which it is responsible.

Comment (Mark Gorney): My experience is essentially the same. I warn my patients at the outset that there is no functional component to be corrected. I tell them that I simply cannot perjure myself when I respond to the letter from the insurance company asking how much of the operation was aimed at restoring function, how much was aesthetic, or whether it was a combined procedure. My answer is always very straightforward. The patient usually will then decide what he or she is willing to pay.

Comment (Eugene Kern): I see primarily noses that have been traumatized, with the result being airway problems; I so state that fact, and I keep rhinomanometric data to support the fact of a breathing prob-

lem. Therefore I don't face the problem of insurance coverage with the frequency of those surgeons who do primarily cosmetic work.

Comment (Mark Gorney): The forms that I give patients indicate that I will not honor requests to falsify reports. I further point out to patients that our integrity is a valuable asset and that insurance companies have profiles on all physicians. Therefore I will do exactly what I think is right, and patients accept that.

Comment (Tom Rees): I prefer to be honest, but this is a very real dilemma we face. About every third patient I see claims to have a deviated nasal septum. We all know the game we are playing, although the third-party carriers are not privy to it at this point. I will not put down SMR or radical SMR on every form, but many surgeons do. This is going to backfire on the hospital, because Blue Shield will begin investigating and will turn the investigations over to Blue Cross; Blue Cross will then demand back payments from the hospital. Thus this is a very practical issue, for which I have no solution. A standard rhinoplasty, in which I do virtually no septal work, except some minor trimming of the caudal septum, cannot be called an SMR.

Comment (Gene Tardy): It is absolutely critical that we be honest. In the Midwest, at least, the insurance companies look very carefully at this. They have a very strong profile on doctors who do this work, and they are interested in knowing who is honest and who fudges a little bit. This situation is going to change in a hurry.

Question: Do you think in the next 5 to 10 years that rhinomanometry will be available in all our offices to clinically evaluate patients before and after operation. Will this be a relevant tool in finding a specific structural problem?

Comment (Eugene Kern): There is no question in my mind that if a significant structural problem exists, rhinomanometry will record an elevation in nasal resistance. This elevation will be important in convincing third-party payors or governmental agencies of the need to operate. But a related problem exists; there are patients with septal problems who have "normal resistance," so resistance is not everything. Septal deformity downstream and recurrent rhinosinusitis or epistaxis can be present without causing an elevated resistance. What rhinomanometry can do is measure nasal resistance so that increased resistance can be documented.

Yet another problem is presented by the patient with a wide-open nose and a decrease in the airway resistance who complains of difficulty in breathing.

Not everyone who complains of difficulty in breathing has an elevation in nasal resistance.

There is no simple answer to this complex problem, but I think rhinomanometry will help you in your patient evaluations, and it is up to you to decide if it is a method you want to use.

Question: Suppose that a patient with a deviated septum complains of nasal obstruction and you do tests to confirm that septal deviation is a component of the nasal obstruction. However, the patient also has a strong allergic history and other factors contributing to this obstruction. What do you tell this patient preoperatively? What is your success rate in giving patients straight noses and improving their airways?

Comment (Jack Sheen): In terms of improving the airway, I have had a fairly good success rate. I certainly do not tell them that they are assured of an improvement, but I tell them their chances for improved breathing are very good. As far as the deviated nose is concerned, I tell patients that improved breathing is the only thing I can guarantee; the nose will not be straight, because I cannot reposition a nose in the midline. I tell them that I can, however, camouflage the nose so that it appears more symmetric and more in line.

Comment (Mark Gorney): If the patient has significant symptoms of allergy, I like to have those cleared up, so I send the patient to a nasal allergist. If there is a significant combined component, I spend a great deal of time warning the patient both verbally and in writing that there is a strong possibility that mechanical problems will persist, that primarily what we are trying to do is straighten the nose, but that there are no guarantees.

Comment (Eugene Kern): I think that an important part of the pre-operative evaluation is the discussion with the patient. Each physician needs to take the necessary time to discuss with the patient what might be achieved and what problems exist. In patients with both mucosal and structural problems, more time is required to explain the possible need for postoperative medical management of the mucosal problems. The mucosa problems may be allergic or nonallergic vasomotor reactions that require evaluation and medical management. I believe it is important to medically evaluate the patient preoperatively, discuss this evaluation in detail with the patient, and then obtain informed consent. Let the patient know that two modes of therapy will be administered: medical and surgical.

Comment (Gene Tardy): I simply tell patients that allergic or nasal hyperreactivity conditions cannot be corrected surgically. I also point out the possibility for mechanical improvement in the space where obstructions can occur because of allergic swelling. Care needs to be taken with the highly allergic patient who has very dark pigmentation beneath the eyes; such patients may very well have hemochromic-breakdown pigment reactions beneath the eyes for a long time after surgery. This reaction should be recognized and pointed out to the patient before the operation so no explanation is necessary later.

Question: The incidence of rhinitis or nasal obstruction for several months after rhinoplasty is about 10%. Does anyone address the fact with patients preoperatively that almost all patients will have nasal obstruction postoperatively? Also, how do you treat postrhinoplasty rhinitis?

Comment (Jack Sheen): I am not sure I understand the question. Are you saying that 10% of patients who have rhinoplasty have an obstruction after the operation?

Comment (Tom Baker): It is generally believed that postoperative obstruction is related to a vasomotor rhinitis phenomenon. In my experience almost all the patients had obstructions of several weeks' duration as a result of crusting and edema internally. Most obstructions clear up, but a certain number with allergic components and emotional components become chronic nasal obstructions after rhinoplasty.

Comment (Jack Sheen): When I finish treatment the patient has no mechanical obstruction, and if there is a medical problem, I send the patient to an allergist.

Comment (Mark Gorney): I see these obstructions from time to time, but usually they resolve spontaneously. I have found turbinaire spray and dexamethasone spray helpful since I began using it several years ago.

Comment (Eugene Kern): I don't see postoperative obstructions very frequently. I do think it is important to determine whether or not eosinophils are present in the patient's secretions and the reason for their existence. If eosinophils are present, these nonallergic patients will respond to topical cortiosteroids, primarily dexamethasone, because these are not absorbed. The dexamethasone controls symptoms in the patient with an inflammatory reaction or rhinitis.

Comment (Gene Tardy): I am sure that fewer than 10% of my patients complain of nasal obstruction after operation. I tell them that they may have what appears to be a common cold for a week or less. I think suturing the septum, as mentioned, and delicate instrumentation, most particularly, in the nose make a big difference in the patients who feel "stuffy." When I used big instruments and did less conservative surgery, I saw more problems. Now that I do more conservative surgery, the incidence of postoperative problems is very small. Last, if you are going to send a patient to an allergist, choose a *sympathetic* allergist who understands immunology and the nose. He is just like the sympathetic psychiatrist who understands cosmetic or aesthetic surgery.

Question: Do you ever use banked homograft cartilage in the nose? Please elaborate on the Iowa experience.

Comment (Gene Tardy): I have never used homograft cartilage and don't plan to. I am a proponent of autogenous cartilage as you know.

The Iowa experience with irradiated cartilage seems to be fairly good, but nonetheless, results of long-term human studies with repeat biopsies are not in yet. There are reports of irradiated cartilage that does in fact absorb. However, why not use autogenous cartilage, since its fate is so well known?

Question: Because the extramucosal technique is extremely difficult to perform technically, wouldn't it be preferable to simply use gentle tissue handling and judicious resection of the upper lateral cartilage and mucosa and, if necessary, carefully tease the mucosa off the upper lateral cartilage and septum?

Comment (Eugene Kern): I try to preserve the mucosa if at all possible, and if I am going to separate the upper lateral cartilage from the septum, I use magnification. I was taught this approach by Vernon Gray about 14 years ago, and I think it has helped my surgical technique; and obviously, it is important to have the planes as avascular as possible.

Question: Do you use an extramucosal technique in all cases? If there is a very high, bony, and cartilaginous hump and there is excess mucosa, do you divide the mucosa? Or do you still try to preserve it? What happens in the redundant mucosa?

Comment (Eugene Kern): No, I don't divide the mucose in all cases. I still try to preserve it. I will separate it. I have never found redundant mucosa to be a great problem.

Comment (Jack Sheen): I also have never found redundant mucosa to be a problem. In fact, it almost serves as a spreader graft. At one time I, transected it, but I found that the lateral cartilage would fall too far medially. Preservation of the mucosa is the preferred procedure from the standpoint of contour.

Question: Are you using the extramucosal technique in most of your primary rhinoplasties?

Comment (Jack Sheen): Yes.

Comment (Mark Gorney): Basically, yes. I try to preserve all the mucosa and hopefully some extramucosal tissues, at least around the valve area. Above that level I find the technique technically difficult, but certainly the initial division of the upper lateral cartilage from the septum should be done extramucosally.

Question: You have stated that in certain deviations and deflections of the upper lateral cartilage in the septum, it is essential to divide the upper lateral cartilage from the septum. Could you comment on that statement. Also, how often do you use the extramucosal technique, and do you feel it is an important one to use?

Comment (Gene Tardy): The only time I divide the upper lateral cartilage from the septum and then divide the underlying mucoperichondrial bridge, which is very important to maintain, is in unusual cases of extreme deviation or deflection. For instance, if there is excessive redundant mucoperichondrium and a huge nose whose hump has been taken down, then the excess mucoperichondrium should be resected. The same is true with vestibular skin and mucosa: The old idea that skin should never be sacrificed is absolutely wrong. In a reduction operation the components of the nose that are in excess are reduced; one of those components is mucoperichondrium or mucoperiosteum, or mucosa. In the past, when noses were perhaps overoperated and a great deal of tissue was taken off the nose, these mucoperichondrial bridges were divided. This is not necessary in today's surgery.

Question: What is the role of external rhinoplasty and when would you use it?

Comment (Gene Tardy): External rhinoplasty is an *approach* to the nose just as transcartilanginous resection or delivery is an approach. It is not a technique. I think the pendulum has swung too far; some surgeons are now doing almost everything from an external rhinoplasty approach, something I just can't understand. This approach gives you ambidextrous capability if you like to work with both hands. It gives you binocular vision in the nose, if you like to have that. Nonetheless, I restrict the use of the external approach. I use it to repair large septal perforations that I can't handle otherwise. (Most septal perforations don't need repair.) I use it for nasal tumors that require resection and all cleft lip/nose complex problems. I also use an open approach for the patient with a severely twisted nose that I feel I must approach from the top through the septum. The last indication for the open approach is to teach residents about relationships of anatomy, in which case I'll stretch my indications. Otherwise I don't think the external approach is the God-given answer to all our problems.

Comment (Eugene Kern): I use it infrequently and primarily in problems of exposing the operative site in severely traumatized noses.

Question: Dr. Tardy, I was impressed with the 75% success rate that Dr. Kern reported in using silicone rubber buttons for septal perforations; it certainly appears to be an easy technique. Do you consider use of that technique before you use a flap to close the septal perforation?

Comment (Gene Tardy): Absolutely. I consider it. It is a simple approach, but it works only part of the time. My main treatment of septal perforations is medical. I treat them with saline, humidity, ointment, and tender, loving care. I prefer to avoid surgery in septal perforations. When for some reason the perforation must be repaired and obturation is not successful, and if I am convinced that the patient is not a "picker" or a cocaine user with a factitious perforation (and I am appalled at the number of middle-class people who use cocaine), then I prefer reconstruction with the sublabial myomucosal (for small perforations) or the sublabial composite myomucosal-cartilage flap. Since the prime reason for failed repairs of septal perforations is insufficient blood supply in the host bed, it makes good sense to effect repair with a regional flap that carries its own blood supply.

PART
X

COMPLICATIONS
OF RHINOPLASTY

Antibiotic Prophylaxis, Epistaxis, and Nasal Packing

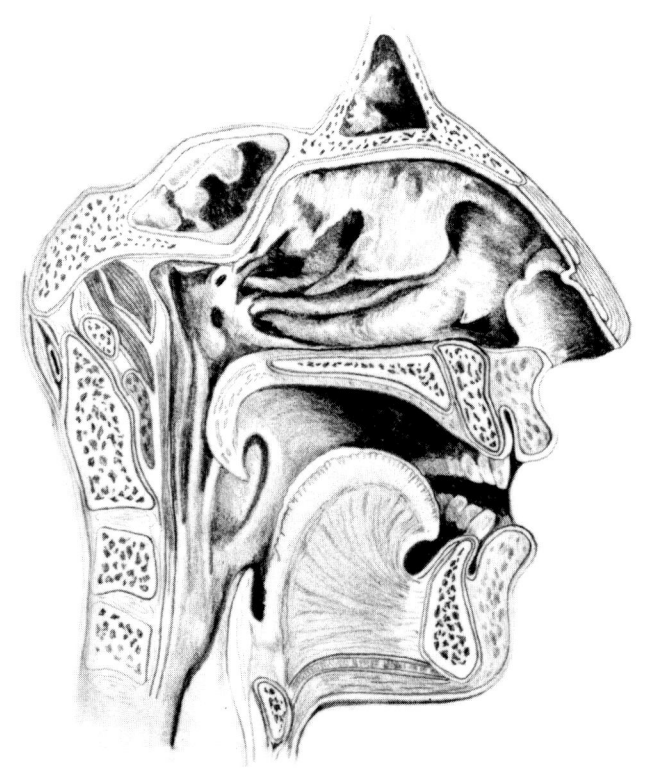

32

The Use of Antibiotics in Nasal Surgery

Nicolas Tabbal

The nasal cavity constitutes a vast reservoir of microorganisms. Under normal circumstances, these bacteria rarely cause local or systemic infections, even after rhinoplasty. The abundant vascularity of nasal tissues contributes significantly to the low incidence of infections following nasal surgery.

Occasionally, periosteitis is noted as an area of swelling and tenderness over the dorsum or along the osteotomy site. It is usually caused by a low-grade infection of bone dust and generally responds well to antibiotics. Another source of potential infection is a hematoma, which may go unrecognized until the nasal splint is removed. Treatment of this problem should be agressive and directed toward prevention of nasal skin loss. The thorough removal of bone debris, evacuation of the blood clot, and application of a well-fitting nasal splint help avert these local wound problems.

When discussing postrhinoplasty infection, however, what comes to mind instead of these local wound problems are the few case reports that have been published in the literature describing some grave and sometimes fatal infections following a rhinoplasty. A wide variety of septic conditions (for example, toxic shock syndrome) have been reported after prolonged packing following submucous section. However, most of the involved patients had some predisposing conditions to infection unrelated to the rhinoplasty itself. One patient with unrecognized mitral valve prolapse developed staphylococcal endocarditis. Another with arteriovenous malformation of the face died of cavernous sinus thrombosis. The venous drainage of the nose is pe-culiar in that it drains directly into the cavernous sinus through the ophthalmic veins and indirectly through small veins that arise from the pterygoid plexus. This peculiarity probably accounts for the spread of infection in the patient just mentioned.

A survey in 1975 of nearly 1,400 plastic surgeons revealed that one surgeon out of four administered antibiotics before a rhinoplasty.[1] A similar study among otolaryngologists revealed more widespread use. A high incidence of bacteremia should justify such use. Numerous other procedures are associated with a high incidence of bacteremia. For instance, dental manipulation is associated with a 59% incidence. Posterior nasal packing has been reported to cause bacteremia in nearly 12% of the cases.[1]

It is logical to assume that since the nasal fossa is such a reservoir for microorganisms, a certain incidence of bacteremia following rhinoplasty should be expected. This hypothetical conclusion, however, was found inaccurate in a study that investigated the incidence of bacteremia during rhinoplasty in 52 healthy adults who were not given preoperative antibiotics.[2] Nasal cultures that were taken preoperatively indicated that 80% of the patients had *Staphylococcus epidermidis* present, whereas 25% were silent carriers of *Staphylococcus aureus*.

Preoperative nasal and blood cultures were obtained from all patients. Blood cultures were also obtained 5 and 15 minutes after osteotomy, since it is the most traumatic step in the procedure and is most likely to cause bacteremia. A positive blood culture was obtained in only one patient, and the organism found was *S. epidermidis*. However, this was believed to be a contamination problem rather than true evidence of bacteremia.

The logical assumption from this study is that rhinoplasty rarely, if ever, causes bacteremia. Surgeons who believe that antibiotics protect patients from unusual infections following this procedure should weigh the potential toxicity of these medications against the extremely low risk of systemic infections. Susceptible patients suffering from cardiac valvular disease should be covered with broad-spectrum antibiotics preoperatively, but in all other conditions this routine is of questionable merit.

REFERENCES

1. Krizek, T.J., Koss, N., and Rosson, M.C.: The current use of prophylactic antibiotics in plastic and reconstructive surgery, Plast. Reconstr. Surg. 55:21, 1975.
2. Slavin, S.A., and others: An investigation of bacteremia during rhinoplasty, Plast. Reconstr. Surg. 71:197, 1983.

33

Epistaxis

Harvey Caplan

Epistaxis can be a most frightening and disturbing occurrence for the patient who has had surgery. Significant epistaxis occurs in approximately 1% of the patients during routine nasal surgery. However, an orderly approach to surgical preparation and management can make this infrequent complication a minor unpleasantness.

HISTORY

One of the first measures to obviate this complication is obtaining a thorough history. A family or personal history of excessive bleeding during menses or following routine surgery, trauma, or dental work should not be ignored. Similarly, the surgeon should be aware that, particularly among Hasidic Jews and some other ethnic groups, factor VIII antigen deficiency, or von Willebrand's disease, is not rare. This disorder can be difficult to detect through routine preoperative testing. Should this condition be suspected from the history, consultation with a hematologist is mandatory, since a routine coagulogram may not reveal the disorder.

A normal partial thromboplastin time (PTT) does not necessarily rule out such problems. I prohibit aspirin in my patients for at least 2 weeks before surgery and for 2 weeks postoperatively. Alcohol also affects the PTT and is included in this restriction; alcohol potentiates the bleeding time when taken with aspirin. A recent nasal infection or other upper respiratory tract infection also can increase the incidence of epistaxis and is cause to postpone the surgery.

SITES OF BLEEDING

One should be aware of the common sites of bleeding. Tip incisions can bleed and commonly do so for 24 hours after surgery. Along the incision, the nasal roof between the upper-lateral cartilage and the septum is also a common site.

During surgery it is important to elevate tissues en bloc, especially in the subperichondrial or subperiosteal level. Dissection in a superficial plane injures larger blood vessels, which may retract and start bleeding 5 or 6 days postoperatively.

The purpose of using *medial osteotomies* is to allow joining of the nasal suture line after the bony hump has been removed. The medial osteotomy is made in a Y-shaped manner. In other words, it diverges from the septum toward the frontonasal suture line. If performed in a lateral direction, the osteotomy is not likely to involve the vessels high on the dorsum of the septum, which can cause severe bleeding if injured.

When flaps are sewn after a *septoplasty* or *submucous resection,* mattress sutures should be used to approximate the tissues accurately. In my experience, amputation of the inferior turbinates can result in severe epistaxis; thus turbinectomy should be undertaken with great caution.

Treatment

Fortunately, routine measures stop most bleeding. Administration of fresh plasma can be helpful in treating patients with bleeding dyscrasias by providing fresh anticoagulant factors.

Using a stretcher bed is desirable in managing a nosebleed in a hospital because this bed can be locked in place. Dependable operative illumination is mandatory for accurately locating the bleeding. A fiber optic headlight is an excellent light source that can give proper visualization. Reliable nasal suction apparatus is necessary for clot removal. Often the bleeding occurs in the intercartilaginous incision, with continuous oozing behind the clot. The application of a pledget containing adrenalin will often control the bleeding after complete removal of the clot.

Sedation of the patient with appropriate doses of meperidine (Demerol) or morphine helps control the stress that bleeding induces and the blood pressure, which often rises. *Topical anesthesia* is very important during packing or cauterization because the nose is probably very sensitive. An epistaxis tray with electrocautery equipment should be available. The tray should also contain a balloon catheter to use in case posterior pressure be necessary.

Meticulous suturing of the nasal flaps using a small, straight septoplasty needle with 5-0 catgut and through-and-through mattress sutures will coapt the mucosal flaps after submucous resection (bleeding from between these flaps is not uncommon). I favor cellulose nasal tampons as packing material.

SECONDARY AND REVISIONAL RHINOPLASTY

Bone and Cartilaginous Framework Deformities

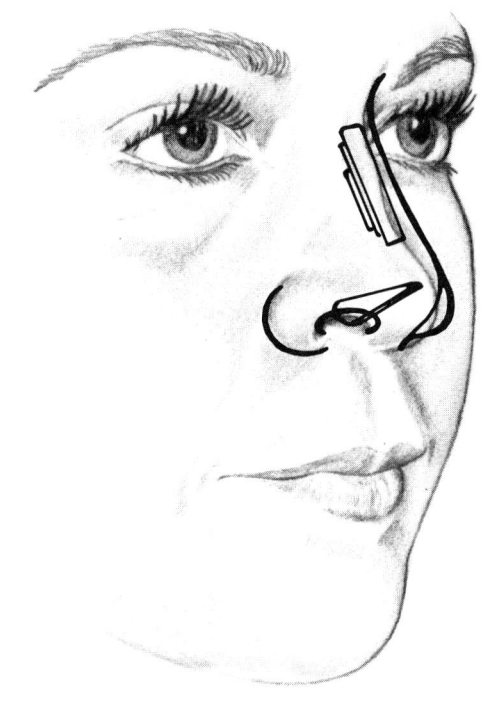

34

Secondary Rhinoplasty: Basic Considerations

Thomas Rees

Candidates for secondary rhinoplasty must be selected with care and only after careful evaluation by the surgeon. The patient satisfaction level does not always match the surgeon's evaluation of the surgical result. The physical problem is often complicated by considerable emotional and psychological overlay. Occasionally patients are seen who have had multiple procedures. In fact, I recall a patient from the clinic at the Manhattan Eye and Ear Hospital who had approximately 32 operations on her nose. Patients with multiple procedures are sometimes victims of their own sense of perfection. They may be classified as "insatiable cosmetic patients," and the surgeon should be aware that such a patient might be seen in his consultation. Of course, the procedure can be inexpertly performed, or a complication can occur that leads to the necessity of secondary surgery. The inexperienced surgeon can easily fall into a trap with patients who "want just a little bit more done." It is very tempting to think that he or she can perform a small correction and solve the problem, when in fact the problem may be complicated by emotional overlay that is not immediately apparent. My advice to the surgeon beginning his or her career regarding secondary rhinoplasty patients who were operated on by another surgeon is to go slowly and evaluate the patient very thoroughly.

Timing is all important in performing secondary rhinoplasty. There are no hard and fast rules, but I rarely perform a secondary procedure on my own patients until at least 6 months (usually 1 year) after the primary operation. I might add here that, in the best of surgical hands, secondary surgery of the nose will be necessary in approximately 5% to 10% of patients. Often the secondary procedure is minor such as trimming a cartilage point in the tip or rasping a small dorsal bump. Many small problems that would seem to require revisional surgery often disappear as the edema and wound reaction subside. Minor defects disappear, so the surgeon should not hurry to return the patient to the operating room. Some patients apply considerable pressure on the surgeon to perform a secondary correction before the nose has completely healed. Such pressure can easily cause a less-experienced surgeon to agree to operate again, hoping to alleviate the problem. The early repeat operation can result in additional edema, scar tissue, and wound reaction, compounding the problem even further and eventually requiring more surgery. The surgeon must persevere in waiting until he feels that the tissues are ready for further surgical intervention.

If you are the "new guy in town"—the surgeon with the youngest practice, inevitably some of the first patients that come to your office will be dissatisfied secondary rhinoplasty patients. No one else has satisfied these patients, and it is unlikely that you will either, no matter how well you succeed technically. Remember that in the eyes of the patient and his or her friends, it is the last surgeon's result that is evaluated. His skill is judged by what is seen. Clearly, if the task of reshaping a "crucified nose" is impossible, it is best to refer the patient to another surgeon who specializes in this type of problem and who usually practices in a major institution.

The surgical principles of secondary rhinoplasty are simply a reaffirmation of the basic principles of reconstitution of the skeletal structure and the covering envelope. Sometimes it is possible to achieve this goal by rearranging existing tissues, but more often in complicated secondary cases, tissue augmentation (especially cartilage grafts from the septum or concha of the ear) is required to achieve the goal. Lining grafts of skin may also be required in treating stenosis of the nares, and composite grafts have a definite place in full-thickness repair of the tip, alae, and columella. Reconstitution of the nasal skeleton must provide the framework for the skin cover and tip elements. The remainder of my discussion concerns the osteocartilaginous structure of the vault.

INFRACTURE

Failure to obtain or maintain an adequate infracture of the lateral nasal walls is a common vault problem in postrhinoplasty patients. This problem is slightly more complicated than might be expected, especially in view of the recent computerized axial tomography (CAT) studies of Dr. Rollin Daniel who has shown how rarely the infracture performed during surgery maintains its position with the passage of time. The full implication of his work is not yet known, but it is indeed interesting. The early pioneer surgeons in rhinoplasty often did not even attempt to infracture the nasal bones. They only removed the offending dorsal hump to improve the profile, a procedure that was considered quite enough at the time. Later it was realized that this open roof should be closed and that the only way to perform the closing and therefore the narrowing of the nose was deliberately to fracture the nasal bones where they joined the maxilla and to displace them medially.

Narrowing the nose can be difficult in a patient with thick nasal bones, particularly at the radix, or in a patient with a very wide vault and increased width of the pyriform aperture. A thick web of bone at the radix can sometimes be punched out with a sharp Kazanjian forceps, or a sliver of bone on either side can be cut with a sharp osteotome to allow room for medial displacement of the lateral elements.

Removal of hump

The patients in Figure 34-1 demonstrate removal of the hump without infracture. A lateral osteotomy, which corrected the problem in these patients, was performed as deep in the angle as possible, using a small 3-mm osteotome just along the frontal process of the maxilla. This solution may not always suffice in patients in whom the hump is very large and the bones are thick or in patients with a significantly high septal deviation.

Closing the open roof and achieving a narrow appearance in these patients often require some other maneuver, namely a graft (usually of septal cartilage) to close the open roof or a replacement of the trimmed and modified hump as championed by the late Tord Skoog. If the surgeon is contemplating using a cartilage graft to close the open roof in a secondary problem, it is important to ascertain preoperatively whether or not the cartilaginous septum has been removed during a previous surgery. If so, he must make other plans—possibly to harvest a graft from the ear, in which case permission must be obtained from the patient. Sometimes the impression is given that septal cartilage is present when it is only present to a small degree from regrowth; thus the "pin test" is helpful. A needle or a pin is forced through the cartilaginous septum during examination to determine the resistance and relative thickness of the cartilage. Cartilage that is regrown but attenuated can readily be determined by the surgeon after he has a little experience. This test avoids the embarrassment of discovering during surgery that insufficient cartilage exists to provide a graft of suitable size.

Septal deviation

It is very important to conduct a thorough examination of the internal nose before surgery, especially in secondary patients. A quick look with a pocket light will not suffice. The membranes should appear shrunken, and the interior should be examined using a good headlight or spotlight. Anatomical details must not be overlooked in a patient with a secondary problem. Noting details can determine the difference between success and failure in such cases. For example, examination may show a high-dorsal deviation of the septum that will surely interfere with medial displacement of the bone on that side during secondary infracture. Various maneuvers can be used to prevent this situation. The dorsal septum can be lowered below the level of the nasal bones. I sometimes insert a small 2 mm osteotome transcutaneously and fracture the ethmoid plate when it is displaced. Of course, such a technique is predicated on the presence of the required supporting elements of the septum. The ethmoid plate can also be fractured with a Goldman bar. If the nose is crooked, the surgeon must do whatever is necessary to straighten it as much as possible. The septum clearly has a great deal to do with the effectiveness of the infracture (Figure 34-2). Sometimes the nasal bones come into place during surgery but, after a few weeks, drift laterally again. CAT scans (Daniel)

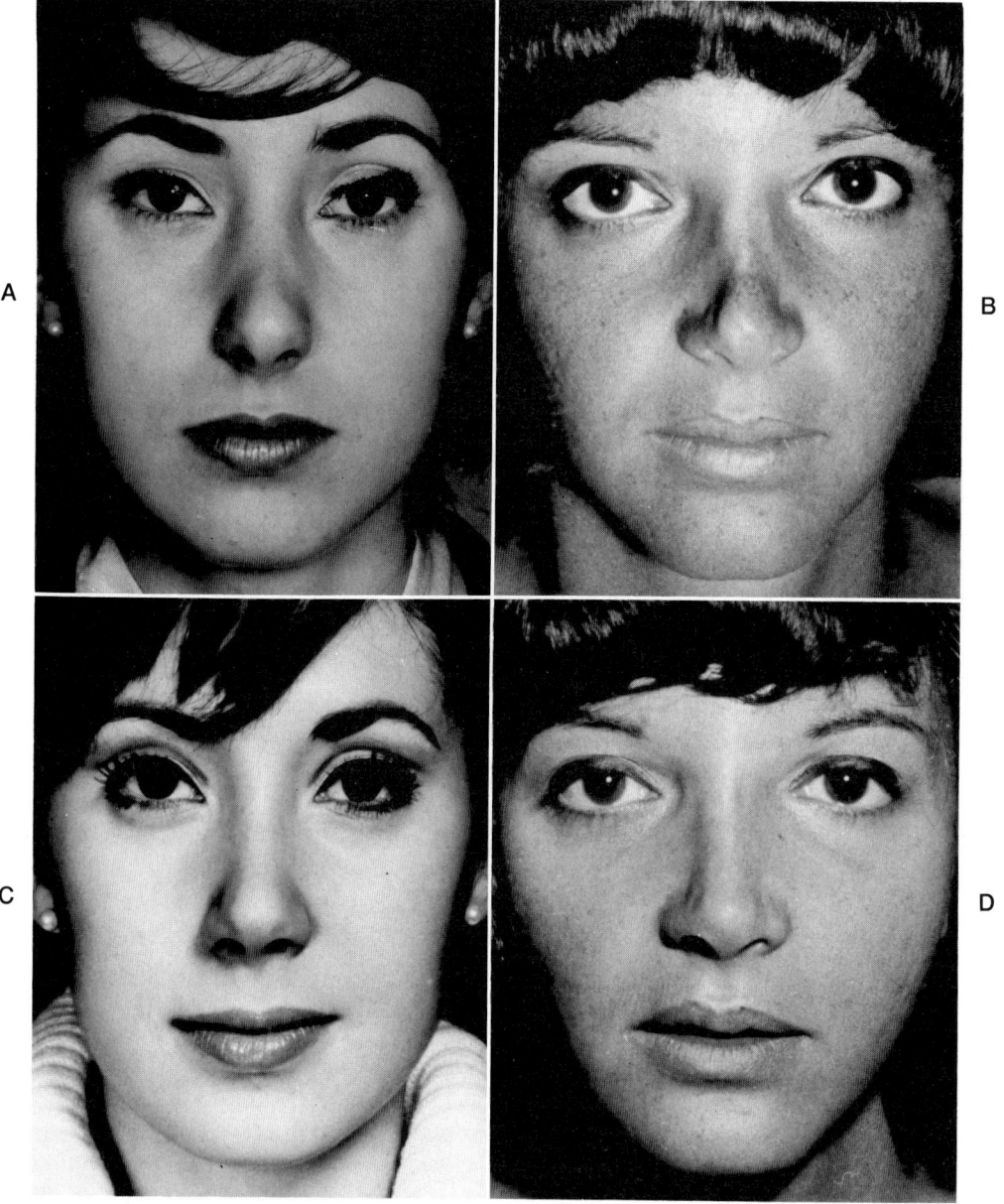

Figure 34-1. Both of these young ladies had primary rhinoplasty in which only the hump was removed. Lateral osteotomies and infracture were not performed. Secondary surgery required only lateral osteotomy and infracture to achieve the result. **A** and **C** are preoperative photographs, and **B** and **D** are postoperative photographs. No dorsal augmentation was required in either patient. (From Rees, T.D.: Aesthetic plastic surgery, Philadelphia, 1980, W.B. Saunders Co.)

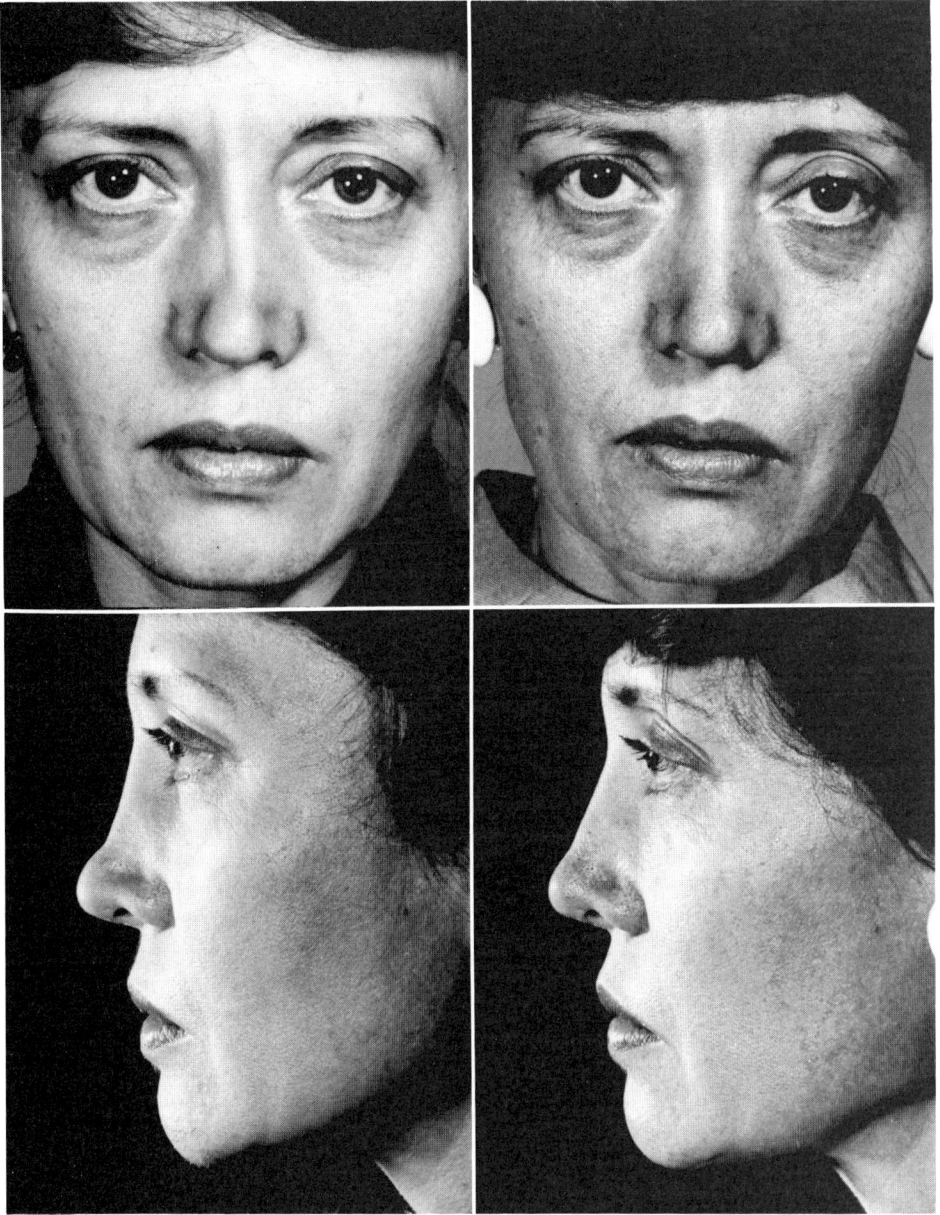

Figure 34-2. Patient after primary rhinoplasty. The surgeon failed to identify a marked septal deviation during his preoperative examination. The result was not only an open roof, but the deviated septum became very obvious, and it was impossible to obtain an infracture because of the septal blockade. During surgery the entire septum was mobilized, an infracture was performed, and a dorsal "filler" graft of septal cartilage was used. (From Rees, T.D.: Aesthetic plastic surgery, Philadelphia, 1980, W.B. Saunders Co.)

confirm this clinical impression. If this drifting occurs on only one side, a high septal displacement to that side is often the culprit.

Stripping the periosteum

It is not a good idea, at least early in the operation, to strip the periosteum from the nasal bones because we can never be exactly sure what is going to happen during infracture. Should comminution of the bones occur—a not uncommon event—and the periosteum has been stripped from the nasal bones, they literally have no support, and both bones can drop into the pyriform aperture, resulting in a saddle nose just as if a midface fracture had occurred. Asymmetrical removal of the hump is a useful technique in patients with externally deviated noses; the unequal infracture can then result in a relatively straight-looking dorsum. The hump is removed through an oblique cut because one bone must travel further medially than the other. Another very useful technique in removing the large hump that is displaced to one side or another is the Skoog technique to which I referred previously. These large humps can be removed and replaced in the midline into a more central position after remodeling the skeletal structure of the hump itself. This technique is discussed elsewhere in this book (see the chapter about the osseocartilaginous vault).

Stairstepping

Any discussion of infracture must include the problem of "stairstepping," the obvious groove deformity that sometimes results after rhinoplasty, especially if the lateral osteotomy has been made too high on the lateral walls of the nose (Figure 34-3). The exact location of the lateral osteotomy has been discussed a great deal, and controversy still exists as to exactly how and where this cut in the bone should be positioned. There are advocates of the "high-to-low cut," the "high-to-high cut," and so forth. I believe much of this discussion is somewhat fanciful. What is important is to make the lateral osteotomy as low as possible and through the thick bone of the frontal process of the maxilla. If I feel that the osteotome is penetrating the bone too easily, indicating that the bone is thin rather than solid, I know that I am placing the cut too high. A "stairstep" deformity results from these high osteotomies and is an unattractive stigma of a rhinoplasty. In some patients the angle formed between the frontal process of the maxilla and the sidewall of the nose is more obtuse than in others. In these patients it may not be possible to avoid stairstepping altogether.

Saddle-nose deformity

Many years ago I learned the hard way—from experience—that it is unwise, and indeed risky, to perform a classic Killian-type radical submucous resection along with a rhinoplasty in which a significant dorsal hump is removed. All that may be left for support of the septum and, in large measure, the vault in these patients is a fragile dorsal and caudal strut. During the course of the procedure, injury can easily occur to the remaining dorsal strut, fracturing it completely, in which case the entire remnant of the septum, as well as the nasal bones, may collapse into the pyriform aperture. This situation is similar to what occurs in patients with severe midface trauma. If such a calamity occurs during surgery, the only method I know for salvaging the situation and restoring projection of the nose is to treat it as a traumatic case. The remnants are brought forward and fixed in position with through-and-through wires tied over plastic buttons or lead plastic. If this immediate treatment is not successful and a saddle nose results, reconstruction with a dorsal augmen-

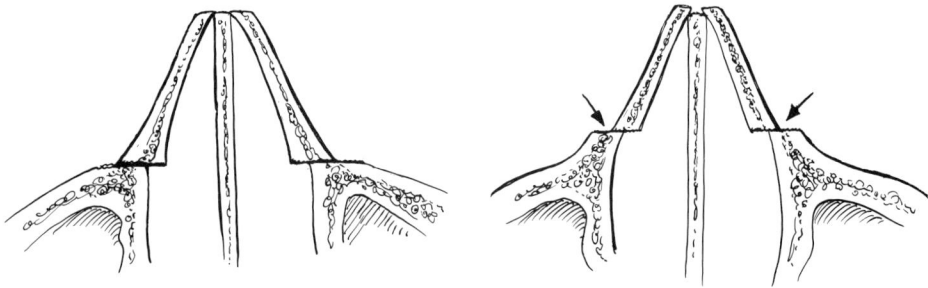

Figure 34-3. The lateral osteotomy should be made as deeply in the nasomaxillary angle as possible through the thick part of the frontal process of the maxilla to prevent a stairstep deformity. (From Rees, T.D.: Aesthetic plastic surgery, Philadelphia, 1980, W.B. Saunders Co.)

tation using cartilage or bone may be required at a subsequent time.

Another, and certainly more common, cause of postoperative saddle-nose deformity is overzealous removal of the hump (Figure 34-4). Most surgeons have given up the use of nasal saws for hump removal for this reason. Sharp osteotomes and rasps are much safer than saws and permit more gradual hump removal with much better control by the sur-

geon. Should it be recognized by the surgeon at the time of surgery that he has removed more hump than intended, the obvious solution is to replace the hump after sculpting it to the desired size and shape, a method similar to that of Skoog. If the hump is insufficient or in too many pieces, a septal cartilage graft or even an auricular cartilage graft should be used.

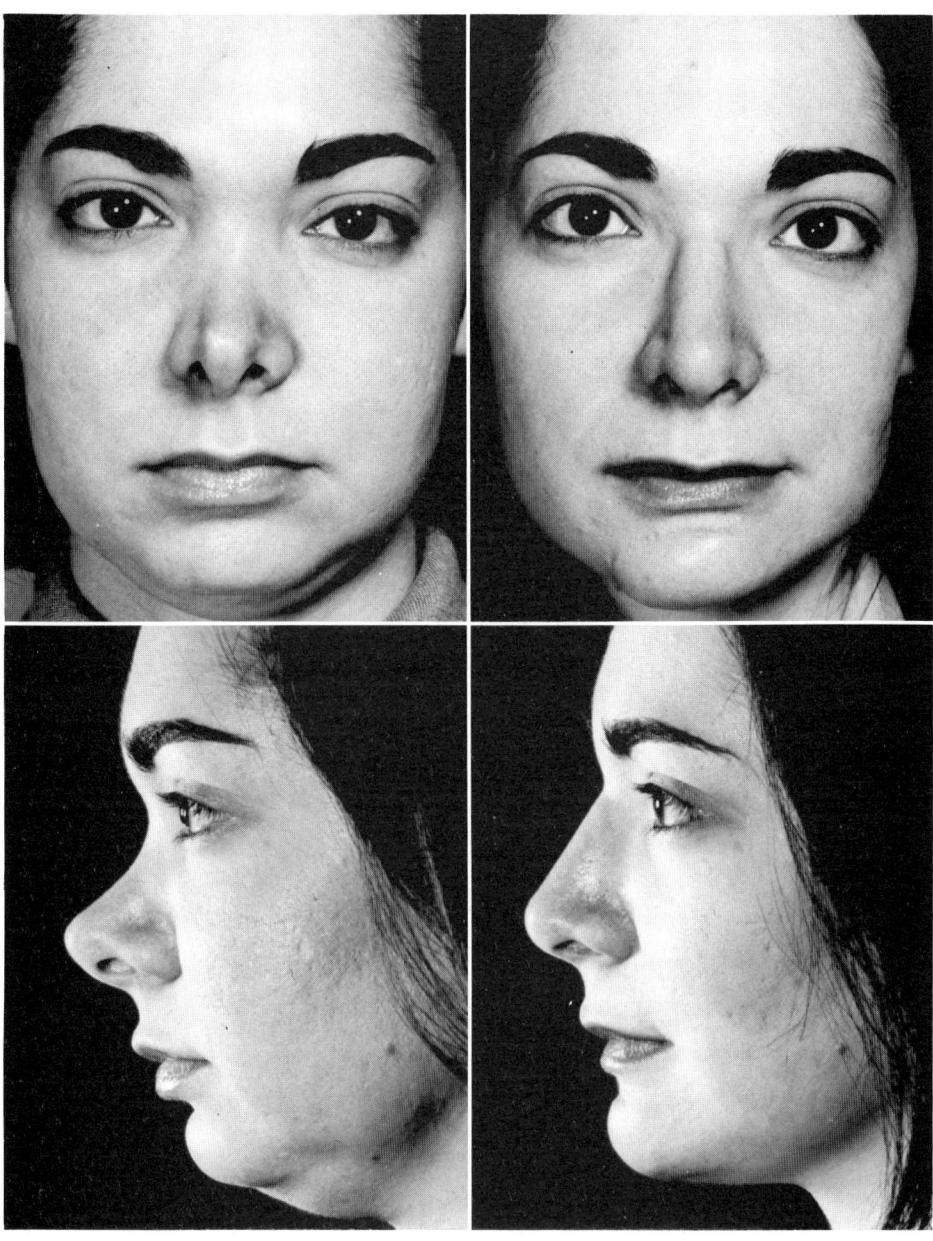

Figure 34-4. Overresection of the dorsal hump by the saw technique. Reconstruction was achieved using a generous iliac bone graft. Overcorrection of the dorsum is avoided best by using osteotomes or sharp rasps. (From Rees, T.D.: Aesthetic plastic surgery, Philadelphia, 1980, W.B. Saunders Co.)

EXCESSIVE SHORTENING

I believe the most difficult secondary problem to solve in rhinoplasty is correction of the nose that has been overly shortened. Typically the columella is retracted, and the upper lip appears long and curtainlike. These problems are often impossible to correct to my satisfaction or that of the patient. Composite grafts have a limited effectiveness in achieving nasal lengthening, and grafts to augment only the nasal skeleton are not sufficient, because there is almost always a concomitant shrinkage of the soft tissues. Overshortening is one of the unsolved problems of revisional rhinoplasty.

CONCLUSION

During recent years, better and better results have been achieved through secondary rhinoplasty mostly because of a change in concept. Most surgeons engaged in this work now recognize that most patients with severe secondary nose problems require augmentation of one sort or another, not simply revision of existing tissue. This concept has, in my mind, significantly improved our results.

35

Secondary and Revisional Rhinoplasty

Wolfgang Mühlbauer

Corrective rhinoplasty is among the most frequent aesthetic plastic surgical procedures performed. It is not known exactly how many secondary rhinoplasties produce unaesthetic results. The percentage of failures is inversely proportional to the experience and skills of the surgeon.

A rising number of patients are requesting secondary and revisional surgery. We have a moral obligation to accept our own patients, but how do we handle someone else's failures? The natural reaction would be to send these patients back to their first surgeon, yet these patients distrust the original surgeon and are looking to another for help. Accepting such a patient for a second, third, or fifth revision means risking your own good reputation because it becomes increasingly tough to achieve a satisfactory final result. If the patient remains unhappy, he or she tends to forget the previous surgeons and blames you for the final result.

CONCEPTS OF REVISIONAL AND SECONDARY RHINOPLASTY

A "surgical nose" is an unnatural-looking, disharmonic nose on which surgery has obviously been performed. A natural deformity has been converted to a surgical deformity.

During revisional rhinoplasty the careful analysis of the deformity and its causes is even more important than during a primary case. I always ask the patient about the name of the previous rhinoplastic surgeon because I know most of my colleagues and their personal techniques. My goal is the same as during primary rhinoplasty—namely, recreation of a nose that appears natural, functions naturally, and blends harmoniously with the other facial features.

My concepts of revisional and secondary rhinoplasty are rather simple and are listed according to priority as follows:
1. Rearrangement of structures and tissues
2. Reduction of structures and tissues
3. Augmentation of structures and tissues
4. Reconstruction of structures and tissues

Although the problems can not be standardized, I relate the problems to the various components of the nose, analyse them, and offer appropriate solutions.

Osseus dorsum problems

Minute irregularities of the osseous dorsum after hump removal may be smoothed by rasping only. A sterile surgical brush is useful in cleaning the rasp between strokes.

Greek profile

A Greek profile is the result of a too-shallow hump removal performed without sculpturing the nasofrontal angle properly. This angle may be carved with a fine osteotome and/or a sharp rasp (Figures 35-1 and 35-2).

Secondary hump

A secondary hump is usually the consequence of incomplete removal and rarely is caused by callus formation, yet this term serves well as an explanation to the patient about this undesired result. It is one of the rare instances in which early revision for complete hump removal is advisable to keep the patient from becoming angry and pursuing litigation.

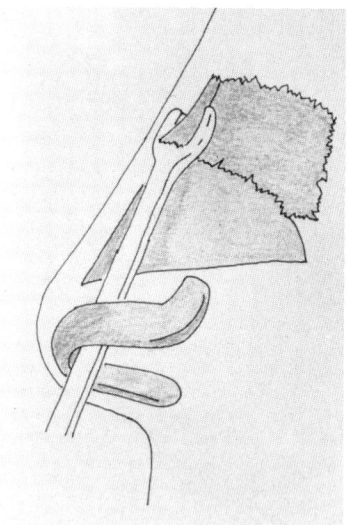

Figure 35-1

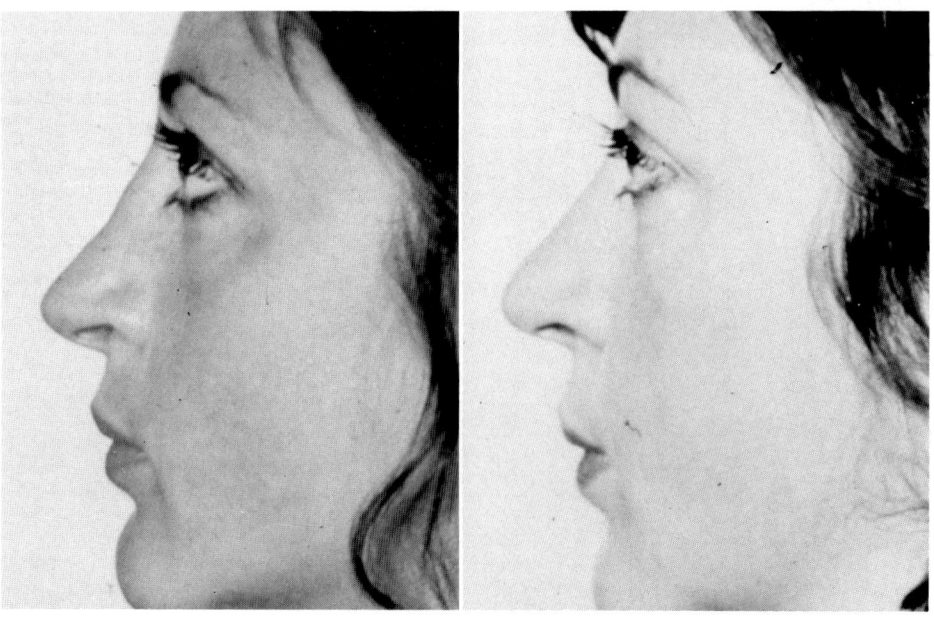

Figure 35-2

Ski-jump nose

Many girls (15 to 18 years old) who have suffered from a large hump nose desire the extreme opposite—a cute little turned-up baby nose. As honest surgeons we should resist these expectations and counsel the patient to accept a more pleasing and harmonious feature. However, a ski-jump nose may result inadvertently from overreduction of the dorsum, mainly in the osseous part. If this result is recognized during the primary procedure, part of the hump may be replanted with fibrin glue. For a secondary case I usually augment the deficit with auricular cartilage from the concha that is trimmed with a scalpel and sometimes shaped in addition with a cartilage-squeezing forceps. Warping is rarely a problem, nor is absorption. See the representative case (Figure 35-3) before, during, and 6 years after implantation of the conchal cartilage.

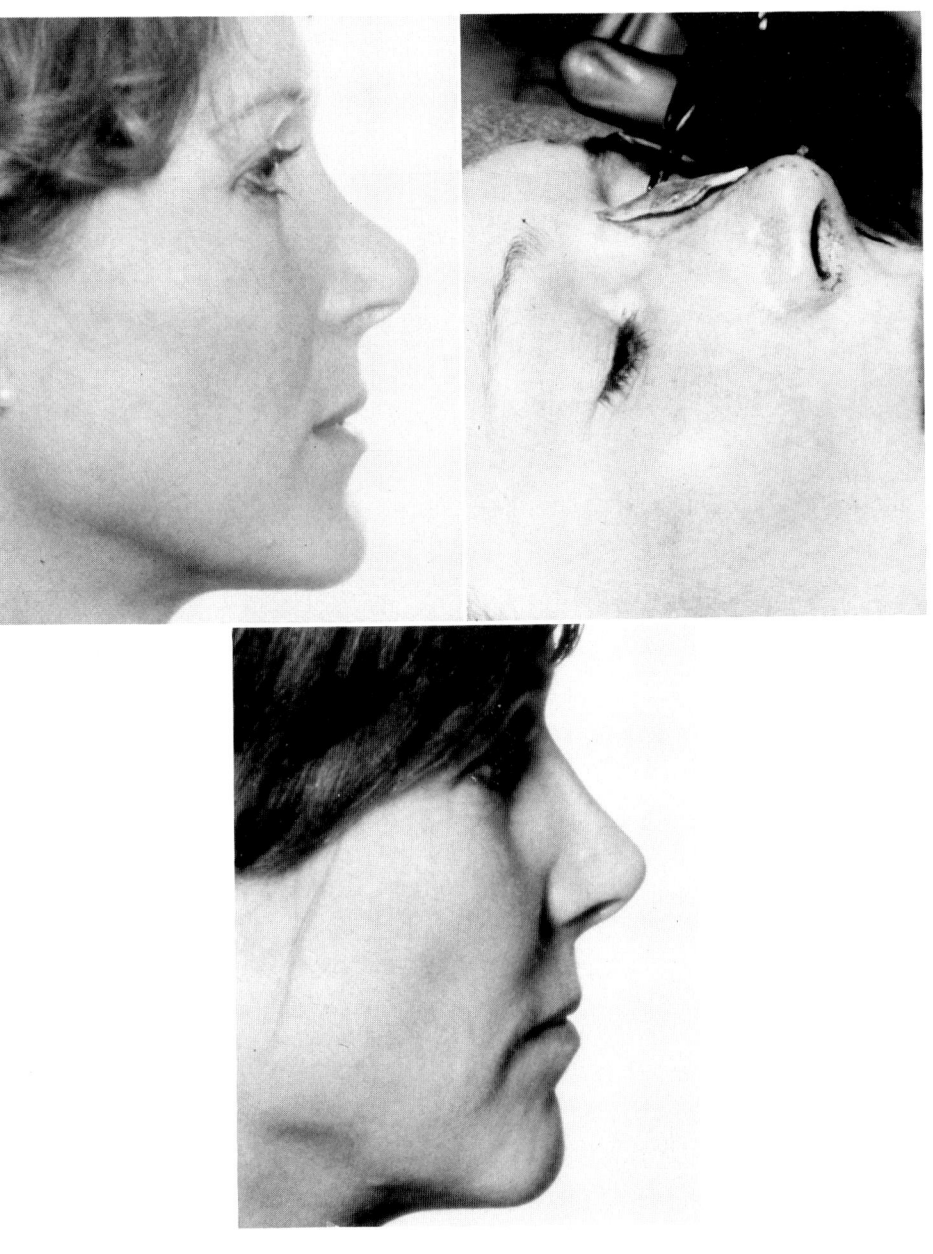

Figure 35-3

Osseocartilaginous junction

Frequently I see patients with obvious depressions at the junction of the osseous and cartilaginous nose. It is a telltale sign of a crude rhinoplasty technique in which the osseocartilaginous junction is disarticulated and the upper-lateral section is pushed partly inside the nasal cavity.

In late cases the repositioning of the structures fails because of scarring, so the camouflaging technique of placing onlay cartilage grafts around the piriform aperture using fine slivers from the septum must be used (Figure 35-4). The result in this model (Figure 35-5) has remained stable for 2 years.

Saddle nose

I will discuss only iatrogenic saddle noses as a result of a radical submucous resection (SMR) or hump removal. Minor and moderate cases may be dealt with through hump shifting or augmentation with an auricular graft. More pronounced or excessive saddle noses with telescoping of the cartilaginous nose into the nasal cavity need a firm support and expansion. It is best to insert an L-shaped graft of autogeneous rib at the osseocartilaginous junction to get bony contact with the remaining nasal pyramid and some mobility through the cartilage in the cartilaginous nose.

My department has used merthiolate-preserved cadaver rib cartilage for over 20 years with equally good and stable results in patients with saddle noses. From histological studies we have learned that the banked cartilage either is revitalized by the host's chondrocytes or is stabilized as a firm structure by necrobiotic calcification.

Although I personally do not like using silicone struts in the nose, I had to reposition one in a young girl after deviation from the midline. The strut has remained in position and without reactions for a follow-up period of 1 year.

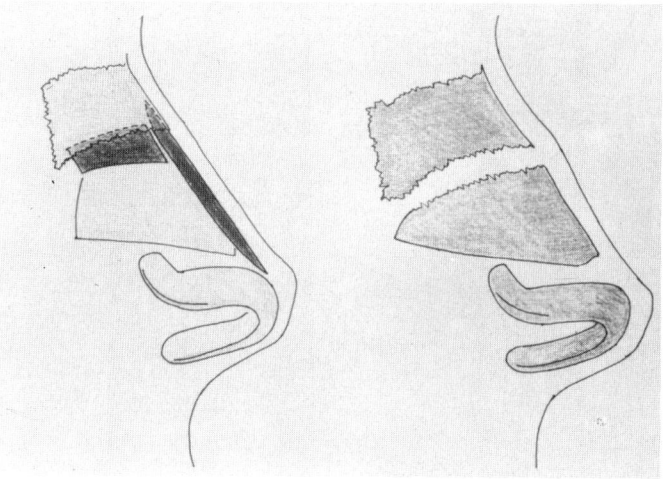

Figure 35-4

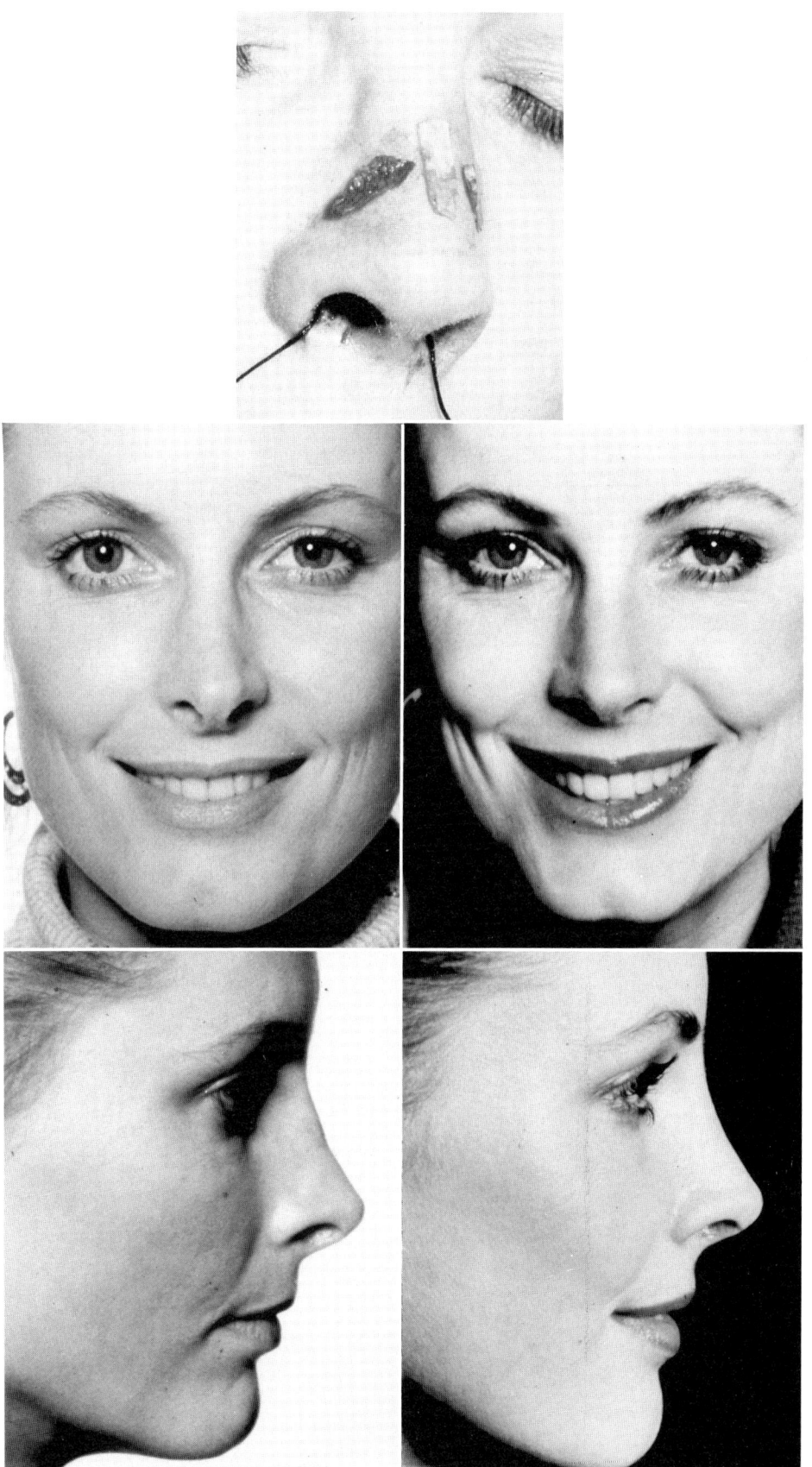

Figure 35-5

Cartilaginous dorsum

The firm supratip prominence is caused either by the remaining dorsal edges of the upper-lateral cartilages that are not kept flush with the rest of the dorsum or that are pushed medially too much or by the dorsal septum that is not trimmed enough. The secondary correction must reduce the upper laterals or the septal border.

A true supratip swelling is soft and compressible by the finger and is usually the result of crowding of the skin after excessive shortening of the nose.

Thinning of this type of "polly-beak" deformity, "scar tissue" removal, or further lowering of the supportive cartilaginous structures of the tip does not seem logical and seldom cures the problem. I would much rather reexpand the skin through elevation and elongation of the nose using an appropriate cartilage graft, preferably from the septum (Figure 35-6). Figure 35-7 demonstrates this concept on one of my own cases in which I reduced a long straight nose too much; I recreated a better-proportioned nose in this manner, and it has remained stable for 10 years.

In another case, to underline my point, I tried to thin the subcutaneous tissue under a supratip swelling in a patient who had greasy skin with acne. When I removed the Steri strips from the nasal tip, I found exposed septal cartilage and a skin ulcer where the previous supratip swelling had been. This defect eventually healed through conservative treatment and without major aesthetic or legal consequences.

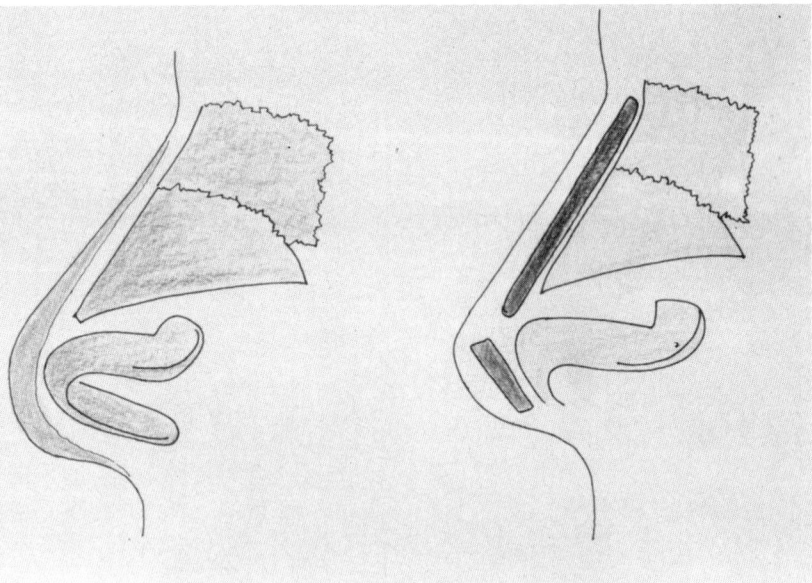

Figure 35-6

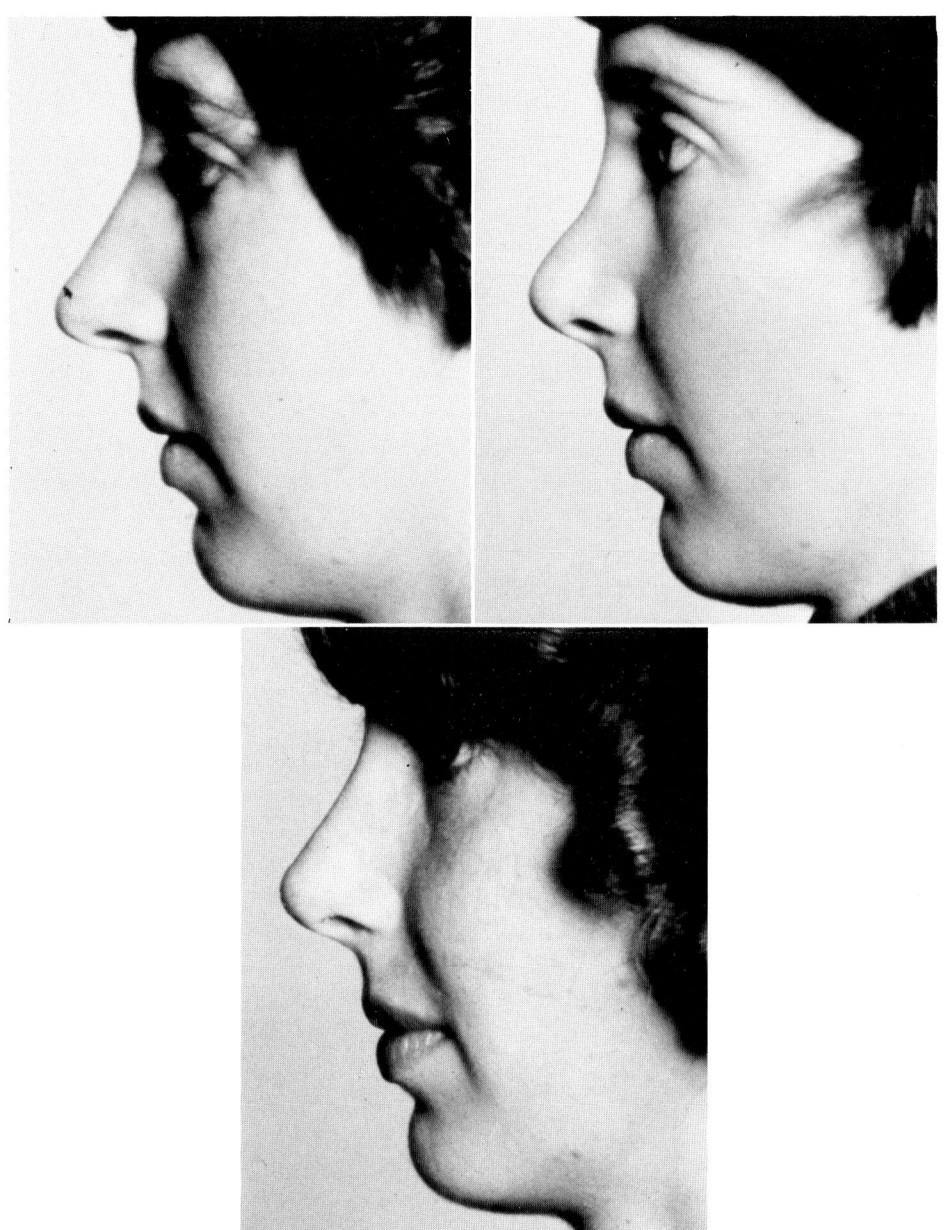

Figure 35-7

Irregular prominent tip

The irregular prominent tip usually results from asymmetrical alar cartilage reduction, a typical mishap that I try to prevent by carefully marking the excisions on my primary rhinoplasty patients.

Correction is achieved through symmetrical reduction of the cartilages, which is performed while it is fully visible. I deliver the cartilages through an intercartilaginous and a rim incision bilaterally.

Acute cartilaginous dome

Transsecting the genu of the alar cartilages between the medial and lateral crura is a widely used technique to achieve a refined triangular nasal tip during primary rhinoplasty. Yet I have seen a number of middle-aged women with sharply pointing tip cartilages shining through the thin skin after the camouflaging soft-tissue layers have gradually vanished. From these cases I learned to respect the continuity of the "cartilaginous domes" and to shape them with partial excisions or, even better, only interdigitating incisions.

To correct this deformity I deliver the alar cartilages and reconstruct a round genu by suturing the medial crus to the lateral crus and softening the edges with little interdigitating incisions.

Boxy tip

The iatrogenic boxy tip is a result of the lateral transsection of the genua of the alar cartilages rather than transsection of the medial part.

The very obvious bifidity has to be corrected in much the same manner used in reconstructing the cartilaginous domes.

Lack of tip prominence

If the tip lacks prominence, its support is too weak because either the alar cartilages were very soft from the beginning or they have been reduced by more than two thirds of their volume. In some cases a simple tip-only graft, well-positioned slightly above the "domes," will suffice and will give the desired definition. More often the lack of definition of the tip is caused by intentional weakening of the tip support by the transsection of the genu of the alar cartilages. The primary rhinoplasty's initially good result gradually deteriorates during the following months and years, with the tip drooping below the line of the dorsum.

In secondary rhinoplasty cases the reerection or augmentation of the tip by using cartilage grafts alone is compromised by the scarred vestibular skin. Therefore, in addition I lower the nasal dorsum to achieve the desired definition of the tip.

In the patient in Figure 35-8 the nose was also narrowed for further refinement. The follow-up period has been 6 years.

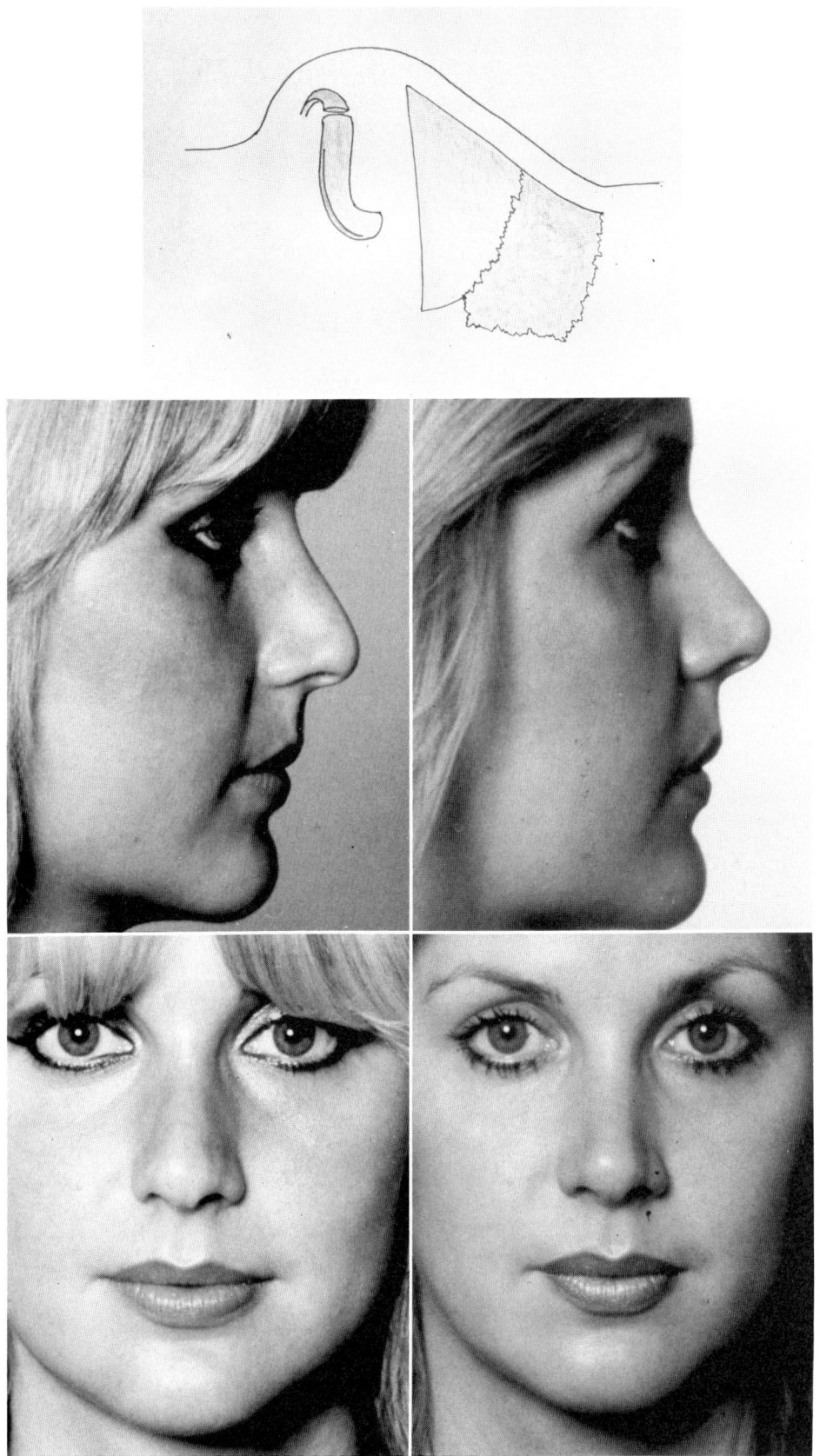

Figure 35-8

Collapsed tip

Excessive resection of the alar cartilages and the caudal septum such as is sometimes done for bulky tips may result in a complete collapse of the tip with functional stenosis of the nasal entrance. Usually too much lining has been sacrificed simultaneously, so the tissues of the entire nasal tip have shrunk.

Reconstruction is extremely difficult. I could achieve a moderate aesthetic and functional result with a "mushroom graft" composed of cartilage of the two auricular conchae to support the tip and to bring the columella forward and downward as shown in Figures 35-9 and 35-10.

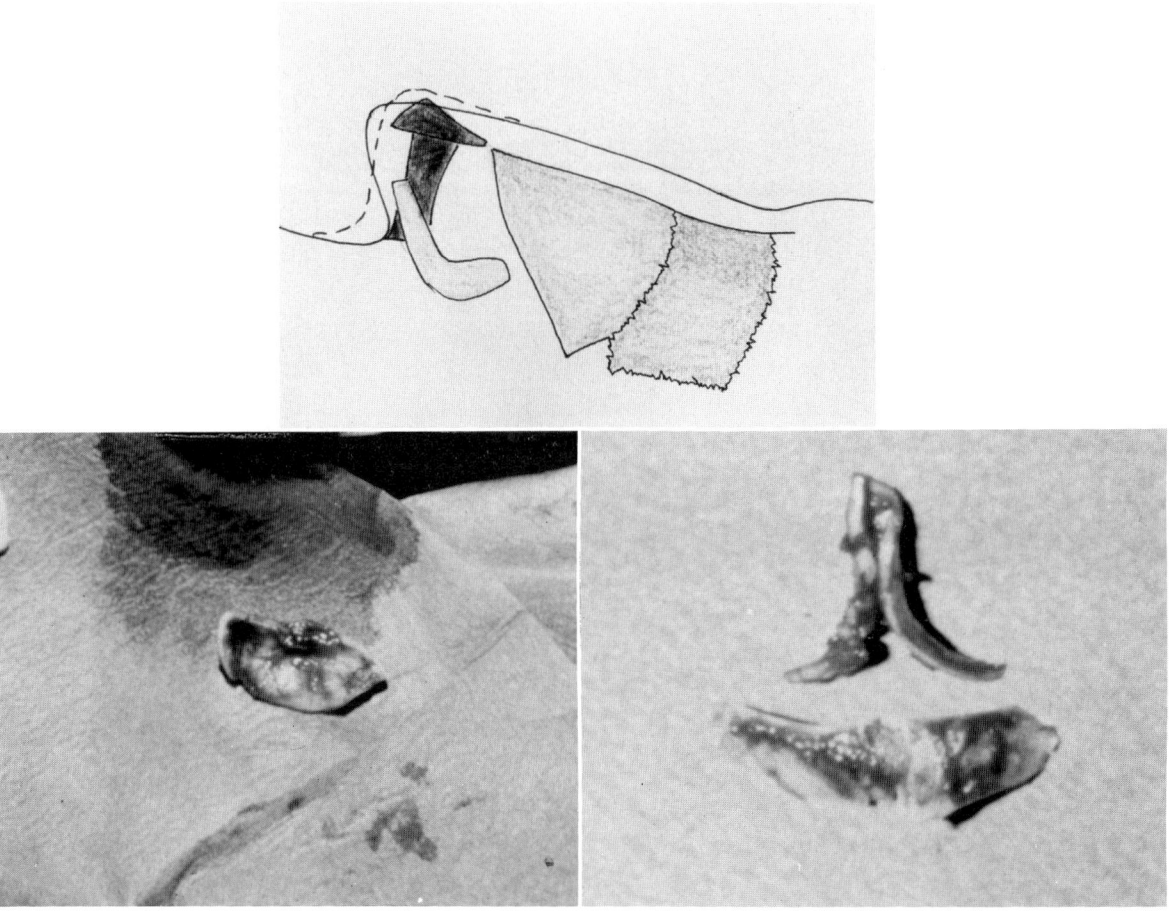

Figure 35-9

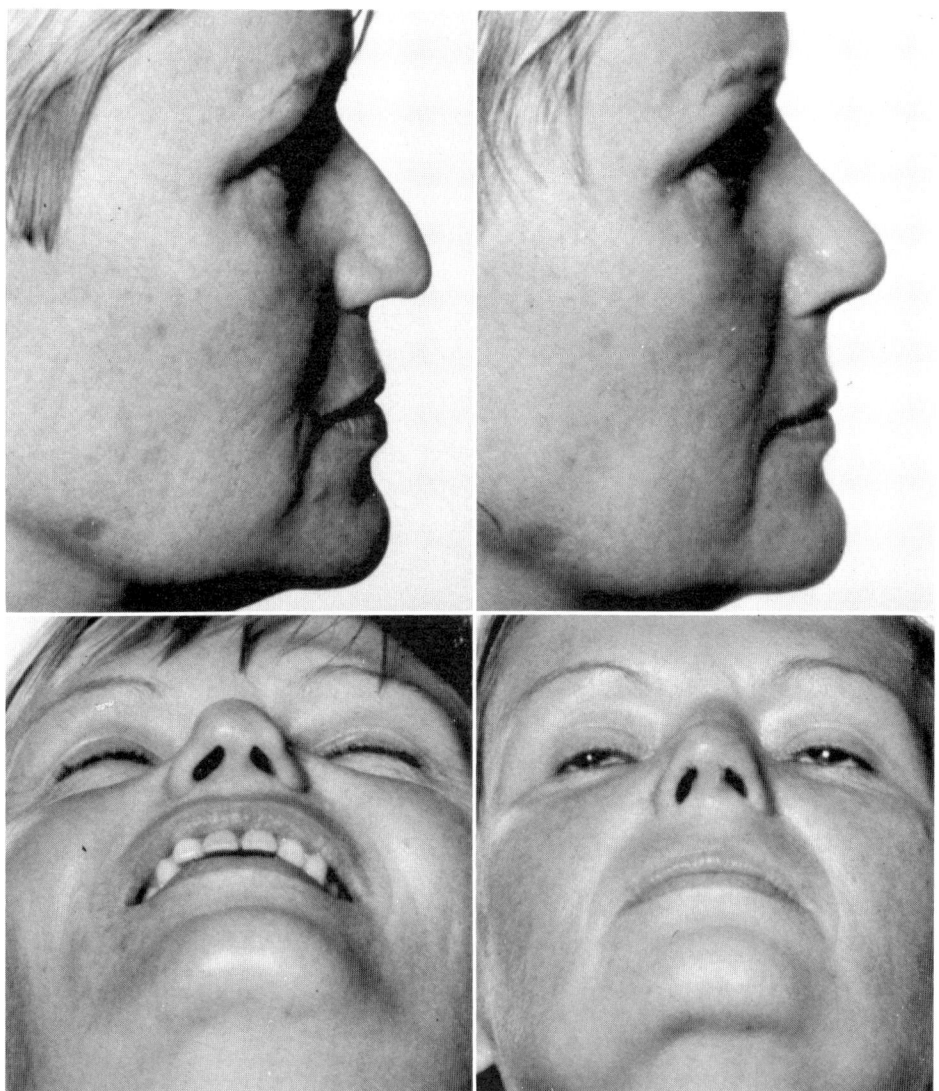

Figure 35-10

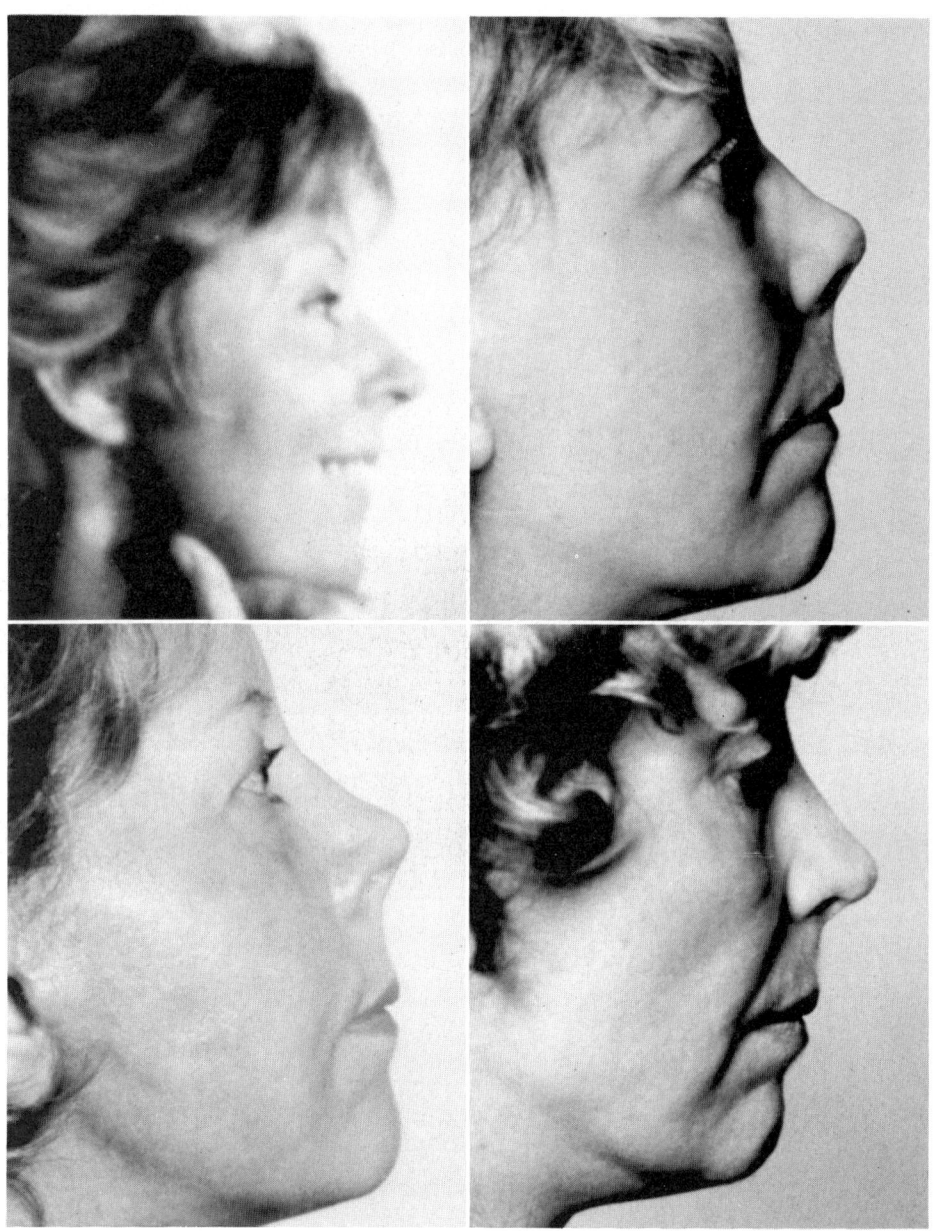

Figure 35-11

Shortened nose

A patient's long nose had been shortened excessively, resulting in a ridiculously tiny turned-up nose and a relatively too-long lip. Because the entire face was a surgical battlefield, I persuaded the unhappy patient to wait for 6 months and to lengthen and soften the nose through manual massage. The waiting period and the "physiotherapy" gave approximately 50% of the final result that was achieved after I did only extensive submucosal dissection and loosening of the tissues (Figure 35-11).

Another patient needed microsurgical revision and grafting of the ophthalmic and temporal branch of the right facial nerve for treatment of upper-facial palsy—the unfavorable result of a rather brutal simultaneous facelift and rhinoplasty (Figure 35-12).

The excessive reduction of a hypertrophic hump nose resulted in a foreshortened broad nose. The secondary correction consists of augmentation of the alae with auricular composite grafts, elongation of the septum with a cartilage graft to the columella, tip grafts for more definition, shortening of the iatrogenic elongated upper lip through eversion of the vermilion, narrowing of the nostril through an alar base excision, and narrowing and elevation of the bony nasal pyramid through a lateral osteotomy and infracture.

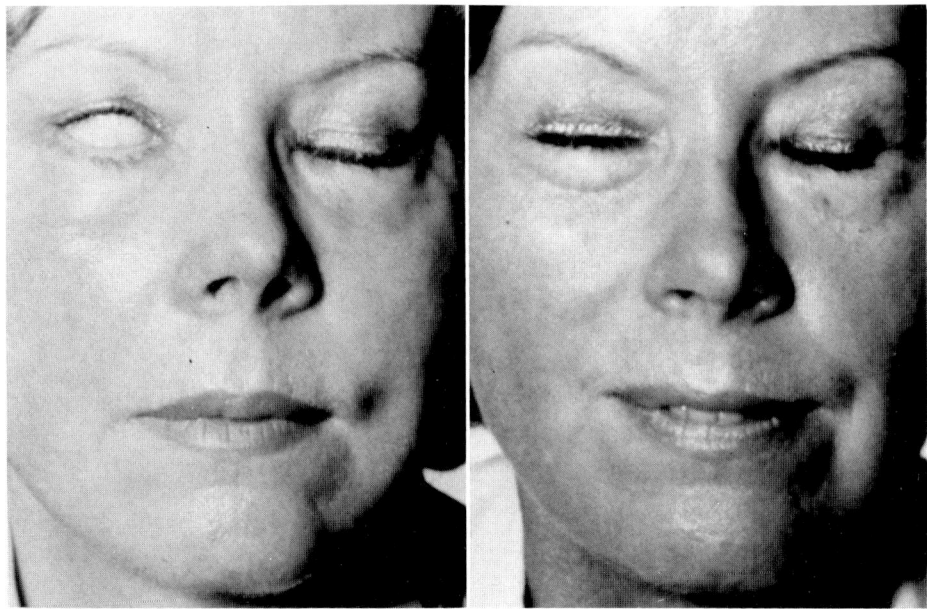

Figure 35-12

The narrow nose

The narrow nose is a rare case to come across for secondary correction. It is caused by excessive infracture of the lateral walls. The nose looks sharp—like a sword in the middle of the face. The nasal airways are somewhat impaired, as is the normal drainage from the frontal sinuses.

To correct this problem in a patient I first recreated the normal width of the nasal pyramid through osteotomy and outfracture and then covered the "open roof" with a large auricular conchal graft that was fixed firmly in place using fibrin glue (Figure 35-13). For better harmony with the sunken-in flaring alae, I added an alar base excision.

The patient in Figure 35-14 wanted the nose she had before her radical primary surgery. I came close to the original and satisfied the patient.

The rhinopsychopath

Finally, I would like to warn you about the "rhinopsychopath," who may have started with a rather sizable hump nose but who never stops asking for another reduction even if there is very little nose left in the face. I have the impression from some of these patients that the nose is overrepresented in the precentral gyrus of the frontal brain. When they look in the mirror, they see not an objective picture but an exaggerated mirror-image of the nose that has nothing to do with reality.

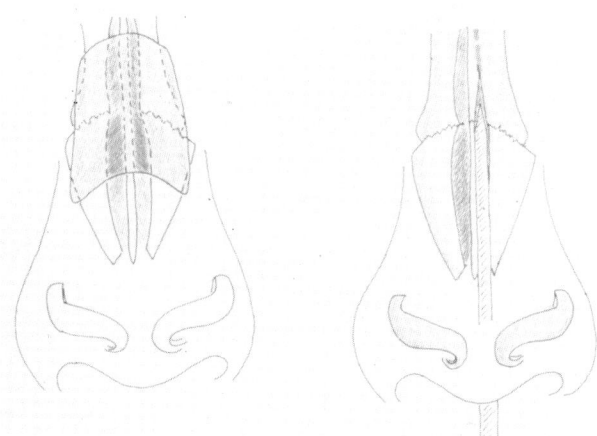

Figure 35-13

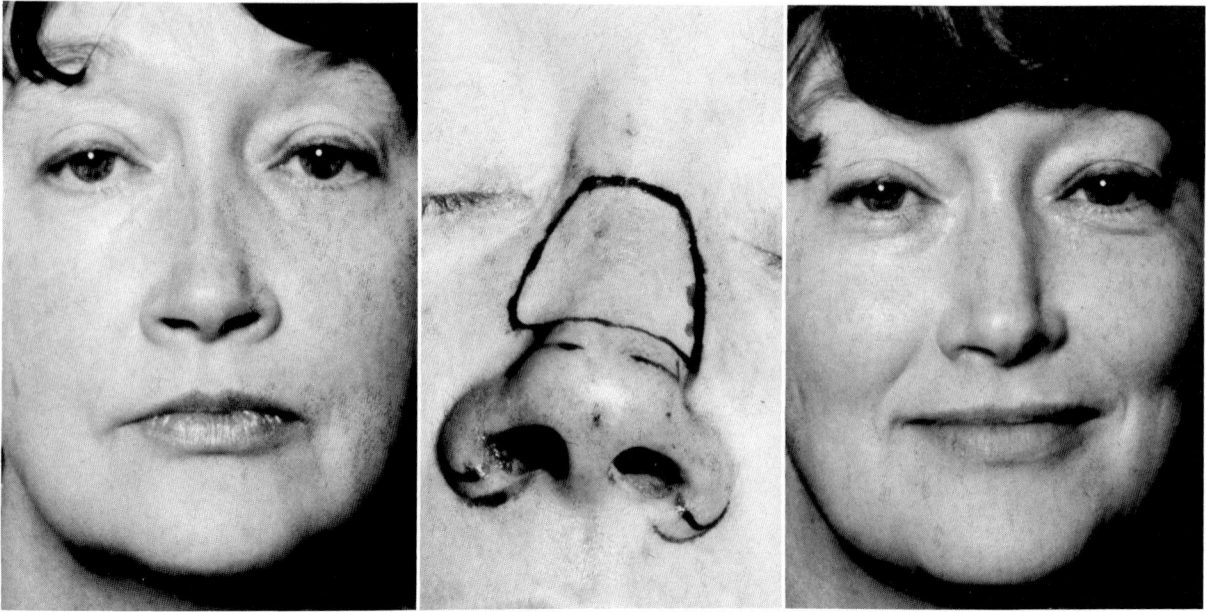

Figure 35-14

36

Rhinoplasty and Profile Plasty: Basic Considerations

Wolfgang Mühlbauer

Profile plasty is an extension of rhinoplasty. It encompasses the correction of the shape of the nose, correction of the upper and lower jaws, remodeling of the contour of the neck, as well as reshaping of the entire neurocranium and viscerocranium through application of the techniques of craniofacial surgery.

Performing rhinoplasty and profile plasty satisfies some of the essential goals of plastic surgery: form, function, and appearance of a person may be altered to advantage without visible scars. Better appearance usually initiates a positive development of the personality.

Chin dimple

Dimpling of the chin makes a man look energetic yet makes a female look too masculine. It is a soft-tissue problem caused by diastasis of the mental muscles, which may easily be corrected by suturing them in the midline through a vestibular incision (Figure 36-1).

Prominent chin

A prominent chin with eugnathia is caused by hypertrophy of the symphysis of the mandible. It is corrected by reducing the hypertrophic symphysis using an oscillating saw and/or a burr through an intraoral approach. The soft tissue redrapes easily without forming a "double chin." The reduction of the prominent chin results in a much softer appearance (Figure 36-2).

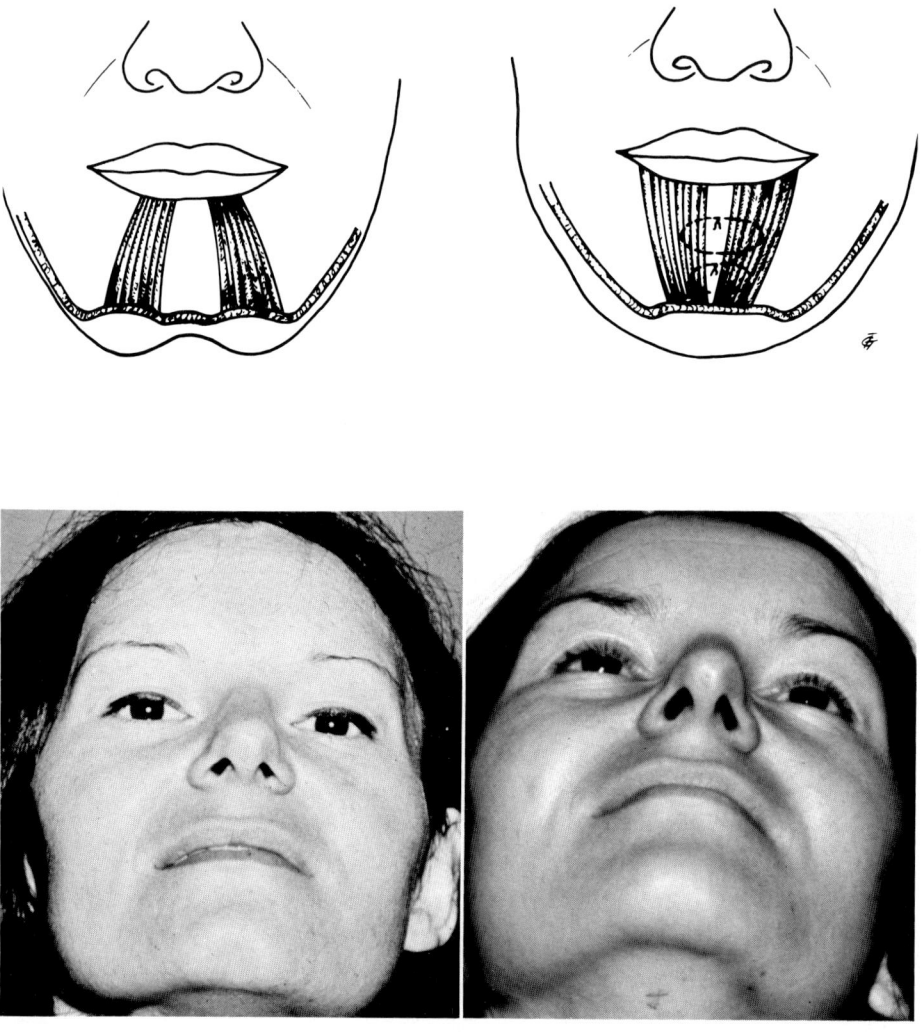

Figure 36-1. Diastasis of the mental muscles may cause a masculine chin dimple. Correction is achieved by correcting the diastasis through a vestibular incision.

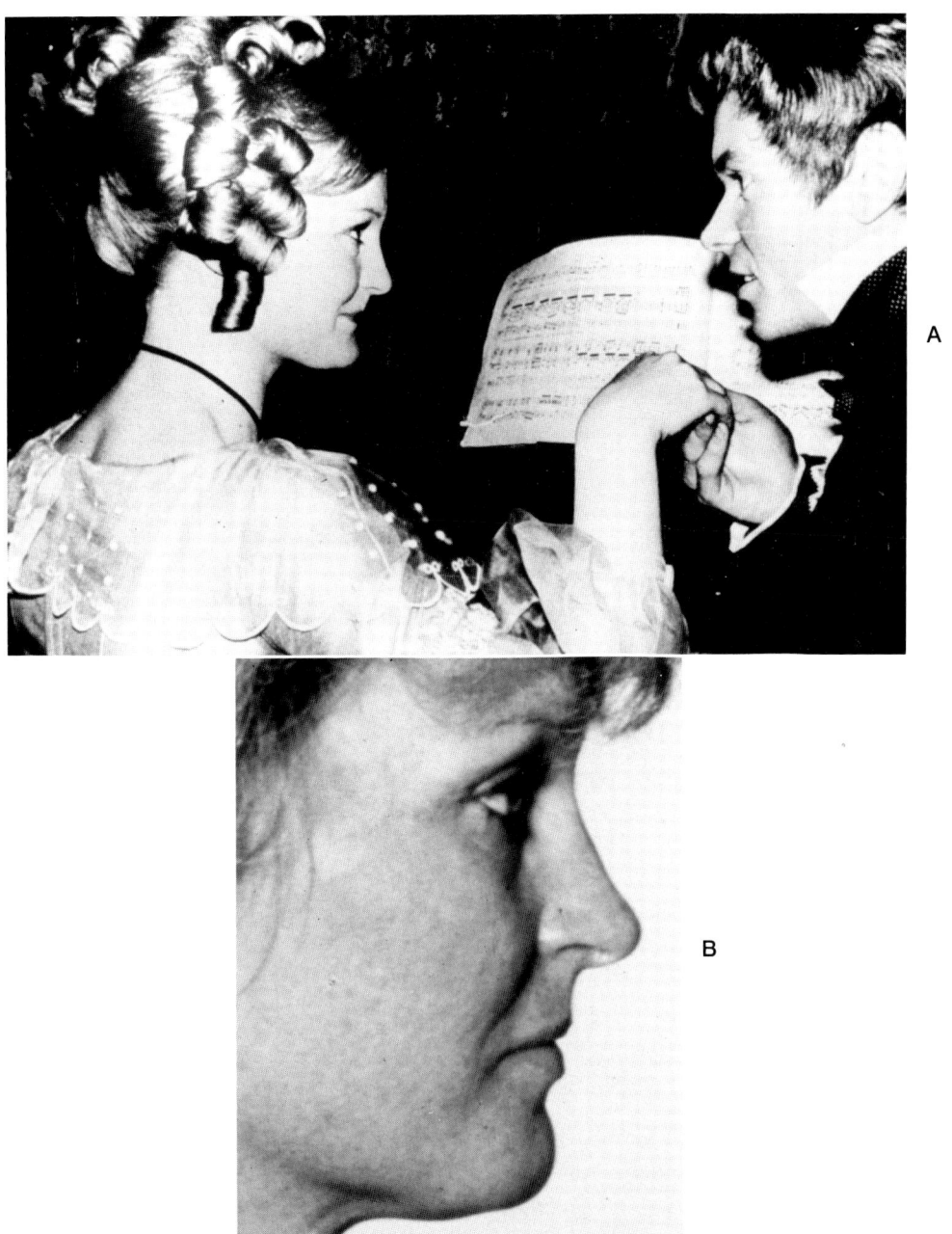

Figure 36-2. A, The prominent chin (hypertrophic symphysis of the mandible) was aggravated on close-up views on the screen. **B,** Reduction of the symphysis by using an oscillating saw through a vestibular incision. No skin excision was necessary.

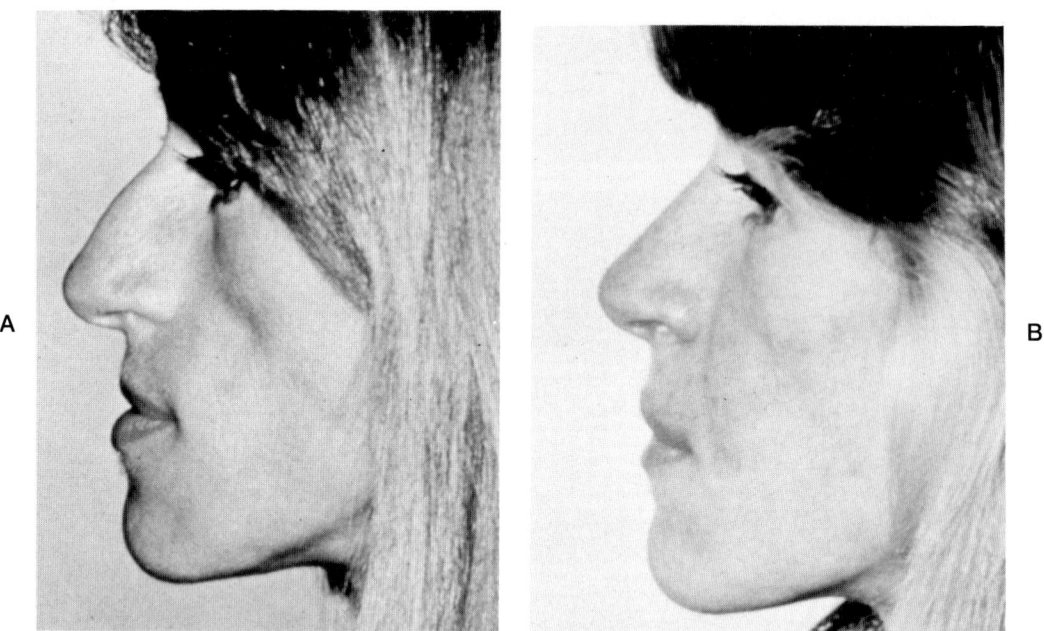

Figure 36-3. A, A 23-year-old woman with sharply edged faced caused by a prominent chin, an acquilinear nose, and a buccal lipodystrophy. **B,** Result 2 years later. Softening of her face through chin reduction, reduction rhinoplasty, and augmentation of the cheeks with collagen.

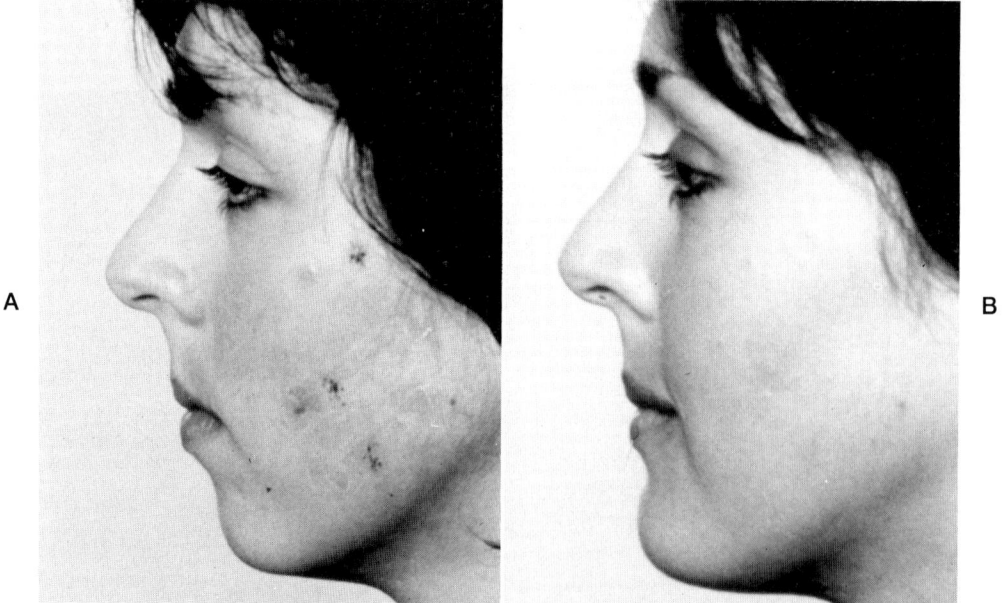

Figure 36-4. A, A 20-year-old with mildly receding chin. **B,** One year after chin augmentation with preformed proplast.

Sharp-edged face

A young woman was sad about her sharp-edged face caused by a prominent chin (with eugnathia), an aquiline nose, and buccal lipodystrophy (Figure 36-3, *A*). The appearance of her face was softened when the mandibular symphysis was reduced, the nose slightly shortened and straightened by a reduction rhinoplasty, and the cheeks augmented with collagen injections on three occasions. The result has remained stable for 2 years (Figure 36-3, *B*).

Receding chin

Patients with a slightly receding chin often request a reduction rhinoplasty; however, what is needed is an augmention of their chin for greater harmony of their profile. In minimal cases I prefer to add alloplastic material such as proplast or preformed silicone to bone or cartilage (Figure 36-4).

Micrognathia

A truly hypoplastic mandible is corrected much better, and usually permanently, by using a horizontal osteotomy and advancement as a so-called genioplasty. Thereby the submental muscles are also pulled forward, and the angle between the chin and the neck is improved (Figure 36-5).

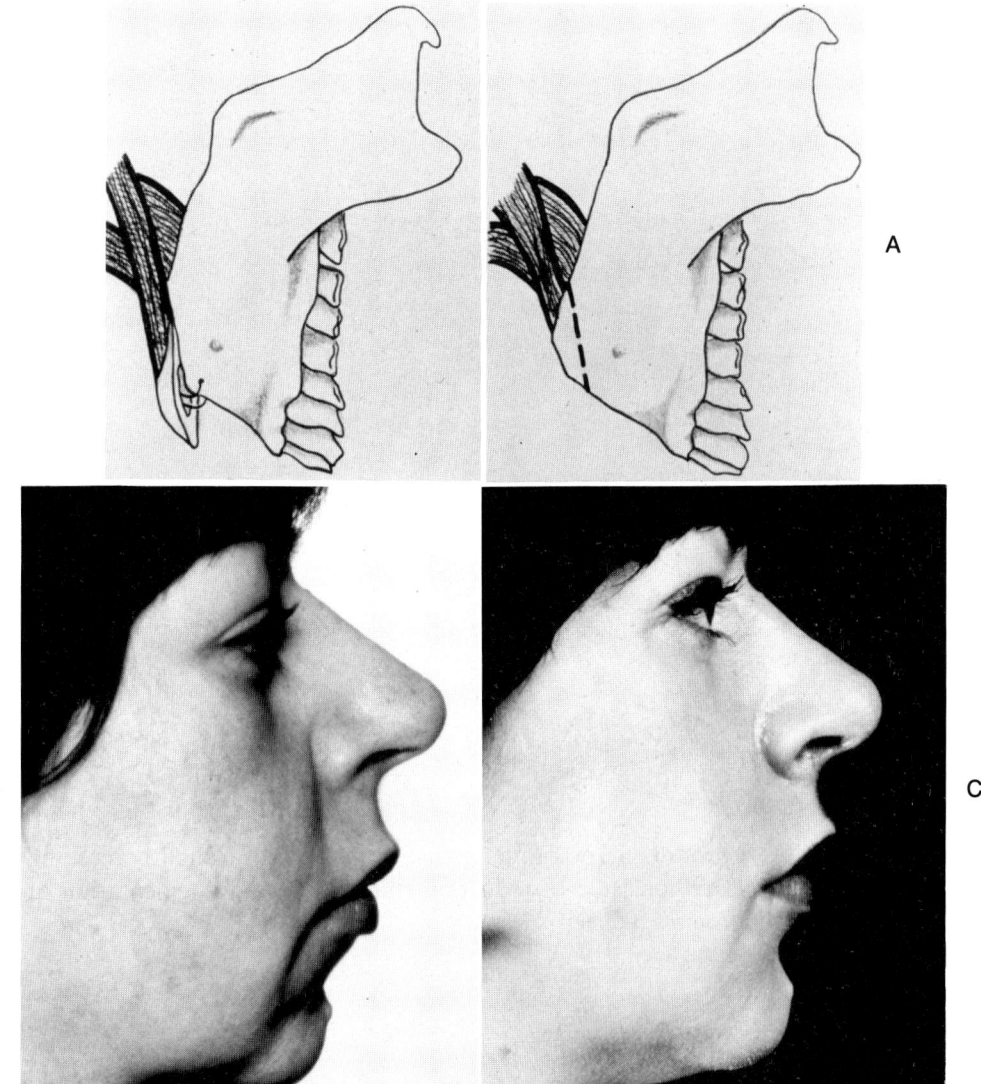

Figure 36-5. A and **B,** Receding chin resulting from hypoplastic mandible. **C,** Correction with horizontal osteotomy and advancement, genioplasty through an intraoral approach.

Prominent nose with receding chin

A prominent, pointing nose is aggravated by combination with a slightly receding chin. Reducing such a large nose provides enough material to augment the chin sufficiently to harmonize the profile (Figure 36-6).

Bird's face

A prominent hump nose combined with a hypoplastic mandible gives the appearance of a bird's face. The material from the nose is usually not sufficient to increase the chin; therefore radical reduction rhinoplasty is combined with a horizontal osteotomy and advancement of the hypoplastic mandible (genioplasty). It is amazing how the genioplasty can positively influence the lips and the oral commissures (Figure 36-7).

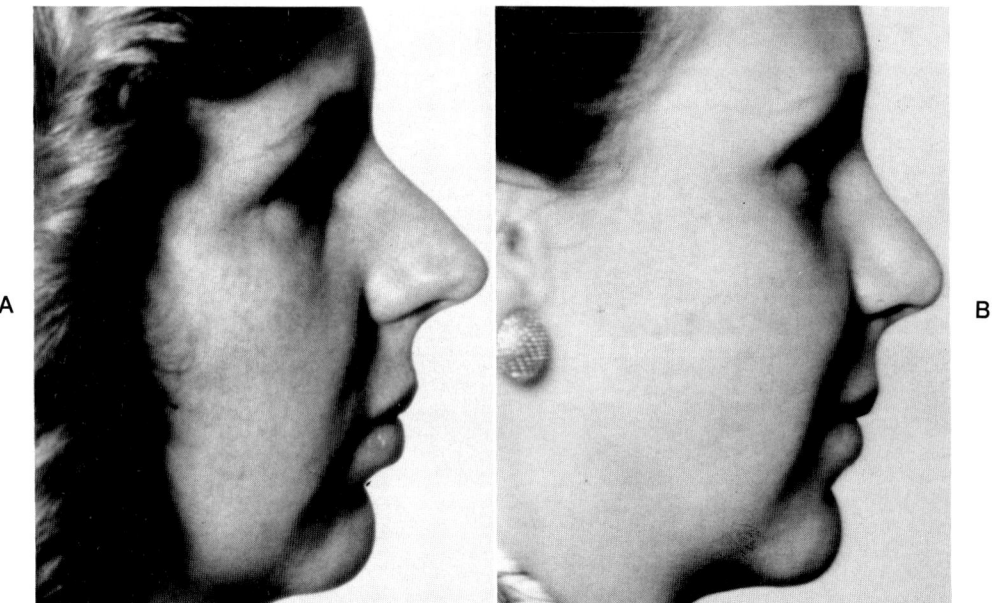

Figure 36-6. A, A prominent, pointing nose is emphasized by a slightly receding chin. **B,** Profile plasty consisted of reduction rhinoplasty and augmentation of the chin with the hump material.

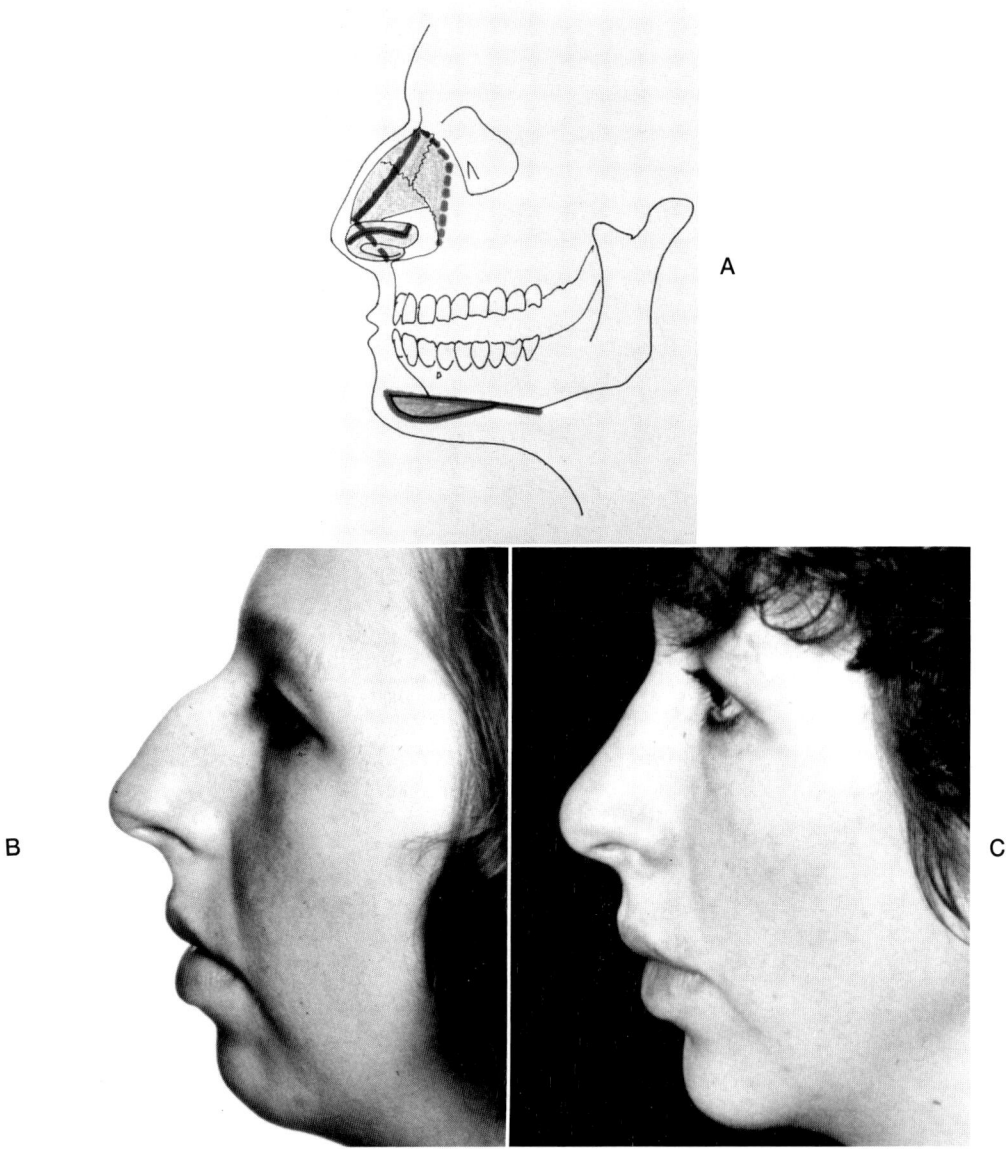

Figure 36-7. A and **B,** Young girl with a bird's face (prominent hump nose with hypoplastic mandible). **C,** The profile plasty consisted of radical reduction rhinoplasty combined with a horizontal osteotomy and advancement genioplasty.

Inca face

I would like to coin a new word for a rare profile anomaly that is the combination of a prominent hump nose, a hypoplastic mandible, and a receding forehead, which provides an appearance favored by the Incas. They produced this profile artificially by wrapping bandages around their babies' foreheads.

The correction of an "Inca face" consists of performing a radical reduction rhinoplasty, horizontal osteotomy, advancement of the mandible, and augmentation of the forehead with pericranium through a coronal incision (Figure 36-8).

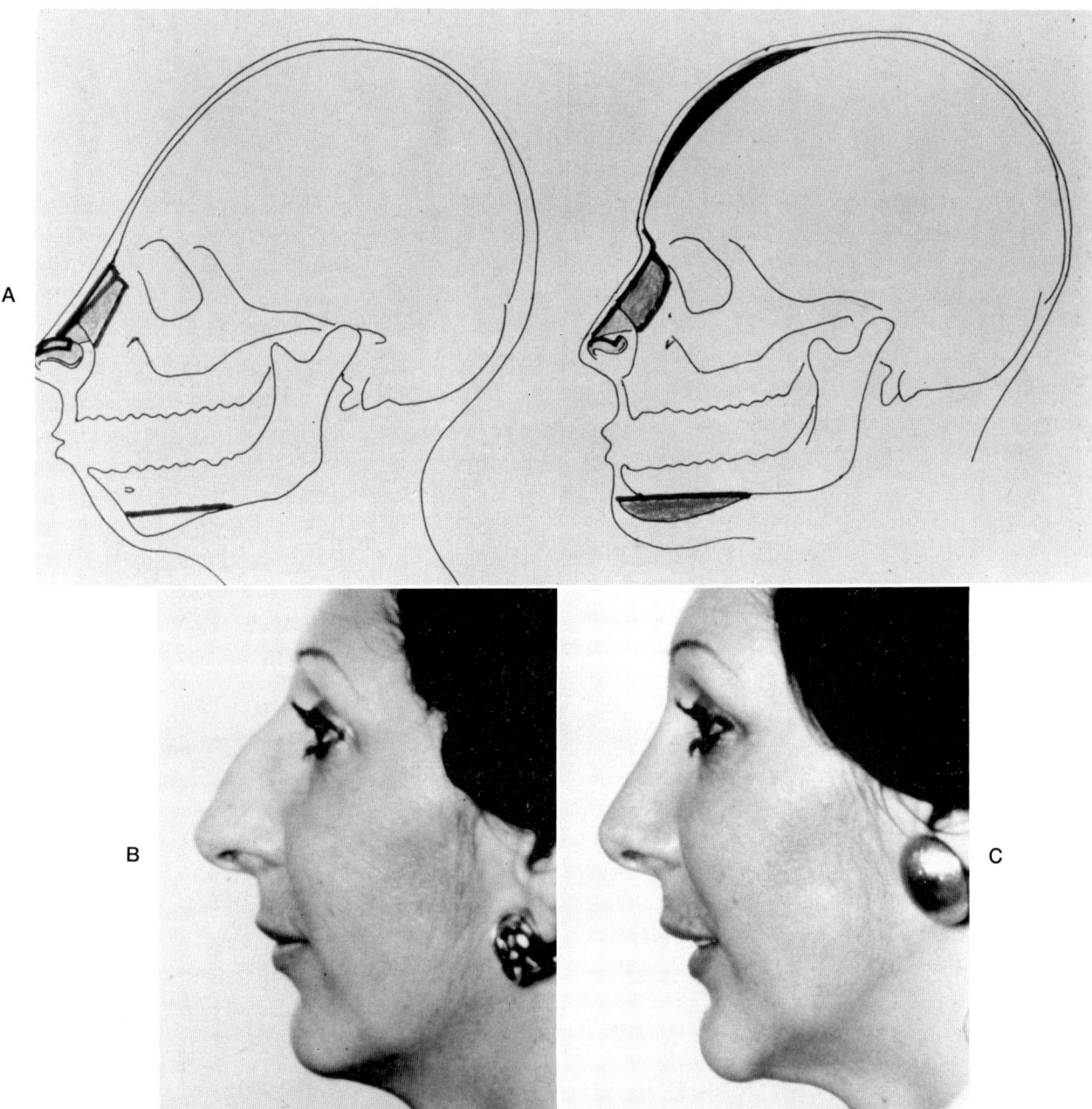

Figure 36-8. A and **B,** Middle-aged woman with an Inca face (combination of a prominent hump nose, hypoplastic mandible, and a receding forehead). **C,** The profile plasty consisted of a radical reduction rhinoplasty, horizontal osteotomy, and advancement genioplasty and augmentation of the forehead with pericranium through a coronal incision.

Long face

Ortiz Monasterio has drawn attention to the long- and short-face syndromes, for which he proposes horizontal osteotomies and reduction or augmentation of the maxilla and mandible as appropriate. These procedures are spin-offs of craniofacial surgery. Although the indication is mainly aesthetic, sometimes the dental occlusion may be corrected as well. I have performed segmental reduction of the maxilla at the Le Fort I level and the horizontal branch of the mandible, along with a moderate reduction rhinoplasty with shortening and straightening of the dorsum (Figure 36-9).

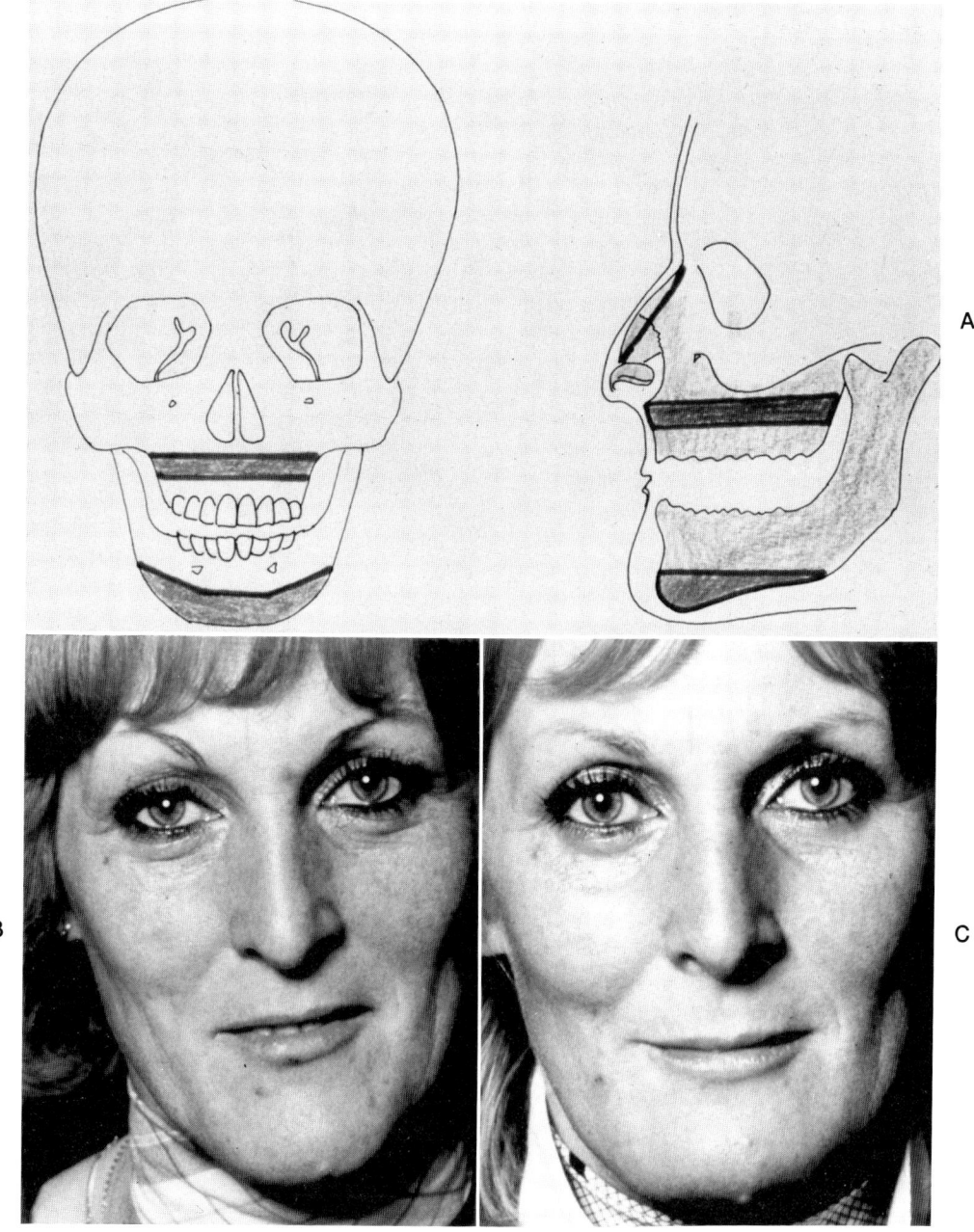

Figure 36-9. A-C, A long face syndrome is corrected through vertical reductions of the maxilla and mandible. A mild shortening of the nose was also performed.

Nasomaxillary hypoplasia (Binder syndrome)

The congenital nasomaxillary hypoplasia (Binder syndrome) produces a so-called dish face with a very flat nose and blocked airways. Moderate cases may be corrected by implantation of an L-shaped bone graft and onlay bone grafts to the maxilla after very extensive submucosal dissection to free the soft tissues. A dramatic change can be achieved (Figure 36-10).

In patients with more severe anomalies the hypoplastic facial skeleton must be cut and advanced at various Le Fort I to III levels in addition to performance of the nasal bone graft.

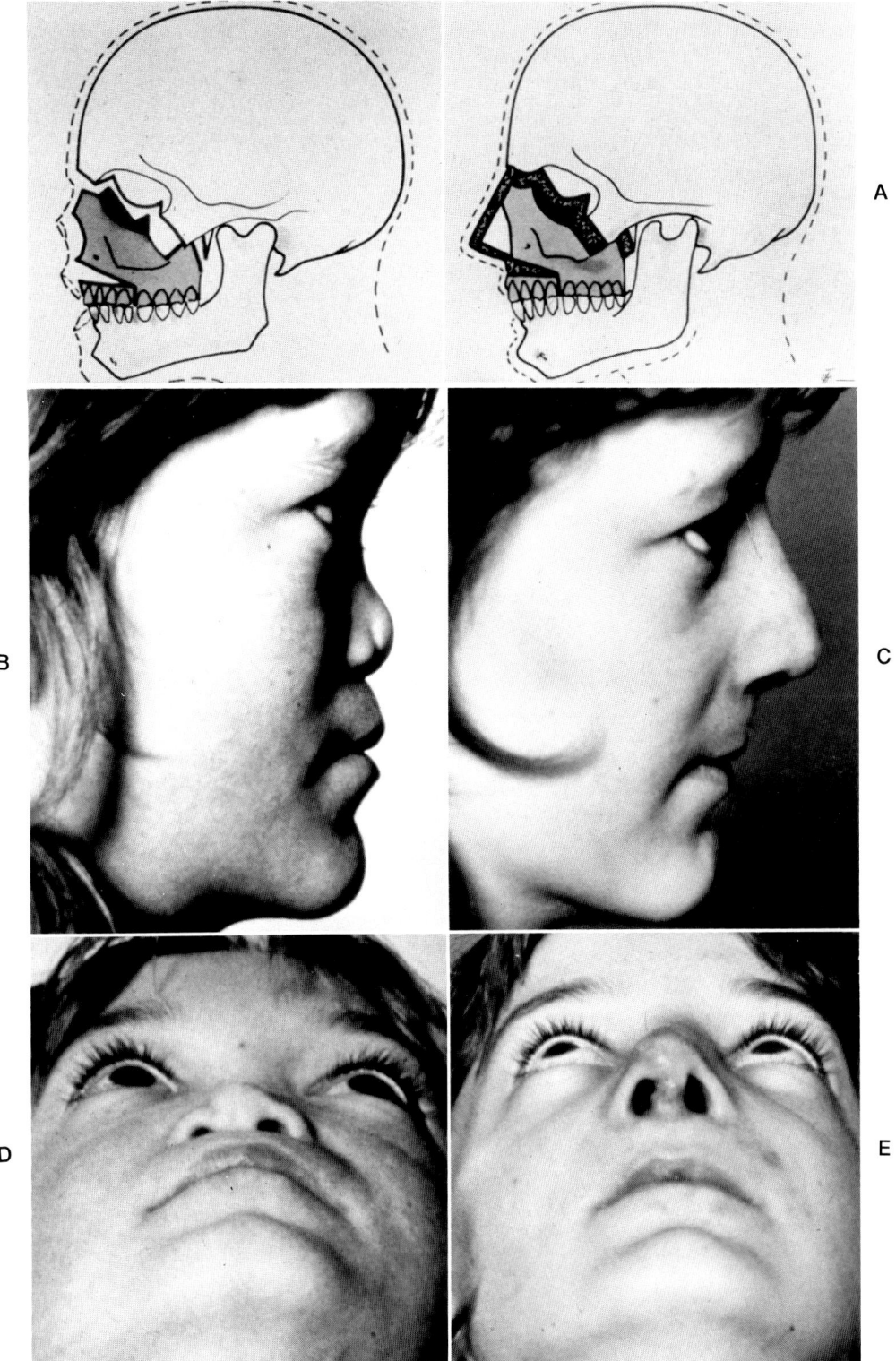

Figure 36-10   A and **B,** Congenital nasomaxillary hypoplasia (Binder syndrome) produces a very flat nose and blocked airways and a dish face. **C,** Correction with onlay bone grafts and maxillary osteotomies and advancement. **D,** The girl at age 14. **E,** Two years later at age 16 (case of Mühlbauer and Marchac).

Craniofacial dysostosis

Even complex craniofacial dysplasias with awkward profiles may be corrected with craniofacial surgical techniques. In many instances the basic reason for these malformations is prematurely fused sutures of the neurocranium and the viscerocranium. Personally I advocate very early (at 3 to 6 months of age) complete osteotomy and remodeling of the neurocranium and the viscerocranium, thereby correcting functional as well as aesthetic deficits simultaneously. So far, the postoperative skeletal growth in many of my surgical infants is near normal during a 5-year (maximum) follow-up period (Figure 36-11).

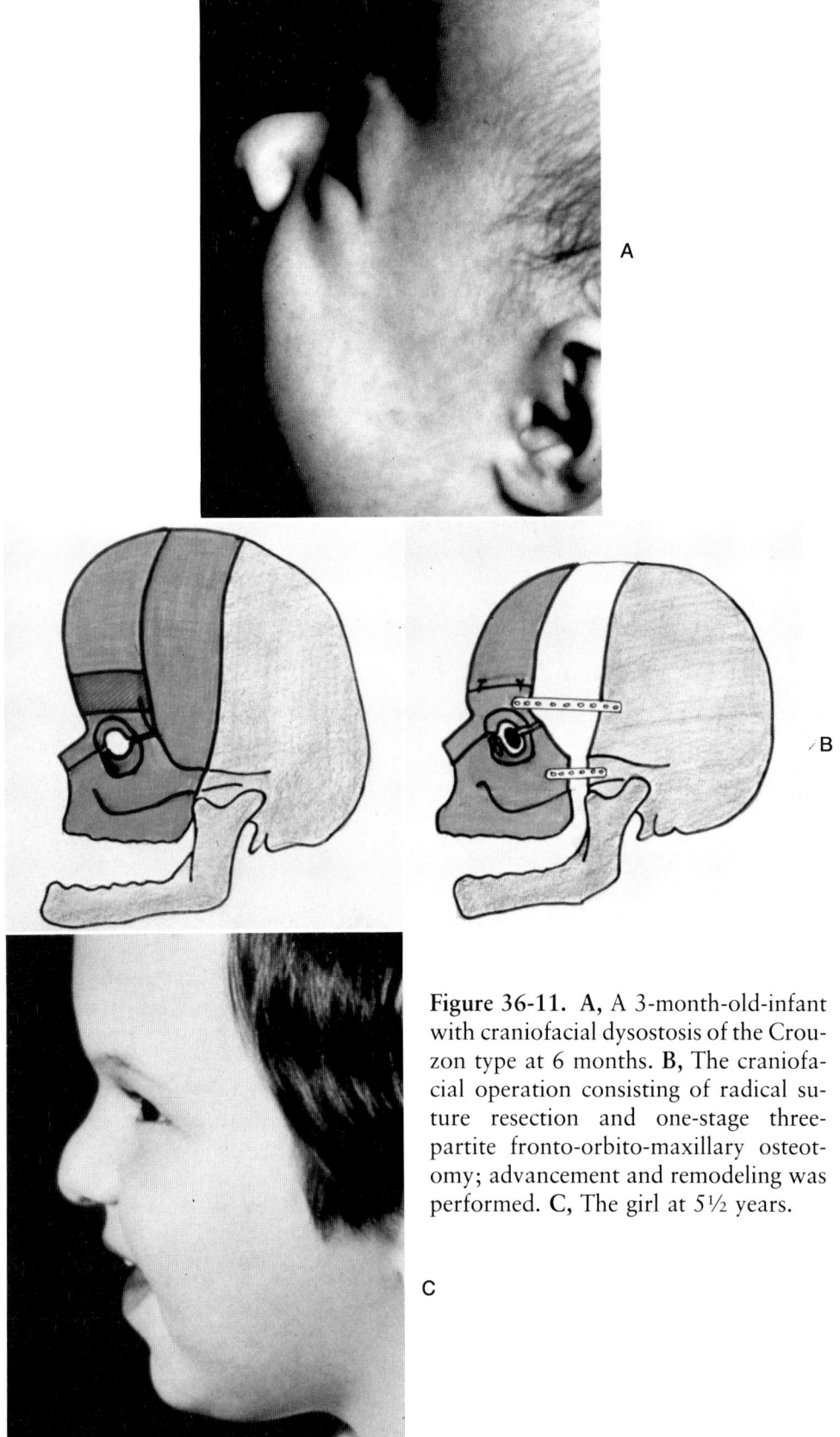

Figure 36-11. A, A 3-month-old-infant with craniofacial dysostosis of the Crouzon type at 6 months. **B,** The craniofacial operation consisting of radical suture resection and one-stage three-partite fronto-orbito-maxillary osteotomy; advancement and remodeling was performed. **C,** The girl at 5½ years.

37

Secondary Rhinoplasty in the Thick-Skinned Nose

Fernando Ortiz-Monasterio, Alvaro Olmedo

The nose can be visualized as a narrow tent in which the support is provided by the septum, the nasal bones, and the upper and lower cartilages. The skin coverage is the canvas. The surface and contour of a tent as well as the protrusion of the supporting framework depend on the thickness of the canvas. When the skin of the nose is thick, it does not adapt to the supporting structures in the same manner as thin skin. The sharp angles of the nasal skeleton and the edges of the cartilages are smoothed or erased by the thick cover and are converted into a round structure. Furthermore, thick skin does not retract as much as the thinner coverage when the size of the skeleton is decreased. In addition, stronger structural support is required to maintain the shape.

Patients with thick-skinned noses often request an aesthetic improvement through rhinoplasty. When the operation is performed by an inexperienced surgeon unaware of the pitfalls of trying to thin the skin, severe secondary deformities may occur. Alas, even in the hands of an expert, secondary deformities may occur in this type of patients. If too much bone or cartilage is resected, the skin will not adapt properly, and the resulting nose will be more bulbous and shapeless than before. If an attempt is made to thin the skin by resecting the subcutaneous fat, two problems may occur. First, if too much tissue is taken from the dermis, the skin will retract and adhere to the underlining skeleton, producing visible irregularities and depressions. Second, when the resection is carried even further, skin necrosis may take place. If only fat is removed, the procedure

is often followed by chronic edema with loss of the initial improvement through the accumulation of scar tissue.[3]

PREOPERATIVE PLANNING

The nasal problems and the personality of the patient should be carefully evaluated. Most of these patients, in spite of careful explanations by the surgeon, still expect a beautifully carved, well-proportioned nose. No effort should be spared in stressing the limitations in general of a secondary procedure and the special problems presented by the thick skin.

The characteristics of the coverage should be carefully evaluated. Some patients have a moderately thick skin, a slight increase in the number of sebaceous glands, and a thick layer of subcutaneous fat. This type of skin is fairly pliable and mobile and adapts well to cartilage grafts. In other patients the subcutaneous fat is practically absent, and the skin itself is extremely thick and very rich in sebaceous glands. It is not rare to find multiple sebaceous cysts and fibrous tissue resulting from chronic acne in these patients. In more severe cases, the quality of the skin suggests incipient rhinophyma. This type of skin is not movable and adapts very poorly to the supporting structures, including grafts.

The shape and irregularities of the supporting osteocartilaginous framework should be carefully assessed.

The objectives of the secondary rhinoplasty are to improve the contour and support of the skeletal framework and to correct skin irregularities.

CORRECTION OF THE NASAL PYRAMID

Findings in the nasal pyramid include dorsal irregularities plus incomplete or asymmetrical lateral fractures. Rasping of these irregularities and resetting inadequate fractures are necessary. However, contrary to what happens in patients with thin-skinned noses, the contour of the dorsum is not greatly improved by this maneuver. Supratip deformity is a frequent result of excessive resection of the nasal dorsum and of subcutaneous scar contracture in the lower third of the nose.

Most of the patients in this group require an augmentation to the dorsum through cartilaginous or bone grafts. No foreign materials should ever be used in these patients. When a limited amount of tissue is required, septal bone and cartilage, when available, are the ideal materials.[4-7] One, two, and even three strips of cartilage approximately 5 mm wide can be obtained to build up the dorsum. This procedure would, however, leave very little cartilage to correct other irregularities (Figures 37-1 and 37-2). Therefore cartilage from the concha of the ear may be used for the same purpose.[1] Correction of the dorsum with ear cartilage does not produce the best result because we find it difficult to produce the proper shape and to avoid postoperative irregularities. Rib cartilage, although easy to carve, has a tendency to buckle secondarily. The same is true for preserved homologs of rib cartilage. Although we use preserved cartilage extensively, we believe that the achieved dorsum is not as good because the irregularities produced by minor absorption may be conspicuous.

When more material is needed to reconstruct the nasal pyramid, we prefer to use bone grafts taken from the ribs or cranium. Rib bone grafts are superior to tibial and ulnar grafts and have less morbidity than iliac bone grafts.

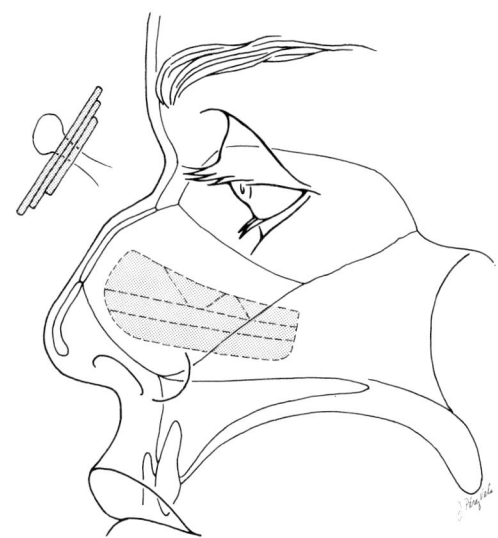

Figure 37-1

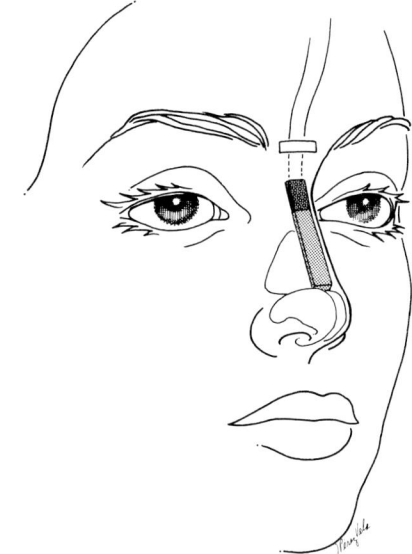

Figure 37-2

Rib grafts are taken through a small incision in the inframammary fold. The periosteum on the external surface of the rib is preserved, and a section 7 to 8 cm long is removed, carefully preserving the integrity of the pleura (Figure 37-3). The preservation of the periosteum on the graft helps early vascularization and prevents absorption of the graft. When tip support is necessary, a second piece of rib cartilage is used to make the short arm of the L. The rib is split longitudinally, leaving the periosteum on the cortical side, which will be placed under the skin, whereas the cancellous side rests on the nasal skeleton. The graft is crushed with Tessier forceps to give it the proper shape and is introduced into the previously dissected area of the nasal dorsum. The use of a cartilage graft in the columella not only provides support but improves the nasolabial angle. The prominence of the tip should be made by the cartilage and not by bone because the latter would be absorbed in a short time. A further touch-up procedure may be necessary at a later date in this type of patient. For this purpose, we store a portion of cartilage immediately under the skin to have it easily available. We have stored cartilage subcutaneously for as long as 12 years in some cases with minimum loss of volume.

To improve tip projection and definition, we insert cartilage directly under the skin in front of the dome. The ideal donor site is the septum when available or the ear concha when the septum has been previously used. One, two, or three layers of cartilage may be used to increase the projection. This cartilaginous graft should not be crushed, and its carving is different from the procedure used for the thin-skinned nose that was suggested by Sheen.[7] We insist on carving slightly elongated triangular pieces, leaving sharp angles that tend to protrude under the skin, since it is impossible to have an exaggerated effect in these thick-skinned noses (Figure 37-4). In some patients, when much larger pieces are necessary, grafts can be made of rib cartilage.

The insertion of cartilage in the columella in front of the nasal spine improves the nasolabial angle and provides support for the tip (Figure 37-5).

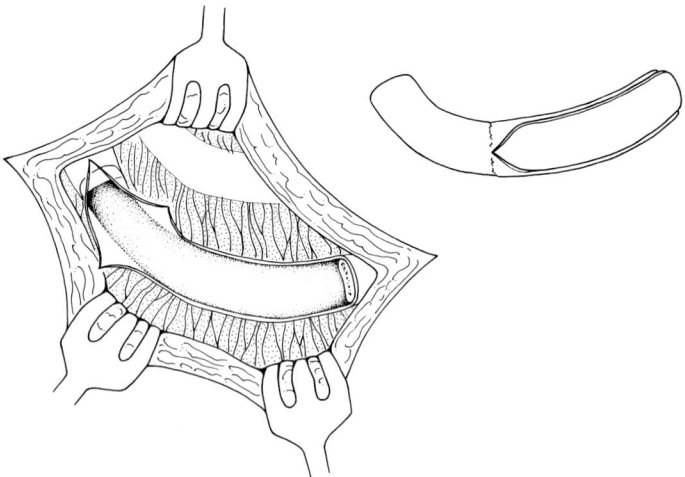

Figure 37-3

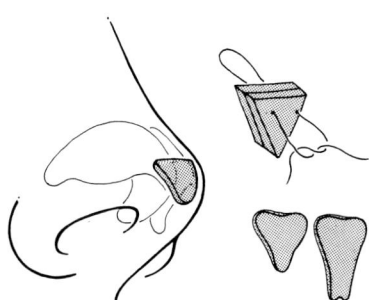

Figure 37-4

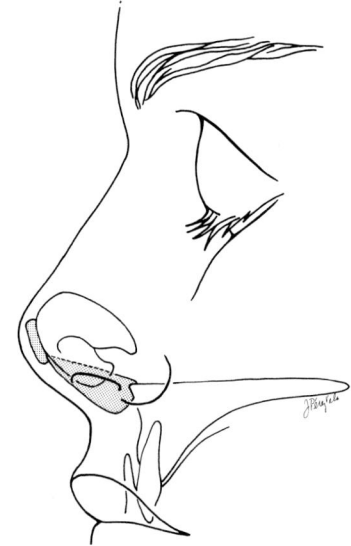

Figure 37-5

SKIN IRREGULARITIES

Depression and irregularities of the skin around the tip and the alae can be corrected by inserting cartilaginous grafts immediately under the skin. The depressions are approachable through a small incision in the nasal mucosa; only the necessary undermining is performed so that a snug pocket is made for the graft. When several areas require correction, the pockets should be separated from each other to prevent displacement of the grafts.

The very thick nasal skin, rich in sebaceous glands, does not yield to surgical correction by any of the previous procedures because of its thickness and lack of flexibility. If this type of skin is considered an incipient rhinophyma, dermabrasion may be used with acceptable results. The procedure should be discussed with the patient, who must understand clearly that temporary skin discoloration and permanent enlargement of the skin pores will occur. The thinning of the skin is performed with a rotary dermabrador with a flat cylinder to produce flat surfaces with some angularity (Figure 37-6). The abrasion should be limited to the lower half of the nose and can be performed simultaneously with a complete rhinoplasty and bone and cartilaginous grafts. The operation requires experience and a clear understanding of its potential problems. It is a helpful procedure to be used only by experienced surgeons.[2]

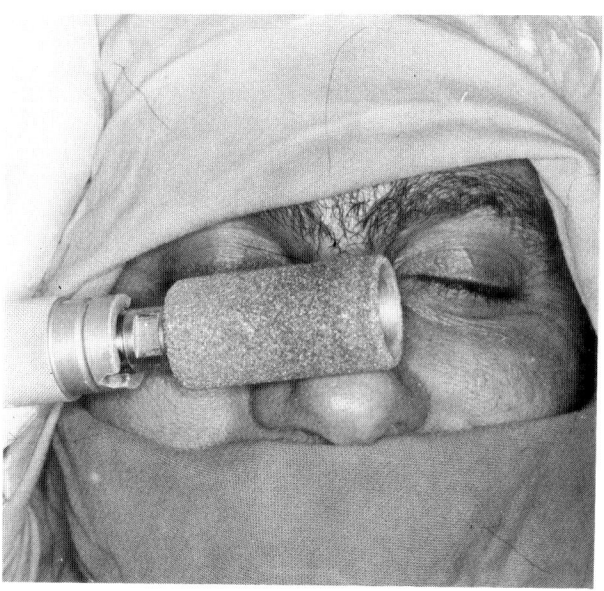

Figure 37-6

CASE REPORTS

Case 1

One year after a rhinoplasty this 40-year-old female came for consultation, requested aesthetic improvement of the nose, and complained of mild breathing problems and occasional pain at the nasal dorsum (Figure 37-7, *A* and *B*). Examination revealed a mentally stable, intelligent patient who was unhappy about the results of an operation that she had hoped would improve her facial appearance.

During nasal palpation, a depression of the bony and cartilaginous framework of the dorsum could be detected. The skin coverage was moderately thick, and the supratip swelling corresponded, not to the prominence of the anterior edge of the septum but to the remaining soft tissues. The flatness of the nose was quite evident, and the loss of continuity of the line extending from the brows to the nasal tip was evident. Intranasal examination revealed no septal deviation. The collapse of the central portion of the roof could be confirmed, and some dryness and crusting was found in the area where the mucosa directly adhered to the skin. The skeletal framework of the septum was intact.

It was decided to augment the dorsum with a multilayered septal cartilaginous graft (Figure 37-7, *E*) to improve the contour, to provide the desired continuity with the forehead, and to separate the skin from the mucosa, thus correcting the open roof and protecting the nasal lining from changes of temperature. It was also decided to use a small cartilaginous graft into the columella to provide support to the tip and to open slightly the nasolabial angle without overexposing the nares.

Transcartilaginous incisions were made on both sides of the nose and were extended to the right side to the base of the columella. The skin was separated from the mucosa at the dorsum, and a narrow tunnel was made to the glabella. Two millimeters of the cephalic edge of the lower laterals were removed on both sides, and the cartilages were dissected free from the skin to allow better skin redraping. A graft, 2 cm wide and 4½ cm long was obtained from the septum, preserving the integrity of the support anteriorly and superiorly. Three strips of cartilage 5 mm wide were carved, cut, and sutured together to form a piece that was flat on one side and convex on the other that would fill the concavity of the dorsum. The graft was inserted and fixed with a monofilm nylon suture passed through the skin at the level of the glabella. The suture was fixed to the skin by Micropore tape. A triangular piece of cartilage 5 mm wide at its base and 2 cm long was introduced into the columella after separating the medial crura from each other and from the nasal spine. The wide part of the graft was left in front of the nasal spine and was fixed with a U suture. No osteotomies were performed.

Postoperative results were excellent. The dorsal contour was restored, and the symptoms related to the open roof disappeared entirely. The refinement of the lower lateral cartilages and the addition of the cartilaginous graft to the columella added an extra element of angularity. Figure 37-7, *C* and *D*, shows the postoperative result 1 year after secondary rhinoplasty. Contour, angularity, and continuity of the line from the brow to the tip of the nose should be noted.

Summary

This was a relatively easy correction because there was enough tissue on the septum to replace the amputated dorsum. In addition, the moderate thickness of the skin allowed a certain degree of angularity. Symptomatic relief was obtained because the open roof was closed, separating the skin from the nasal mucosa.

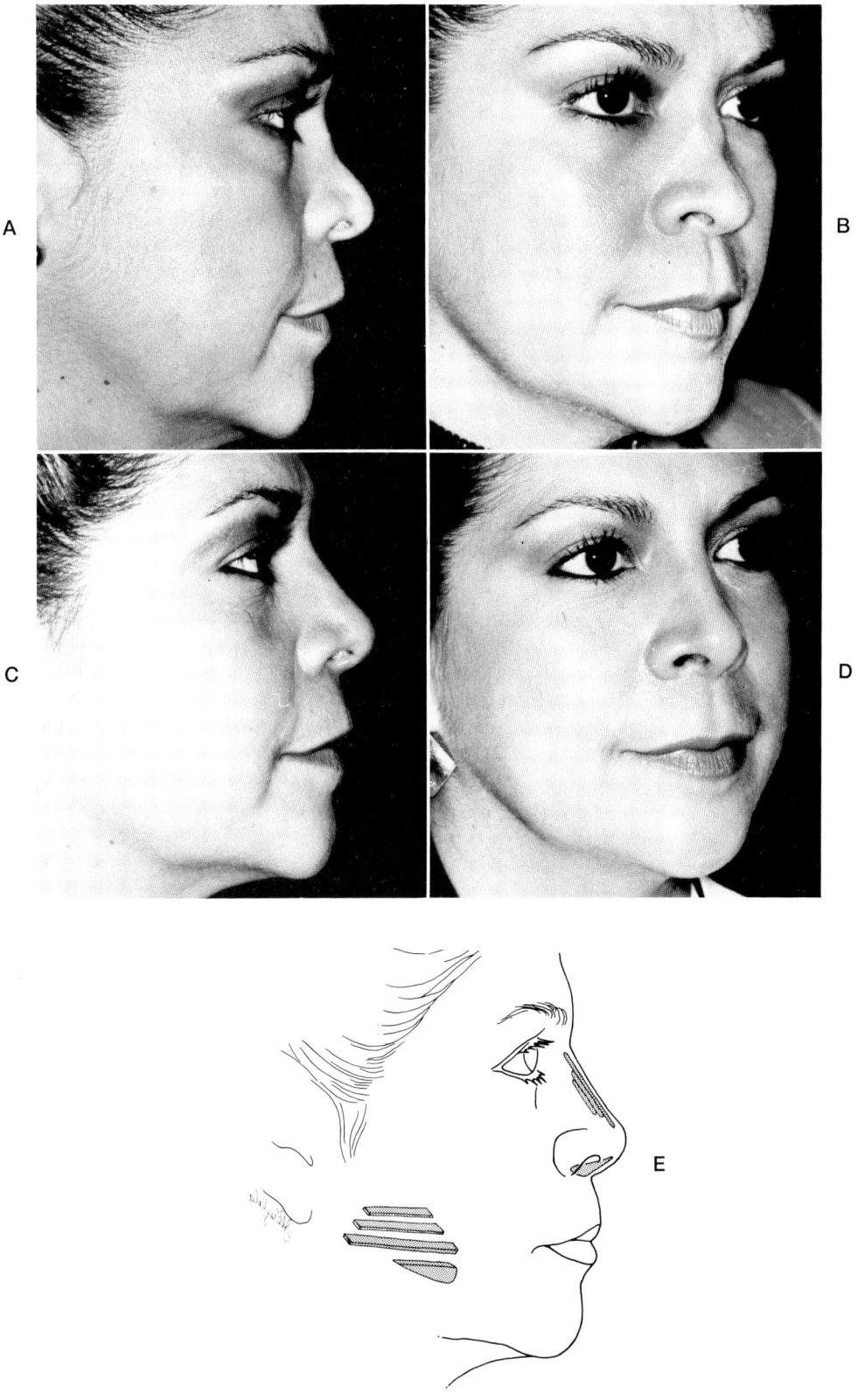

Figure 37-7

Case 2

A 24-year-old female with moderately thick skin had had a rhinoplasty performed 2 years earlier. She disliked having a bulbous tip and a slightly depressed dorsum (Figure 37-8, *A* and *B*). During the examination some irregularities of the dorsum, which were not visible because of the thickness of the skin, were detected, with a minor depression at the center obviously resulting from an excessive resection of the hump. At the nasal tip two depressions were evident on each side of the midline, giving an impression of pinching and emphasizing the roundness of the nasal tip. The slightly hanging effect of the columella was interpreted as a combination of lack of skeletal support and retraction of the scar from the previous operation.

It was decided to use septal cartilaginous grafts to reconstruct the dorsum and to improve the nasolabial angle. Other cartilaginous grafts to give angularity to the tip and to fill the depressions of the alae were also considered (Figure 37-8, *E*).

A cartilaginous graft 4 cm long and 1½ cm wide was obtained fron the septum, thus preserving the integrity of a supporting framework. Through a small intercartilaginous incision a narrow tunnel approximately 6 to 7 mm wide was dissected subperiostially along the nasal dorsum, and a strip of cartilage 5 mm wide and approximately 4 cm long was introduced and left without fixation. Moderate crushing of that cartilage was done to avoid sharp edges. The intercartilaginous incision on the right side was extended downward to the columella, the medial crura were separated from the nasal spine, and a triangular piece of cartilage 7 mm wide and 8 mm long was introduced, with the base located directly in front of the nasal spine and fixed with a through-and-through suture.

A small rim incision was made on the right side at the level of the dome, and a pocket was dissected between the anterior aspect of the lower-lateral cartilages and the skin just large enough to accept a shield-shaped septal cartilage graft as described by Sheen.[7] Finally, through a small stab mucosal incision in each nostril, a small pocket that corresponded to the depressed areas on the alar rims was dissected, and small pieces of crushed cartilage were introduced to fill the defect. The postoperative photographs taken 6 months postoperatively show a satisfactory result (Figure 37-8, *C* and *D*). Continuity of the lines descending from the brows into each side of the nasal dorsum was obtained, and a pleasant carving effect with well-defined angles was obtained at the nasal tip and columella through the use of the cartilage grafts.

Summary

A moderately thick nose clearly illustrates how the reconstruction of the skeletal framework, providing support to the thick skin, enhances angularity and produces a very pleasant effect. This result could not have been achieved by shifting the available tissues of the nose, and there was even less possibility of success by further reducing its size.

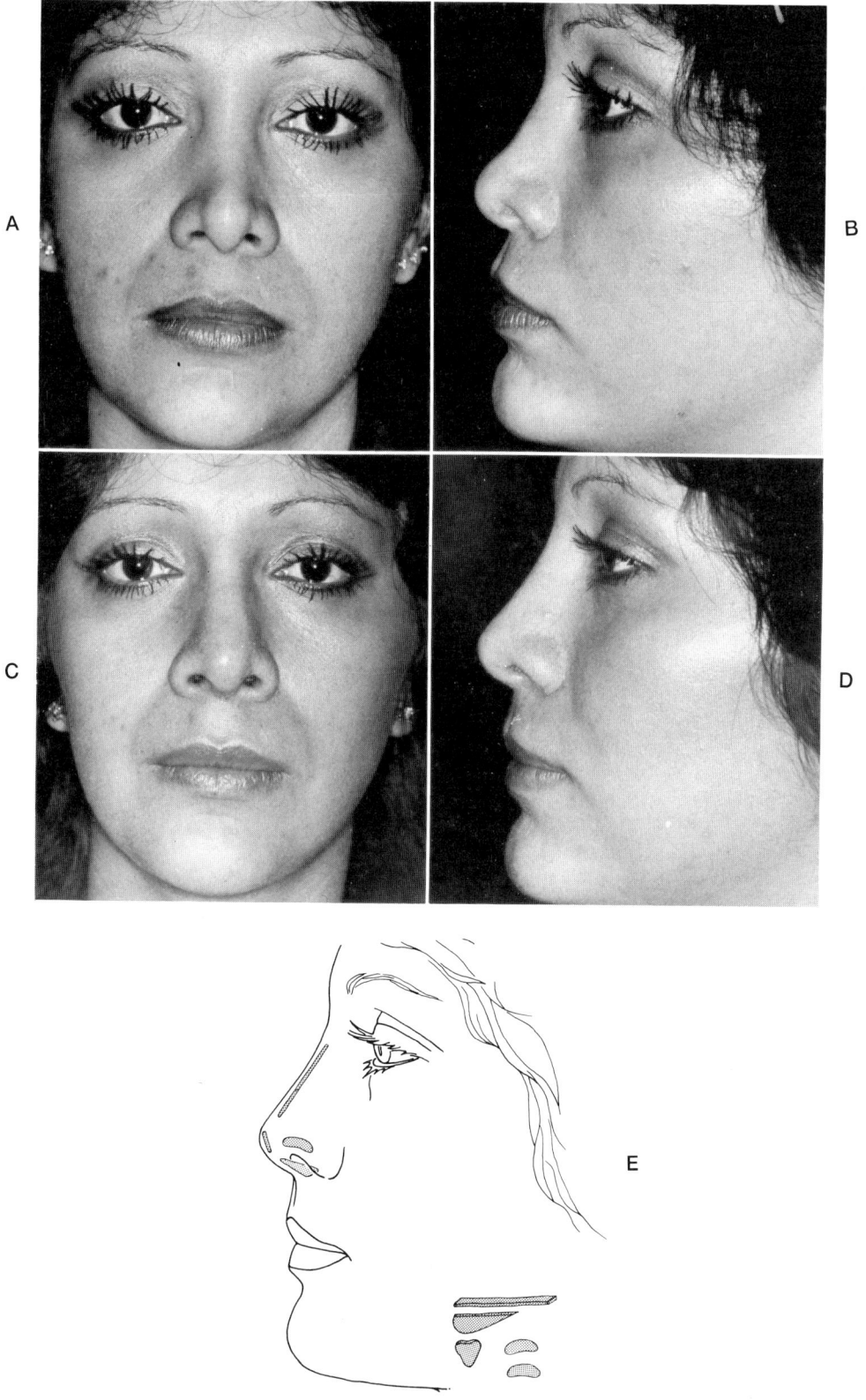

Figure 37-8

Case 3

A 35-year-old female had a rhinoplasty performed 3 years earlier, and she requested correction of the depressed nasal dorsum and the bulbous tip. Before her first operation she had breathing problems, which were apparently corrected by a septoplasty. During examination it was evident that an extremely large amount of nasal pyramid had been removed, including the caudal edge of the septum and the medial edge of the upper-lateral cartilages. The bulbous effect of the tip resulted more from lack of support than from excess of lower-lateral cartilages, although the thickness of the skin in the lower half of the nose contributed to the bulbousness of the tip (Figure 37-9, A and B).

Considering that the septum was not available because of the previous septoplasty and that a considerable amount of tissue was needed to rebuild the dorsum, we decided to use a bone graft taken from the rib. We believe that even if the septum were available, the rib should be used to replace missing skeleton (Figure 37-9, E).

With the patient under general anesthesia, a 4 cm incision was made in the left submammary fold. A portion of the seventh rib approximately 8 cm long was obtained, preserving the periosteum on the superficial side. A small piece of rib cartilage was also removed for use in the nasal tip and the columella. A small intercartilaginous incision was made on each side of the nose, and a tunnel was dissected along the dorsum to the level of the frontonasal angle. The rib was split and shaped using a Tessier crusher to produce the longitudinal contour, and transverse pressure using a Kelly forceps was used to produce a smooth convex cortical side with its periosteum intact. The graft was introduced into the tunnel with the cancellous surface in contact with the nasal skeleton. A small notch had previously been made at the level of the frontonasal suture to fix the graft and to prevent it from sliding upward. No fractures were made on the nasal skeleton, and the nasal tip and columella were left untouched.

The contour of the dorsum was restored as shown in the photographs taken 1 year after the operation (Figure 37-9, C and D). The bulbousness of the tip disappeared when the balance between the dorsum and the tip was restored. There was no evidence of resorption of the bone graft.

Summary

This case demonstrates how reconstruction of the supporting skeletal framework markedly improves the shape of thick-skinned noses. This result can be systematically obtained if a sufficient amount of tissue is transplanted. Our impression is that an adequate correction could not be obtained without strong support and that any attempt to remove more tissue from the lower half of the nose would produce a disastrous effect.

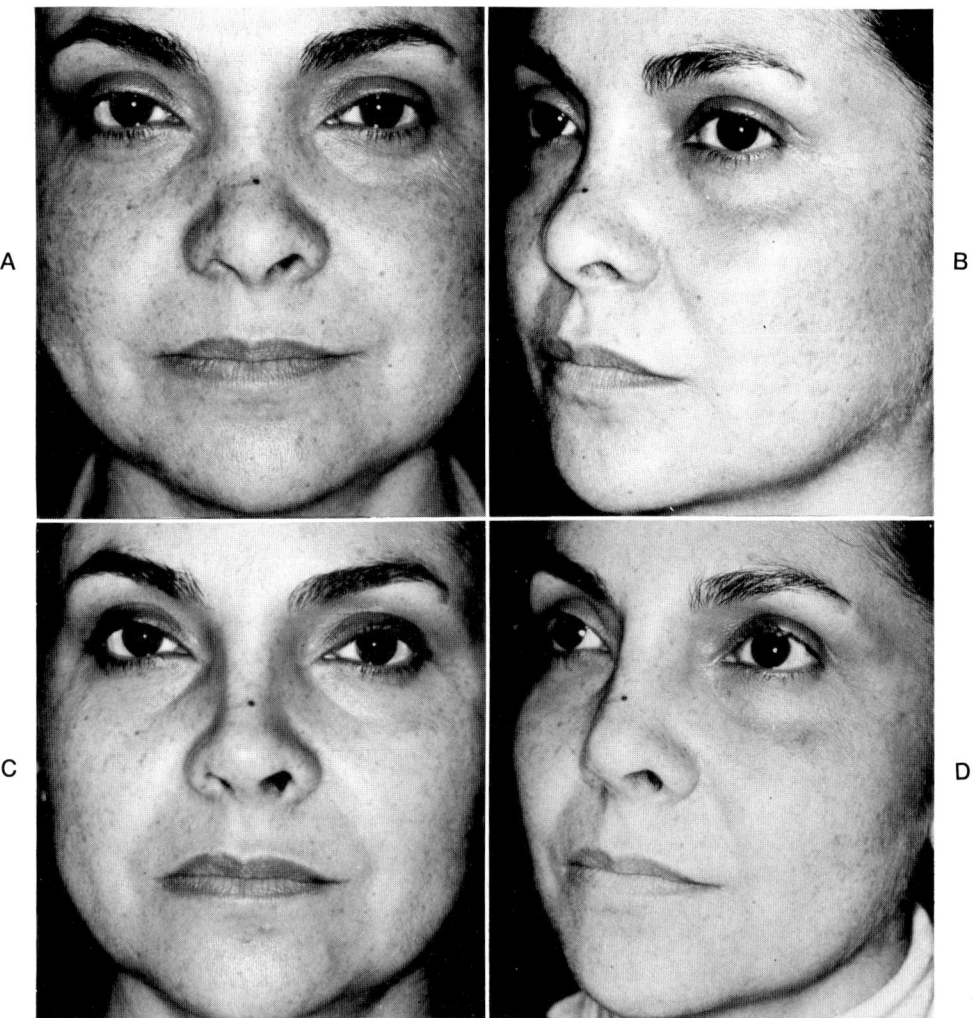

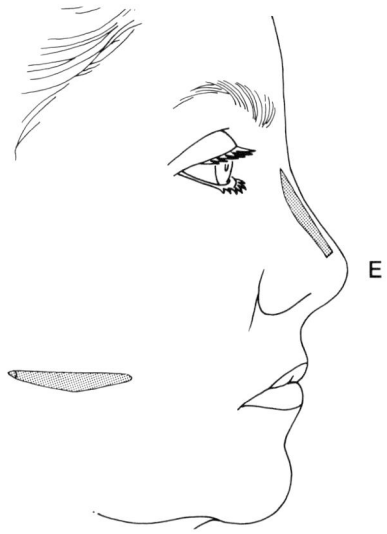

Figure 37-9

Case 4

A 39-year-old female requested nasal correction after three previous rhinoplasties had been performed in the preceding 5 years. Her chief complaints were the lack of projection of the tip, the presence of scars and depressions on the skin of the lower half of the nose, and the destruction of the nostrils, causing breathing difficulties.

Examination revealed that she had an extremely thick nose with little subcutaneous fat but a great number of sebaceous glands. The skin had depressions on both sides of the midline above the alae (Figure 37-10, A-C) and firmly adhered to the underlying tissues. The nasal spine was not palpable, and the lower third of the nose had no skeletal support. The septum had probably been removed during one of the previous procedures. The intranasal examination revealed bilateral circular contractions limiting the airway (see Figure 37-10, B).

Because the amount of fibrous tissue, combined with the lack of elasticity of the skin and mucosa, would require a strong support structure, it was decided to use a rib bone graft for the dorsum and rib cartilage for the tip. Regardless of the fact that not enough material was available at the septum for a graft, we believed that stronger support was needed and could be provided only by using a strut of costal cartilage to improve projection (Figure 37-10, E). We also believed that the use of conchal ear cartilage was not indicated because it lacked the strength to support the tip.

Through a small submammary incision a bone rib graft approximately 8 cm long was obtained from the seventh rib in continuity with a piece of costal cartilage approximately 5 cm long. The rib was split manually with a chisel, preserving the periosteum on the cortical convex part of the graft, which was shaped by means of a Tessier crusher. Through an intercartilaginous small incision a tunnel was made along the nasal dorsum by subperiostial dissection, bony irregularities were shaved with a fine rasp, and the thin bone graft was introduced over the dorsum from the glabella down to the limit of the lower-lateral cartilages. Through an extension of the intercartilaginous incision to the columella the nasal tip was widely undermined down to the level of the nasal spine. A triangular piece of cartilage 3 mm thick and 3 cm long was carved and introduced in the pocket; its wider lower end, which measured approximately 12 mm in width, was set in contact with the nasal spine, and its superior wider end, which measured approximately 5 mm, rested right under the skin of the nasal tip.

Through a small stab incision pieces of cartilage were subcutaneously introduced to fill the depressions of the alae, and Z-plasties were performed on the nasal mucosa to correct the scar contracture on both sides.

Postoperative results were acceptable, considering the severity of the deformity. The contour of the nose was improved, and the nasal tip projection was augmented. Skin depressions were almost eliminated through the use of cartilage grafts (Figure 37-10, D-F).

Summary

This case is typical of the problems occurring in patients with thick skin when an attempt is made to decrease its thickness by removing subcutaneous tissue and supporting structures. In our opinion no procedure other than replacing the supporting structures and filling the depressions with cartilage can be of any help to these patients.

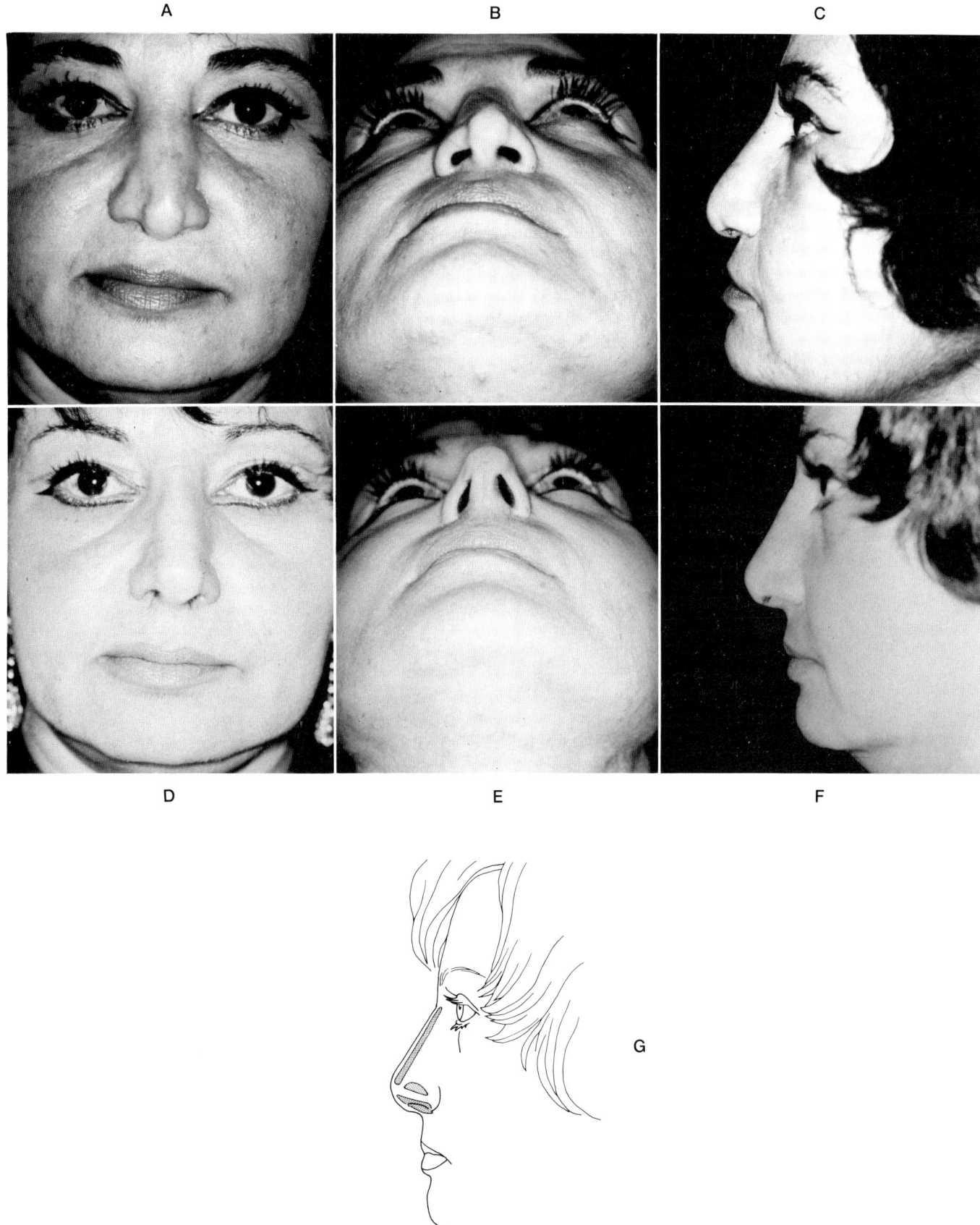

Figure 37-10

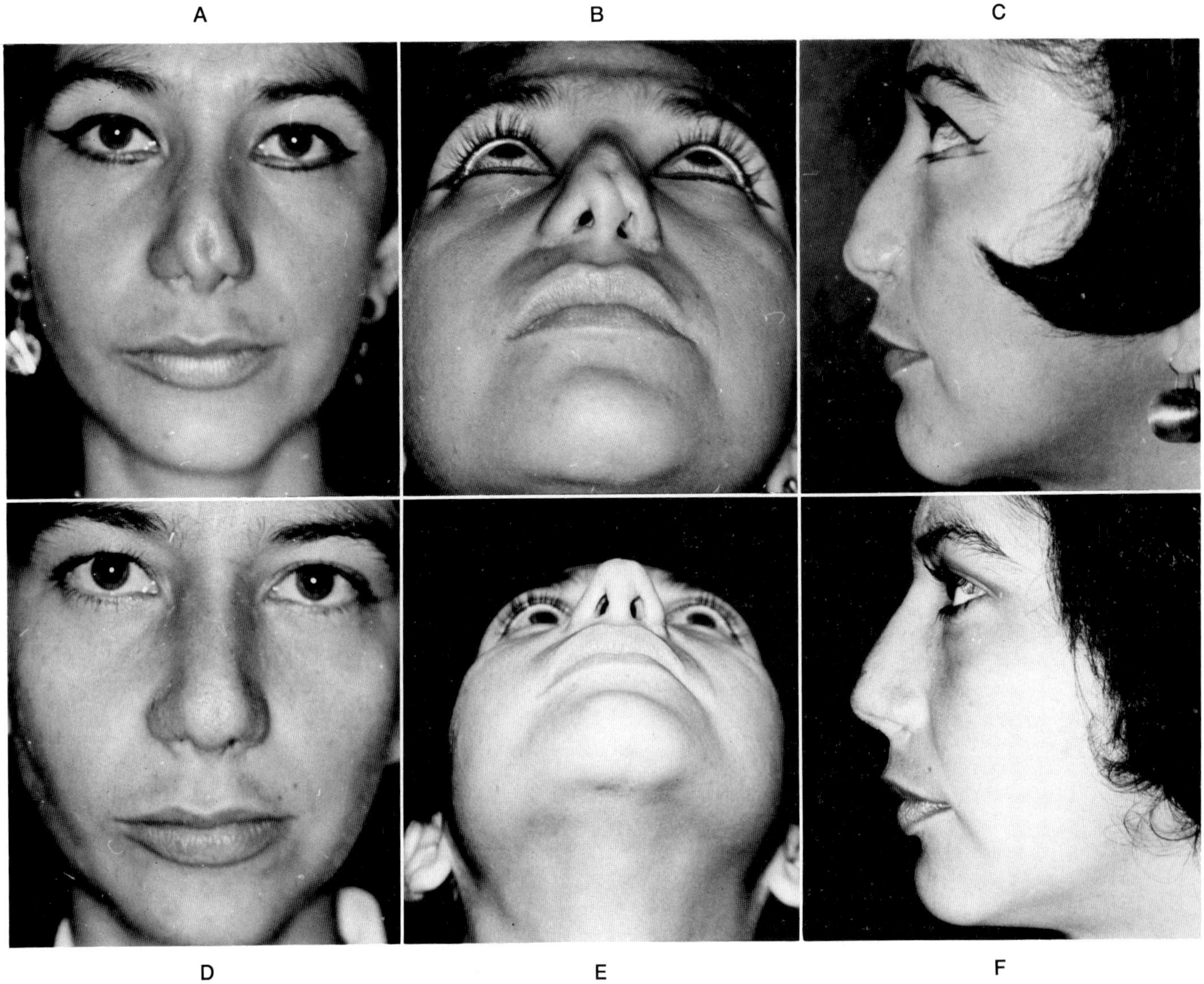

A   B   C

D   E   F

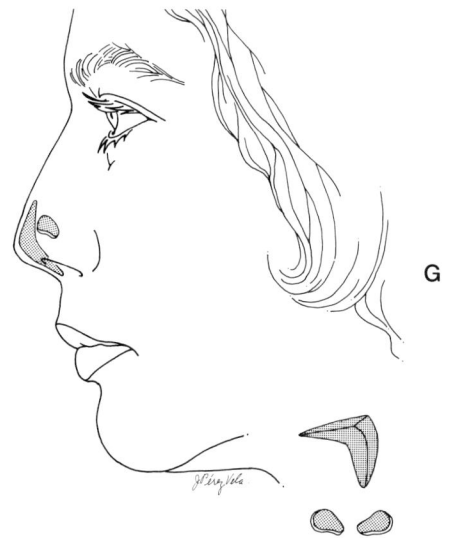

G

Figure 37-11

Case 5

A 21-year-old female requested improvement of a nasal deformity after three previous rhinoplasties. The last two procedures involved the insertion of Silastic implants that extruded on both occasions (Figure 37-11, *A-C*).

When the patient was examined, a depression was noted in the nasal tip with adherence of the skin to the deep structures at the site of extrusion of the Silastic implants. The nasal pyramid was intact. The loss of tip projection was the result of resection of the caudal septum along with the upper and lower cartilages in addition to intranasal scar contracture. The scar tissue around the alar rim caused nearly total vestibular stenosis.

Considering the severe nasal retraction and the need for strong structural support, we decided to reconstruct the nasal tip through a costal graft and to improve the airway stenosis with Z-plasties and composite skin and cartilaginous conchal grafts in the nasal vestibule (Figure 37-11, *G*).

With the patient under general anesthesia, a piece of cartilage was taken from the rib through a small submammary incision. A composite skin and cartilaginous graft was obtained from the concha. The circular scars around the nostrils were opened, and local flaps were elevated to form multiple Z-plasties. The adhesions between the septum and the lateral nasal walls behind the alar rim were freed. The skin around the columella was undermined, and an L-shaped piece of cartilage was introduced with the long segment into the columella and with the short one along the dorsum to create the anterior projection of the tip. The Z-plasties were closed with fine absorbable material, and the composite grafts were sutured to the recipient areas along the internal valve of the nose.

The aesthetic postoperative results for the nose have been satisfactory. The anterior projection of the tip is satisfactory, and the skin depressions have disappeared. There is some improvement of the stenosis of the nostrils, but this result is far from the ideal (Figure 37-11, *D-F*).

REFERENCES

1. Dingman, R.: Use of composite ear graft in correction of the short nose, Plast. Reconstr. Surg. **43**:117, 1969.
2. Ortiz Monasterio, F., López-Mas, J., and Araico, J.: Rhinoplasty in the thick skinned nose, Br. J. Plast. Surg. **27**:19, 1974.
3. Ortiz Monasterio, F., and Olmedo, A.: Secondary rhinoplasty principles of reoperation. Paper presented at Transactions of Seventh International Congress of Plastic and Reconstructive Surgeons, Rio de Janiero, Brazil, 1979.
4. Ortiz Monasterio, F., Olmedo, A., and Ortiz Oscoy, L.: The use of cartilage grafts in primary aesthetic rhinoplasty, Plast. Reconstr. Surg. **67**:597, 1981.
5. Peer, L.A.: The fate of living and dead cartilage transplanted in humans, Surg. Gynecol. Obstet. **68**:603, 1939.
6. Peer, L.A.: Fate of autogenous septal cartilage after transplantation in human tissues, Arch. Otolaryngol. **34**:697, 1941.
7. Sheen, J.H.: Achieving more nasal tip projection by use of small autogenous vomer or septal cartilage graft, Plast. Reconstr. Surg. **56**:211, 1975.

PART
XII

SECONDARY RHINOPLASTY AND SUPRATIP DEFORMITIES

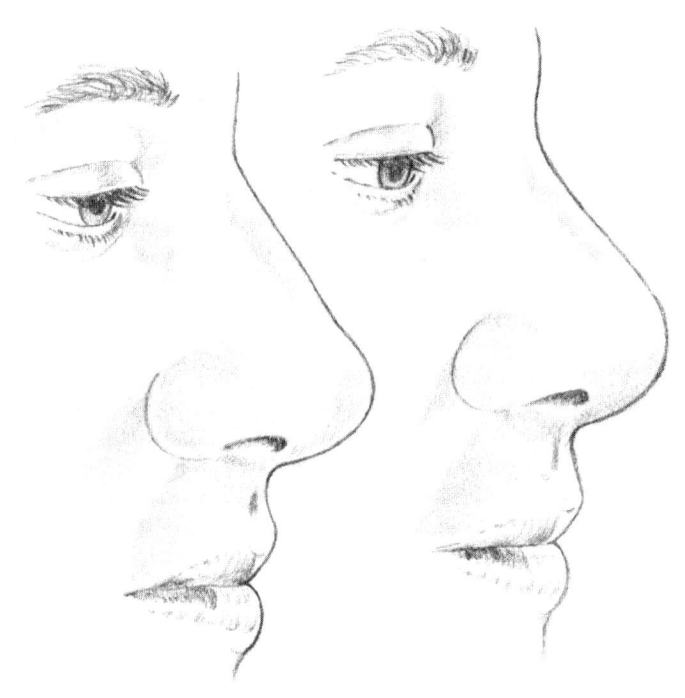

38

The Nasal Cripple

Harvey Caplan

The term *nasal cripple* refers to patients who suffer the stigma of rhinoplasty complications, which are often the result of poor surgical treatment. Some of the problems faced by these patients are as follows:

Tip and columella

Retracted columella
Loss of vestibular skin
Excessive or uneven removal of alar cartilage
Rim incision contractures
Skin contracture and displaced alar crura
Spicules of cartilage, leading to irregularities and bosses

Cartilaginous vault

Inadequate lowering of the ventral septum, leading to postoperative dorsal hump
Avulsed, detached, and denuded upper-lateral cartilages, producing external deformities, indentations, pitting, and intranasal synechiae
Collapsed internal nasal valve
Septal perforations
Upper-lateral cartilage sutured over the cartilaginous dorsum, leading to a secondary cartilaginous hump of the lower dorsum

Bony vault

Excessive bony hump removal with saddling
Open roof with adherent skin
Incomplete lateral osteotomies
Wrongly positioned lateral osteotomies—stairstep deformity
Depressed, irregular, or extracted nasal bones

Nasal skin

Perforations
Shallow undermining with adherence to bone and cartilage
Excessive thinning
Poorly placed wires
Keloids and unsightly external scars

Some of these problems, with appropriate illustrations, will be discussed.

Tip and columella

Since the tip mostly consists of a cartilaginous framework with some subcutaneous fat and a covering of skin and vestibular lining, all manner of deformities can result from surgical invasion of these tissues. Excessive excision is the most common culprit, along with asymmetrical and irregular cartilage excision. Overshortening of the septum can cause a retracted columella, and direct surgical excision of the medial crura can cause scar contractures of the columella.

Unadvisable resection of the vestibular lining, if not carefully repaired, results in various deformities—notably contractures of the tip with depressions, buckling of the alar cartilage, and related deformities.

Cartilage "points" or bossing of the tip may result from transsecting the cartilage through its vertical width or from resection of the lining with scar contracture or both.

Cartilaginous vault

In the area of the cartilaginous vault, inadequate lowering of the dorsal septum can cause a postoperative hump. The skin in the immediate postoperative supratip area is thickest along the nasal dorsum. It is wise to consider this anatomical fact when lowering the septal cartilage and perhaps lower it a bit more to allow for the dipping effect.

A detached and denuded upper-lateral cartilage and its lining can produce external deformities, indentations, pitting, and intranasal synechiae and webs. Septal perforations can also be an unpleasant complication, often resulting from surgical lacerations of the opposing septal flaps or from avascular necrosis.

Bony vault

Step deformities or depressed, irregular, or extracted nasal bones can occur if the surgeon has been overly zealous with rasping the nasal bone. If the pyramid is not fixed, it may suddenly be at the nasal vestibule.

Nasal skin

The nasal skin can also be involved in complications. If it is perforated, a scar, which often is depressed, will result. Shallow undermining causes extra bleeding and excessive thinning of the skin layer. Poorly placed incisions produce irregularities, keloids, and external incisions.

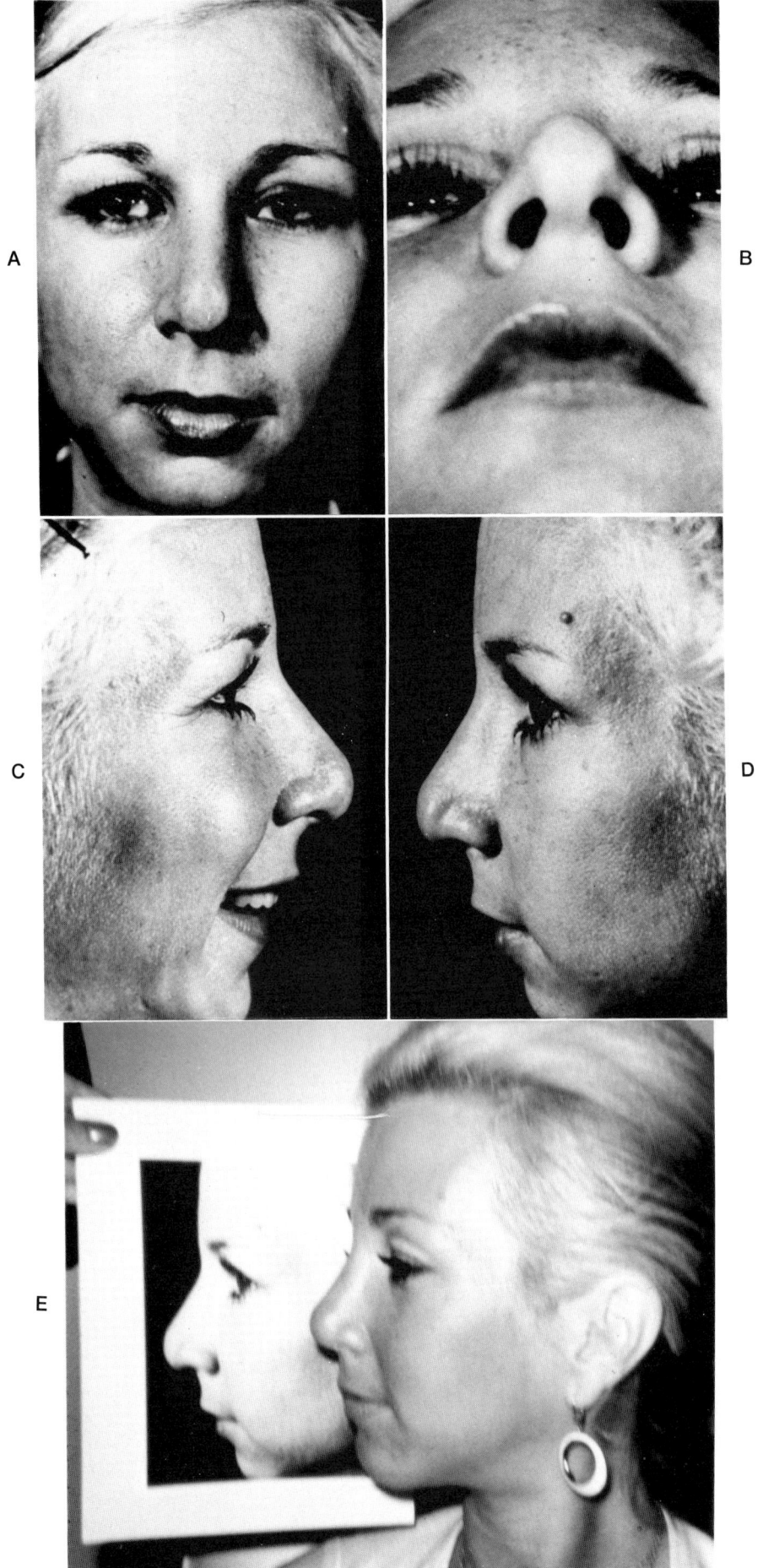

Figure 38-1

CASE REPORTS

Case 1

This patient (Figure 38-1, *A-D*) shows the stigmata of a poor rhinoplasty. The columella is retracted, and an inordinate removal of alar cartilage has produced the chopped-off (surgical amputee) nasal appearance. A collapsed nasal valve also is present. Excessive hump removal had been performed, the skin was adherent, and incomplete lateral osteotomies had caused an open roof. The patient also had a receding chin. Whenever it is desirable to expand the original surgery to include chin implants or other procedures, the surgeon should do so. When indicated, mentoplasty can be added to revisional rhinoplasty to enhance further the patient's self-image. Figure 38-1, *E* shows the result after secondary rhinoplasty and chin augmentation.

Case 2

This patient (Figure 38-2, *A-C*) shows the classic post rhinoplasty "disaster." The defects include an open roof, excessive hump removal, large flaring nostrils, a residual bulbous tip, and a hanging columella. The procedure used involved freeing the nasal skin, performing lateral osteotomies, obtaining cartilage from the septum, and using it as a dorsal graft. A marginal incision was used, and there was, fortunately, enough alar cartilage present to permit carving, thus decreasing the bulbousness of the tip. In addition, some of the alar cartilage was used as a filler to decrease the cleft in the intramedial crurae space; alar wedge resections were also performed. The postoperative result is shown in Figure 38-2, *D-F.*

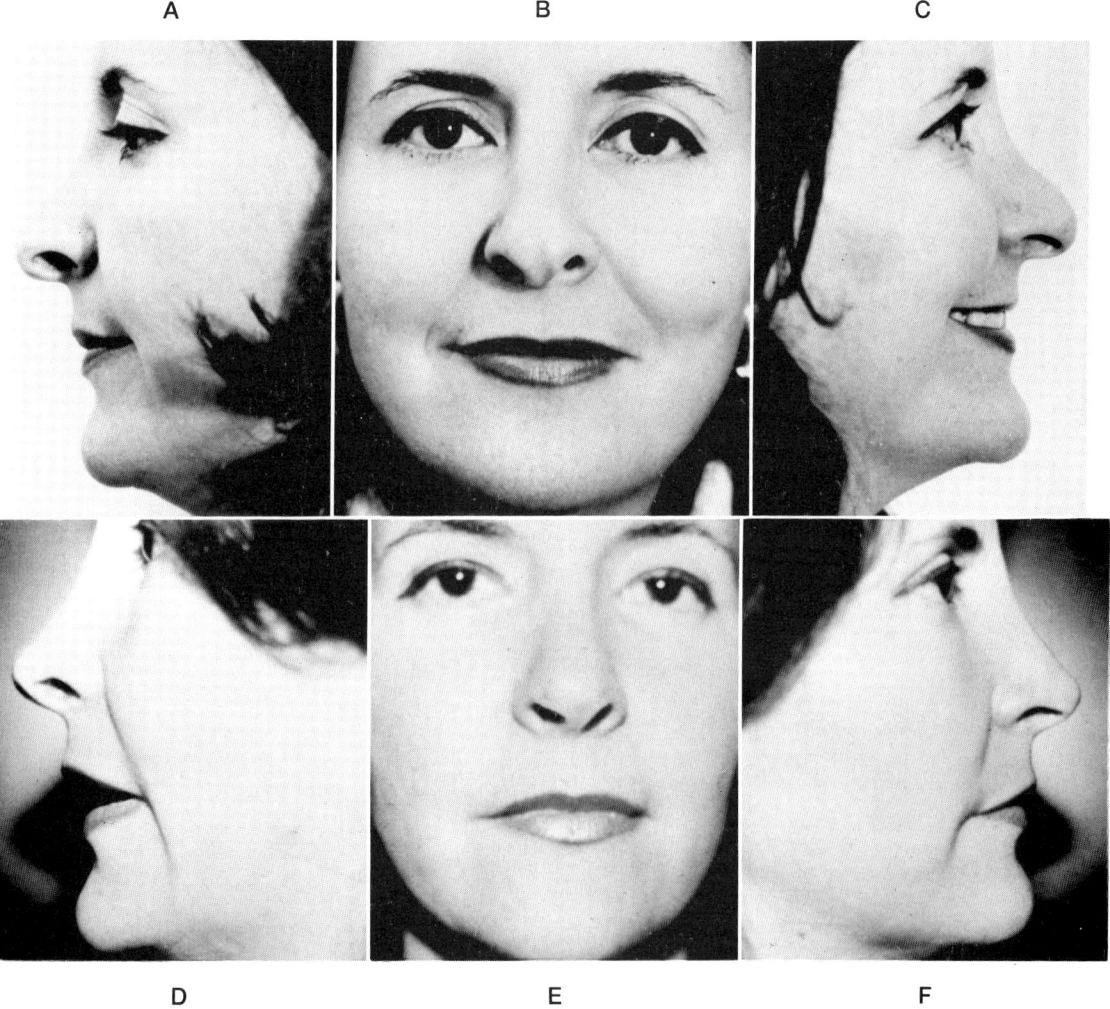

A   B   C

D   E   F

Figure 38-2

Case 3

This patient (Figure 38-3, *A-D*) also shows the surgical stigmata of poor rhinoplasty—excessiv hump removal, an open roof, a retracted columella, and excessive scarring in the supratip area. These defects were corrected. Use of a cartilaginous strut was necessary in the tip. The vestibular skin was cut, and the medial crura were approximated to give more projection. One can be fooled into thinking that the projection in the supratip area is only dorsal cartilage. In most cases removal of excessive scar tissue is required. The open roof was closed through medial and lateral osteotomies and the insertion of residual cartilage as a dorsal filler. A good postoperative result was obtained. The postoperative result is shown in Figure 38-3, *E* and *F*.

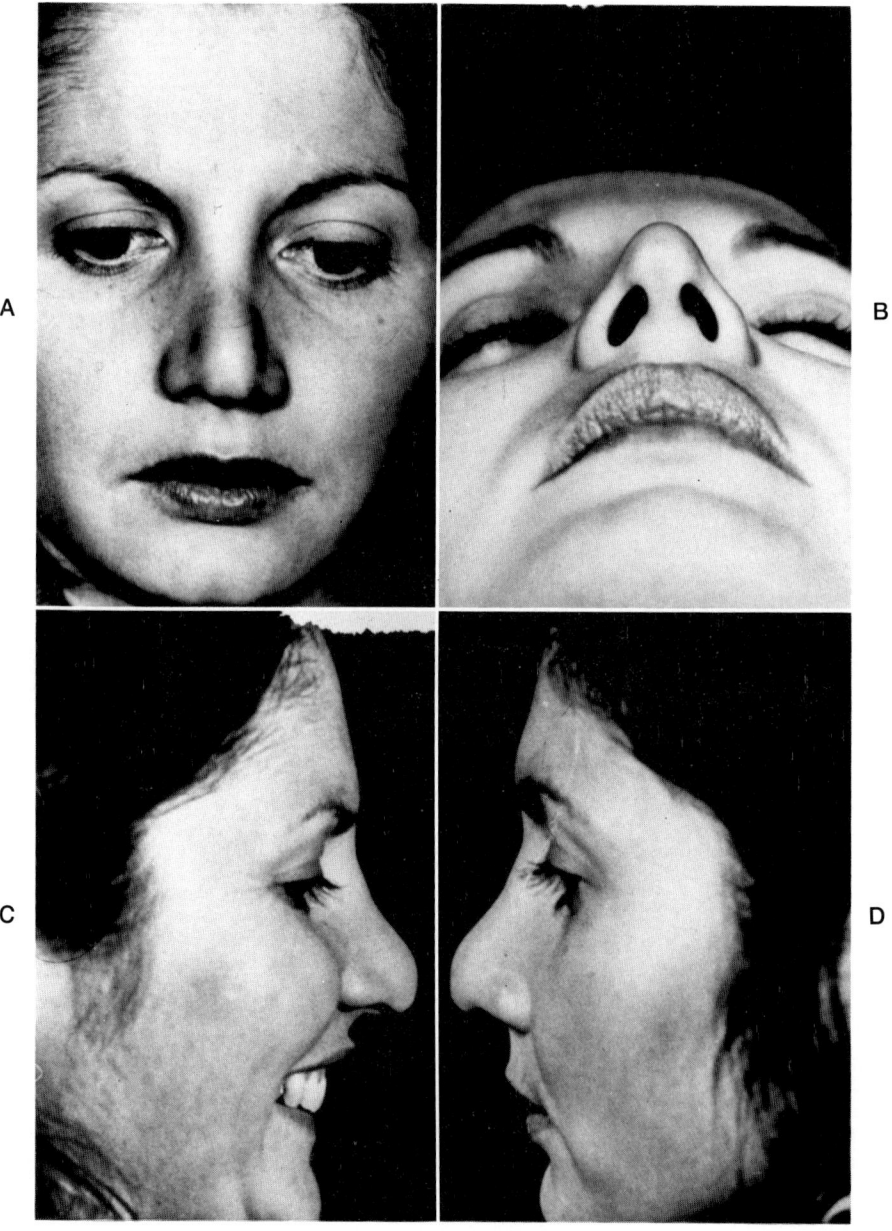

Figure 38-3

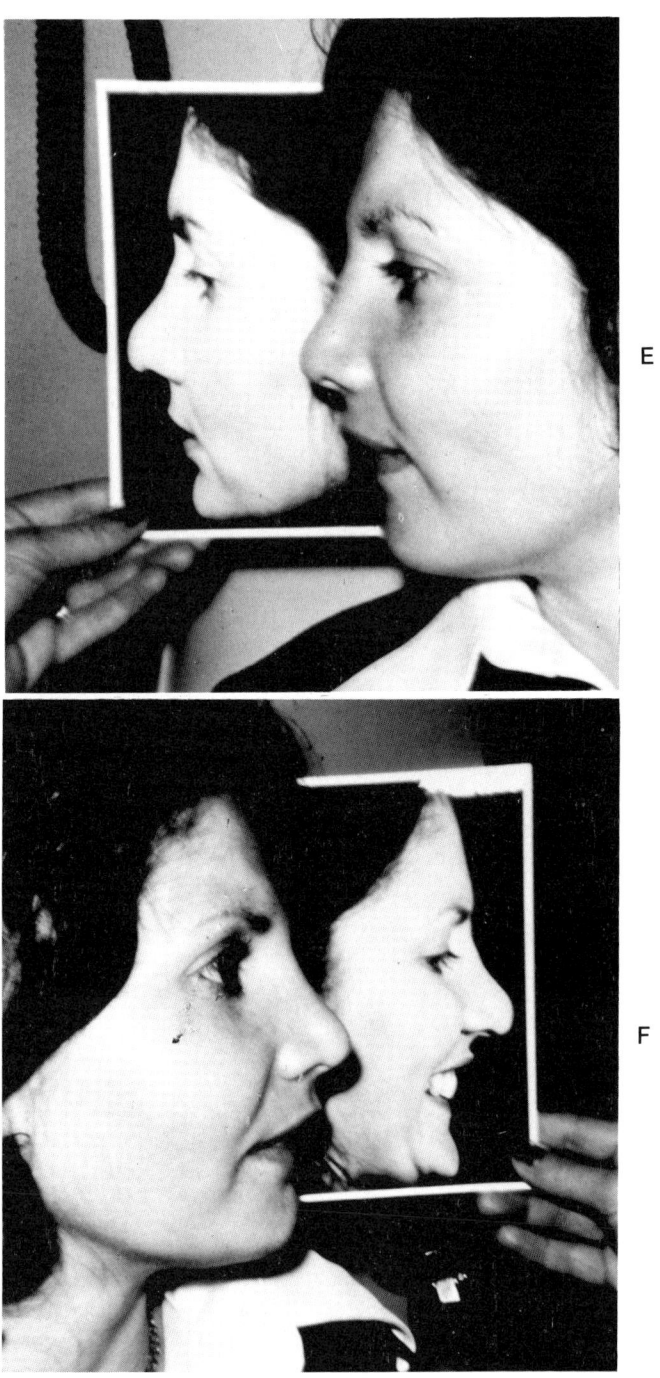

E

F

Figure 38-3, cont'd

39

Secondary and Revisional Tip and Supratip Deformities

Walter Berman

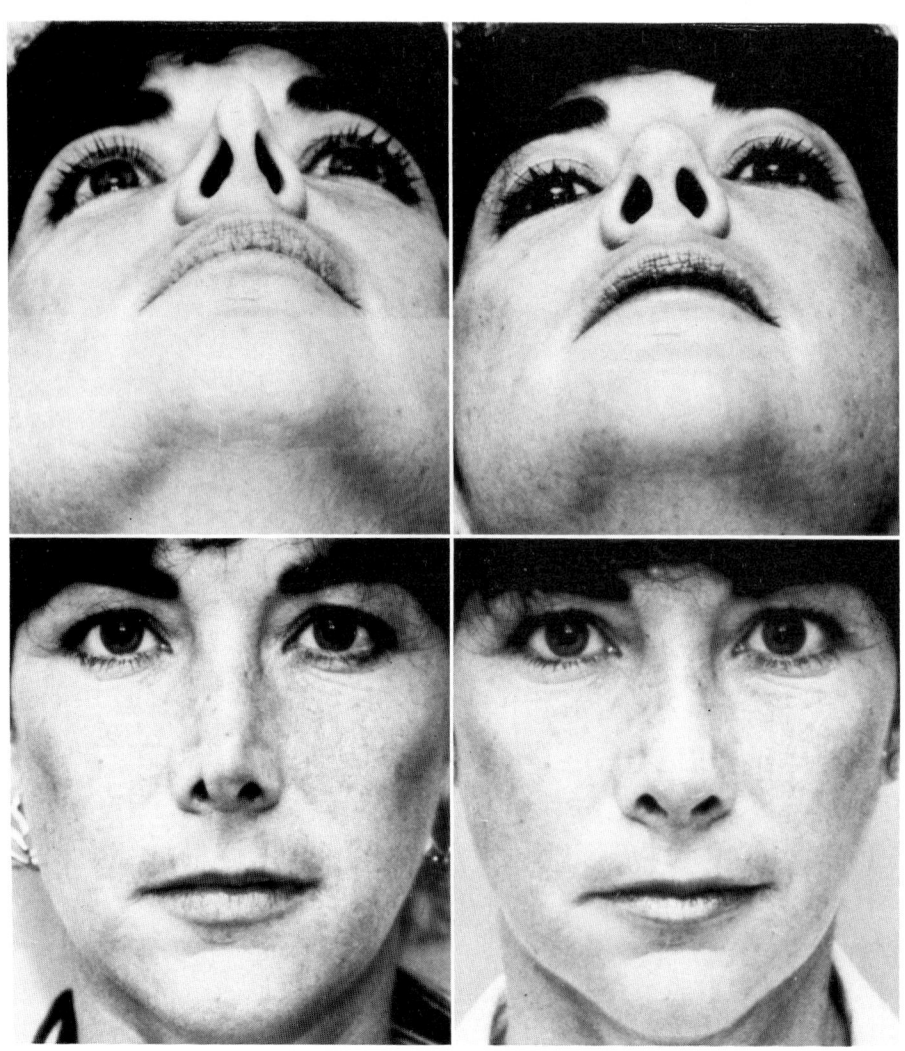

Figure 39-1

A 41-year-old Caucasian female who had a rhinoplasty 22 years earlier was initially seen with a marked loss of supporting lower- and upper-lateral nasal cartilages bilaterally (Figure 39-1, *A-D*). This lack of support had also caused a framework collapse in the valvular areas bilaterally. She experienced great difficulty with nasal respiration, especially inspiration. Excessive tip projection was also present.

Evaluation

This patient needs replacement of tissue deficits, primarily repositioning of existing lower nasal cartilages and insertion of supramid mesh implants. Because of excessive tip projection and its subsequent decrease during reconstruction, adding epithelial lining would not be necessary. The layers of supramid mesh will act as a baton in a sail. They firm the collapsed area without adding excessive bulk, and they cannot be absorbed. This mesh also decreases the "pinch nose" effect and compensates for the valvular collapse on inspiration.

Surgical procedure

Intercartilaginous incisions are placed medially along the inferior (caudal) aspect of the nasal septum to the anterior nasal spine. Marginal rim incisions along the lower-lateral cartilages are then connected to the inter-cartilaginous incisions. During this step the dissection frees the domes and a large part of the adjoining medial and lateral cartilages.

The delivery of the bipedicle chondroplastic flap is facilitated through the use of a single skin hook projecting from the dome inferiorly, and the delivery of the lower-cartilage complex is facilitated through the use of Fomon scissors. With the dome and adjacent cartilages in place, any irregularities are carefully trimmed.

A portion of the medial crural cartilage equal to the proposed tip projection decrease is excised. No vestibular skin is taken. This procedure rotates the old dome into the new medial crural cartilage and creates a new dome from the former lower-lateral cartilage (Figure 39-2).

A small subcutaneous pocket is developed over the internal valve area, and multiple layers of supramid mesh are inserted.

Summary

This case was the product of the performance of an overly zealous rhinoplasty, an occurrence that was all too common several years ago. Cartilaginous and internal valve support deficits were present, along with an external nasal deformity. Surgery consisted of delivery of the lower nasal cartilages, medial rotation of the lateral crus, removal of a segment of medical crus to decrease tip projection. Supramid mesh layers were placed in pockets over the internal valve areas that had collapsed, causing greater stability during inspiration.

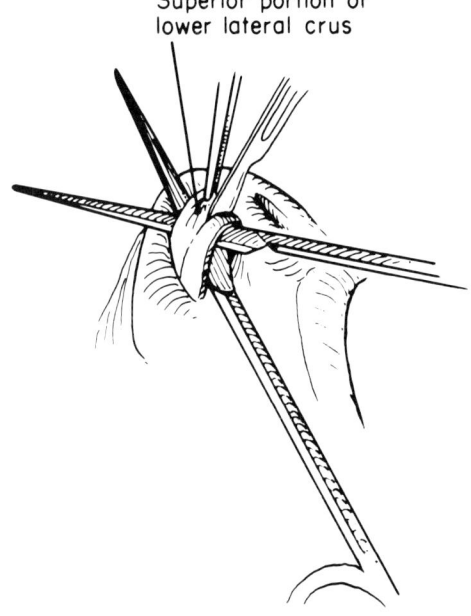

Superior portion of lower lateral crus

Figure 39-2
(From Berman, W.E.: Rhinoplasty, ed. 2, Washington, D.C., 1984, American Academy of Otolaryngology—Head and Neck Surgery Foundation, Inc.)

40

Supratip Deformities

Jack Sheen

Supratip deformity is one of the most common causes of patient dissatisfaction after rhinoplasty. The problem of supratip deformity has plagued plastic surgeons since the time of Joseph. Much has been written about the cause and treatment of this problem. In my experience, much of the information has been incorrect. A supratip deformity is a postsurgical fullness or convexity of the dorsal line just above the nasal tip. This is not the transient supratip swelling that frequently occurs during the immediate postoperative period, but it is a supratip fullness that is definite and persistent. I would like to present a different opinion regarding the cause and treatment of postsurgical supratip prominence.

The Unfavorable Result in Plastic Surgery, edited by Goldwyn,[2] summarized the information available at that time. He listed the common causes of supratip deformity as follows: insufficient lowering or trimming of the dorsal septal border contours, insufficient trimming of the dorsal borders of the upper lateral cartilages, uncontrollable and frequently inherent or inherited thickness of the skin and subcutaneous tissues, a short columella, excessive excision of the domes of the alar cartilages, and inadequate trimming of redundant dorsal septal mucosa.

Some surgeons advocate overreduction of the anterior edge of the septum in patients thought likely to form supratip fullness. Safian wrote of the potential dangers of overlapping side walls.[6] Rees suggested overformation of scar tissue from granulation tissue in the area as a possible cause of supratip deformity.[3] Denecke and Meyer discovered that a hump is unavoidably formed by fibrous tissue as a result of the lateral compression of the dressing if a straight dorsum is left just above the tip at the end of the operation.[1]

Most contemporary writers teach that the principal causative factor of supratip deformity is excessive skeletal tissue in the area of the supratip. Although I do not discount the several causes listed by Rogers[4,5] and others, my experience has shown that they apply only in a minority of cases.

It is my contention that the most common cause of supratip deformity is overreduction of skeletal parts, principally the dorsal edge of the septum. When the dorsal structure is reduced beyond the soft tissue's ability to contrast or drape over the reduced framework, a poorly defined thickened supratip will result. The essence of the problem is the inability of tissues to contract to an overreduced skeleton. Since the generally accepted cause is excessive tissues, it is logical that the prevailing recommended treatments for supratip deformity include a resection of scar tissues, which is also called a thinning procedure or reduction of the dorsal septum. Unfortunately, except in a small percentage of cases, this practice has not had long-term clinical success and, in many cases, has added to the distortion by producing scarring and compounding the essential problem of inadequate skeletal support.

I shared the theory of inadequate resection of skeletal parts until I begin to palpate noses with supratip deformities and found that in many the hump of soft tissue was significantly higher than the dorsal edge of the septum. Therefore, further reduction of the dorsal edge seemed illogical. Palpation of the supratip deformity then became routine in my evaluation of secondary rhinoplasty patients (Figure 40-1).

Many of these patients have supratips that can be compressed below a desirable dorsal line; however, not all patients with supratip deformity have compressible dorsal irregularities. The patient in Fig-

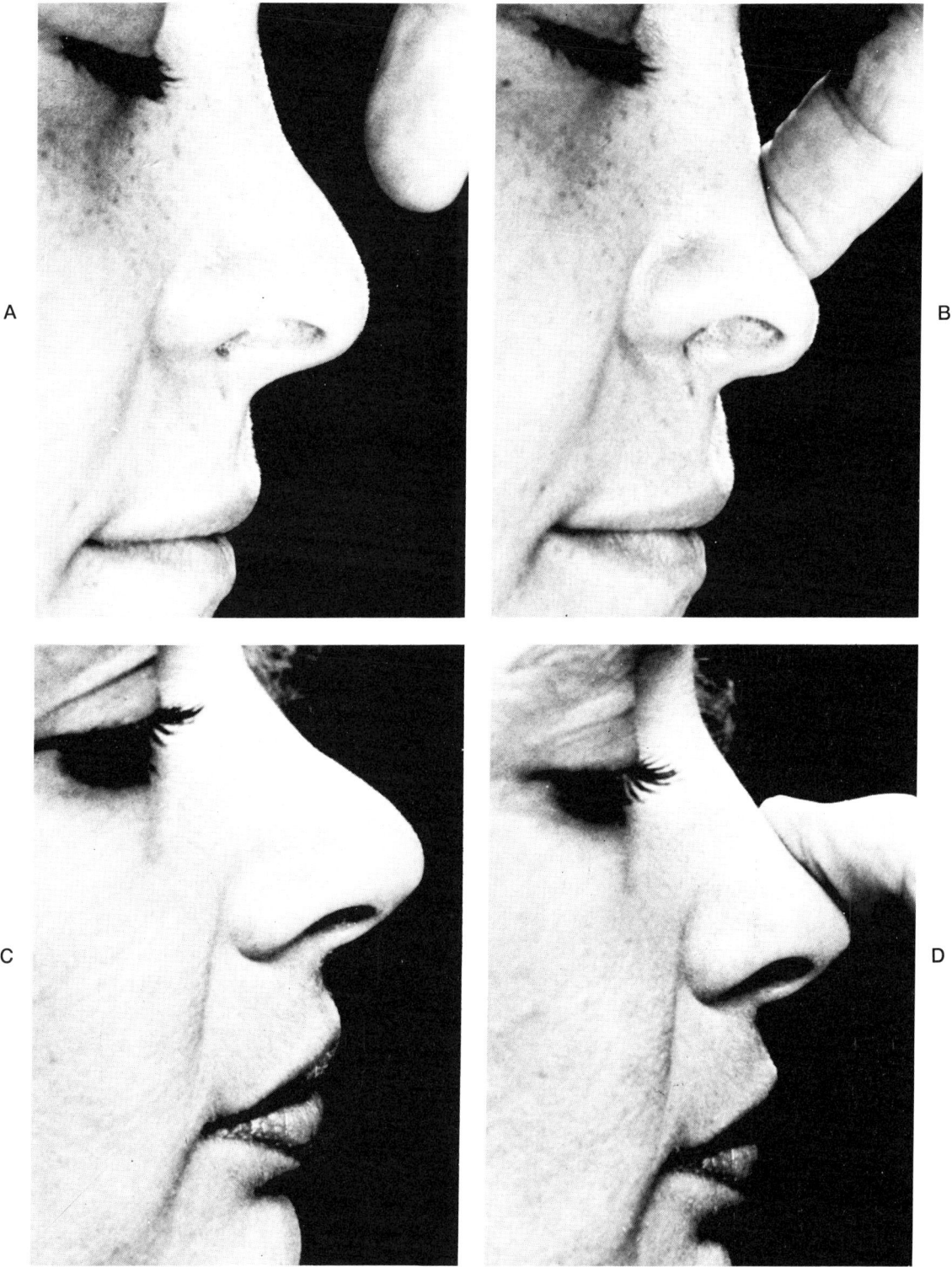

Figure 40-1. A-D, Palpation is the principal means of evaluating supratip fullness. If the tissues are easily depressed to the dorsal edge of the septum, structural deficiency is evident. These soft tissues will not contract down to the reduced skeleton. Further reduction of skeletal support, subdermal thinning, or scar resection is contraindicated. (From Sheen, J.H., and Sheen, A.P.: Aesthetic rhinoplasty, ed. 2, St. Louis, 1987, The C. V. Mosby Co.)

ure 40-2 had one previous surgery on her nose. She consulted many plastic surgeons, most of whom recommended thinning the scar tissue in the supratip. I recommended dorsal augmentation without thinning. A secondary rhinoplasty was performed at the Rhinoplasty Symposium in Miami in January 1975. That surgery demonstrated that the dorsal edge of the septum adjacent to the supratip had been undercut 4 to 5 mm, a familiar but ineffective prophylactic measure to prevent supratip deformity. Surgical correction of this patient's nose was produced by augmenting the supratip with a double layer of cartilage. There was no resection of scar tissue or the dorsal septum. Tip grafting was also done.

I operated on a consecutive series of 100 secondary rhinoplasty patients, 23 males and 77 females. The average age was 28.9 years; the youngest was 16 years old, and the oldest was 67 years old. The average number of procedures per patient was

1.7; the greatest number was 8. The treatment for these patients included 82 dorsal augmentations with or without tip grafts, 8 tip grafts, 7 dorsal reductions and external excisions, five dorsal augmentations, and no supratip thinnings. It is significant that 82% of the patients in this series were treated with dorsal augmentation. Resection of scar tissue was not performed in any of these cases. The successful use of augmentative techniques in the majority of secondary patients in this series would support the opinion that overresection is the most frequent cause of supratip deformity.

The correction of a supratip deformity using augmentation is predictably successful. The following photographs represent a spectrum of patients with supratip deformities; all were treated through augmentative techniques. First, young patients who needed a single operative procedure (Figure 40-3). Next, a case of common supratip deformity. The patient had four previous rhinoplasties; three de-

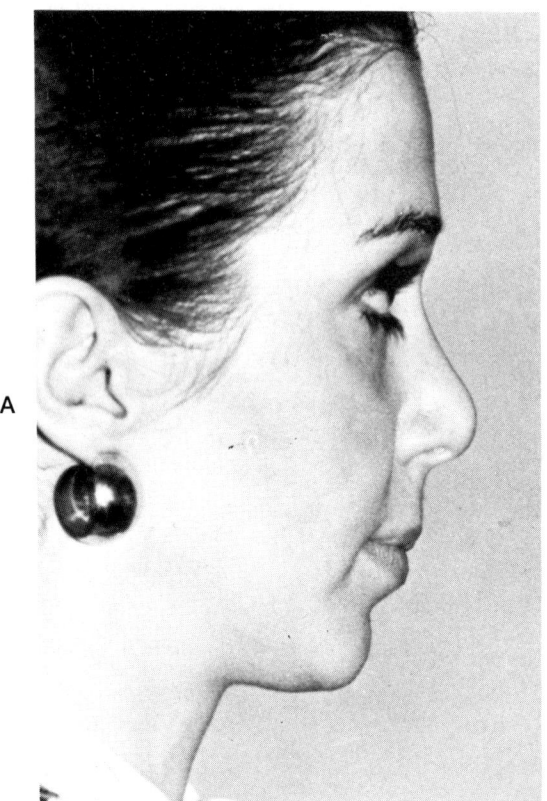
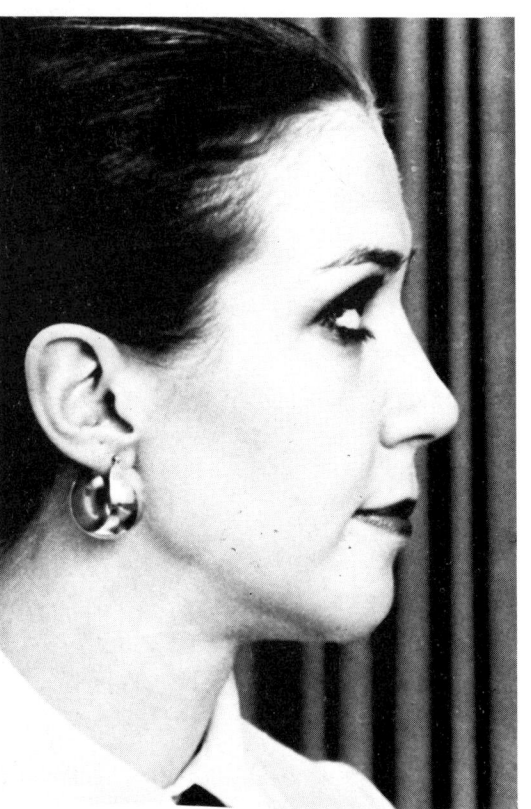

Figure 40-2. **A** and **B,** This supratip fullness was corrected by dorsal augmentation and tip grafting. Additional cartilage was placed under the caudal edge of the graft in the immediate area of the supratip. No tissues were resected.
(From Sheen, J.H., and Sheen, A.P.: Aesthetic rhinoplasty, ed. 2, St. Louis, 1987, The C. V. Mosby Co.)

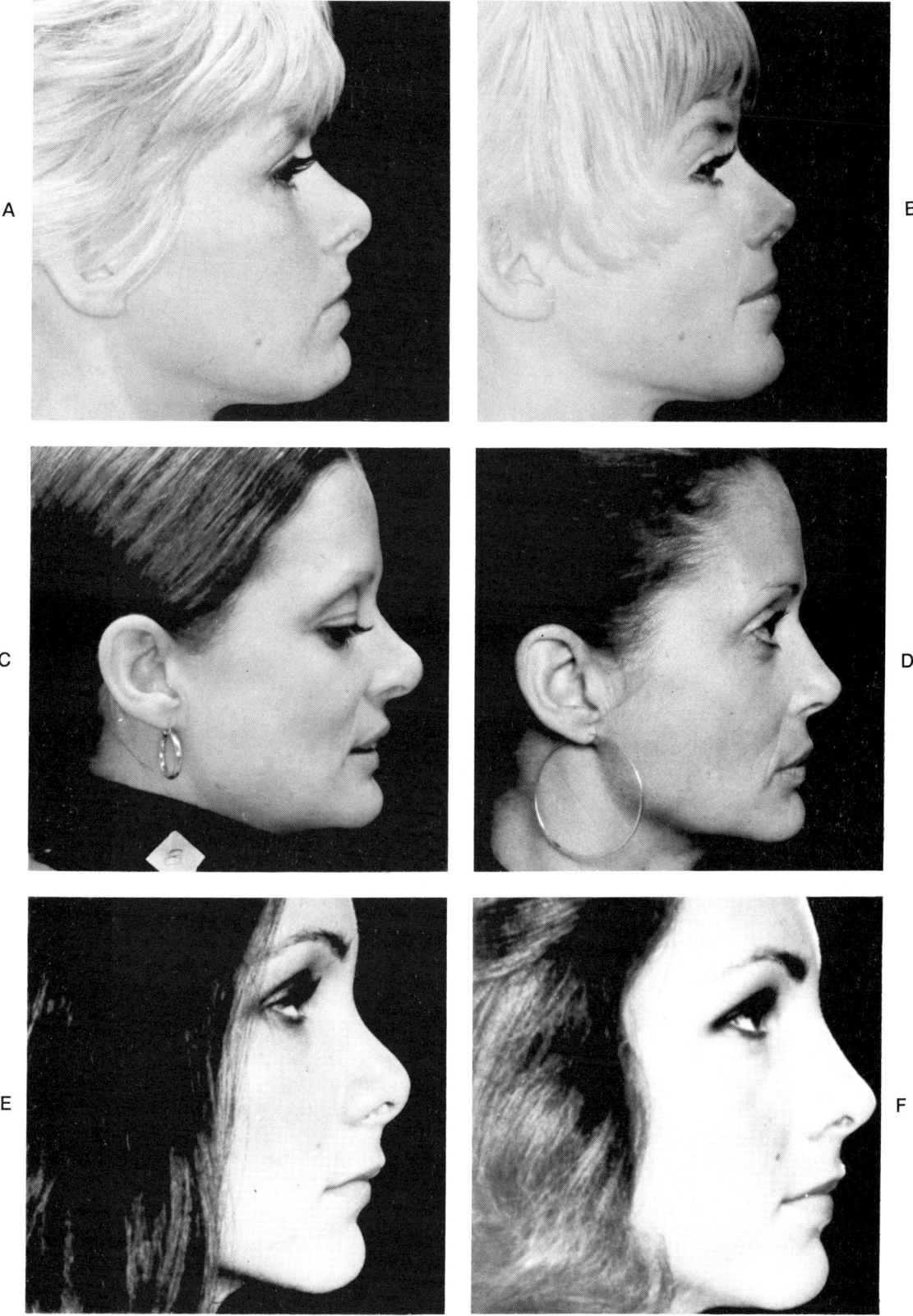

Figure 40-3. A-F, Three patients illustrate common supratip deformity. This is the typical appearance of patients following a classic reductive rhinoplasty. All skeletal elements have been overreduced. These cases required correction of structural deficiency. Dorsal and tip grafts were key to the secondary surgical plan. No tissues were resected. (From Sheen, J.H., and Sheen, A.P.: Aesthetic rhinoplasty, ed. 2, St. Louis, 1987, The C. V. Mosby Co.)

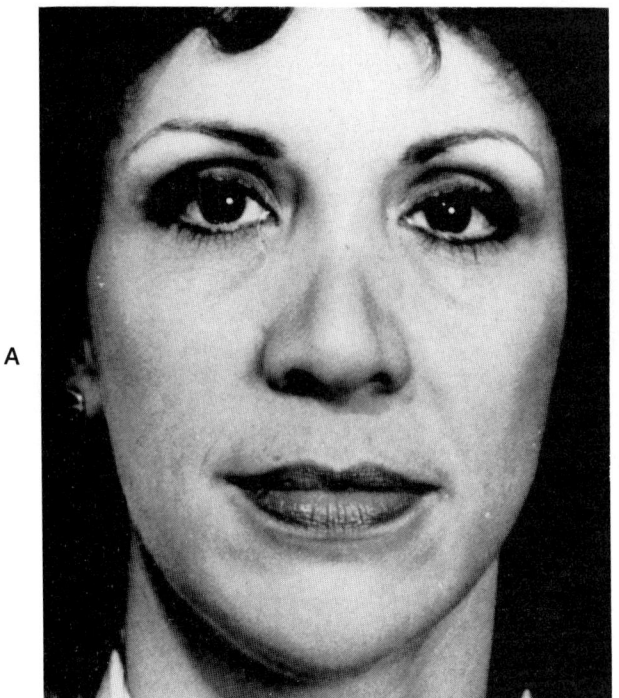
A

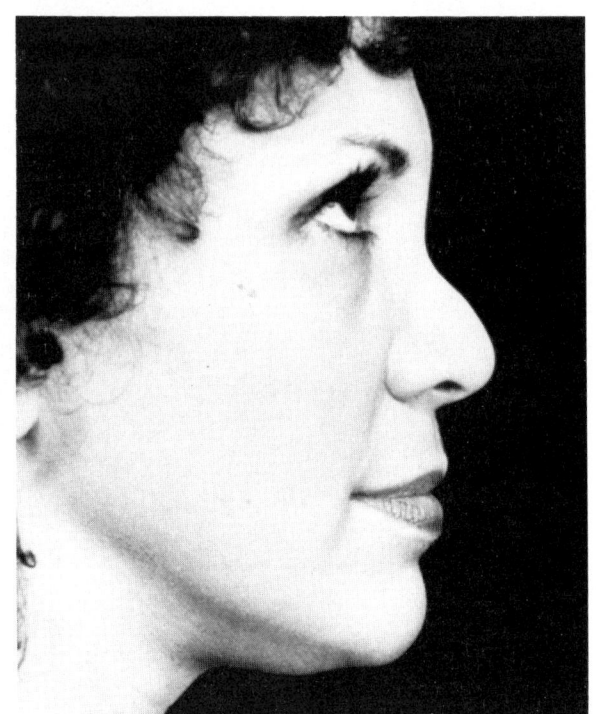
B

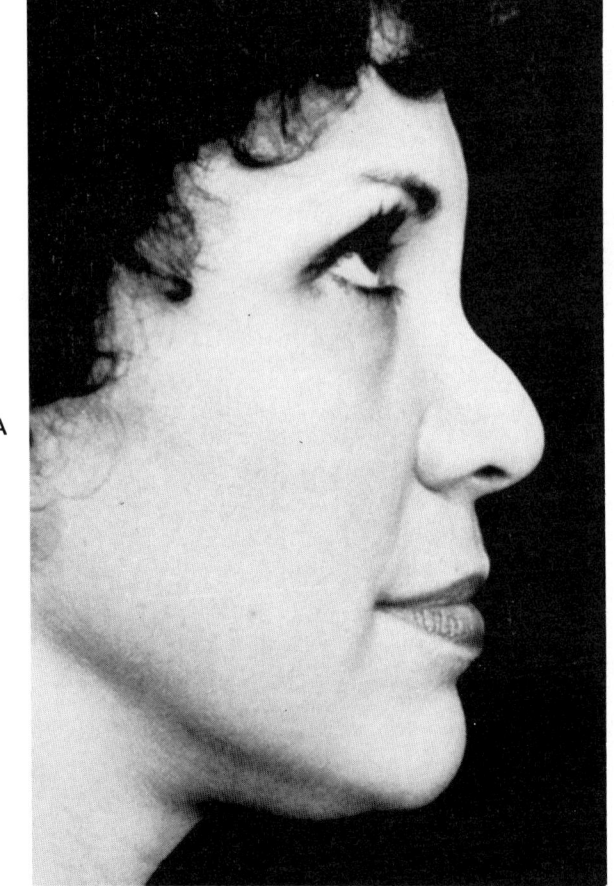
A

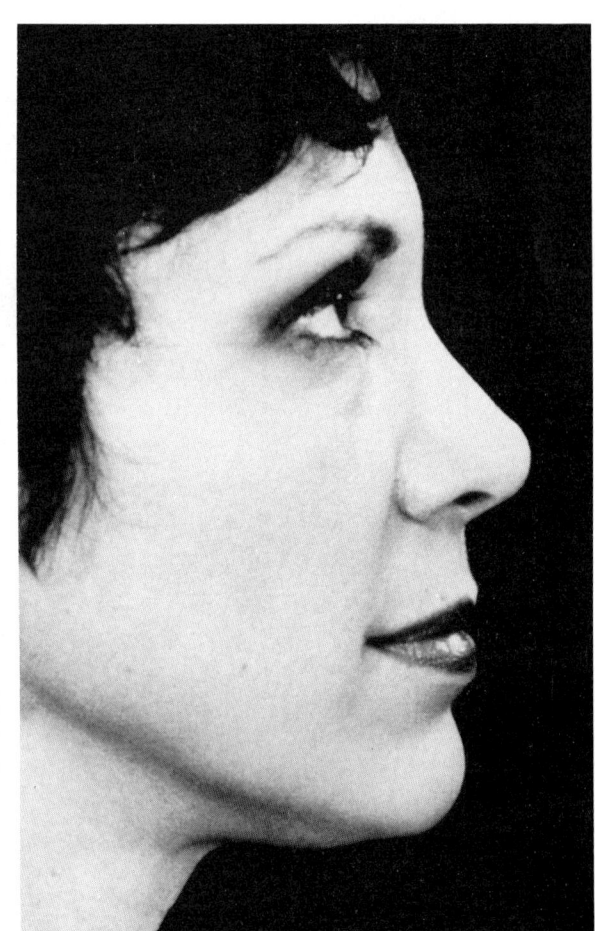
B

Figure 40-4. **A** and **B,** Supratip deformity with collapsed middle vault, low dorsum, and compromised internal valves. Result of four previous rhinoplasties. (From Sheen, J.H., and Sheen, A.P.: Aesthetic rhinoplasty, ed. 2, St. Louis, 1987, The C. V. Mosby Co.)

signed to reduce the supratip fullness (Figure 40-4). She cannot breathe normally through her nose nor wear her eyeglasses. The solution to this problem is not further resection of tissues but augmentation of the dorsum and nasal tip. The postoperative photographs (Figure 40-5) show the pleasing result 2 years after secondary rhinoplasty.

Another type of patient particularly susceptible to supratip deformities is the older patient with redundant and inelastic tissue. These patients have heavy tissues that would certainly resist thinning procedures. Frequently they have been subjected to multiple procedures. The patient in Figure 40-6 had six previous surgeries during which his tissues were thinned. His nose was corrected through external excisions with a dorsal and a tip graft performed in one procedure (Figure 40-7). All of these patients were treated with dorsal augmentation without resection of any skeletal tissue or thinning of the supratip area.

Figure 40-5. **A-D,** Two years after secondary rhinoplasty, supratip deformity has been eliminated by increasing the height of the root, augmenting the dorsum and tip with cartilage, and no tissue resection. (From Sheen, J.H., and Sheen, A.P.: Aesthetic rhinoplasty, ed. 2, St. Louis, 1987, The C. V. Mosby Co.)

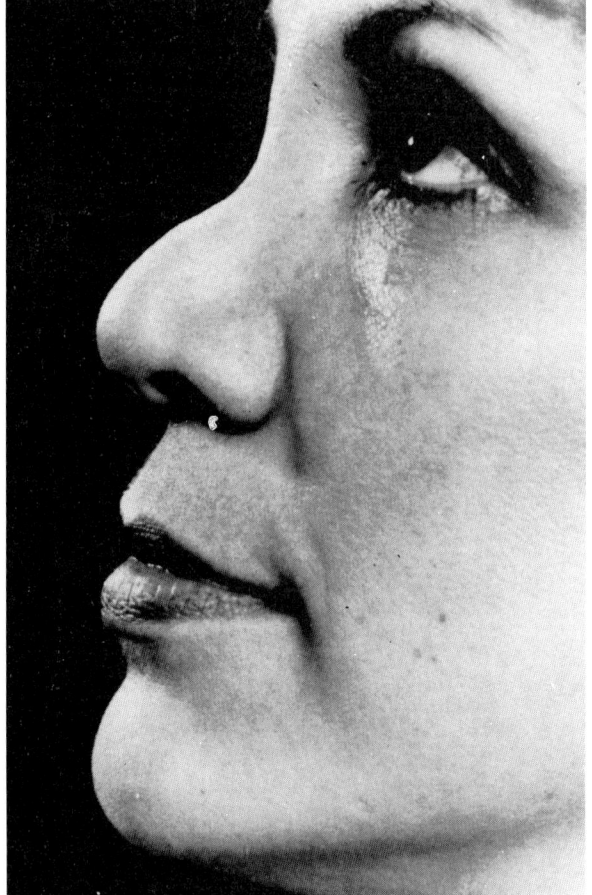

C

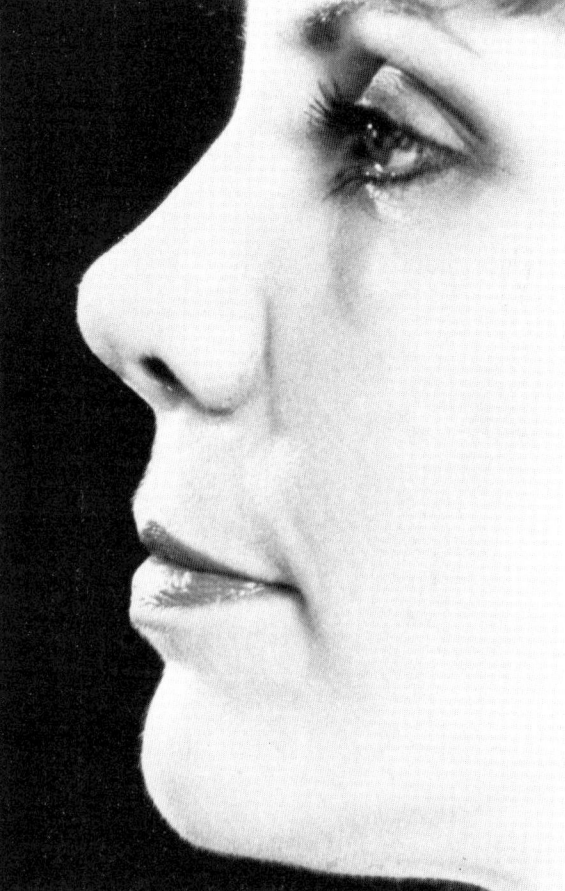

D

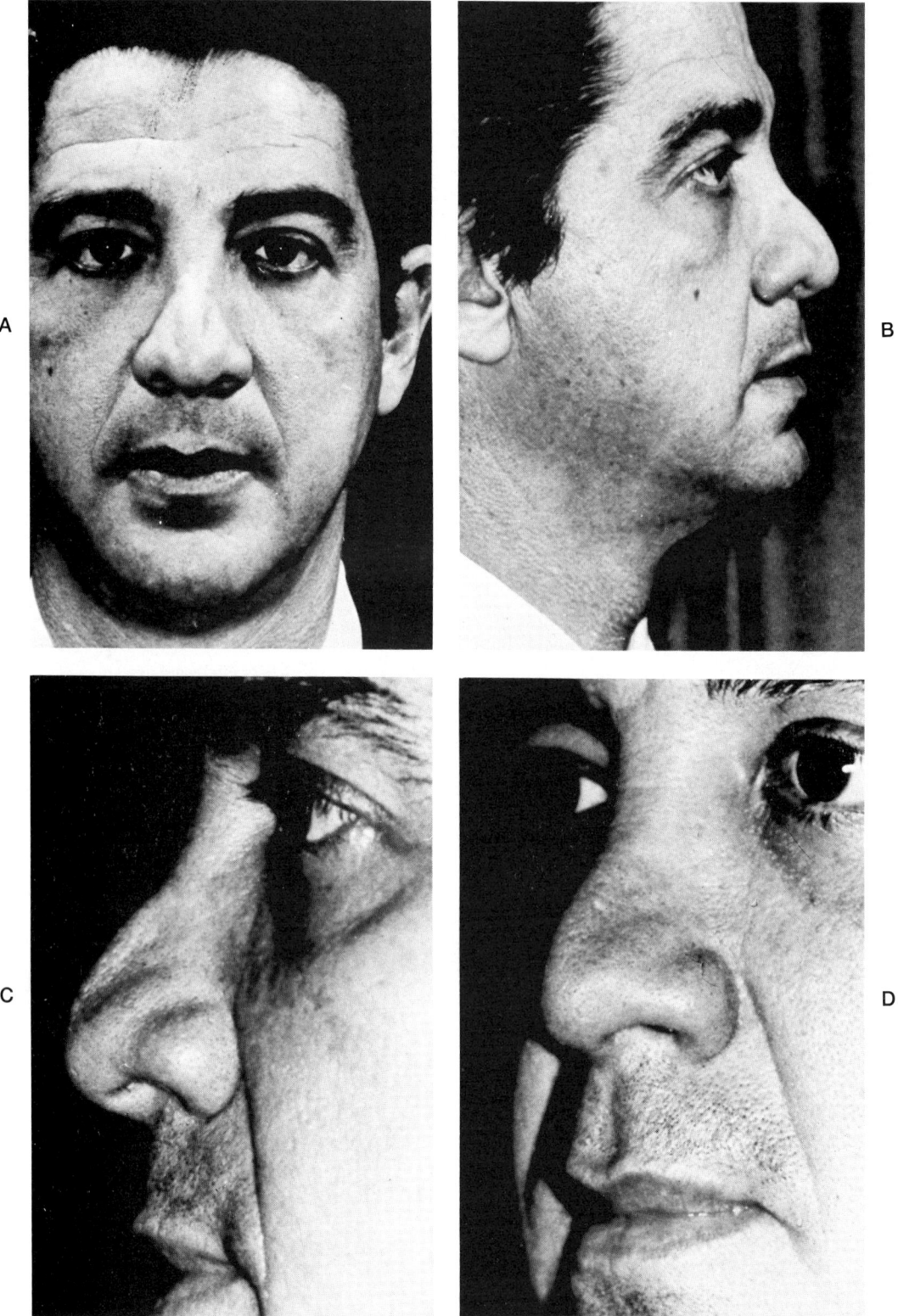

Figure 40-6. A-D, Six operations to thin out and reduce the skin sleeve produced a bulging supratip and deep vertical grooves. This patient required dorsal augmentation and a tranverse external excision. (From Sheen, J.H., and Sheen, A.P.: Aesthetic rhinoplasty, ed. 2, St. Louis, 1987, The C. V. Mosby Co.)

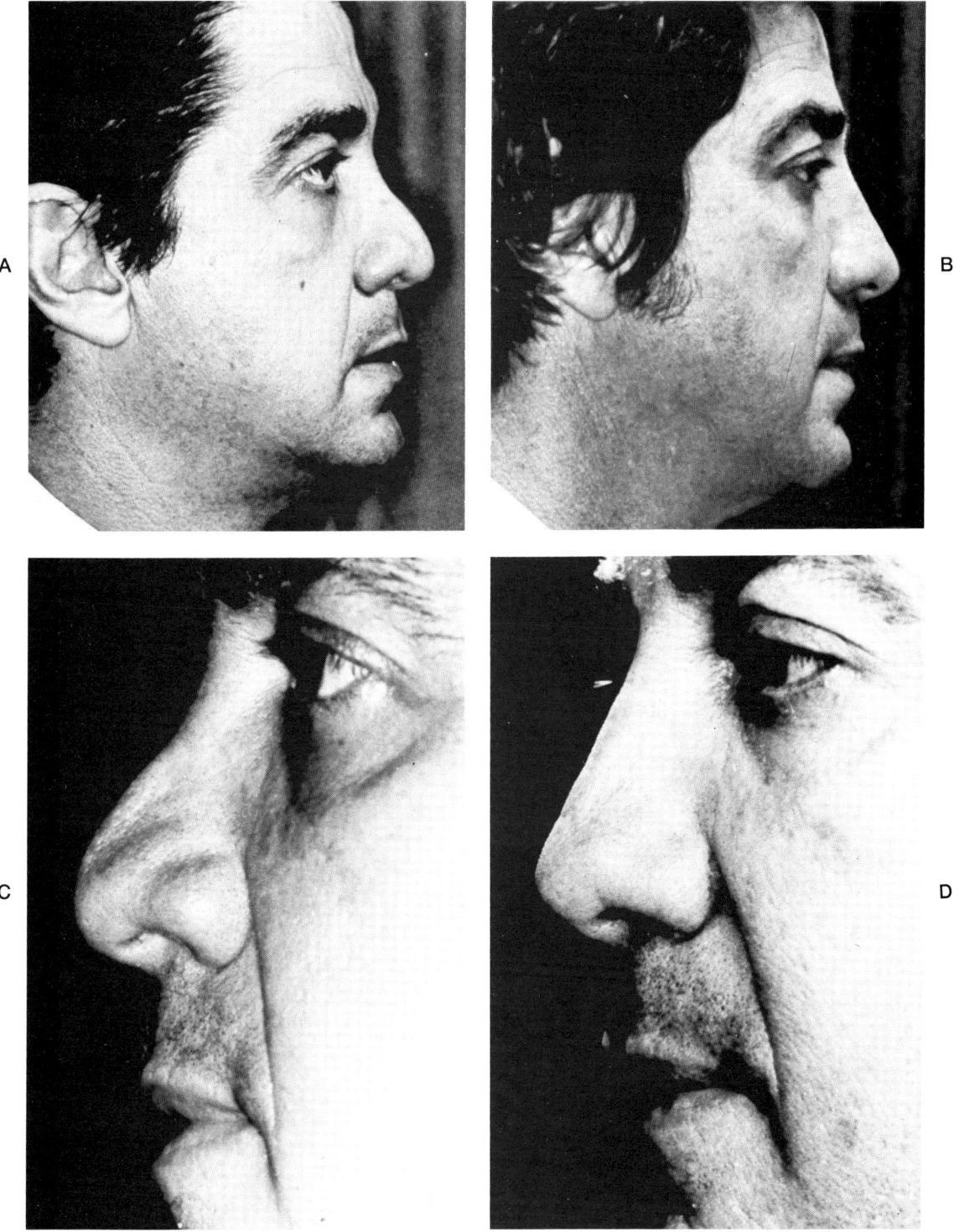

Figure 40-7. A-D, Postoperatively, the vertical grooves are still somewhat visible, but the nose is more natural looking. (From Sheen, J.H., and Sheen, A.P.: Aesthetic rhinoplasty, ed. 2, St. Louis, 1987, The C. V. Mosby Co.)

I believe we should take a closer look at the current thinking concerning the cause of supratip deformity and question the recommended treatment of further tissue resection. I suggest that the most frequent cause of supratip deformity is the overresection of skeletal parts—principally, the dorsal edge of the septum. I recommend using autogenous material to augment the overresected parts and to provide support and contour to the dorsum.

I have performed this procedure for the last 10 years, since I first reported it. My experience with the technique has supported the findings that I had with the initial series of 100 patients. We have to take a serious look at the treatment of this deformity; I continue to believe that the most logical causative factor is, in fact, overreduction of skeletal parts, and the treatment that I recommend is augmentation of the dorsum.

REFERENCES

1. Denecke, H.J., and Meyer, R.: Plastic surgery of head and neck, New York, 1967, Springer-Verlag Co.
2. Goldwyn, R.M.: The unfavorable result in plastic surgery: avoidance and treatment, Boston, 1972, Little Brown & Co.
3. Rees, T.D.: An aid in the treatment of supratip swelling after rhinoplasty. Laryngoscope **91**:308, 1971.
4. Rogers, B.O.: Secondary and tertiary correction of post-rhinoplastic deformities: some dos and don'ts. In Millard, D.R., Jr., editor: Symposium on corrective rhinoplasty, St. Louis, 1976, The C.V. Mosby Co.
5. Rogers, B.O.: Secondary and teritary rhinoplasty. In Transactions of the fourth international congress of plastic and reconstructive surgery, Amsterdam, 1969, Excerpta Medica.
6. Safian, J.: Corrective rhinoplastic surgery, New York, 1935, Hoeber Co.

41

Supratip and Related Deformities

Claus Walter

At the present time nasal corrections to alter the shape and appearance of the nose and in some cases to improve nasal function are the most often performed aesthetic operations in the world. Complications can occur that are caused by the patient's own tissue reaction or by the surgeon's misjudgment in performing the surgery. My comments about problems of supratip deformity and related nasal-entrance deformities are based on my experience with over 1,000 secondary revisions.

Figure 41-1 is a typical picture of a patient with a supratip deformity. This deformity is caused by overresection of the lower-lateral cartilages; thus the remaining tip cartilage is suspended by only the dorsal border of the septal cartilage. If the nasal dorsum is shortened and lowered in these cases, the patient will come back saying, "It was fine for the first half year, and then my nose assumed the appearance it had before the last intervention." The skin retracts; therefore the nasal cartilages of the tip are pulled downward even more, and basically the same deformity reappears.

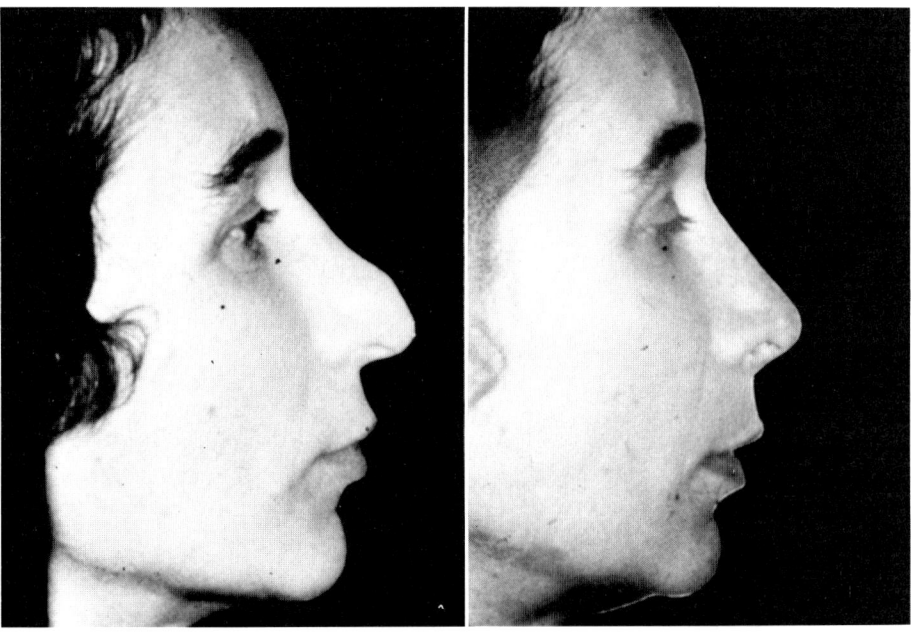

Figure 41-1. Polly-beak after rhinoplasty and postoperative appearance after correction.

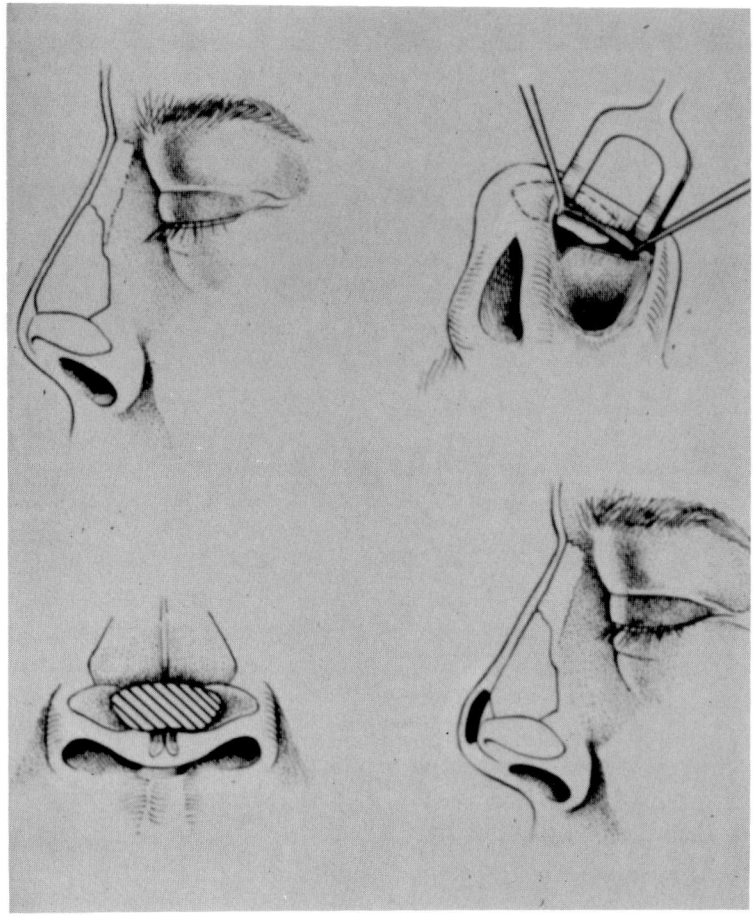

Figure 41-2. Cartilage insertion to raise nasal tip.

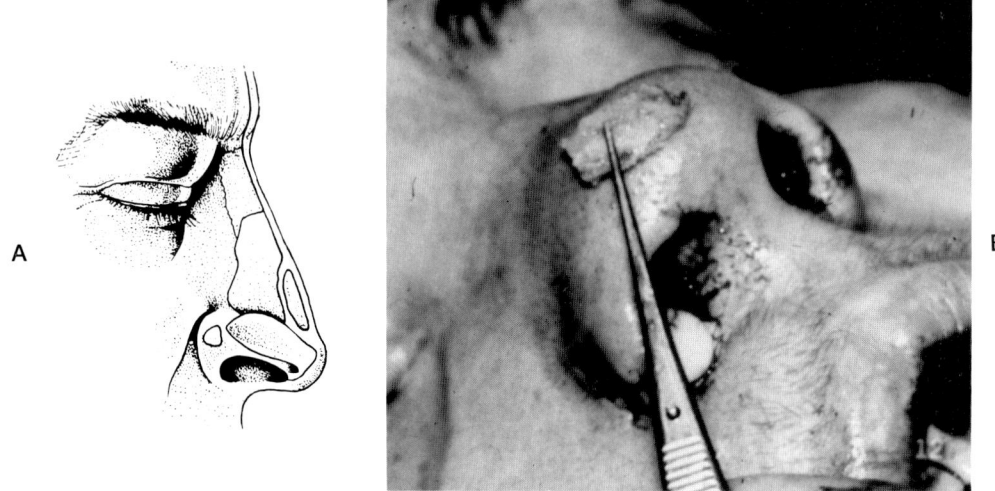

Figure 41-3. A, In cases of postoperative saddling, piece of auricular or septal cartilage is used to replace defect. **B,** Cartilage is inserted to raise nasal tip. (A, From Walter, C.D.: Secondary nasal revisions after rhinoplasties, presented by the Committee on Reconstructive Plastic Surgery at the seventy-ninth annual meeting of the American Academy of Ophthalmology and Otolaryngology, Dallas, Oct. 6-10, 1974. (J. Otorhinolaryngol. Relat. Spec. **80:** Nov./Dec. 1975.)

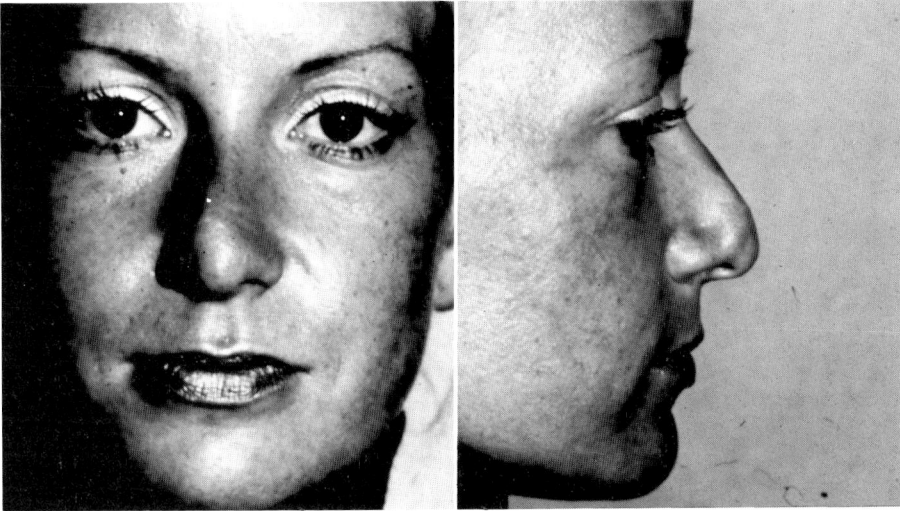

Figure 41-4. Preoperative photographs after two rhinoplasties.

To correct this deformity the surgeon must decide whether to shave the septal dorsum or to raise the tip. I favor the Goldman technique and augment the medial crura with some cartilage. Sometimes excess cartilage is left in the lateral portion of lower-lateral cartilages and can be excised and used for reimplantation into the center of the tip. The surgeon must be careful, however, not to cause an alar collapse by taking away too much. A very thorough preoperative evaluation is therefore mandatory (Figures 41-2 and 41-3).

The preferred areas for harvesting cartilage are the septum and the ears. If the preoperative examination reveals that enough support is in the lower-lateral cartilages, the surgeon can safely remove cartilage on the dorsal border of the septum in conjunction with tip correction and correction of the medial part of the upper-lateral cartilages, which often have not been trimmed sufficiently, producing the polly-beak (Figures 41-4 and 41-5).

If, in addition, the nose has been overshortened, it also needs lengthening. This procedure is only possible through insertion of a composite ear graft to give cartilaginous support and epithelial lining. It is important to excise a small rectangular piece of cartilage and mucosa on the dorsum of the septum before inserting the composite graft to lock it on the dorsum of the septum. This step prevents any cephalad sliding of the graft. The skin portion of the graft must be divided vertically to be able to suture the skin parts of the graft to the surrounding mucosal parts on each side (Figure 41-6). In this way the nose can be lengthened.

Occasionally cartilaginous and mucosal trimming is necessary to obtain a good tissue approximation. In a few cases this procedure alone fails to achieve the desired result. Then it is necessary to place a baton or a strut into the columella to elevate the tip and to replace these overly resected lower-lateral cartilages (Figure 41-7).

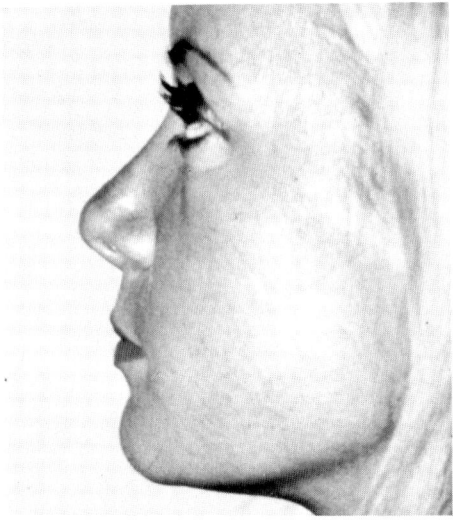

Figure 41-5. Postoperative photograph.

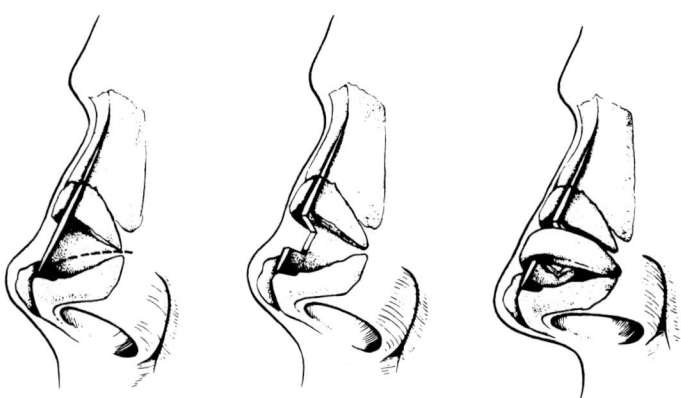

Figure 41-6. Placement of composite graft for correction of a distorted tip. *Left,* incision; *center,* cartilage resection of cranial part of septum; *right,* location of graft. (From Walter, C.D.: Composite grafts in nasal surgery, Arch. Otolaryngol. 90:624 Nov. 1969)

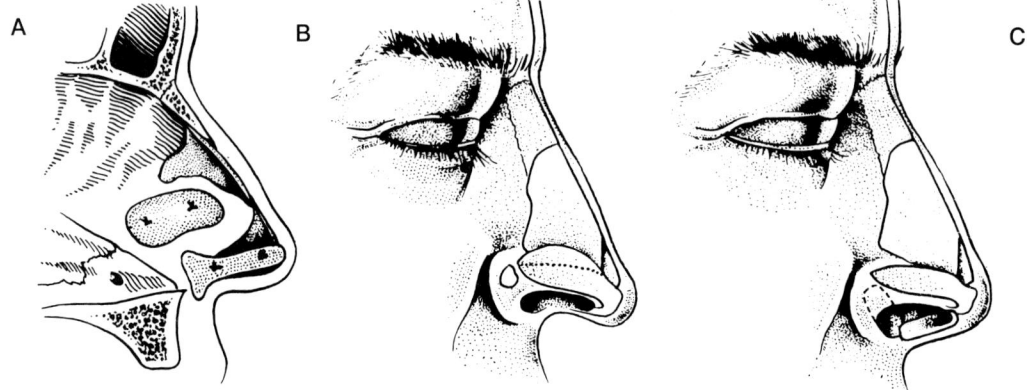

Figure 41-7. A, Replantation of cartilage after extensive septal cartilage excision with retraction of columella, producing hanging tip. Cartilage is specially shaped to compensate for missing anterior nasal spine. **B,** Cranial portion of lower-lateral cartilages is inserted into nasal septum to counterbalance postoperative tendency to contract in region of nasal spine. **C,** Additional cartilage is needed to keep nasolabial angle well-stabilized. (From Walter, C.D.: Secondary nasal revisions, Trans. Am. Acad. Opthalmol. Otolaryngol. 80:520, Nov./Dec. 1975.)

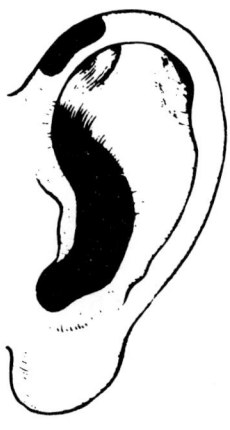

Figure 41-8. Donor sites for composite grafts.
(From Walter, C.D.: Composite grafts in nasal surgery, Arch. Otolaryngol. 90:623, Nov. 1969.)

The needed composite graft is taken from the anterior aspect of the concha since its cartilage has a curvature that corresponds to the nasal cartilages and its skin is closely attached, facilitating handling of the graft (Figure 41-8).

A retracted columella can be corrected in a different way. By excising the inferior crus at the junction with the helix, perfectly matching cartilage is obtained that resembles the medial crura. The skin portion of the graft is divided vertically to obtain a graft perfectly suited to duplicate the area of colu-

mella. Depending on the size of the graft, a transfixion of 50% the membranous septum must be performed. By pulling the freed columella caudally, the resulting tissue gap is the site for the insertion of the composite ear graft. In patients and secondary nasal tip and supratip deformities with nasal scarring, two options for taking auricular composite grafts are available. The anterior conchal skin is attached very tightly to the cartilage, facilitating handling. Furthermore, the cartilage curvature and skin match the lower-lateral cartilages (Figures 41-9 to 41-12).

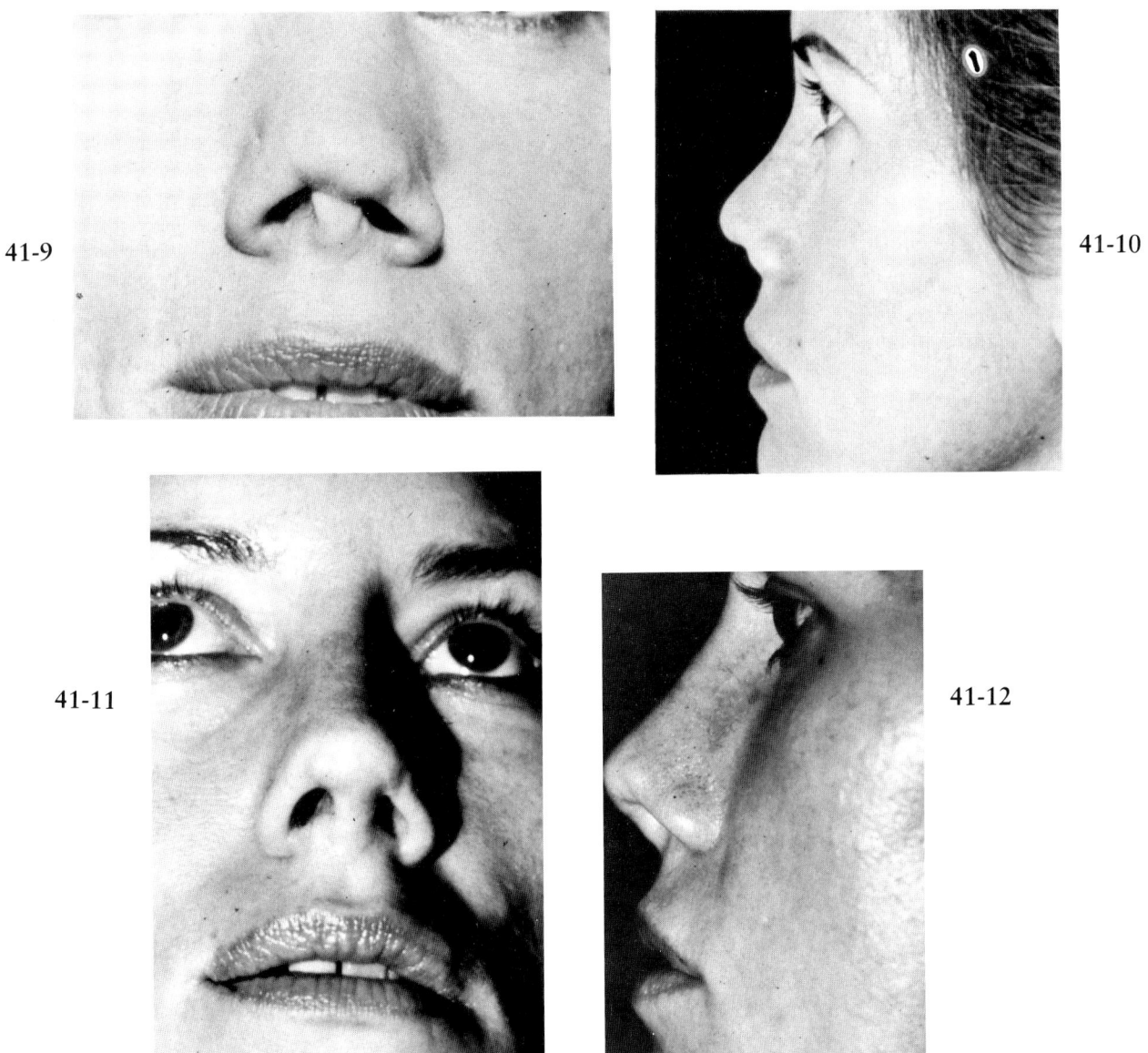

41-9

41-10

41-11

41-12

Figures 41-9 to 41-12. Preoperative and postoperative appearance after three previous rhinoplasties.

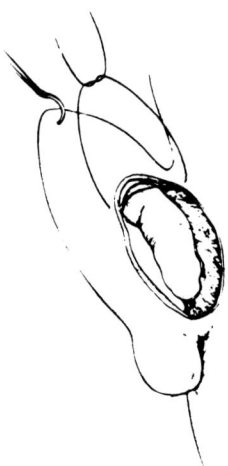

Figure 41-13. Construction of a postauricular island flap. (From Walter, C.D.: Composite grafts in nasal surgery, Arch. Otolaryngol. 90:623, Nov. 1969.)

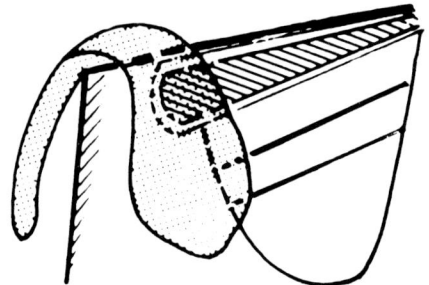

Figure 41-14. Placement of composite graft from either septum or ear for correction of alar collapse. (From Walter, C.D.: Composite grafts in nasal surgery, Arch. Otolaryngol. 90:624, Nov. 1969.)

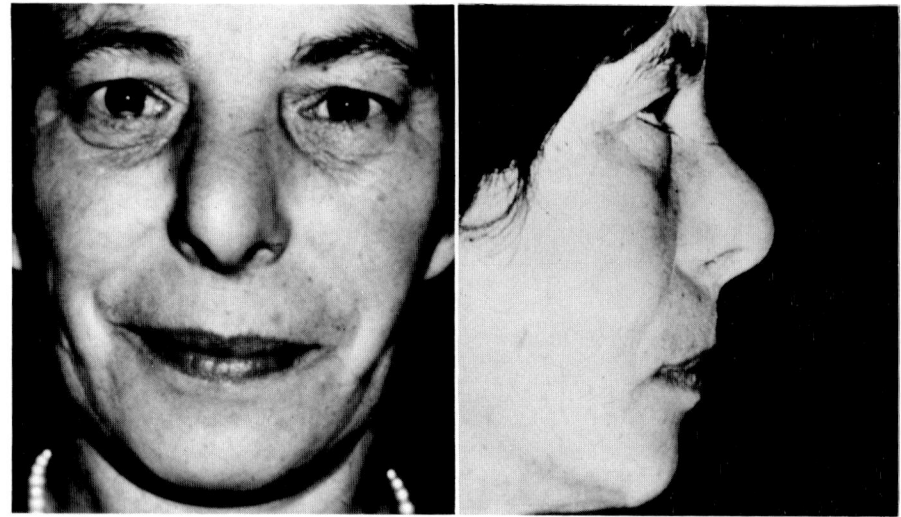

Figure 41-15. Preoperative photographs after two rhinoplasties.

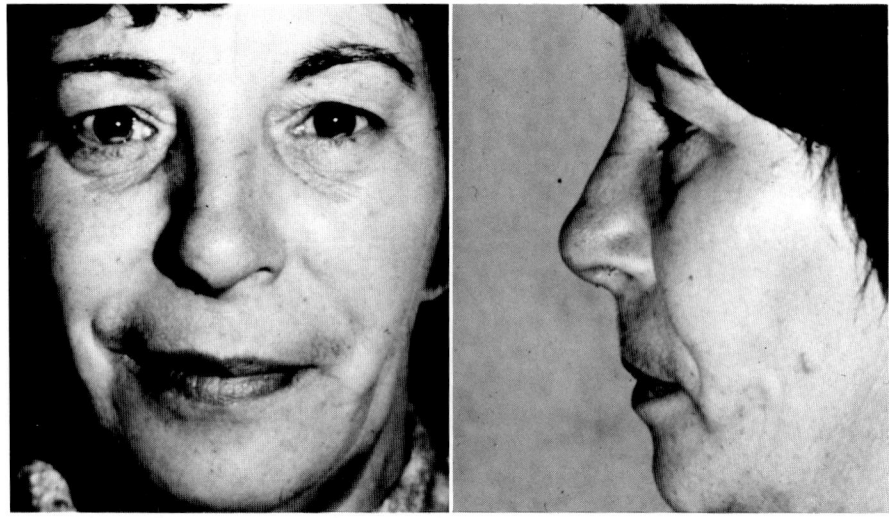

Figure 41-16. Postoperative photographs 1 year later.

The anterior donor site is easily closed from the mastoid area. At the postauricular-mastoidal junction an incision is made through the skin. Through a circular incision a postauricular island flap is created, which is rotated on a subcutaneous pedicle forward into the anterior conchal defect, giving a perfect match. The postauricular skin is closed directly (Figure 41-13). I use this type of graft also if there is too much scarring in the inner valve area (Figure 41-14).

The composite graft can be trimmed as needed. Sometimes just a small strip of skin is left on a larger piece of cartilage or the reverse. Bilateral obstructions or supratip deformities require a saddle graft over the septum. This graft can extend into the nasal dorsum or downward into the tip of the nose. I do not use packing with too much ointment on it because the ointment can enter the suture line and cause irritation. Telfa is better suited as packing.

In cases of too much tissue excision on the dorsum and the lower laterals the physician is confronted with a supratip deformity resulting from nonresected upper laterals. It is important to determine the high point of the nasal dorsum. Is it the height of the bony dorsum and tip, or is it the height of the unresected upper laterals (Figures 41-15 and 41-16). Depending on the case, either cartilage must be inserted from the rib or ear (I prefer autogenous material) or the dorsum must be trimmed.

BIBLIOGRAPHY

Rees, T.D., Krupps, S., and Wood-Smith, D.: Secondary rhinoplasty, Plast. Reconstr. Surg. 46:332, 1970.

Walter, C.: Composite grafts in nasal surgery, Arch. Otolaryngol. 90:622, 1969.

Walter, C.: Secondary nasal revisions after rhinoplasties, Trans. Am. Acad. Ophthalmol. Otolaryngol. 80:519, 1975.

Point & Counterpoint
PARTS X, XI & XII

Question: Several years ago it was suggested that incisions separating the upper-lateral cartilage from the septum are a probable cause of supratip deformity. Dr. Caplan, I know that you separate the upper-lateral cartilages from the septum in almost every rhinoplasty that you do. Since we're talking about controversy, I'd like to invite your comments, and then I'd like to hear from Dr. Tardy who says that he almost never does separate them.

Comment (Harvey Caplan): I have done probably 7,000 to 8,000 rhinoplasties by separating the upper laterals from the septum. I don't think I'd still be doing them if I were getting supratip deformities.

Comment (Eugene Tardy): My contention is not with those surgeons who do something and get good results because they are men who would not be doing these procedures if their results were poor. My contention is that this should be an anatomical operation. I see no point in doing things that are unnecessary. I see great virtue in maintaining anatomy that's there for a reason. I regularly see problems from cases that are performed in which there is radical separation for no reason. These problems include excess scarring, nasal valve deformities, lateral wall pinching, supratip scar deformities from trapping, and infarction of divided mucosa.

Question: Do you ever inject steroids into the supratip deformity, and if so, how much and at what intervals?

Comment (Thomas Rees): Yes, but I don't do it nearly as often now as I did when I reported it. There are patients who have a little persistent edema of the supratip. I will inject them with triamcinolone, rarely more than two or three times, beginning at approximately the fourth week when edema is at its maximum. The key here is minute doses of triamcinolone. If you inject large doses (for example, 10 mg) or use 40 mg/ml doses, you can cause considerable subcutaneous atrophy. The steroid should be diluted. I use a tuberculin syringe and inject 2 mg at the most. I think it is effective in many patients.

Question: Do you use antibiotics for routine rhinoplasty patients? Also, should the mouth and the nose be considered separate bacterial zones with different potential infection rates?

Comment (Jack Sheen): With a routine rhinoplasty I do not use antibiotics. However, when I use grafts, I do prescribe a prophylactic antibiotic. I use erythromycin—1 g/day.

Question: After a minimum hump removal and infracturing, a slight hump sometimes remains and is sometimes quite obvious. Do you see this problem, and how can it be avoided?

Comment (Eugene Tardy): Sometimes it's intentional. If we look at aesthetics, the ideal nose probably has a very slight profile convexity. Most patients like a straight profile, but it is a matter of finding out what the patient wants. I do see an occasional bony excrescence in my patients that I think is the result either of the failure to remove sufficient bone with a rasp or of new bone formation. On occasion there is a patient who, 8 or 10 weeks after surgery, begins to show a little fullness or prominence at the dorsal portion of the nasal bone. A 16-gauge needle can be used to penetrate through the skin, do a little scraping, and aspirate what looks like soft bone. This procedure is done only occasionally, but it might save two or three little revisions later.

Question: Do you charge for your own secondary rhinoplasties?

Comment (Harvey Caplan): I do not charge for my own secondary work.

Comment (Thomas Rees): I charge if a patient comes back to me 10 years later and says, "I really want *this* now. I had *that* before, and now I want a little of *this*." This request is not because of a surgical fault but is because the patient wants a little different style. In this situation I will charge them but not the full fee. Otherwise, I don't charge for my own secondaries.

Question: How do you handle the situation in which a colleague from your own town who has done a rhinoplasty and is in trouble wants your help? How do you handle the charges for that patient?

Comment (Thomas Rees): In my experience a lot of patients who come for secondary rhinoplasty expect to pay. They are not always totally unhappy with the first surgeon. The answer to your question as to whether or not to charge for a secondary when the primary was done by a trained colleague is difficult and must be determined on an individual basis.

Question: When you see a patient that was first operated on by another surgeon, do you pick up the telephone and call the first surgeon to discuss the fact that the patient has consulted you? Do you think it proper for the first surgeon to pay the fee for the secondary surgery?

Comment (Jack Sheen): When I was younger, more idealistic, and not doing so many secondary rhinoplasties, I did call the first surgeon. Sometimes I even called the second and third surgeons. But I got so much heat, hostility, and inaccurate information that I stopped. Now probably 50% of my practice is secondary rhinoplasty, and I have an established approach to managing these patients. I spend a great deal of time with them explaining the problems of rhinoplasty in general and their problems in particular. I usually say something like this, "This is a very complex and demanding procedure; the doctor who did your surgery did a good job, but good results cannot be guaranteed because of the pitfalls associated with this surgery." I have approximately 500 secondary rhinoplasty consultations per year, and I receive at least two letters a week from attorneys, which I don't answer because I cannot support litigation. Also, I do charge all patients who come to me for secondary rhinoplasty.

Comment (Thomas Rees): I just clarified my thinking on this. It is not incumbent on the first surgeon to pay the second surgeon. That is totally unethical and out of the question. If the patient has a problem with the first surgeon, that is a separate problem. If that surgeon wants to pay or return the fee, that's acceptable and ethical, but I think it would be totally out of the question to ask the first surgeon to pay the second one under any circumstances.

Question: You advocate reducing the lower-lateral cartilages through delivery through a rim or a bucket-handle type of incision. When you put in a tip graft after delivery of the lower-lateral cartilages, how do you prevent the graft from moving?

Comment (Jack Sheen): The whole trick is to insert the graft as the very last step in the procedure. I suture all of the incisions—the intercartilaginous, the lower-lateral incision on the opposite side—and finish absolutely everything. At least 90% of the time I can fix the grafts just by setting them in place and then putting my little contour grafts anteriorly and posteriorly. I then very carefully apply the tape dressing. With the occasional patient who has a severe tip problem, I put a mattress suture through the tip, fixing the graft or the several grafts combined with the mattress suture. I pull the suture forward and hold it as I place the tape dressing on the nose.

Question: Has anyone seen postrhinoplasty skin infections or superficial ulcerations beneath a nasal dressing? They are not a result of pressure necrosis but are secondary to accumulation of sebaceous material in thick nasal skin. Any advice on predictability and treatment?

Comment: Superficial infections or infected sebaceous cysts can be a problem with patients with thick, seborrheic skin. When I anticipate this problem, I simply remove the dressing early—on the third or fourth day.

Comment (Eugene Tardy): I've never had a necrosis over the dorsum, but I've seen situations where I think I undermined too superficially in thin skin. I have a colleague who sent me a slide of a serious necrosis following hematoma over the nose combined with a tightly adherent splint.

I'd like to make another point in this regard about secondary and revisional rhinoplasty. I think there comes a time (even though the nose is a very forgiving organ) when you have perhaps one more shot to do the work reasonably well and you're dealing with a lot of scar tissue and poor blood supply. This is precisely when you need to be very careful about the possibility of necrosis. My splint is very simplistic. I cushion the dorsum of the nose with a layer of gelfoam. If there is going to be an expansion, the gelfoam will help to accommodate some of it. It also aids in removing the splint without disturbing the skin.

Comment (Thomas Rees): I had one patient who sloughed some of her dorsal nasal skin from a hematoma that went unrecognized under the splint. The hematoma unquestionably converted to an abscess. It looked hideous, but I waited and waited. She developed a through-and-through fistula into the nasal cavity, which gradually shrunk as it contracted. Six months later, I was able to close it while it was viewed under magnification with fine sutures.

Question: Exactly what is the function of the nasal splint? Some surgeons don't even use a splint.

Comment (Eugene Tardy): Primarily, the function of the nasal splint is to facilitate adherence of the elevated skin to the new framework. Secondarily, it protects the damaged nose from husbands, boy friends, and children. Finally, it reminds the patient that something's been done and he or she needs to be careful.

Question: Do you think the results on most people would be the same, provided they didn't manipulate the nose or do stupid things?

Comment (Eugene Tardy): I like compression over any area that's been dissected to create a pocket. I like compression over the chin when I do a chin implant, and I think it does reduce edema and swelling. I think it reduces some pain and discomfort as well. So any part that needs to heal is in better shape if it is splinted.

Comment (Thomas Rees): I think there are two reasons for splinting. One is to get the skin flap to adhere and keep a pocket from forming during the first 24 hours postoperatively. The other one is to keep the patient away from the mirror for the first week.

Comment (Jack Sheen): I agree with Dr. Rees's and Dr. Tardy's reasons for splinting. Also, during the first week, the splint is effective in maintaining the position of the bones by preventing lateral distraction caused by edema.

Comment (Harvey Caplan): I think of splinting as a protective measure; that's all.

Question: Can you ever remove a bony hump or a cartilaginous hump and not do osteotomies?

Comment (Harvey Caplan): No.

Comment (Jack Sheen): I don't agree. I frequently omit osteotomies when there is good reason for it. If you have a bony pyramid that is in good proportion to the base, an osteotomy is contraindicated. You can remove a dorsal hump, reroof the dorsum, and get an absolutely superb nasal contour, in good balance, without osteotomy. Also, in the older patient who has to wear heavy glasses, the need to support these glasses is extremely important. So if I see a person of 60 or 70 who wears heavy glasses and who has a dorsal hump and thin osteoporotic bones, then I know if I fracture these bones, I'll probably get a comminution, which would overly narrow the nose and would make wearing glasses impossible for the patient. In such cases, I forgo osteotomy.

Question: Do you put a graft in it?

Comment (Jack Sheen): Yes, you would have to place a graft to reroof the dorsum.

Question: Why would you be adverse to just closing the gap and making sure that the skin doesn't adhere to an open roof by doing an osteotomy?

Comment (Jack Sheen): It makes it too narrow. I hate narrow noses.

Comment (Harvey Caplan): I think there's a soft osteotomy and a hard osteotomy. It depends on how you approach it. A soft osteotomy is accomplished when the lateral osteotomy does not stay in a horizontal line but curves gently upward to meet the area where the nasal frontal suture occurs. So you don't have to go around and huff and puff and crack the bones in.

Dr. Sheen is saying don't do the osteotomy, just stick a piece of cartilage in there, and go into the septum and start removing the septum. How long does it take to do an osteotomy, and how difficult is it to do an osteotomy? I think we've created a certain amount of fear about osteotomies. There isn't anything complicated about an osteotomy.

Comment (Jack Sheen): I want to assure my colleagues that I am capable of doing an osteotomy. I think, however, that it is an advantage to the patient, both functionally and aesthetically in certain cases, not to do an osteotomy, but to reroof.

Question: What can be done with postoperative telangiectasis?

Comment (Eugene Tardy): The argon laser reduces them very nicely.

Comment (Jack Sheen): Telangiectasis over the dorsum is caused by a decreased superficial blood supply to the dermis. This certainly is a condition where an ounce of prevention is worth a pound of cure. Frequently, telangiectasis is present when alloplastic material has been placed beneath the skin, thereby isolating the dermis from its underlying blood supply. Similarly, when the dorsal skin is elevated superficially, without periosteum, telangiectasis can result. I think it is extremely important to preserve as much tissue as possible over the dorsum and to elevate the periosteum whenever possible.

Comment (Thomas Rees): In nine out of 10 patients with these telangiectases, whether they're on the eyelids or on the neck after a facelift or a rhinoplasty, you'll find that they were present preoperatively and were only exacerbated by surgery. So I disagree with Jack. I think that any disturbance of the skin, whether it's at the periosteal level or anywhere else, is going to bring out a natural tendency in that patient toward broken vessels. I'm delighted to hear about the laser success because electrocoagulation of these vessels with a needle is not always successful.

Question: Dr. Tardy showed his ear cartilage grafts for the dorsum, and it looked as though he were laying in strips, some with and some without fascia around them. I think that Dr. Sheen frequently folds them and sutures them together.

Comment (Eugene Tardy): I have modified my technique a little bit. When I do roll the ear cartilage, now I will score it longitudinally so I will get an actual break in the contour. I only occasionally wrap it, and I wrap it for two reasons. One, I want the contour to simulate the anatomical dorsal edge, and two, I gain some height. In other words, if you wrap it tightly you'll get a narrower, higher augmentation. I fill the cavity of the graft with as many tissue scraps as I can find. The only problem I've had with some of these grafts later on is flattening so that the lateral edges of the graft are visible. So I've been careful to score the dorsal side. If laminated septal cartilages are used, I prefer to stabilize their relation to one another with sutures. In Europe they use fibrin glue in a number of cases, and I hope that sooner or later we'll have fibrin glue, which is a wonderful kind of adhering material with which to put cartilage together.

Question: What about harvesting fascia?

Comment (Eugene Tardy): Fascia is available in abundance. A great deal can be harvested through a 1 inch (or less incision in the temporal scalp. The otologist does it every day to build new eardrums. There's a rich source of both superficial and deep, thick temporalis fascia, which can be laminated and layered. It forms an excellent cushion over the dorsum either to contour defects or to fill in the boat of the cavum concha graft that's lying like a saddle over the nose. The problem is that it tends to furl and to roll, making it difficult to work with. If you can take a piece of gel foam and layer a little moist fascia over it, it forms a nice little implant.

XIII

ETHNIC VARIATIONS IN RHINOPLASTY AND AUGMENTATION RHINOPLASTY

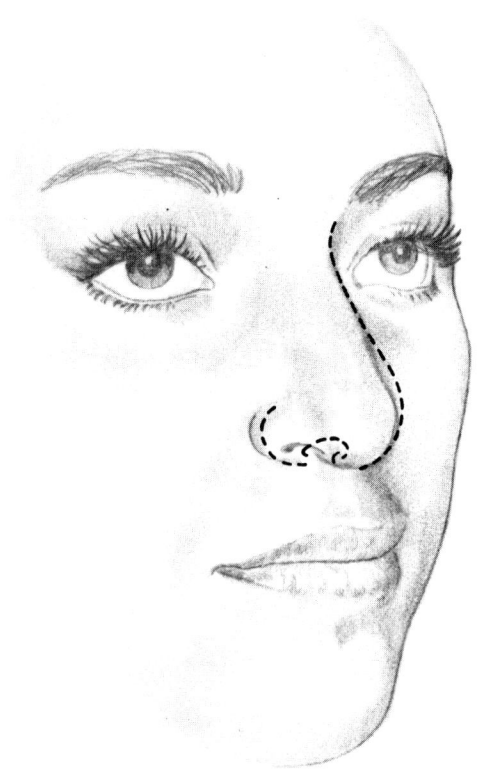

42

Rhinoplasty for the Mestizo Nose

Fernando Ortiz-Monasterio, Alvaro Olmedo

Aesthetic rhinoplasty was originally conceived as a procedure to remove some portions of the nose to decrease its size and to change its shape. The photographs from the early writings of Joseph, the father of aesthetic rhinoplasty, show individuals with gigantic noses who obviously represented the majority of the patients requesting aesthetic rhinoplasty in those days.[4] This concept of removing tissue, sometimes leading to catastrophic multilations, has been gradually replaced by a more conservative approach with greater respect for the integrity of the nasal structure. Increasing popularity of plastic surgical procedures has also prompted a vast number of people with small noses that do not conform with the accepted aesthetic standards to request an aesthetic rhinoplasty.

The nose is responsible in great part for the character of the face. Its size and shape vary among the different ethnic groups, giving to each particular race its own facial features. The visual information provided by newspapers, magazines, cinema, and television has reached almost every corner of the earth, promoting an Occidental look and disrupting long-established aesthetic values. A Caucasian nose with a straight dorsum covered by thin skin, separated from the forehead by a shallow groove, and joining the upper lip at a 90-degree angle has been accepted as the standard of beauty for the nose. People from all parts of the world with all colors of skin and entirely different racial characteristics are requesting surgical procedures to adjust their noses to the accepted aesthetic standards.

Mestizo in ethnological terms means a mixture of races. For the American continent the mixture is composed of European, Amerindian and black African races. The percentage of each particular race varies in the different countries of the Americas, depending on the type and the date of their colonization, the grade of development of the original inhabitants, and the importation of African slaves during subsequent centuries.[2]

The noses of descendants of Caucasians and blacks have some characteristics in common with the descendants of Caucasians and Indians. Both of them have a small skeletal framework, rather thick skin, and underdeveloped upper- and lower-lateral cartilages. In many respects the criteria for correction is the same. There are, however, other differences in the facial skeleton, the texture of the skin, and the position of the dental arches between the two groups. Our experience has mainly been with the correction of the mestizo nose found in the mixture of Caucasians and American Indians.

CLINICAL FEATURES

The Euroindian mestizo face is broad with a prominent malar eminence and an increased bizygomatic distance in relation to the vertical dimension. The convexity angle is slightly larger than in the average Caucasian, which means that the nasal spine is located more anteriorly in relation to the face; this effect is increased by the procidentia of both dental arches. The chin may be slightly receding, enhancing the general impression of convexity.

Framed by a wide face, the nose is relatively small, the dorsum is slightly convex with a very small osteocartilaginous hump, and the base is wide in relation to its limited anterior projection. The nostrils are moderately large with a tendency toward appearing more horizontal that is produced by the

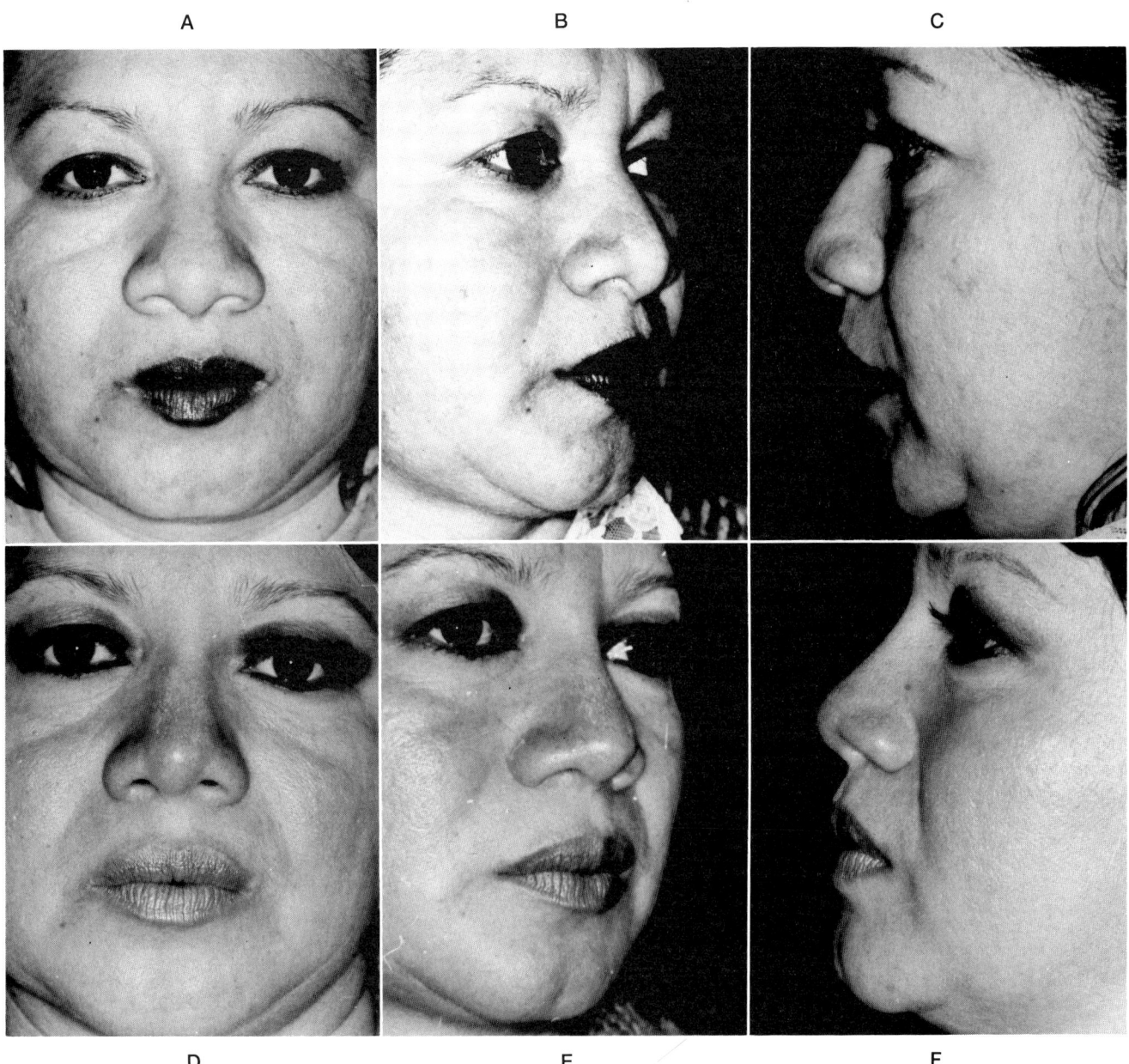

Figure 42-2

Case 3

A 15-year-old female, with many of the classic features of the mestizo nose somewhat exaggerated by microgenia, requested improvement of her nose and lower face. She complained about the drooping nasal tip and the receding chin. Examination revealed a fairly small nose with moderately thick skin, minimal dorsal hump, and limited anterior projection of the tip. The nasolabial angle was 80 degrees. There was prominence of the upper and lower dental arch, with good dental occlusion and a very evident microgenia (Figure 42-3, *A* and *B*).

We decided to do an augmentation rhinoplasty in combination with a sliding osteotomy of the lower edge of the mandible (Figure 42-3, *E*).

With the patient under general anesthesia a minimal resection of the hump was performed in combination with the insertion of a cartilage graft approximately 2 cm long and 8 mm wide into the columella, with its widest section in front of the nasal spine. Another triangular piece of cartilage was inserted in front of the dome of the alar cartilages at the tip of the nose, and the pyramid was narrowed using lateral and medial osteotomies. Through a lower-vestibular incision, the mandible was degloved and exposed, preserving the integrity of the mentalis nerves on each side. With an air-driven saw, a horizontal osteotomy was made at the symphysis, extending posteriorly on each side to approximately 8 cm from the midline. The free lower segment was advanced 12 mm, maintaining contact with the body of the mandible, and was fixed with wire sutures.

Postoperative results showed a considerable improvement of the facial profile. The position of the chin in relation with the forehead, the nose, and the dental arches was greatly improved, as were the nasolabial angle and the anterior projection of the nose (Figure 42-3, *C* and *D*).

When one deals with this type of problem, it is important to visualize the whole face and not only the nose. It is our impression that when microgenia is severe (as it was in this patient) and the dental occlusion is normal, a sliding osteotomy produces more natural results than a Silastic implant. The insertion of a cartilage graft in the columella improves its relationship with the upper lip, opening the nasolabial angle without exposing the nostrils. The cartilage graft to the tip contributes some angularity.

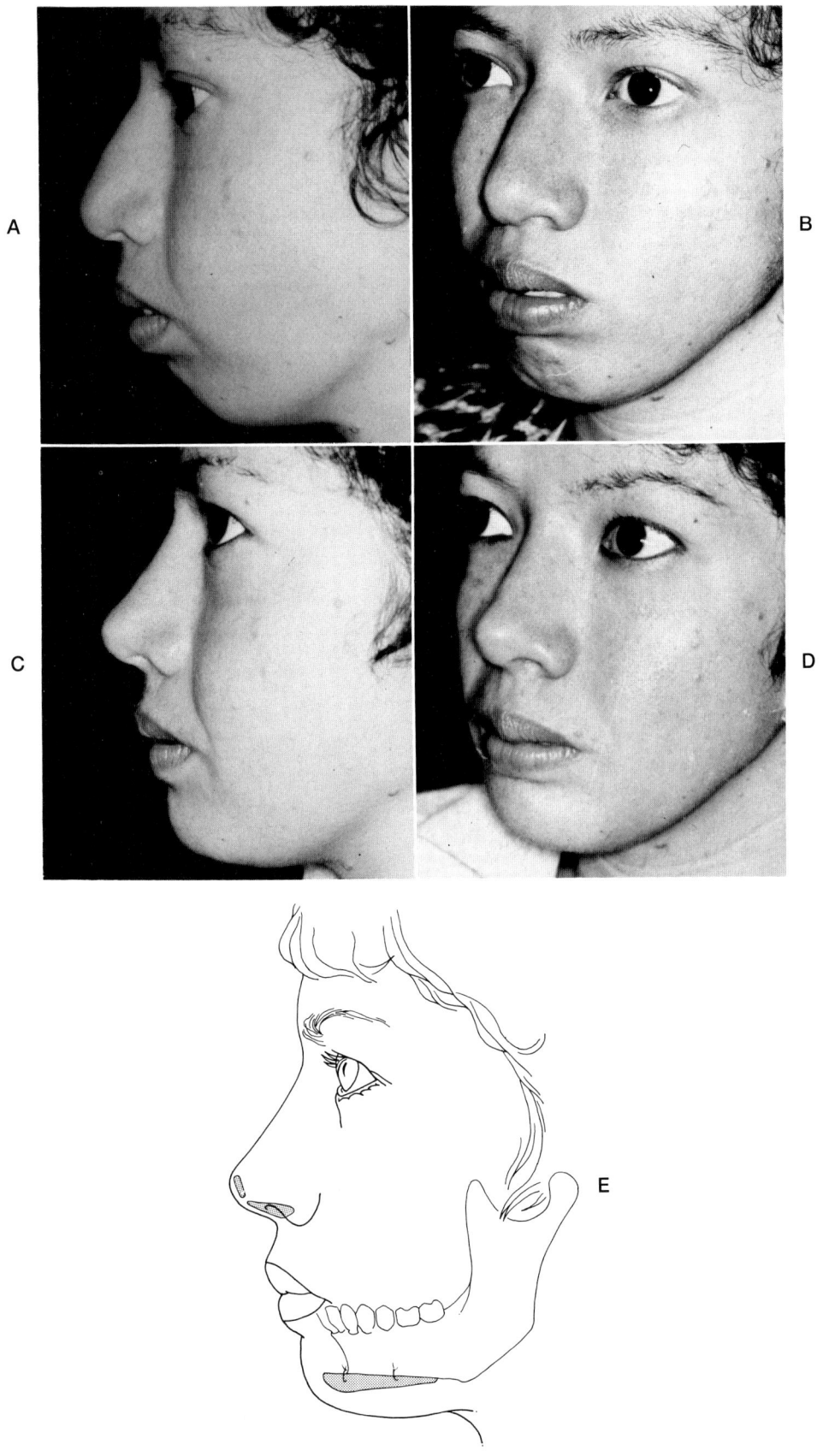

Figure 42-3

Case 4

An 18-year-old female with a typical mestizo face requested an aesthetic correction of her nose. Examination revealed a small nose with a well-defined osteocartilaginous hump, an acute nasolabial angle (resulting from dropping of the tip and from the anterior projection of the dental arch), and limited anterior projection of the nasal tip (Figure 42-4, A-C).

We decided to remove a minimum amount from the dorsum, to increase anterior projection of the tip, and to rotate the alar cartilage to move the tip superiorly while simultaneously advancing the base of the columella (Figure 42-4, G).

With the patient under general anesthesia, a cartilaginous graft was obtained from the septum. A minimal amount of bone was resected from the dorsum with a rasp, and a small section of the cartilaginous hump was resected using the No. 11 blade. A triangular graft of cartilage was introduced in the columella with its base downward in front of the nasal spine. The lower-lateral cartilages were dissected from the skin, and the mucosa was shifted superiorly. Through a small rim incision a triangular piece of cartilage was inserted between the skin and the apex of the medial crus to increase the anterior projection of the tip.

This case illustrates the importance of resecting the absolute minimum from the hump and increasing anterior projection at the tip to obtain a straight nose and also illustrates the use of a columellar cartilaginous graft to improve the nasolabial angle when the superior dental arch is very prominent (Figure 42-4, D-F).

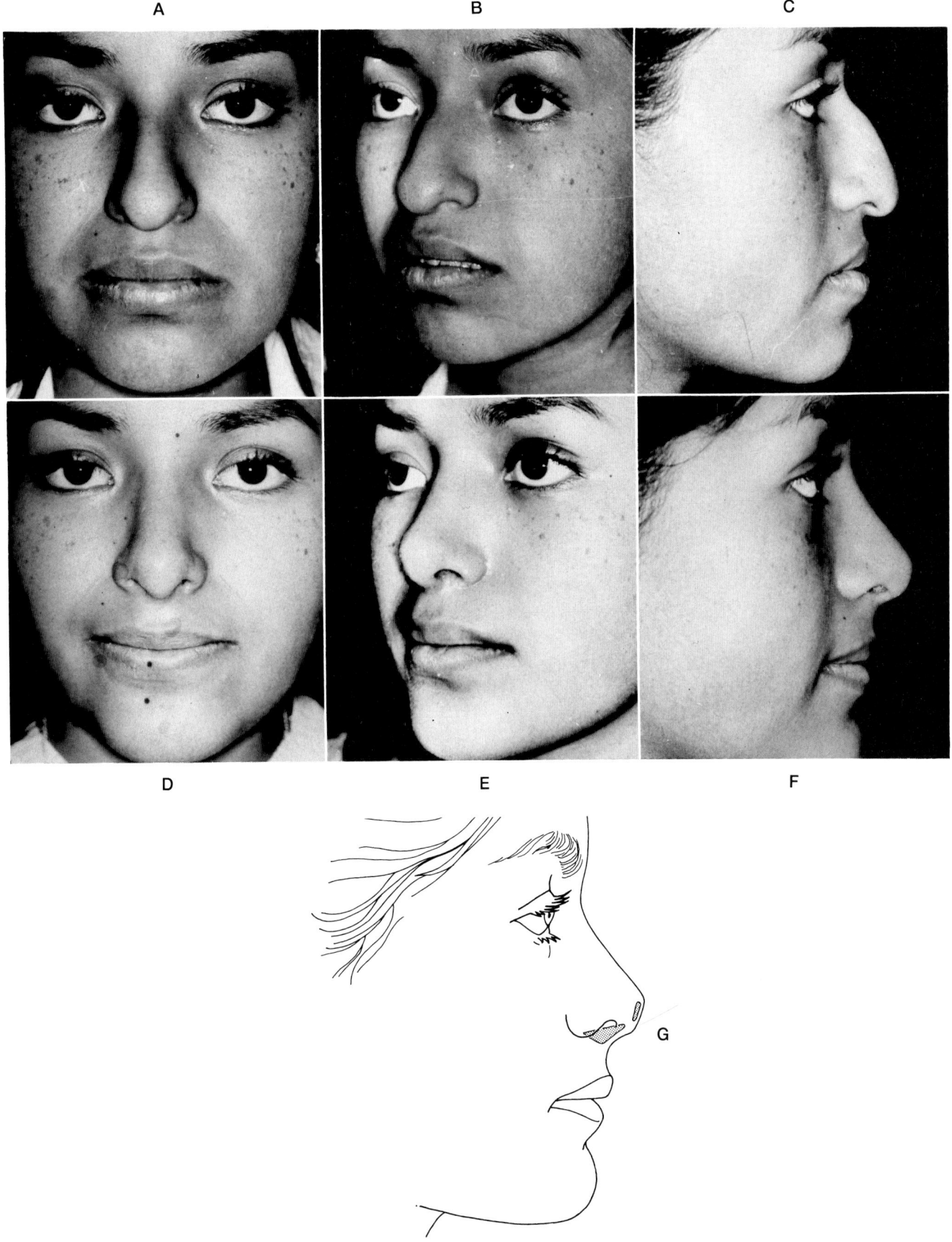

Figure 42-4

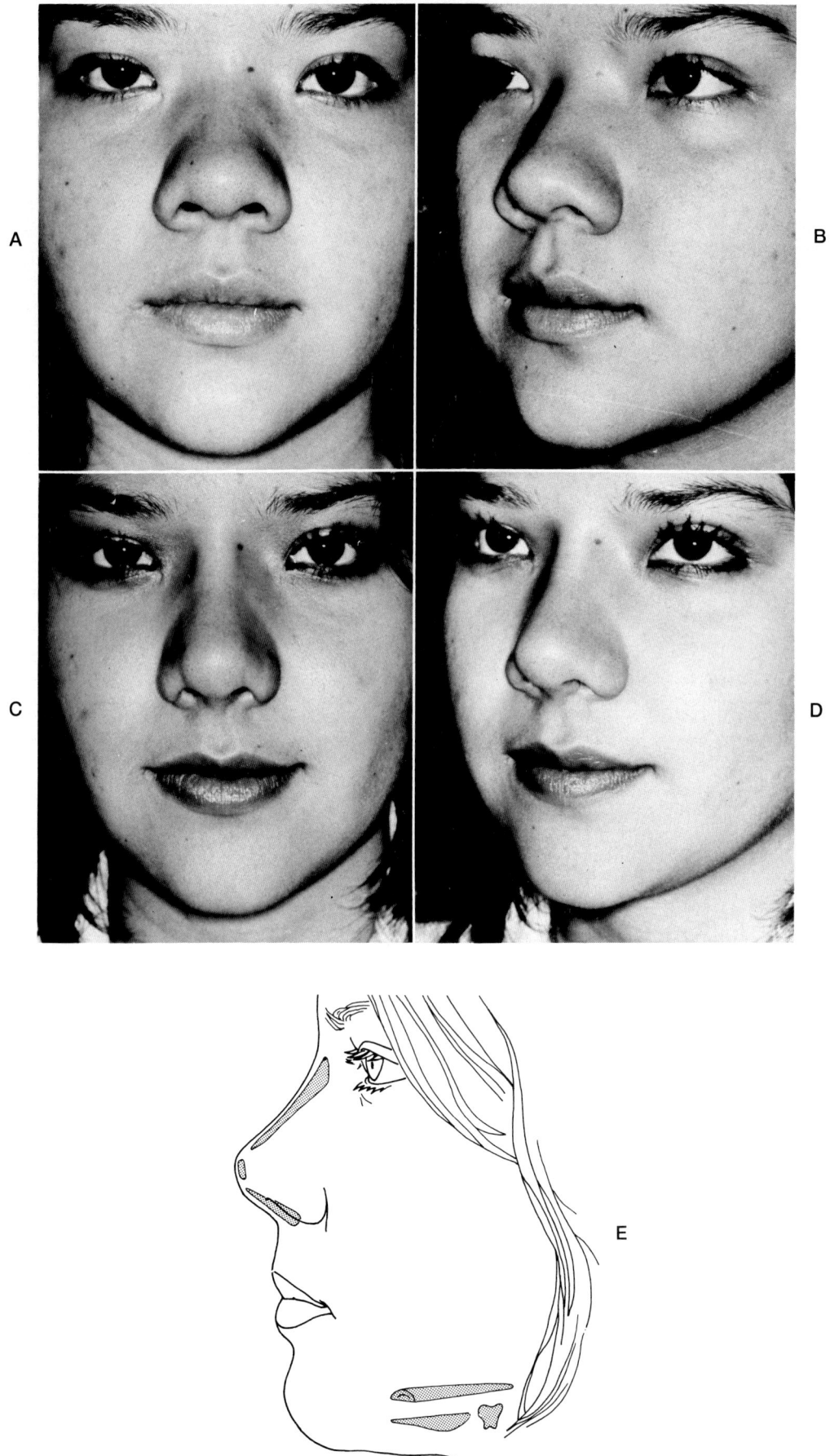

Figure 42-5

Case 5

A female had a relatively small nose covered by fairly thick skin. The dorsum was low, and the lower half of the nose was very wide and was poorly supported by a weak cartilaginous framework. The base of the nostrils was broad, and the columella was receding as a result of the lack of projection of the caudal edge of the septum. Viewed laterally the lower edge of the alae almost hid the columella (Figure 42-5, *A* and *B*).

We decided to increase the projection of the dorsum with a bone graft, to narrow the alar base, and to add projection to the columella and to the tip (Figure 42-5, *E*).

With the patient under general anesthesia, a rib bone graft 6 cm long was obtained through a small submammary incision, preserving the periosteum on the external side. A piece of rib cartilage 4 cm long was also taken from the same area. The rib was split, and the graft was shaped using a Tessier bone crusher to conform the dorsum from the glabella to the caudal edge of the upper-lateral cartilages. A cartilaginous graft was introduced in the columella to provide support and to open the nasolabial angle; a second piece of cartilage was introduced through a small rim incision at the nasal tip to increase the anterior projection of the nose and to produce some angularity. This graft was triangular in shape with sharp edges. A 7 mm wedge was removed from the base of the nostrils on each side, and the skin and wound edges were sutured directly.

Postoperative results were satisfactory. Adding the bone graft to the dorsum improved the relationship between width and height of the nose, giving a much more refined aspect. This procedure was combined with the wedge resection of the alar base and the insertion of cartilaginous grafts in front of the nasal spine and at the nasal tip to help camouflage the skin thickness and to provide some angularity (Figure 42-5, *C* and *D*).

REFERENCES

1. Aufricht, G.: Rhinoplasty and the face, Plast. Reconstr. Surg. **43**:219, 1969.
2. Borah, W., and Cook, S.F.: El mestizaje en la historia de Iberoamérica, Cultura, México, 1962. Instituto Panamericano de Geografía e Historia.
3. Caronni, E.: A new method to correct the nasolabial angle in rhinoplasty, Plast. Reconstr. Surg. **50**:339, 1972.
4. Joseph, J.: Nasenplastik und donstige Gesichtsplastik, Leipzig. 1931, Verlag von Curt Kabitzsch.
5. Ortiz Monasterio, F., and Olmedo, A.: Rhinoplasty on the mestizo nose, Clin. Plast. Surg. **4**:89, 1977.
6. Ortiz Monasterio, F., Olmedo, A., and Ortiz Oscoy, L.: The use of cartilage grafts in primary rhinoplasty, Plast. Reconstr. Surg. **67**:597, 1981.
7. Sheen, J.H.: Achieving more nasal tip projection by use of small autogenous vomer or septal cartilage graft, Plast. Reconstr. Surg. **56**:211, 1975.

43

A Clinical Assessment of Alloplastic Materials in Secondary Rhinoplasty

Jack Sheen

Simplicity and expediency have prompted many surgeons to use alloplastic material for correction of postsurgical nasal deformities, especially if they have used it successfully in primary rhinoplasty. The tissues of the nose after surgery, however, differ from unoperated tissues because of scarring, decreased vascularity, and thinning of the skin. These factors increase the complication rate, because compromised tissues are less tolerant of a foreign body. When these impaired tissues fail to support an implant, patients are frequently told that their bodies have "rejected" the implant. This statement implies that the patient is somehow responsible for the failure. I suggest that it is the surgeon's responsibility to carefully evaluate key factors (such as stress on poorly vascularized tissue, which determines success or failure in implant acceptance) before placing alloplastic material.

Alloplastic material does provide a simple, fast, and seemingly efficient method of reconstruction when compared with autogenous grafts, which involve an additional surgical procedure to obtain graft material, extra operating time and skill, and sometimes less impressive immediate results. Thus surgeons may be seduced into thinking, "It's worth a try; if the implant extrudes later, we can use autogenous grafts then." Meanwhile, the patient looks astonishingly good, with minimal morbidity, and is therefore full of praise and gratitude. This image of the happy, thankful patient may be the last the surgeon sees or remembers, since by the time complications develop, the patient may have moved to other places and/or other physicians.

Defending the use of alloplastic materials, surgeons have said that their complication rate is low. To that I must make three points: (1) there are no statistically valid data that define the complication rate; (2) many patients with complications do not return to the original surgeon so that that surgeon's impression of the complication rate may be grossly inaccurate; and, most important, (3) the rate of complications is insignificant compared to the irreversible tissue destruction that results in permanent deformity to the patient. Any complication rate, however small, cannot justify a procedure that is potentially disfiguring to patients when a better alternative is available—the patient's own tissues.

CASE REPORT

The patient is a 23-year-old model with a history of three previous operations on her nose. The last procedure was performed just 6 months before my initial consultation. A large silicone implant had been used to augment the overreduced nasal skeleton. Shortly after surgery, because of apparent redness, she was treated for 3 months with antibiotics. No culture had been done. A persistent redness and tenderness were most severe on the caudal third of the nose.

Figure 43-1 shows the patient as she appeared at my first consultation. The nose was short, with a rounded, poorly defined, fluctuant nasal tip, which was covered by very thin, translucent skin. A palpable large, single prosthesis extended from the radix to the tip, then down the columella to the maxilla, giving the nose an unnatural, rigid texture. The thick arm of the prosthesis distorted the columella and the membranous septum, making it impossible to evaluate accurately the caudal support. Internally, the valves were narrow. The septal partition was flaccid.

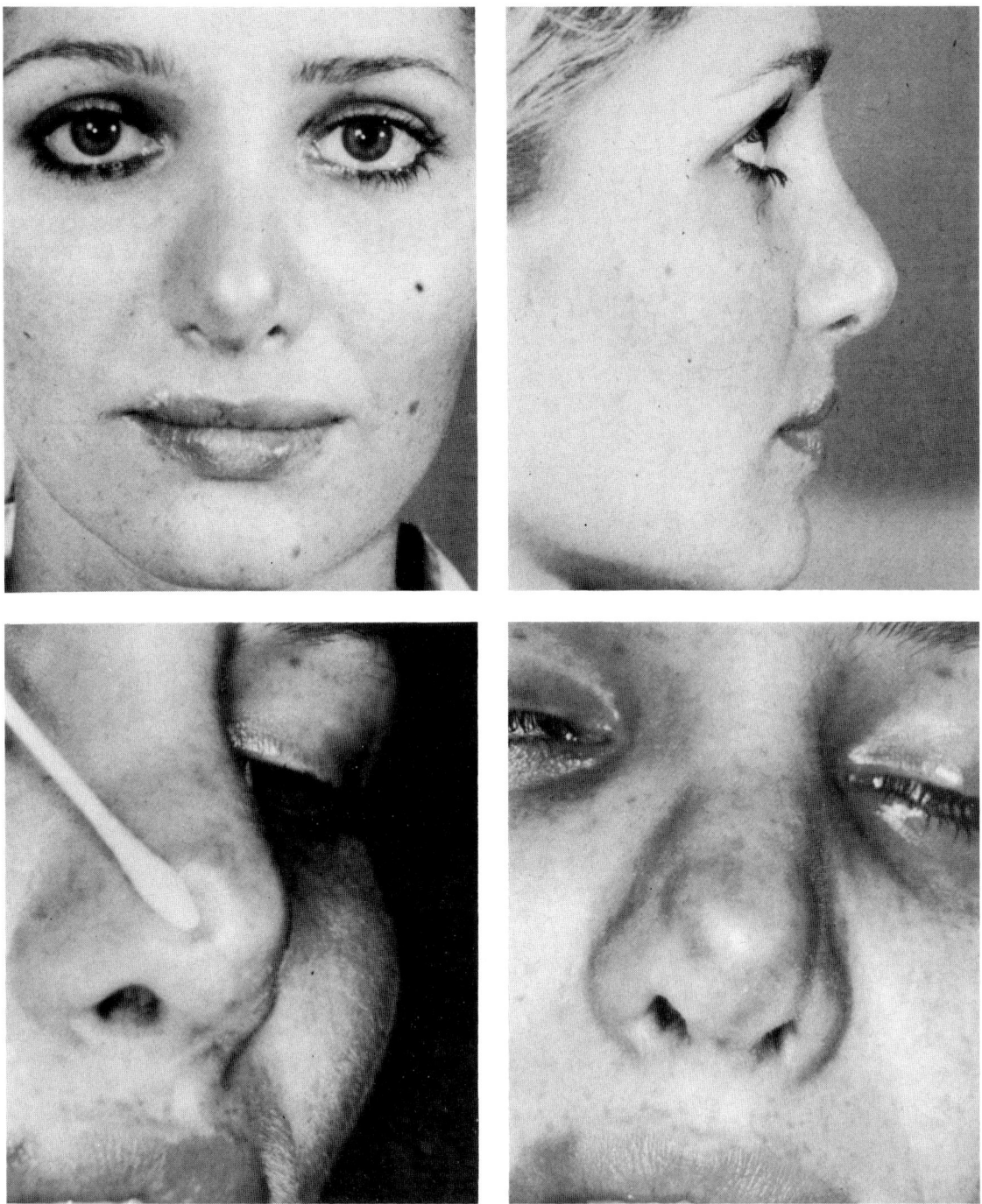

Figure 43-1. Patient 6 months after implantation of silicone prosthesis. The nose is red and swollen; the nasal tip is fluctuant. (From Sheen, J.H., and Sheen, A.P.: Aesthetic rhinoplasty, ed. 2, St. Louis, 1987, The C. V. Mosby Co.)

Surgical approach

It was immediately apparent that the alloplastic prosthesis must be removed if the remaining tissue of the tip was to be salvaged. Tissue had been lost subsequent to infection and to the pressure of the leading edge of the prosthesis, which eroded most of the lobular part of the nasal tip. The area of tissue thinning appeared as a well-defined line of demarcation between the normal and attenuated tissues. The tip was slightly discolored; when palpated, it felt much like a blister under tension. Extrusion was imminent. My first and most important duty was to inform the patient of the following: (1) the antibiotic had failed to stop the process of erosion, and if left alone, the prosthesis would soon erode through the nasal tip; and (2) following extrusion or surgical removal of the prosthesis, the tip would be distorted, and there would be a striking reduction in the overall size of the nose.

After two additional surgical consultations, she agreed to the proposed two-stage plan—first, immediate removal of the implant and, second, if possible, reconstruction with autogenous grafts at least 1 year later, depending on the condition of her tissues.

Surgical procedure

The procedure was done with the patient under general anesthesia. Approximately 3 ml of 1% lidocaine (Xylocaine) with epinephrine was used as a field block, causing spontaneous rupture of the tip with extrusion of purulent material (Figure 43-2). An incision was made at the caudal border of the lower-lateral cartilage, was carried into the membranous septum, and was extended towards the prosthesis. The tissues were gently spread with scissors until the silicone prosthesis was visible. It was grasped by forceps, and the inferior portion of the columellar part was delivered through the wound (Figure 43-3, A). This step was followed by delivery of the remaining dorsal part (Figure 43-3, B). There was some resistance because of tissue ingrowth through perforations in the prosthesis. These tissue bands were severed by sharp Joseph scissors.

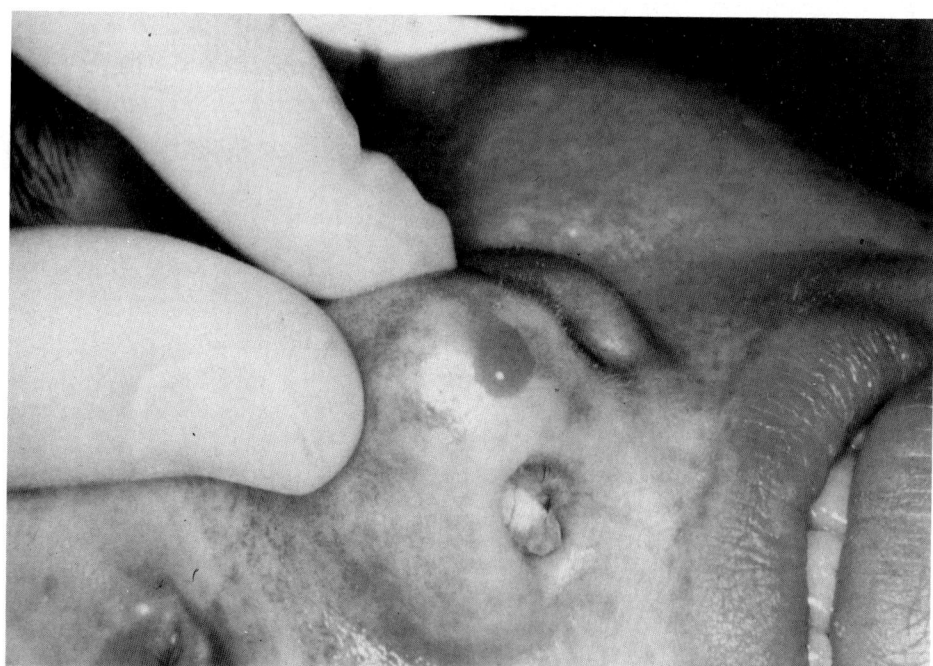

Figure 43-2. Patient just before surgical removal of implant. Spontaneous rupture of the tip, exuding pus. (From Sheen, J.H., and Sheen, A.P.: Aesthetic rhinoplasty, ed. 2, St. Louis, 1987, The C. V. Mosby Co.)

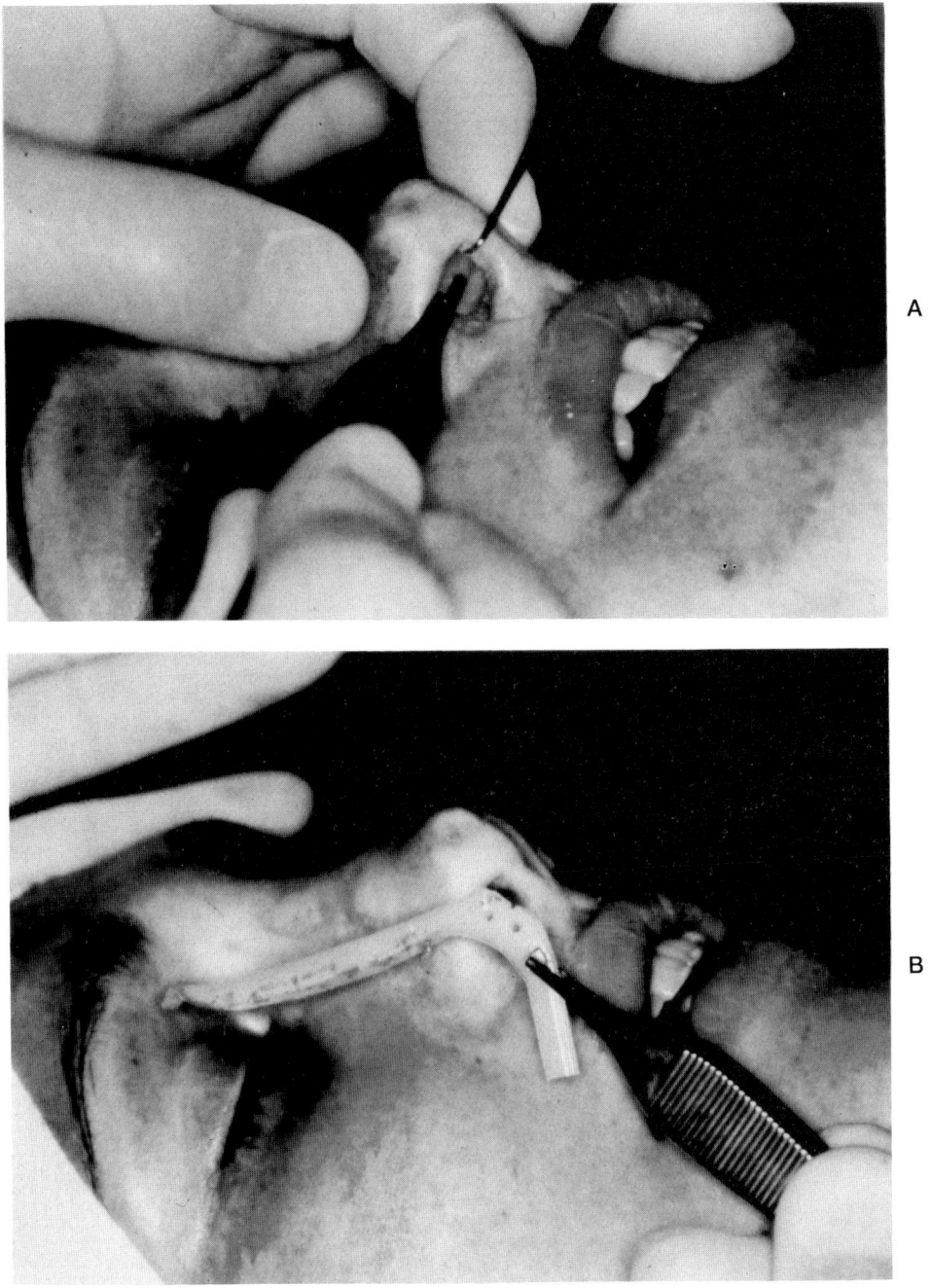

Figure 43-3. A, Removal of inferior arm of silicone implant. **B,** L-shaped, perforated, silicone implant. (From Sheen, J.H., and Sheen, A.P.: Aesthetic rhinoplasty, ed. 2, St. Louis, 1987, The C. V. Mosby Co.)

Following the removal of the prosthesis, the tissues over most of the nose conformed to the remaining skeleton without difficulty. The tip, however, became extremely distorted as the thin skin cover crumpled without the support of the prosthesis and the fluids (Figure 43-4). Cultures were taken, the wound was irrigated, and a dressing was applied.

Postoperatively, her course was uneventful except for persistent drainage from one of the crevices in the tip, which lasted for 1 week after removal of the dressing, that is, for 2 weeks after surgery. Exploration of the sinus tract produced another small piece of silicone (Figure 43-5). After removal of this final implant, healing was uneventful. Thus the patient began the 18-month wait before autogenous reconstruction could take place (Figure 43-6).

Discussion

This case illustrates one of the most important arguments against the use of alloplastic materials in the nose: the possibility of irreversible tissue damage following implantation of alloplastic material. Not only is autogenous material readily available for use as grafts—a fact that in itself puts into question any justification for implanting alloplastics—but also the problems associated with alloplastic implants in the nose are numerous and common. In revisional rhinoplasty, they are often especially serious and disfiguring.

The most common problems, all of which this patient demonstrated, include the following:

1. Thinning of the superficial tissues under tension as they are pressed over the edges of the prosthesis. The foreign implant is isolated from the body and acts as a barrier between the overlying tissue and the supporting tissue.
2. Ingrowth of blood vessels laterally, producing a web of telangiectasis as the tissues attempt to revascularize.
3. Mobility of the implant with a "rocker" effect—the ends of the implant press in opposite directions.
4. Complaint by the patient that the nose is always cold.
5. Translucence of the dorsum when viewed with cross lighting.

Despite all these problems, the second stage of correction was performed, using autogenous ear cartilage. There were no complications.

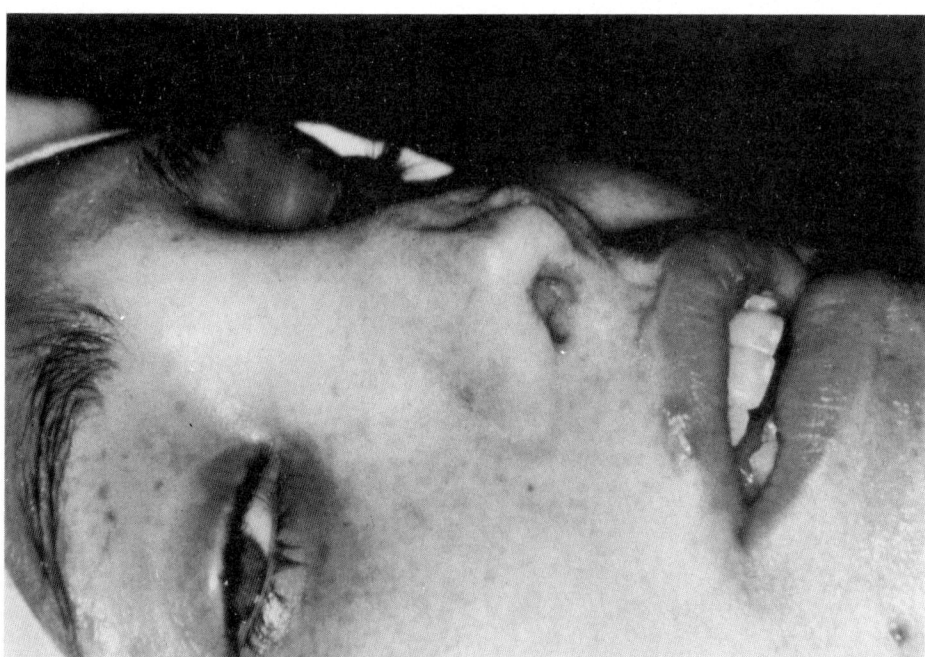

Figure 43-4. After removal of silicone implant, the overlying tissue is extremely thin and distorted. (From Sheen, J.H., and Sheen, A.P.: Aesthetic rhinoplasty, ed. 2, St. Louis, 1987, The C. V. Mosby Co.)

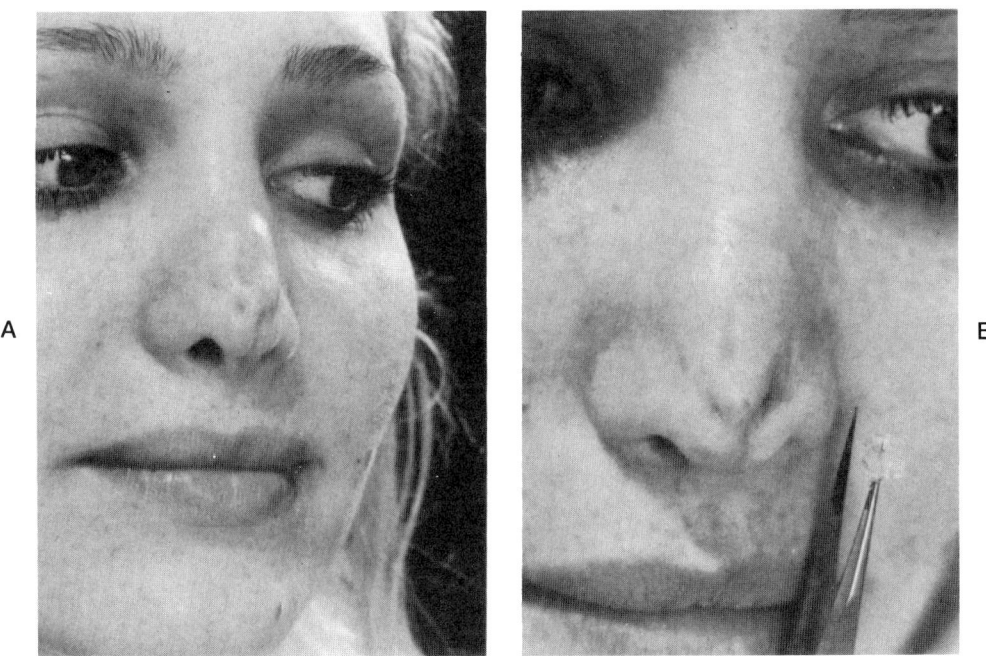

Figure 43-5. A and **B,** Two weeks after removal of implant. A remaining small silicone implant is discovered in the tip. Note dimpling and distortion of tip, resulting from tissue destruction. (From Sheen, J.H., and Sheen, A.P.: Aesthetic rhinoplasty, ed. 2, St. Louis, 1987, The C. V. Mosby Co.)

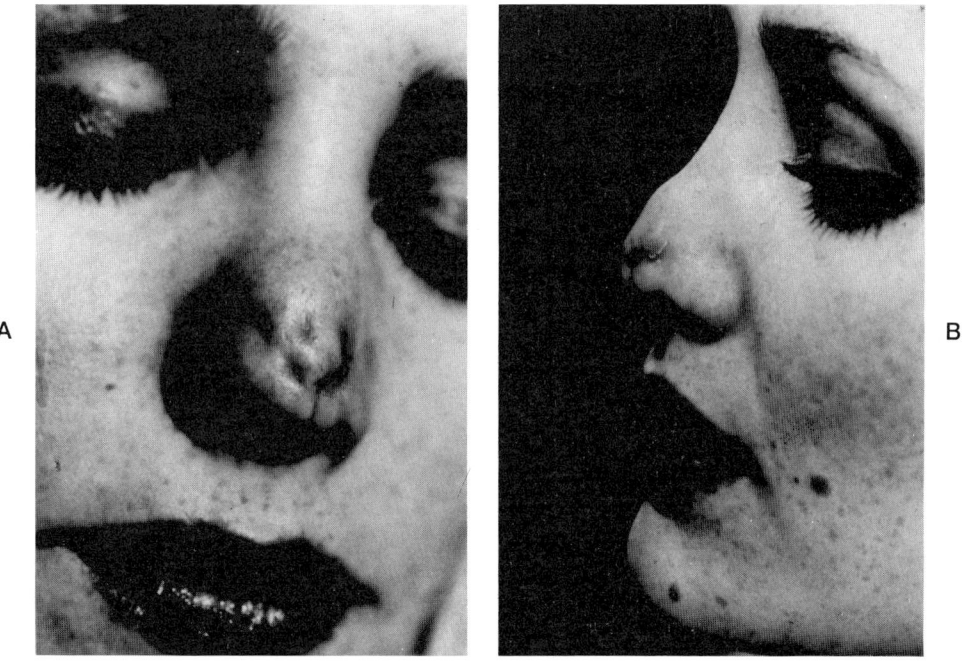

Figure 43-6. A and **B,** One week after removal of remaining silicone implant. Her recovery was uneventful. (From Sheen, J.H., and Sheen, A.P.: Aesthetic rhinoplasty, ed. 2, St. Louis, 1987, The C. V. Mosby Co.)

Point & Counterpoint
Part XIII

Question: How much do you undermine in placing an autogenous graft?

Comment (Jack Sheen): It depends on where I am placing the autogenous graft. For a dorsal graft, I undermine a minimum pocket to contain the graft. For a tip graft, the pocket is usually much larger so that the tissues of the tip will drape properly over the tip graft.

Question: If allografts are so bad, why does the Food and Drug Administration (F.D.A.) permit their continued production and use?

Comment (Eugene Kern): Sometimes we have to question the wisdom of government.

Question: Would you comment on Dr.Robert Flower's experience using alloplastic material for primary rhinoplasty in Orientals and your feeling about it?

Comment (Jack Sheen): My feeling about the use of alloplastic materials in the nose is that it is, at best, a matter of expediency. I think that not only the rate of complications but the tissue destructive nature of those complications should discourage the use of alloplastics, especially when autogenous material is so readily available.

Comment (Fernando Ortiz-Monasterio): I would like to comment on that question also. I have checked very many of the noses done by the Japanese using alloplastic material. They have done a fantastic number. They do the procedure in just a few minutes like any other thing, and they get many good results for two reasons. First, they seek to improve the dorsum just a little bit, and second, they are magnificently fine surgeons. They do very careful work. My contention is that Silastic comes out because of tension. It is very well tolerated. In fact, it is so well tolerated that there is no fibrous tissue formed by the body and the Silastic goes through eventually. If you wish to produce a little more angularity and a more protruding tip, obviously it is going to come out. The reason it stays in the chin or in the breast is because no tension is there.

Comment (Daniel Baker): I tried to emphasize that in our experience with Silastic implants in the black nose that we had no problems. There were only 11 cases in our series, and the selection of the patients and the size of the implant were judicious. We certainly have seen numerous problems with extrusion and problems with the Silastic implant. In most of those cases, the implant has been too large or has been placed in a traumatized nose or a secondary rhinoplasty.

Question: Dr. Baker, you didn't really mention the time frame of that series you presented.

Comment (Daniel Baker): Those patients were studied over a 15-year period, and all of our Silastic implants were in place for more than 1 to 1½ years.

Comment (Jack Sheen): I have seen patients with very late extrusions of silastic implants—more than 15 years following insertion. I have seen so much damage to patients as a result of alloplastic implants that I cannot justify their use, particularly when we have, literally, a viable alternative.

Question: Is there any place for reduction of tissue bulk in the tip through external skin excisions?

Comment (Fernando Ortiz-Monasterio): I have had a lot of experience with external skin incisions in grafts. In children, the external incision eventually becomes an almost invisible scar. I don't like to use it in adults except in very exceptional circumstances, since the scars are never very good there.

Comment (Eugene Tardy): I do think there is a place for external skin excisions. I agree that you should avoid them if possible. But I have a series of patients who had incredibly bad soft-tissue polly-beaks, in whom the skin, perhaps during the splinting, has been pulled together and the cast has accentuated that and in whom the skeletal framework has been badly overreduced. On occasion, those patients (and most of them are male) can gain not only a nice aesthetic result but also the loss of a very terrible appearance by using a simple fusiform excision right down the center of the nose. If you create incisions right down the center of the nose, repair them carefully, and add a little dermabrasion later, that scar becomes acceptably inconspicuous. It is a compromise. All rhinoplasty is compromise. You trade one thing for another and in those people in whom a terribly grotesque soft-tissue polly-beak abnormality exists, direct excision can be an acceptable answer. I also use direct skin excisions near the root of the nose in aging patients with rhytids created by redundant skin. This "rhytidorhinoplasty" leaves acceptably inconspicuous scars when incisions are properly sited.

PART

XIV

NASAL SURGERY IN OLDER PATIENTS AND IN CHILDREN

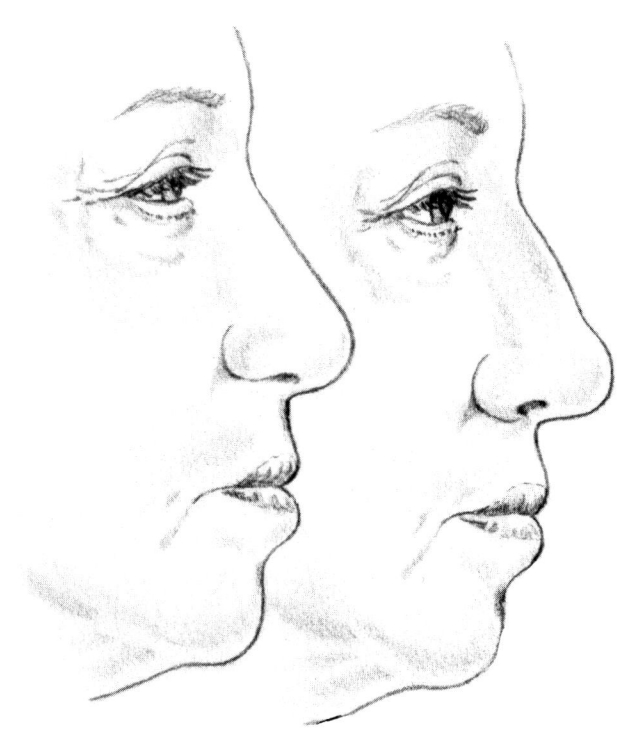

44

Acute Nasal Trauma

Eugene B. Kern

The nose is the most frequently injured facial structure.[1-5] Accurate diagnosis of the injury is possible only when a complete history is recorded and a thorough physical examination is performed.[1-4,6] Essential aspects of the history should include the exact cause and time of the injury and a record of the presence of pain, obstruction to nasal breathing, and epistaxis. The presence of epistaxis indicates that the injury has been severe enough to lacerate the nasal mucosa.

Examination of the external nasal structures (Figure 44-1) should include palpation of both the bony and the cartilaginous nasal pyramid to detect the presence of deformities, crepitus, and abnormalities in mobility. Photographs must be taken to document deformities, ecchymosis, abrasions, edema, external lacerations, and the extent of the facial damage. The internal nasal examination requires use of a head lamp or head-mirror lighting, suction, mucosal vasoconstriction, and topical anesthesia.[3] Thorough visualization of intranasal structures is mandatory. Special attention should be given to the most common posttraumatic problems: mucosal tears, fractures and dislocations of the septum, and septal hematomas.[3-10] The sequelae of these conditions—including septal abscess, necrosis of septal and pyramidal cartilage, and permanent distortion of the nasal architecture leading to nasal airway obstruction or cosmetic deformities (or both)—have been well documented.[2-10] If the internal structures of the nose are not examined, the effects of external nasal trauma may be overlooked. The primary care physician rather than the specialist usually manages the nasal injury in the emergency room. It is important that all the physicians responsible for the care of the acute nasal injury are competent in performing intranasal examination regardless of their specialty.

The purpose of this chapter is to review the care given to the patient with an acutely injured nose in an emergency room setting. From this data we can draw some basic principles for management of the acutely injured nose so that permanent functional nasal breathing disturbances and cosmetic deformities can be avoided or at least minimized.

To determine what really happens to the patient with acute nasal trauma, a random sampling of the charts of 250 patients was undertaken. Three distinct groups of patients with nasal trauma were evaluated. The patients were seen in the emergency room of two hospitals in Rochester, Minnesota, during the period 1970 to 1975. Group 1 included 100 children, 1 to 12 years of age. Group 2 included 100 adults older than 21 years of age; the intent was to determine whether treatment of the adult population varied from that for children. Group 3 was composed of 50 patients of all ages with roentgenographically documented nasal fractures; these patients were included to determine the influence of a confirmed nasal fracture on methods of examination and treatment.

All patients suffered blunt trauma to the face or nose severe enough to warrant physician evaluation in a hospital environment. Patients suffering simple lacerations of the nose or face by a sharp object were excluded from this study. Also excluded were patients with extensive traumatic injuries in whom thorough examination of the nose at the initial evaluation in the emergency room was not reasonable because of the presence of more severe or potentially life-threatening injuries. The patients were examined by resident physicians from various acute care spe-

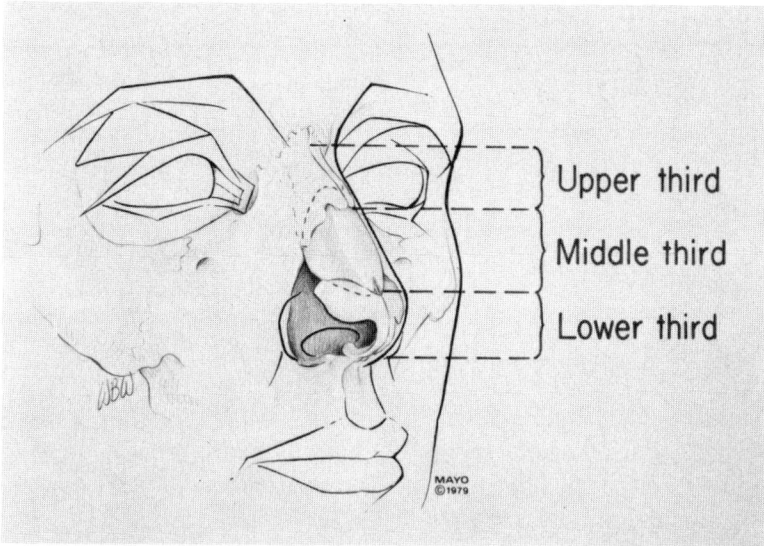

Figure 44-1. Nasal structures. Upper third is bony pyramid, composed of nasal bones and frontal process of maxilla. Middle third is cartilaginous pyramid, consisting of upper-lateral cartilage (roof cartilage) that overlies nasal septum. Lower third is lobular cartilage (alar cartilage). (From Kern, E.B.: Surgery of the nasal valve. In Sisson, G.A., and Tardy, M.E., editors: Plastic and reconstructive surgery of the face and neck, vol. 2, New York, 1977, Grune & Stratton, Inc.)

cialties during the emergency room rotation of their residency programs and not by otorhinolaryngology residents or staff consultants.

History

The precipitating event was a fall in 67% of the children in Group 1. The blunt trauma was sufficient to cause laceration of the nasal skin in 45 of these 100 patients. The presence or absence of epistaxis, which usually indicates the presence of a mucosal tear, was recorded in only 31% of these children.

Trauma in the adult patients in Group 2 was caused primarily by vehicle accidents, sports injuries, and fighting. External lacerations were present in 52 of these 100 patients. The presence or absence of epistaxis was recorded in only 28% of these adults.

The causes of the fractures in patients in Group 3 were mainly the same as the precipitating events listed for patients in Groups 1 and 2. The presence or absence of epistaxis was noted in only 39% of these patients.

Physical examination

An intranasal examination was recorded in only 20 of the 100 pediatric patients in Group 1, in 22 of the 100 adult patients in Group 2, and in 21 of the 50 patients with nasal fractures in Group 3 (Table 5). The external nose was palpated in 49% of the children in Group 1 and in 67% of the adults in Group 2.

Roentgenographic examination

A roentgenogram of the nose was taken in 51 of the 100 children in Group 1; among this group, there were only two fractures, both in older children (ages 10 and 11 years). In 58 of the 100 adults in Group 2, nasal roentgenograms were taken; a fracture was discovered in 18 persons.

Treatment

Emergency room treatment of the nonfractured nose usually was limited to closure of external lacerations and supportive measures such as application of ice packs. In the separate group of 50 patients who had roentgenographically documented fractures (Group 3), 23 fractures were severe enough to warrant reduction. Five of these 23 patients were treated in the operating room, only one of whom had an intranasal examination before the operative procedure! In the 18 remaining patients, reduction of the fracture was performed in the emergency room. Only 9 (50%) of these 18 patients had an intranasal examination before dismissal from the emergency room.

TABLE 5. Frequency of intranasal examination

Group	Number of patients	Description of group	Intranasal examination recorded on chart (%)
1	100	Pediatric patients	20
2	100	Adult patients	22
3	50	Fracture patients*	42

*Roentgenographic evidence of fracture of the nasal pyramid.

Definitive treatment should be instituted before edema and bruising occur or after they subside. Intranasal hematomas should be evacuated to avoid septal abscess, saddle nose deformity, and/or septal perforation. Fractures of the septum must be reduced and stented to obtain optimum healing. External lacerations must be repaired, and intranasal lacerations of the mucosa require diagnosis and repair. Intranasal plastic septal stents are inserted to prevent post-operative mucosal adhesions. The nose is "put to rest" by packing it, thereby sparing the mucosa the desiccating effects of dry inspired air. A frank discussion with the patient and/or parents is paramount, because a secondary operative procedure may be required at some point in the future.

DISCUSSION

The present study demonstrates that adequate nasal examination is not being performed in the emergency room. The primary reasons for inadequate evaluation may be the physician's lack of expertise in rhinologic examination and a failure to recognize that the complications and sequelae of nasal trauma can be very disturbing or serious to the patient. In this study inspection of the intranasal structures—the most important part of the examination—was accomplished in only 20% of the 100 pediatric patients in Group 1 and, although theoretically easier, in only 22% of the 100 adult patients in Group 2. Among the 50 patients sustaining sufficient trauma to produce a fracture of the nasal bony pyramid (Group 3), the internal nasal structures were examined in only 21 patients (42%).

Several authors have maintained that roentgenographic documentation of nasal fractures is much less useful than is clinical evidence of structural deformity.[1-4,7,8,11] DeLacey and others[11] reviewed 100 roentgenograms of nasal injury and pointed out that the roentgenographic studies contributed nothing to the management. Management should be based solely on the history and the physical examination, including the evaluation of the septum and the rest of the intranasal contents. Most childhood nasal injuries involve the cartilaginous portion of the nasal pyramid and are not evident on roentgenograms. This is especially true in young children who normally have short nasal bones. The present study substantiates this finding. The only roentgenographically documented nasal fractures in the 51 patients in Group 1 who had roentgenograms taken were in two older children with well-developed nasal bones. Roentgenographic examination, therefore, should be strictly an adjunctive technique used to determine the extent and severity of the injury. The history and the physical examination of the external and internal nasal structures should not be supplanted by x-ray studies. A negative x-ray report should *never* be used as a substitute for a good examination. Septal injury can be diagnosed only by a complete intranasal examination.

In the treatment of the displaced nose, closed reduction has long been advocated as a safe and effective method of management.[1] To the rhinologist, however, it is evident that this approach is acceptable only in the most minimally traumatized nose.[3,6,9] Severe trauma to the external nasal pyramid usually results in septal injuries as well.[5] The nasal septum is the single most important structure for determining both the functional and the cosmetic aspects of the nose. An external nasal deformity usually cannot be treated adequately without concurrent evaluation and correction of pathological changes in the nasal septum.[8] In the series of cases reviewed, 18 patients had closed reductions, only 9 (50%) of whom had an intranasal examination at the time of the reduction.

Intranasal structures, including the septum, must be examined before initiation of primary treatment. Open reduction is the most acceptable treatment for severe nasal septal injury. Prompt evacuation of a septal hematoma is necessary to avoid sequelae. Adequate drainage removes pressure and restores nutrition to the septal cartilage. A hematoma with no other sign of septal injury can be incised and evacuated, and internal nasal packing can be introduced to prevent the recurrence of hematoma. Packing should remain in place for approximately 5 days to allow healing to begin adequately. With the presence of a foreign body such as a nasal pack, antibiotics are also given to prevent infection. An external splint and taping are applied to prevent a dorsal hematoma, to reduce edema, and to provide adequate protection to minimize pain and discomfort. The patient should be instructed to look for any signs of increasing pain, fever, tenderness, or swelling, and the patient should be reexamined 24 hours later.

In patients with septal dislocation or fracture, the septum must be explored surgically and reconstructed as necessary, with procedures dictated by the extent of the injury.[3,6,9] Septal and external fractures must be exposed and realigned during the same operation so that the nose can be reconstructed in the controlled operating room environment to promote uncomplicated healing and to avoid nasal functional (respiratory) and cosmetic sequelae.[10]

In children with nasal injuries, it may be necessary to examine the nose with the child under general anesthesia. As in the adult, the pediatric patient should have the septal and external reconstruction that is necessary to prevent functional and cosmetic nasal deformities, although rhinoplasty, including tip cartilage modification, should not be performed in the child. When cartilage is lost, whether through hematoma or abscess, it is replaced with fibrous tissue. Scar retraction and loss of support of the lower two thirds of the nose result in a nasal saddle deformity, a retracted columella, and widening of the base of the nose.[12] Early traumatic absence of the cartilaginous septum may also cause maxillary hypoplasia.[13] Minor injuries of the septal bone or cartilage may arrest or stimulate growth.[12,14] Scar tissue can cause buckling or twisting of the septal cartilage. Cartilaginous overgrowth can occur in its membranous envelope, with later bending and resultant nasal airway obstruction. Pirsig and Lehmann[15] demonstrated that the long-term reaction of growing septal cartilage to trauma was incomplete regeneration of cartilage. Regeneration was often unidirectional and thus caused deviation of the nasal septum. In adults or children who have difficulty breathing, a septal deformity secondary to such a minor childhood injury may be found. The degree of deviation does not have to be great to cause significant airway symptoms. A thick, slightly angulated or dislocated septum can cause narrowing of the anterior region of the nose, and this narrowing can be the difference between adequate or inadequate breathing.[16]

The idea that nasal surgery in children causes subsequent facial deformities is not totally correct. Pirsig[17] reported about a series of 261 children who underwent nasal septal reconstruction for nasal obstruction, and no arrest of nasal growth occurred after surgery. Fear that surgery performed on the growing septum will result in retardation or abnormal growth of the nasal pyramid is not justified. Present surgical treatment of septal injuries is not the radical "submucous resection" of septal structures; rather, the current surgical concepts are based on the principles of functional reconstruction, which inlcudes realignment and replacement of septal skeletal structures. Any nasal injury, if left untreated, can in itself cause a subsequent deformity. An intact nasal septum in childhood is necessary for normal facial development. Repeated facial trauma in the child should raise the suspicion that this is a battered child.[3]

SUMMARY

Obviously, patients with extensive traumatic injuries or even potentially life-threatening injuries need them managed before their nasal injuries receive definitive treatment. However, an aggressive examination of patients with nasal injuries is advocated, regardless of the apparent severity of the injury; otherwise, functional and cosmetic complications can result. We who have treated these patients have seen both breathing and cosmetic disturbances following nasal trauma. In the pediatric population it may be necessary to bring the patient to the operating room to examine and assess the intranasal structures adequately. To provide optimal care, every physician caring for patients with acute nasal trauma should become proficient in obtaining the history and in conducting the physical examination. The history should include an inquiry about previous nasal trauma or pathological conditions and should provide an estimate of posttraumatic nasal airway obstruction and a determination of the amount of blood loss (epistaxis). The examination should include thorough palpation of both the bony and cartilaginous portions of the external nasal pyramid. Intranasal examination is mandatory. The internal nasal structures can be examined adequately only with appropriate lighting that allows complete visualization and the use of both hands for suction and manipulation. Mucosal vasoconstriction and topical mucosal anesthesia are usually required to perform adequate evaluation, including palpation of the intranasal structures when warranted. Photographs of the injury should be taken in all patients with nasal trauma. Roentgenographic examination does not supplant the history and the physical examination (especially the intranasal examination) in the management of the injured nose. A negative x-ray report is *never* a substitute for a complete intranasal examination. Nasal surgery on the already injured nose will usually not retard or disturb growth any more than the initial trauma. Treatment of the complications of nasal injuries is more difficult than providing adequate initial management.[18] Only with an accurate diagnosis during the initial examination can appropriate treatment be instituted in the patient with an acutely injured nose.

ACKNOWLEDGMENT

I wish to thank my colleagues, David M. Barrs, M.D., Robert J. Carpenter III, M.D., and Kerry D. Olsen, M.D. for their contributions to this work.

REFERENCES

1. Cottle, M.H.: Nasal surgery in children, Eye, Ear, Nose & Throat Month. 30:32, 1951.
2. De Lacey, G.J., and others: The radiology of nasal injuries: problems of interpretation and clinical relevance, Brit. J. Radiol. 50:412, 1977.
3. Drumhell, G.H.: Acute nasal trauma, Int. Rhinol. 8:161, 1970.
4. Facer, G.W.: Management of nasal injury, Postgrad. Med. 57(6):123, 1975.
5. Fry, H.J.H.: The pathology and treatment of haematoma of the nasal septum, Br. J. Plast. Surg. 22:331, 1969.
6. Goode, R.L., and Spooner, T.R.: Management of nasal fractures in children: a review of current practices, Clin. Pediatr. 11:526, 1972.
7. Hadley, R.B.: Nasal injuries in children, Int. Rhinol. 6:93, 1968.
8. Hinderer, K.H.: Fundamentals of anatomy and surgery of the nose, Birmingham, Alabama, 1971, Aesculapius Publishing Co.
9. Hinderer, K.H.: Nasal problems in children, Ear Nose Throat J. 57:116, 1978.
10. Jordan, L.W.: The management of acute injuries of the nasal septum, Laryngoscope 77:1121, 1967.
11. Jordan, L.W.: Acute nasal and septal injuries, Eye Ear Nose Throat Mon 53:508, 1974.
12. Kemble, J.V.H.: The importance of the nasal septum in facial development, J. Laryngol. Otol. 87:379, 1973.
13. Olsen, K.D., Carpenter III, R.J., and Kern, E.B.: Nasal septal trauma in children, Pediatrics 64:32, 1979.
14. Pirsig, W.: Septal plasty in children: influence on nasal growth, Rhinology 15:193, 1977.
15. Pirsig, W., and Lehmann, I.: The influence of trauma on the growing septal cartilage, Rhinology 13:39, 1975.
16. Schultz, R.C., and deVillers, Y.T.: Nasal fractures, J. Trauma 15:319, 1975.
17. Sputh, C.B.: Experiences with nasal injuries, Int. Rhinol. 8:171, 1970.

45

Cleft-Lip Nose

Fernando Ortiz-Monasterio, Alvaro Olmedo

Great progress has been made in the last 3 decades in the treatment of clefts of the lip and palate. In the hands of an experienced surgeon, a satisfactory lip should be obtained in all patients with unilateral clefts and most cases of bilateral clefts. Normal speech can be achieved using palatoplasty in approximately 80% of the patients, and secondary procedures should repair the velopharyngeal incompetency in another 11%. Good orthodontics can prevent or correct maxillary collapse and can produce normal dental occlusion.

Technical improvements have been less impressive concerning the nasal deformity. Many patients with good labial and palatal repair have a distorted nose that remains as a stigma of the congenital malformation. On the other hand, an adequate nasal correction performed simultaneously with the primary lip repair can result in acceptable, nearly symmetrical noses in most infants.

Innumerable techniques have been described for the secondary correction of the cleft-lip nose. We present our experience with the secondary correction of the cleft-lip nose using two different technical approaches: the external skin incision and the intranasal operation. Our observations are related mainly to the unilateral cleft deformity.

CHARACTERISTICS OF THE CLEFT-LIP NOSE

The nasal deformity in cleft-lip patients affects all the anatomical elements of the nose and the paranasal area as part of the congenital anomaly and also as a result of the shifting of tissues and the scar formation produced by primary lip surgery. The nasal pyramid is always deviated and asymmetrical, the piriform fossa is depressed on the cleft side, and the whole midface may be retruded. Septal deviation is present in all of the patients.

The nasal tip is asymmetrical because the dome of the lower-lateral cartilage is less prominent on the cleft side. In many patients there is marked drooping of the tip, resulting from the binding effect of a short hemicolumella and the anomalous position of the alar cartilage, which is usually smaller and located in a more inferior position. Its curvature does not correspond to the normal side, resulting in alteration of the dimension, the size, and the shape of the nostril. The base of the nostril is too wide and is crossed by a scar that extends into the nasal floor. Oronasal fistulae are common. The alar-cheek junction is sloped and is displaced laterally.

TIMING OF SURGERY

Many children who had good labial and palatal repair performed in infancy have a typical cleft nose that severely affects facial aesthetics and represents an emotional burden on the patient during the critical growth years. In spite of its crippling physiological effect, the correction of the nasal deformity has traditionally been postponed until growth is completed, usually after puberty, because of the assumption that early surgery would interfere with nasal growth.

Experience obtained from caring for children with severe nasal injuries and from the long-term observation of patients in whom major craniofacial surgery, including the nasal and paranasal areas, was performed during infancy, has demonstrated that early surgery, when properly performed, will not alter nasal development.[6] Our own series of complete rhinoplasties, which included medial and lateral osteotomies, cartilage repositioning, and conservative septoplasty performed before the patients reached puberty, shows normal nasal growth.[5] Since that series was performed, we have operated on a large number of children between 6 and 9 years of age with no alteration of nasal and facial development.

For these reasons we believe that rhinoplasty for the cleft nose should be done early near age 6 or 7 years, even if a minor secondary correction might be necessary at a later date.

TECHNIQUES FOR SURGICAL CORRECTION

The correction of the nasal skeleton in the patient with a cleft nose does differ from the conventional aesthetic rhinoplasty. A conservative technique with minimal resection of the osteocartilaginous hump must be used. In children no tissues are resected from the nasal dorsum, and the mobilization of the nasal bones is limited to the minimum. A "green stick" fracture is made, slowly luxating the nasal bones from the frontonasal suture, which acts as a hinge. Perfect stability of the skeleton is maintained in this manner.

Performing conservative surgery of the septum is important, and the subpericondral dissection is limited to the distorted segments. The inferior edge of the septum is repositioned on the midline. Resection of tissues is avoided, the deviated bony segments are fractured and mobilized, and gentle crushing of badly deformed cartilage is performed in situ.

Tip correction

The correction of the nasal tip requires elongation of the hemicolumella, repositioning of the alar cartilage, and shifting of the alar base on the cleft side. These procedures are combined with conventional tip refinement maneuvers on the normal side and frequently with the insertion of cartilaginous grafts to the tip and to the columella.

The correction of the nasal tip is achieved through an external skin incision or through an intranasal approach. External incisions of different types have been used extensively in the past to obtain alar symmetry.[1-3,9,10] Early in this century, Joseph proposed placing an incision on the midline of the columella and extending it on a curved line across the lower-lateral cartilage on the cleft side.[4] This procedure was later modified by Berkeley, who extended the incisions on the lip to make the correction of the cleft of the lip and the nasal deformity simultaneous.[1,2] We have used the external nasal incisions extensively for the primary correction of clefts as well as for secondary rhinoplasties.[9]

For the nasal correction the incision is made vertically along the midline of the columella from the nasal spine to the level of the dome of the alar cartilages. At the base of the nose the incision is curved laterally and is continued parallel to the nostril on the cleft side for 3 to 4 mm (Figure 45-1, A and B). Superiorly the incision is also curved laterally, following the cephalic edge of the abnormal alar cartilage to the base of the alae. A second parallel incision is made at the mucocutaneous junction of the columella on the cleft side, extending superiorly along the mucosa on the intercartilaginous fold. It continues inferiorly into the nasal floor parallel to the incision on the skin for a few mm; then the two are connected by a small deep cut across the rim. One half of the columella and the complete alae are elevated as a flap composed of skin, cartilage, and mucosa and based laterally at the alar base. The alar cartilage is sutured to the corresponding cartilage on the other side in a slightly overcorrected position. The skin and the mucosa of the columella are sutured in their new, more-elevated position, and a small ellipse of skin is resected from the nasal incision along the alae to elevate the rim into a position symmetrical with the normal side. The shape of this skin resection depends on the lateral position of the alar tissues. The cephalic edge of the alar cartilage is sutured to the lateral cartilage in its new position, and the skin is closed (Figure 45-1, C and D). A defect that corresponds to the superior rotation of the tissues remains at the base of the columella. The insertion of the base of the alae to the nasal floor is freed and advanced medially to fill the defect, simultaneously improving the shape of the nostril and narrowing the alar base. A small redundancy of skin may be observed on the lip and can be corrected by a small wedge resection of the superior portion of the scar from previous lip repair.

The refinement of the nasal tip on the normal side is performed in a conventional fashion through an intercartilaginous or transcartilaginous incision according to the preference of the surgeon (see Figure 45-1, B). If necessary, a triangular cartilaginous graft is introduced through a small rim incision to enhance tip definition.

The transcutaneous approach is a simple procedure that permits a relatively inexperienced surgeon to perform correction of a rather complex deformity. Its main limitation is that the elongation of the hemicolumella and the elevation of the nasal dome are performed entirely at the expense of the medial crus, whereas the lateral portion of the alar cartilage remains untouched. The incisions are visible for a short period of time; after a few months, they are hardly visible even when performed in young adults. We have used this procedure in pa-

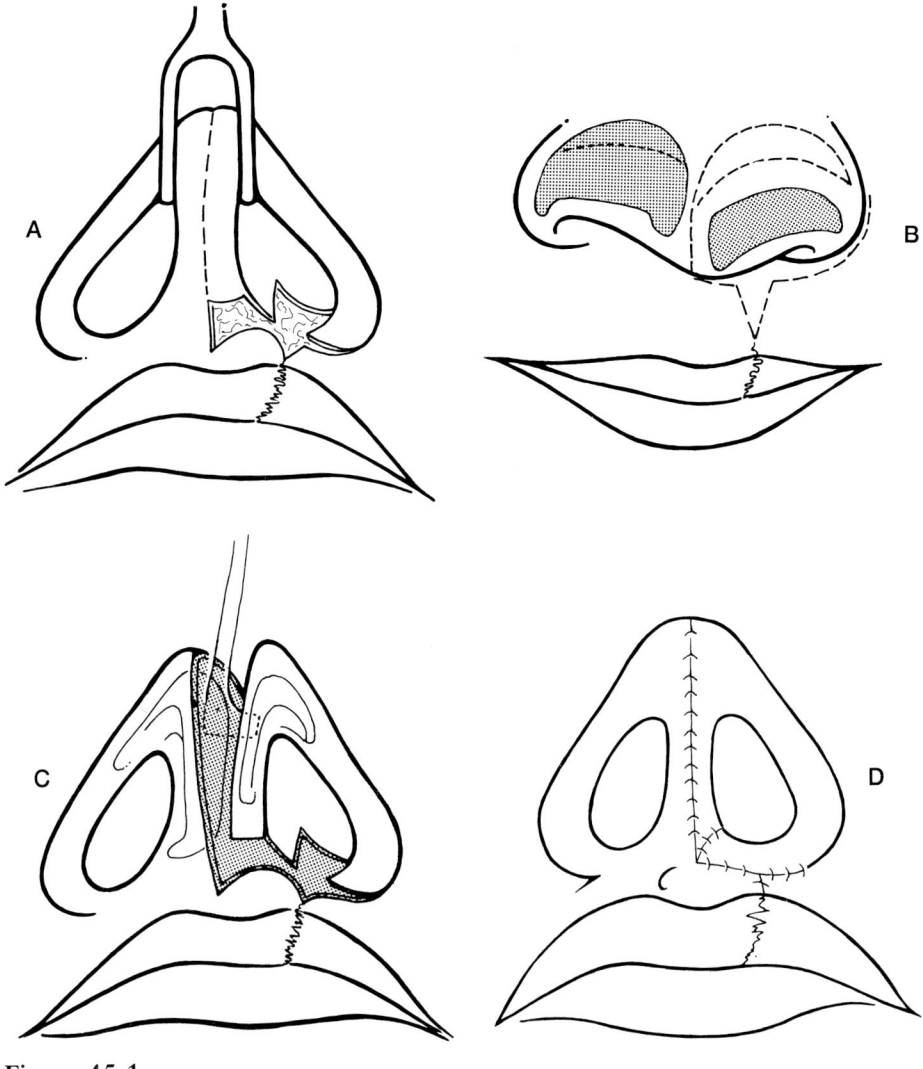

Figure 45-1

tients with light skin and with dark skin, and the aspect of the scars is excellent in all of them. Many of these patients have been examined from a normal conversation distance, and it is difficult to detect the scars (see Case 1).

Intranasal approach

For the intranasal approach, a conventional intracartilaginous incision is made in the mucosa, extending superiorly along the columella to the base of the nostril (Figure 45-2, *A*). A second incision approximately 1 cm long is made along the rim of the alae (Figure 45-2, *B*). The alar cartilage is dissected free from the skin and from the mucosa all along its length, from the dome to its lateral attachment at the alar base (Figure 45-2, *C*). The cartilage remains attached to the skin, and the mucosa re-

mains attached only to the columella. At this point, a small resection of the cephalic edge of the cartilage may be performed in adult patients when necessary, and the whole cartilage is slid medially to form a more prominent dome that corresponds to the normal side. The cartilage, in its new position, is sutured to the corresponding part of the cartilage of the normal side, taking care to remove the fat tissue between the domes to have a more symmetrically narrow tip and to prevent a relapse of the deformity (Figure 45-2, *D*). Two or three sutures of monofilament nylon are passed from the skin of the nose through the alar cartilage and the mucosa and back to the skin of the nose to maintain the position of the cephalic edge of the cartilage (Figure 45-2, *E*). These sutures are maintained under slight tension and are fixed only with tape to avoid unnecessary marks on the

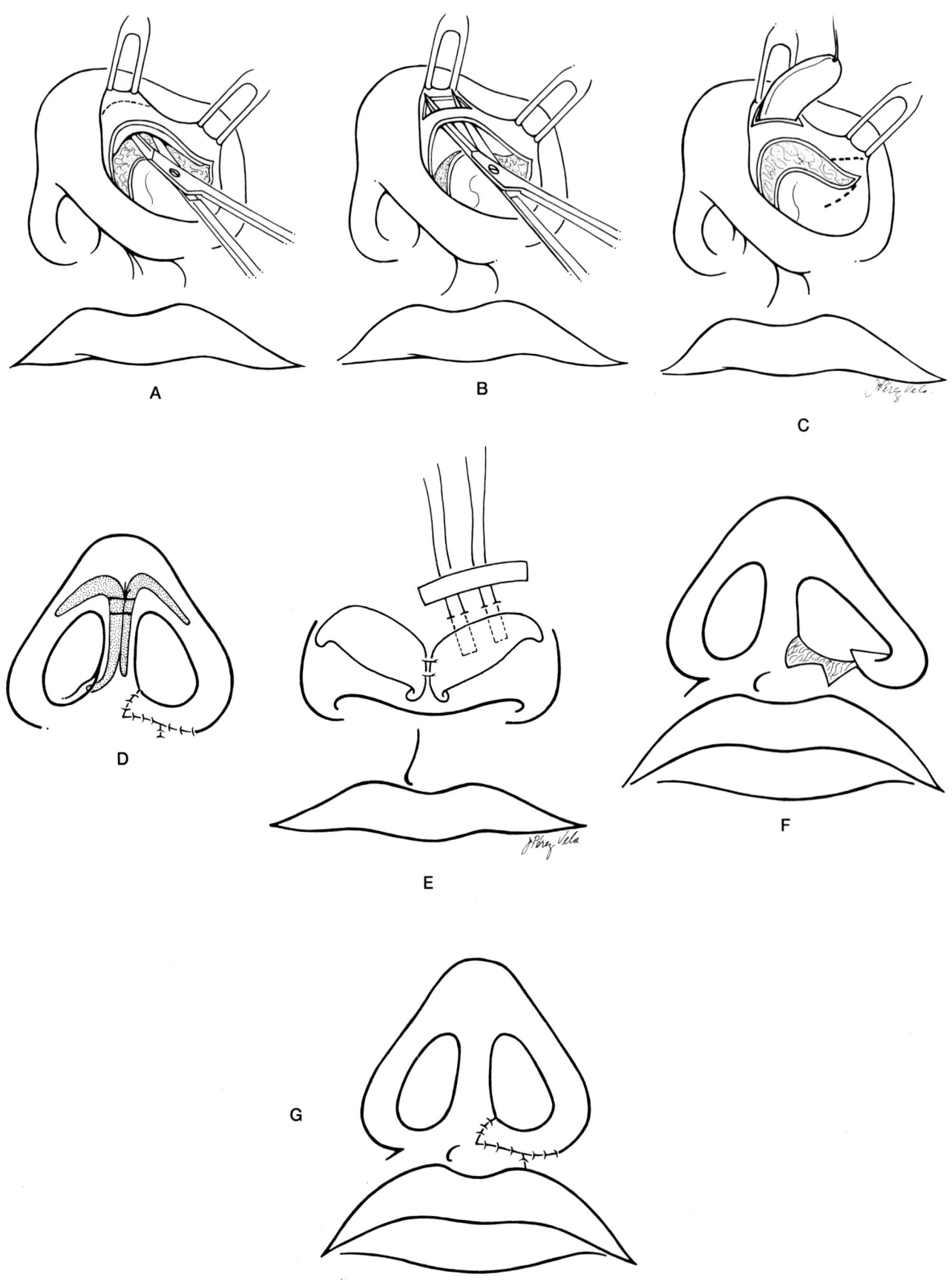

Figure 45-2

skin. It is necessary to free the insertion of the alar base at the nostril to move the base medially to narrow and to shape the nostril (Figure 45-2, *F* and *G*). Finally, a small Z-plasty is performed intranasally to correct the oblique band located laterally in the alar mucosa (see Figure 45-2, *C*).

Excellent results can be obtained with the intranasal approach, and we personally prefer this procedure both for early primary correction and for secondary rhinoplasty in clefts. It demands more experience and skill, but, in our opinion, it is the procedure of choice. We believe also that the medial displacement of the lateral crus of the alar cartilage to elevate the dome produces a more normal anatomical result than the elevation of the hemicolumella (see Case 2).

Cartilaginous grafts

In spite of all our efforts perfect nasal tip symmetry may not be achieved in all patients. This outcome can be improved by the use of a cartilaginous graft introduced through a small rim incision. A pocket is dissected between the anterior aspect of the alar cartilages and the skin, corresponding to the more anterior projection of the tip. A varying degree of projection and angularity can be obtained, depending on the shape and thickness of the graft as has been demonstrated by Sheen and others.[8] When the skin of the nasal tip is thick (as is fairly common in patients with clefts), we prefer to use a triangular graft with sharp angles to produce a better definition and to camouflage the skin thickness. Our choice of the donor site for the cartilage grafts is the septum; the ear concha is our second choice. Occasionally a rib cartilage may be used when stronger support is required. We do not hesitate to use cartilaginous grafts in young children to obtain symmetry. Grafts taken from the ear concha are preferable for the early age group.

In patients with complete clefts a depression is found at the piriform area on the cleft side. It is not uncommon also to find some hypoplasia of the maxilla on both sides. When dental occlusion is adequate, this depression of the midface can be easily corrected by using a cartilaginous graft in the depressed areas, unilaterally or bilaterally (see Case 3). For this procedure we prefer the use of a semilunar piece of rib cartilage 6 to 8 mm thick, carved 1½ to 2 cm long and 1 to 1½ cm wide, placing its concave edge corresponding to the lateral edge of the piriform apperture.[7] This graft may be introduced through a small incision in the buccal sulcus or through the nasal mucosa. A pocket is dissected subperiostially, large enough only to recieve the graft. Sometimes it may be necessary to pass one stitch of monofilament nylon through the skin to maintain the graft in position. The skin suture is fixed to the surface with Micropore tape (Figure 45-3).

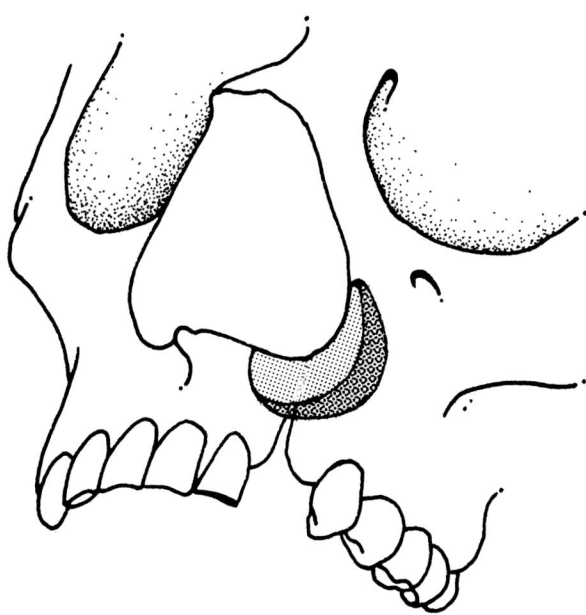

Figure 45-3

CASE REPORTS

Case 1

A 2-month-old patient had a wide cleft of the lip and palate (Figure 45-4, *A*). The immediate result after primary correction showed asymmetry of the nasal base, shortening of the hemicolumella on the cleft side, and the usual location of the irregularities of the nostrils' contour. The deformity persisted during the growth period (Figure 45-4, *B*).

When the child was 11 years old, we decided to do a complete rhinoplasty, including elongation of the hemicolumella on the cleft side, correction of the nasal floor, septoplasty, and medial and lateral osteotomies.

Based on our experience with similar cases that were followed for many years in whom we found that performing early osteotomies and complete rhinoplasty does not interfere with growth, it was decided to do a complete rhinoplasty. The external incision in the columella and the lower dorsum was chosen to obtain elongation and symmetry of the nostrils.

With the patient under general anesthesia, a midline columellar incision was made, extending to the upper border of the lower-lateral cartilages and laterally to the alar base on the cleft side. This incision was combined with an intercartilaginous incision on both sides that was extended along the mucocutaneous border of the columella on the cleft side. The hemicolumella was therefore freed entirely from the nose and elevated as a flap to the proper position (see Figure 45-1, *A*). After trimming the upper edge of the lower-lateral cartilage on the normal side, the medial crura were sutured together in a slightly overcorrected position, and a small ellipse of skin was removed from the alae on the cleft side (see Figure 45-1, *B* and *C*).

The nasal septum was dissected subpericondrally and was replaced over the nasal spine. Gentle crushing of the cartilage was performed to provide an adequate correction of the airway. The base of the alae on the cleft side was freed from the lip for approximately 1 cm and was rotated medially into the defect left by the elevation of the hemicolumella; thus the excessive width of the nostril on the cleft side was corrected (see Figure 45-2, *F* and *G*). Conventional medial and lateral osteotomies were performed without any resection of the hump.

Postoperative results were satisfactory. Acceptable symmetry was obtained at the nasal base, at the dorsum, and at the tip (Figure 45-4, *C*). The patient has been followed for 7 years after the operation without any alterations of the original results. The nasal growth has continued in proportion with the face. The scars on the skin of the columella and the tip of the nose are not visible from a normal conversation distance.

This case illustrates the excellent results obtained through skin incisions in the columella and the tip of the nose, which are almost invisible in all the patients after a few years, regardless of the color of the skin. This does not imply that the skin incision should be used in all cases, but we think it is preferable for surgeons with limited experience to elongate the columella, leaving a minimum scar on the skin rather than to damage the delicate alar cartilages. It should also be emphasized that performing early conservative rhinoplasty at age 11 years or even much before does not interfere with the growth of the nose and midface.

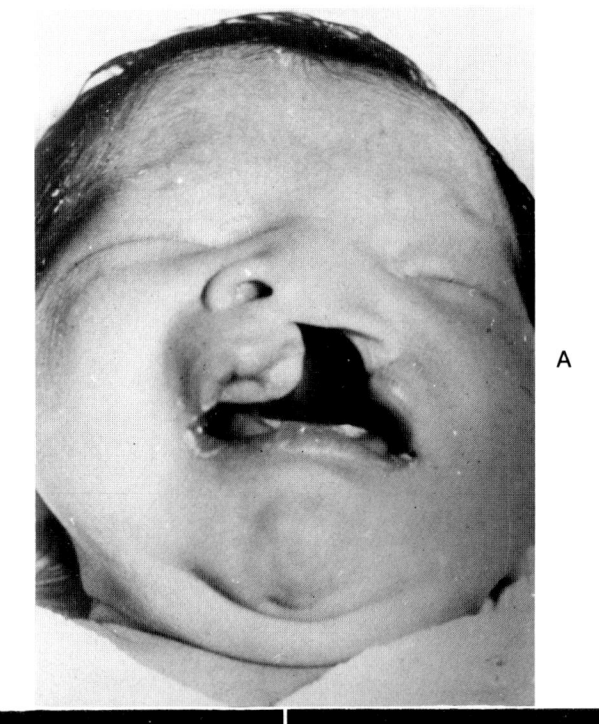

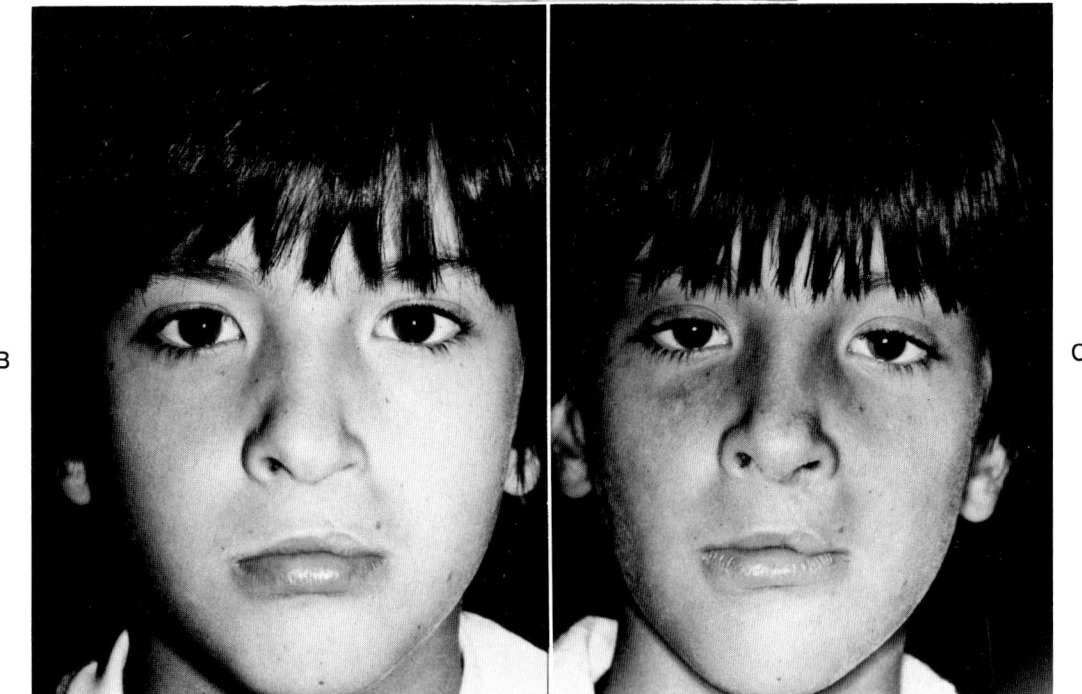

Figure 45-4

Case 2

A 16-year-old female came for secondary rhinoplasty because of a cleft-lip deformity. An elongation of the hemicolumella and recontouring of the alar dome had been performed on the patient many years before through an external incision along the midline of the columella and the lower dorsum and had left an almost invisible scar (Figure 45-5, A and C).

We decided to do a conventional rhinoplasty through an internal incision, including a cartilaginous graft to the tip.

Through a transcartilaginous incision a minimum resection of the hump was performed, and a 3 mm strip was removed from the cephalic edge of both lateral cartilages. A conservative septoplasty was performed, obtaining a small piece of cartilage to use as a graft for the nasal tip. The tip graft was carved in the form of a shield as suggested by Sheen[8] and was inserted through a small rim incision in front of the dome of the lower-lateral cartilages at the nasal tip. Lateral osteotomies completed the procedure.

Postoperative results have been satisfactory. There is a good improvement of nasal symmetry, although it is not perfect, but the general proportion with the face, the relationship with the supraorbital ridge and the forehead, and the impression of angularity are satisfactory (Figure 45-5, B and D).

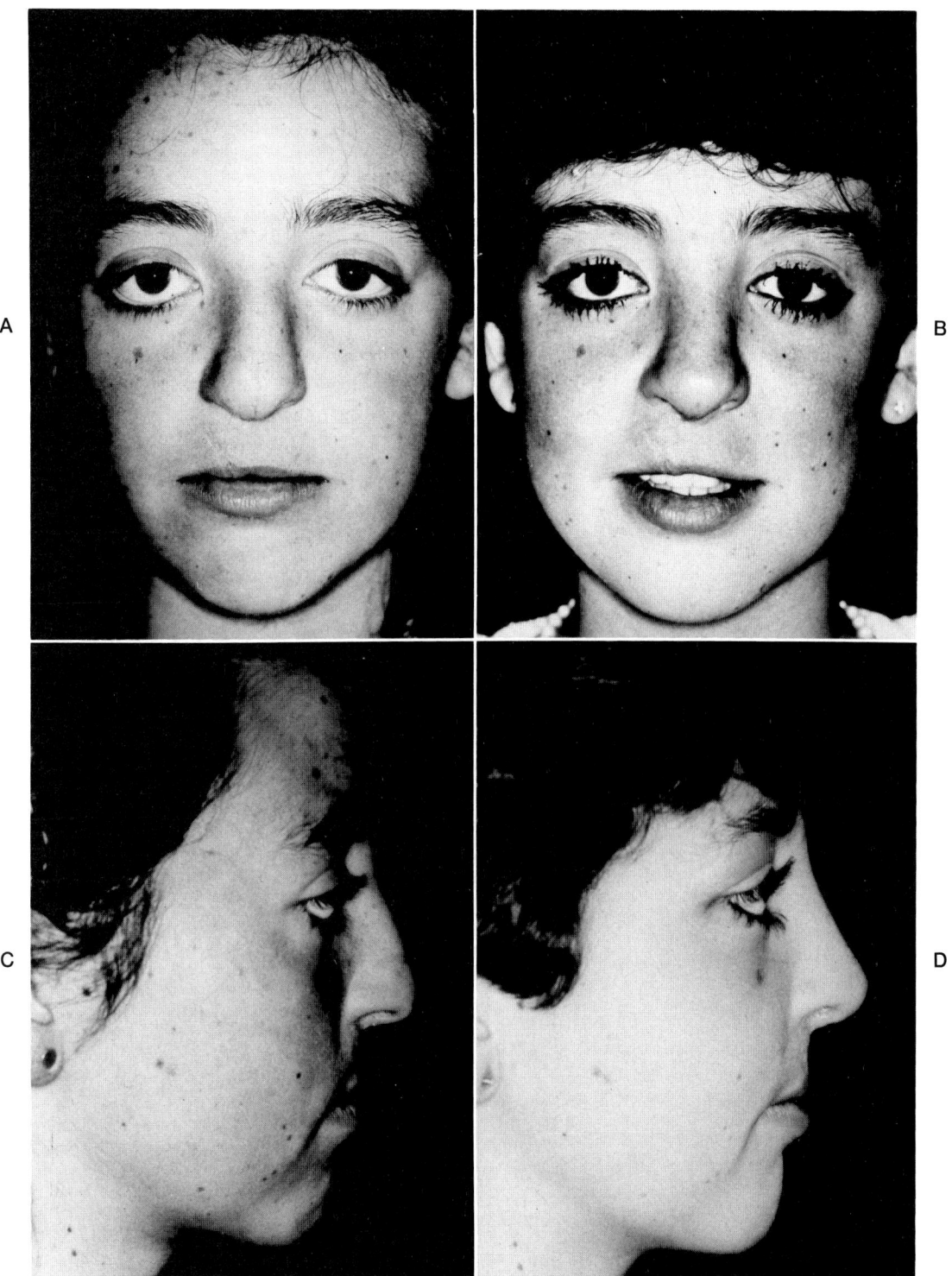

Figure 45-5

Case 3

A 15-year-old female requested secondary correction of her nose related to her cleft lip and palate deformity. This patient had the typical asymmetry of the nasal tip with deviation of the nasal pyramid combined with a moderate recession of the middle third of the face at the level of the alveolar ridge and the piriform fossa (Figure 45-6, *A-C*).

In most cases of hypoplasia of the middle face related to a cleft deformity we prefer to do a Le Fort I osteotomy and advance the maxilla to restore dental occlusion and facial convexity. In this particular case, because of the condition of the teeth, the presence of fistulas in the hard palate, and the amount of scarring resulting from previous surgical attempts, we believed the osteotomy was not indicated. To improve the contour of the piriform fossa we decided to use a cartilaginous graft (see Figure 45-3).

Tip cartilaginous grafts were obtained from the chest wall through a submammary incision. A minimum resection of the hump was performed with a rasp, and the alar cartilage was dissected on the cleft side using an intercartilaginous and rim incision. The lateral crus was freed entirely from the skin and the mucosa and was slid medially to obtain projection of the tip that was symmetrical with the normal side. A piece of cartilage 2½ cm long and 4 mm wide was introduced into the columella to improve the nasolabial angle and to give projection to the tip. Another triangular piece of cartilage was inserted at the nasal tip to increase anterior projection. Finally, through an incision in the buccal sulcus a semicircular piece of cartilage 2 cm long and 1 cm thick was introduced around the edge of the piriform apperture on both sides.

Postoperative results have been satisfactory (Figure 45-6, *D-F*). The nasal symmetry was greatly improved as were the projection and the facial profile.

This case illustrates the multiple uses of cartilaginous grafts to improve angularity and projection of the nasal tip and also to correct depressions in the paranasal area when facial osteotomies are not indicated.

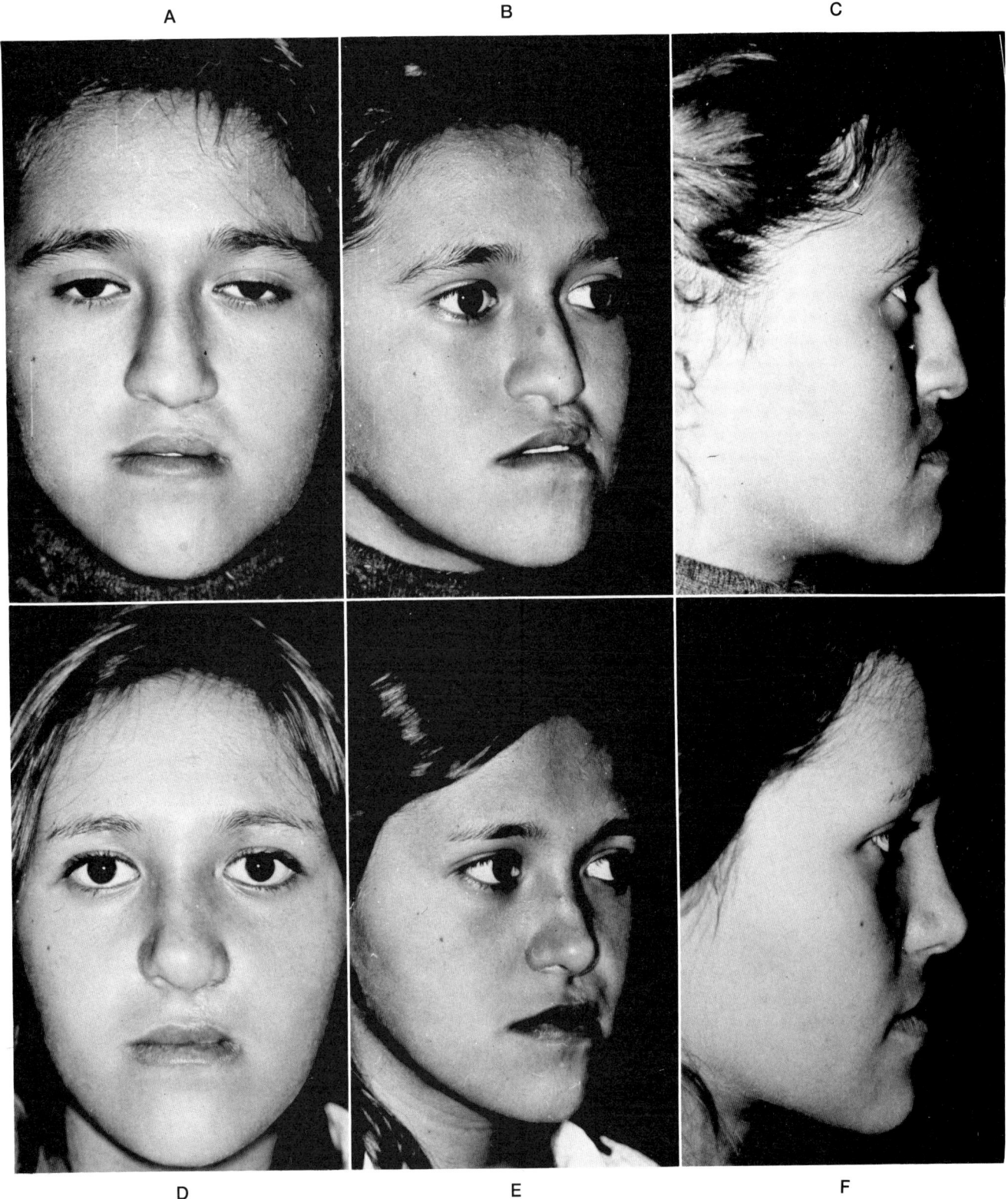

A   B   C

D   E   F

Figure 45-6

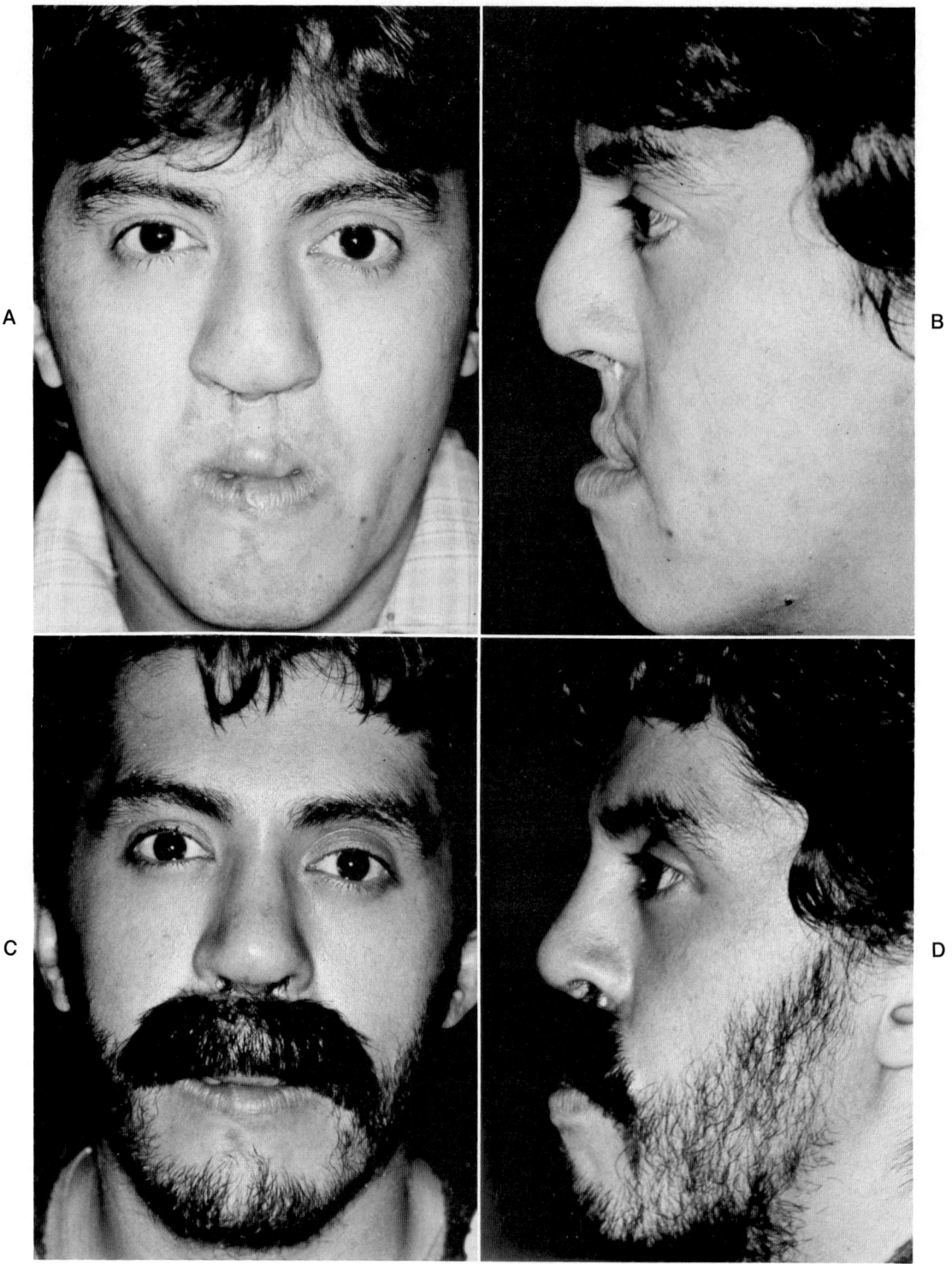

Figure 45-7

Case 4

A 20-year-old male who had a poorly repaired bilateral cleft of the lip and the palate requested correction of his nose. He had had multiple surgical procedures on his lip and palate, including an Abbe flap performed elsewhere. As is typical in bilateral cleft cases, the nose was reasonably symmetrical with a short columella, a broad nasal pyramid, and excessively horizontal nostrils (Figures 45-7, *A* and *B*).

It is well known that scars on the upper lip are never invisible. Scars resulting from repeated surgical procedures present a more difficult aesthetic problem. Although an improvement of the nasal shape can be obtained, the final result with a lip in that condition can be very frustrating especially in a male for whom makeup is impractical and on whom the presence of hair on the skin makes the scars more evident. We decided to perform a conventional rhinoplasty, to elongate the columella, to provide support to the tip, and to replace the skin on the upper lip.

With the patient under general anesthesia, the intercartilaginous incisions were extended down to the base of the columella and into the upper lip so that a segment of the central skin was left attached to the base of the columella, which was entirely separated from the septum and was relocated in a higher position. An elongation of approximately 7 mm was obtained, leaving a raw area in the upper lip. A strip of septal cartilage was inserted in the columella to increase its projection and to provide support to the tip. Septoplasty and medial and lateral osteotomies were performed in a conventional manner, and a small wedge resection of the base of the nostrils completed the nasal part of the procedure. A previously delayed bipedicle scalp flap based on the temporal arteries was rotated down in the fashion of a bucket handle and was used to resurface the entire upper lip after resecting the skin of the area. Two weeks later the two ends of the flap were cut at the nasolabial fold and were replaced in their original site on the scalp.

The shape of the nose and the coverage of the scars on the upper lip have been satisfactory (Figures 45-7, *C* and *D*).

This case illustrates the need for elongation of the columella and the need to give cartilaginous support to the tip simultaneously with the columellar elongation to obtain permanent improvement of the anterior projection of the nose. This is also another example of the need to analyze not only the nose but the face as a whole.

REFERENCES

1. Berkeley, W.T.: The cleft lip nose, Plast. Reconstr. Surg. 23:567, 1959.
2. Berkeley, W.T.: Correction of the unilateral cleft lip nasal deformity. In Grabb, S.W., Rosenstein, S.W., and Bzoch, K.R., editors: Cleft lip and palate, Boston, 1971, Little, Brown and Co., Inc.
3. Dibbell, D.G.: Cleft lip nasal reconstruction, Plast. Reconstr. Surg. 69:264, 1982.
4. Joseph, J.: Nasenplastik und sonstige gesichtsplastik, ed. 2, Leipzig, 1931, Curt Kabitsch.
5. Ortiz-Monasterio, F., and Olmedo, A.: Corrective rhinoplasty before puberty, Plast. Reconstr. Surg. 68:381, 1981.
6. Ortiz-Monasterio, F., Fuente del Campo, A., and Carrillo, A.: Advancement of the orbits and the midface in one piece, combined with frontal repositioning, for the correction of Crouzon's deformities, Plast. Reconstr. Surg. 61:507, 1978.
7. Ortiz-Monasterio, F., Olmedo, A., and Ortiz-Oscoy, L.: The use of cartilage grafts in primary aesthetic rhinoplasty, Plast. Reconstr. Surg. 67:557, 1981.
8. Sheen, J.H.: Achieving more nasal tip projection by use of small autogenous vomer or septal cartilage graft, Plast. Reconstr. Surg. 56:211, 1975.
9. Velasquez, J.M., and Ortiz Monasterio, F.: Primary simultaneous correction of the lip and nose in the unilateral cleft lip, Plast. Reconstr. Surg. 54:558, 1974.
10. Wilkie, T.F.: The "alar shift" revisited, Br. J. Plast. Surg. 22:70, 1969.

46

Reconstruction of the Postcleft Nasal Deformity

Mark Gorney

Despite increased attention to the nasal complement of primary cleft-lip reconstruction, the repair of the secondary cleft-lip/nasal deformity is a challenging and often frustrating undertaking. The literature is full of techniques. Their success is inversely proportional to the severity of the deformity.

SURGICAL OBJECTIVES

Regardless of method used, the reconstructive surgeon's plan of treatment should seek to obtain the closest approximation to normalcy through the fewest surgical stages with the fewest possible donor site deformities, always taking into account the normal ethnic variables in nasal form. For example, in the Oriental individual, the need to achieve nasal-tip projection is less important than in the Caucasian. A horizontally oriented nostril is more accepted as normal in the black nose.

For a unilateral deformity, the goal should be to achieve symmetry with the normal side. For the bilateral deformity, the goal should be to achieve more tip projection and more dorsal height.

In my opinion, it is virtually impossible to achieve an approximation of normalcy in the significantly deformed nose without the addition of extrastructural materials or movement of skeletal segments. The source of these materials and their relative advantages and disadvantages are discussed (Figure 46-1).

TIMING OF SURGERY

It is well known that the nose undergoes a rapid, although late, growth spurt during puberty and early adolescence. The cute "button nose" suddenly begins to take on adult form somewhere between the ages of 11 and 14 years. Girls usually mature physically much earlier than boys. Not only is there a rapid change in size and shape but also in skin thickness. Suddenly the familial genes that have been lying dormant assert themselves very emphatically, and not always with a welcome end-product.

All this change is caused not so much by the growth of the nasal bones, but by the sudden upsurge of the nasal process of the maxilla. This is the route through which the osteotomy chisel must pass during reconstructive rhinoplasty. In addition, the growth center in the lower portion of the septal cartilage should be spared during the early years of development.

During this period of life, a young person undergoes radical changes, emotionally and hormonally. Although emotional maturity has no linear relationship to age, the key to success in *any* nasal surgery is not physical but emotional maturity. Psychological stability is the sine qua non of successful surgery and should be given greater weight. For these reasons it is preferable to postpone these operations until the nose has achieved its full growth, which generally occurs at approximately 13 to 15 years in girls and 14 to 16 years in boys.

Nonetheless, the caring surgeon is often caught in a crunch. In some children, postcleft deformities carry with them a heavy component of emotional liability. It is not easy for a stigmatized child to develop normally at a time in life when peer approval is so desperately needed. Thus a fine balance of judgment is needed in coming to a decision about whether to postpone the surgery and risk permanent psychological scars or to operate early and possibly compromise the eventual results.

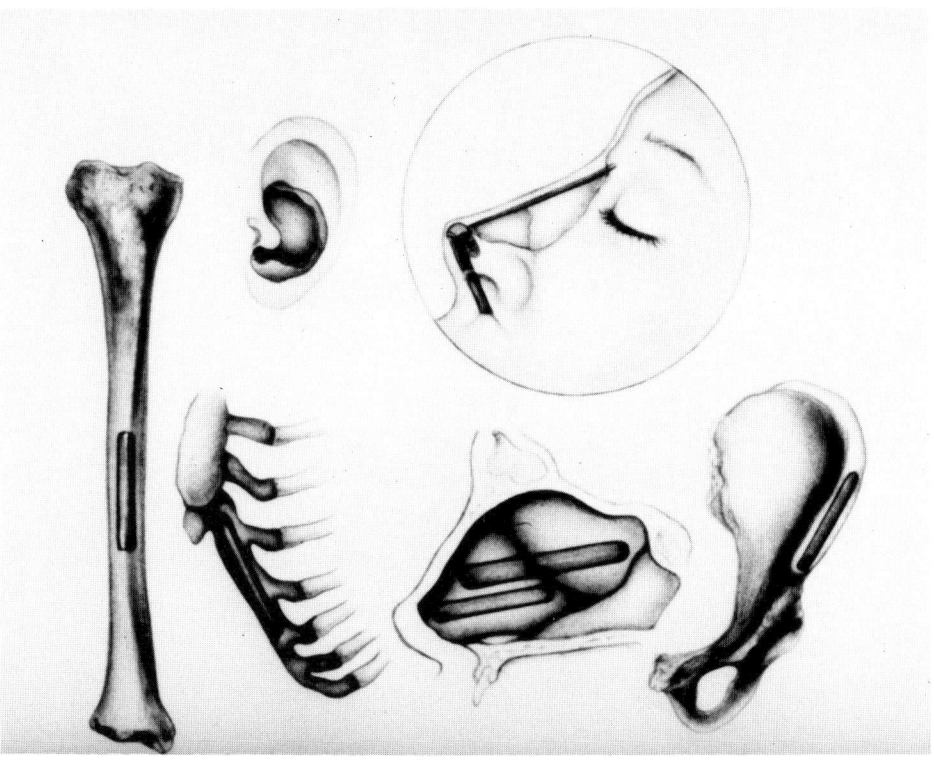

Figure 46-1. Sources of structural material. (From Stark, R.B.: Plastic surgery of head and neck, Edinburgh, 1987, Churchill Livingstone, Inc.)

PATHOLOGICAL ANATOMY

The typical unilateral deformity consists of 10 identifiable components, which may exist in varying degrees. These are shown in Figure 46-2, *A-D*.

The bilateral deformity (although the septum may not be deflected) has three additional problems:

1. The columella is very short.
2. There is a marked lack of nasal-tip projection as a result of displaced and/or inadequate alar cartilages.
3. Both nostrils' axes are oriented much more horizontally than vertically.

Underlying fundamental deformities of the maxillary framework often must also be addressed. Although they are beyond the scope of this chapter, there is no doubt that dramatic improvements can be achieved with recently developed craniofacial surgical techniques.

To resort to a simple analogy: If one were foolish enough to construct an A-frame cabin on uneven ground and an earthquake occurred that split the underlying ground and dropped the ground away under one wall, the whole house would sag on that side. The main bearing-wall (the septum) that divides the house in two would also twist badly. Obviously, the house cannot be rebuilt properly until the sagging support is shored up.

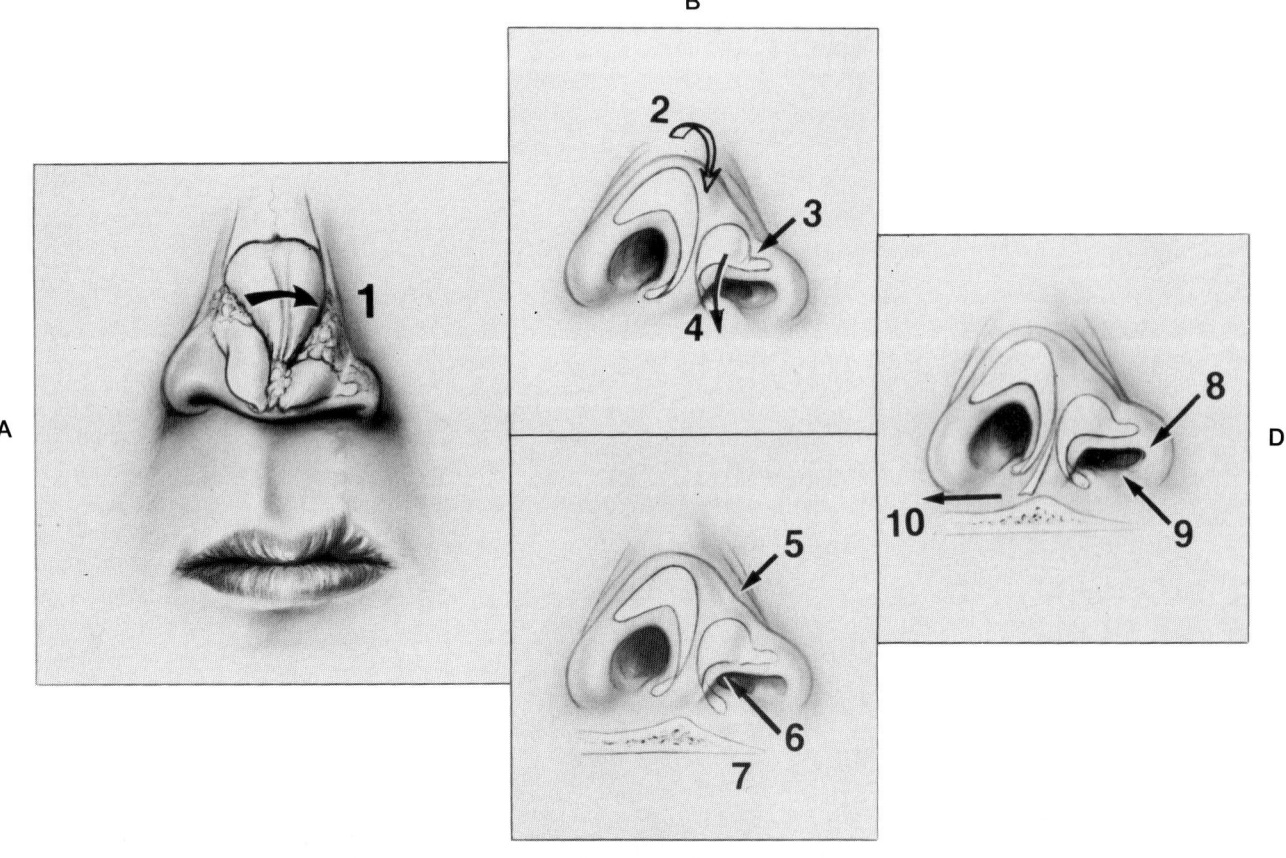

Figure 46-2. A, *1*, Septum deviates. **B**, *2*, Dome is displaced ventrally; *3*, lateral crus is abnormal—buckles or protrudes into nostril; *4*, anterior edge is tipped caudally. **C**, *5*, Tendency is toward bifidity; *6*, angle between lateral and medial crura is obtuse; *7*, bony platform is deficient. **D**, *8*, Lateral angle is acute; *9*, alar base is wide—deficient sill; *10*, columella deviates to normal side. (From Stark, R.B.: Plastic surgery of head and neck, Edinburgh, 1987, Churchill Livingstone, Inc.)

REPAIRS
Anatomical rearrangements through external incisions

The deformed nostril can be approached through external skin incisions that extend onto the dorsal skin of the nostril, and the deformed portion is rotated chephalad as a "unit" of skin cartilage and sometimes mucosa. The principal proponents[1-5,10,11,17] of this approach do not consider the external scar a drawback and show many excellent results with well-healed, acceptable, but, nonetheless, visible scars on the columella and dorsal skin of the nasal tip. It is my belief that if there is any way to achieve my stated goals without an external scar, no matter how unobstrusive, it is preferable to do so even if it is technically more difficult.

Anatomical rearrangements through internal incisions

To correct postcleft nasal deformities, various intranasal or nostril-margin incisions can be used to expose the abnormal cartilage. The cartilages are then rearranged into quasinormal relationships, and they are held in position with a variety of fixation techniques, either to the upper-lateral cartilage directly above, to the contralateral upper-lateral cartilage, or to the normal opposite alar dome. Good results have been shown by numerous surgeons.[6,9,13,18-22] These procedures avoid an external scar, and the early results are pleasing. Nonetheless, most of them depend on suture fixation alone. With the passage of time, these types of repairs tend to show significant loss of improvement.

Anatomical rearrangments through internal incisions with additions of structural support elements

A combination of incisions can be used to reposition or equalize the existing cartilages of the nasal tip, but, in addition, the repair can be reinforced with other autogenous structural supports or onlays, which have been used by numerous surgeons.[6-8,12,14-16]

Some surgeons show gratifying results using alloplastic materials. In my experience, alloplastic materials, no matter how well-fabricated or innocuous, eventually cause more problems than they are worth, and many eventually extrude.

STATE OF THE ART

Current thinking about postcleft nasal deformity may be characterized as follows:

1. If the deformity is minimum, modified tip rhinoplasty techniques, along with reduction of the normal side and mobilization of the abnormal one to a more superior medial position, may be sufficient.

2. When the structural elements of the tip of the nose are largely present but are malpositioned, they can be arranged through inconspicuous incisions inside the rim of the nostrils. If external support is to be added, it is more easily done through an "elephant trunk" exposure—lifting up the skin of the columella to expose the entire tip anatomy. A barely visible scar will be left at the base of the columella.

3. If external scars are to be avoided and if the deformity involves some underdevelopment of the maxillary support on the cleft side, surgical repair must be designed around the addition of adequate structural support for the nasal tip. This support should preferably be autogenous cartilage or bone. If the maxillary support is mildly deficient, an onlay bone graft may suffice. If it is significantly deficient, a maxillary advancement with or without bone graft, should be considered.

THE UNILATERAL DEFORMITY

For the past 12 years I have tried various combinations of techniques to repair the unilateral deformity. In the mid 1980s I settled on the following approach, which has stood the test of time.

If the surgical plan calls for structural materials, they are obtained first (except for septal cartilage, since the nose is a bacterial "zoo," anyway). The preferred donor source whenever possible is the nose itself. However, the septum is often twisted, inadequate, or insufficient. The preferred source then is the cranium or the anterior tibia for bone and the ear for cartilage. The ear has amazing potential as a donor site for a minimal secondary deformity. I prefer not to invade the rib or the pelvis if avoidable because of increased morbidity.

The structural anatomy of the nasal tip is easily accessible through incisions just inside the nostril rim. If these incisions are extended down the sides of the columella and are joined across the base, careful dissection of the skin of the columella (the elephant trunk) will reveal the anatomy and the relationship of all the parts with startling clarity (Figure 46-3, *A* and *B*).

If significant asymmetry or disparity exists, it can be addressed directly. In the unilateral deformity the normal alar cartilage has a lateral crus significantly wider than the opposite side. To correct that asymmetry, the "relative excess" on the normal side is resected and saved for later use (Figure 46-4, *A*). After dimensional parity has been achieved, the degree of positional disparity on the cleft side can be assessed and corrected in one of several ways. If the end of the lateral crus curls into the nostril and the genu is displaced inferiorly, it may have to be dissected, scored, and reattached in a more normal placement on the next higher stable point. This point may be the dome of the opposite side or, more likely, the lowest point of the opposite normal *upper*-lateral cartilage. Either way, this repositioning is much more likely to achieve permanent results and much more dramatic improvement if a stabilizing strut of cartilage is installed between the medial crura. This strut must set on the maxillary spine (or what passes for one). It must be thin enough not to make the columella too wide, yet strong enough to act as a support. Stability can be achieved by making it wide enough (in the dorsoventral dimension). If this strut is allowed to protrude above the level of both alar domes, it will project under the skin as an abnormal white bump that does indeed look like the top of a tent pole. Even if one hoists both domes well above the tip of the strut and fixes them through both domes and the strut itself, in time that bothersome tent pole protrusion may become visible. In addition, there commonly is insufficient material with which to build enough definition to achieve a semblance of normalcy of the nasal tip.

Both problems, strut camouflage and tip projection, can be corrected by fabricating a cartilaginous tip graft. Preferably, it should be composed of septal cartilages. If this cartilage is not available, the most dependent and deeply curved portion of conchal ear cartilage will suffice (Figure 46-4, *B*).

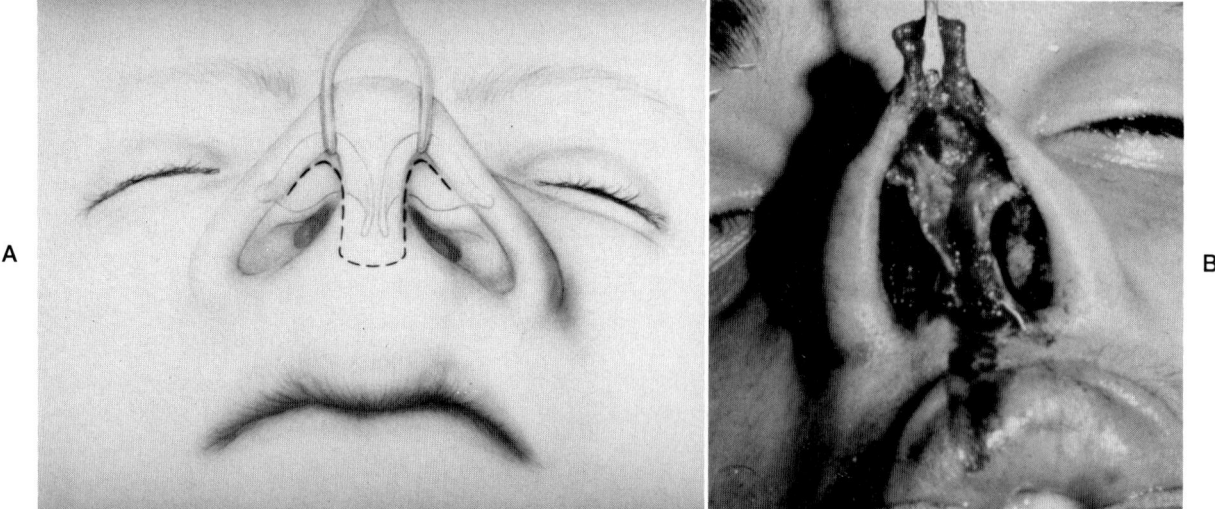

Figure 46-3. A, Modified Rethy or "elephant trunk" incisional design. **B,** Intraoperative exposure of pathological anatomy. (From Stark, R.B.: Plastic surgery of head and neck, Edinburgh, 1987, Churchill Livingstone, Inc.)

The tip graft must be accurately sutured in position, and, once again, this procedure is most easily done when the whole tip assembly is exposed through an elephant trunk approach.

The nostril floor must be managed so that it matches the width and altitude of the opposite side. If there is sufficient soft-tissue coverage, an onlay bone graft will do. If the deficiency is profound, a maxillary reconstruction must be considered.

Often there is no nostril "sill," and the nostril base is "flattened" with no perialar crease. It is difficult to reconstruct this small but important detail. Dibbell[8] has come close to reconstructing it with a small flap lifted out of the nasolabial crease. Based on the ala itself and curled around to simulate the nostril sill, this flap also rounds out the alar base.

Once the tip of the nose has been balanced, the problem of the nasal pyramid must be addressed. If there is adequate structural integrity, standard osteoplastic rhinoplasty with midline and lateral infracture osteotomies serve well. If, after correcting the tip deficiency, the nasal pyramid appears inadequate, often a dorsal graft of sandwiched septal cartilages or bone graft must be used (Figure 46-5, A-E).

THE BONE GRAFT

If a bone graft is necessary, either to build up an inadequate profile, bridge a supratip depression, or camouflage a crooked nose, it must come from either the cranium, the tibia, or the pelvis. Of these three donor sites, the traditional one has been the pelvic anterosuperior spine. I prefer the anterior upper third of the tibia. It is easily accessible, its ridge is a good imitation of a nasal dorsum, the morbidity is minimal, and the donor site scar is quite acceptable. In addition, the graft can be harvested with the patient under local anesthesia and sedated. The same can be said of the ulna, but removal of a large graft can weaken the arm, and the donor site is sometimes obvious. The external table of the cranium is an excellent and easily accessible donor site, which leaves no visible scar, and for a columellar strut it is excellent material. It also serves well for dorsal onlay grafts, except it may curve the wrong way, requiring turning the graft over and putting it with the external surface down. Fixation and, above all, the crucial bone-to-bone contact may be less than optimal.

Once harvested, the graft must be fashioned so that it will be stable. Although all bone grafts will undergo significant resorption with time, clearly bone-to-bone contact will promote direct healing, stability, and longer duration. To maximize such contact I fashion my grafts with a "keel" on the undersurface (Figure 46-5, B and C). This keel fits directly in the midline osteotomy, thus giving the desired contact, stability, and profile elevation.

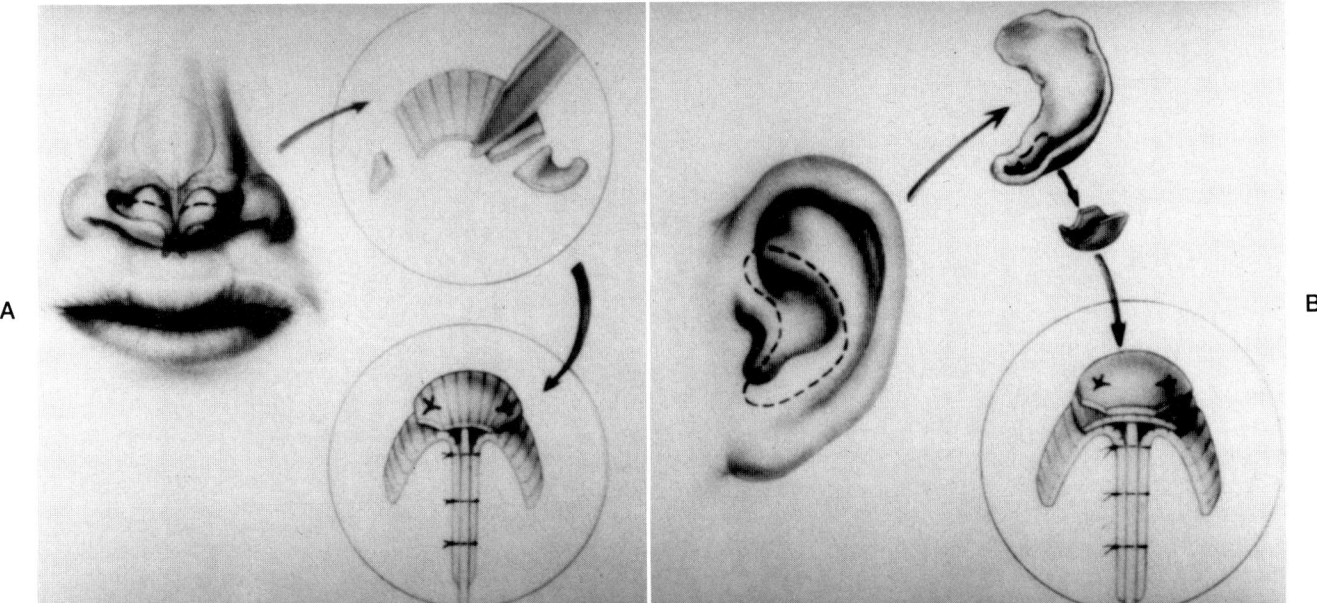

Figure 46-4. A, Relative "excess" from dorsal aspect of alar cartilages used for cap. **B,** Deepest portion of conchal ear graft used for cap. (From Stark, R.B.: Plastic surgery of head and neck, Edinburgh, 1987, Churchill Livingstone, Inc.)

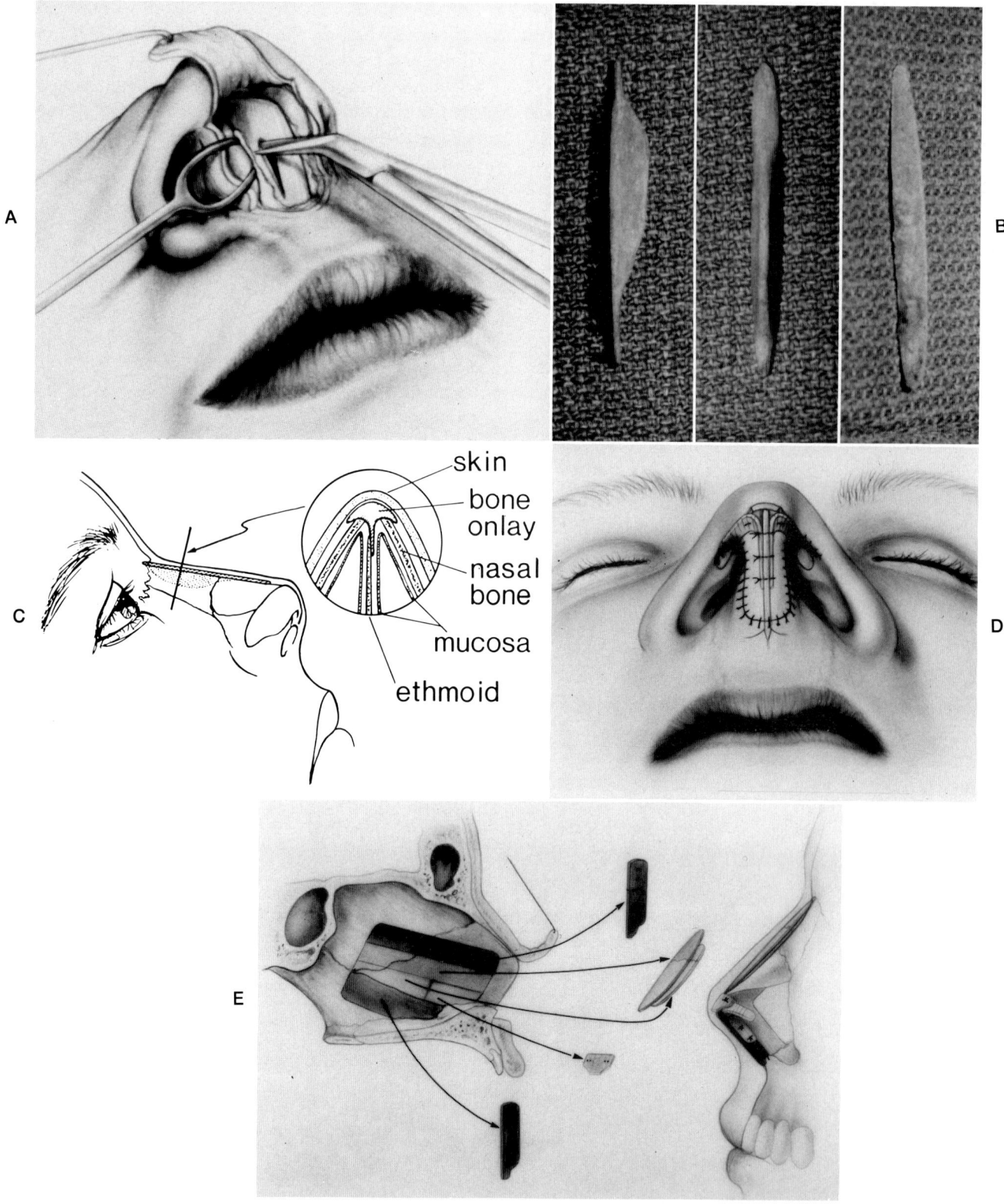

Figure 46-5. A, Direct exposure of septum to harvest cartilage graft through original incisions. **B,** Lateral, inferior, and superior views of keel graft, which may be fabricated from cartilage or bone. **C,** Fitting keel graft between nasal bones for direct contact and fixation without sutures. **D,** If septal cartilage graft is sufficient, distribute as shown. **E,** Final structural assembly at end of procedure. (From Stark, R.B.: Plastic surgery of head and neck, Edinburgh, 1987, Churchill Livingstone, Inc.)

SUMMARY

The postcleft nasal stigma can be a psychologically crippling deformity that challenges the reconstructive surgeon's imagination. Rewarding improvements can be achieved through a direct open approach. Repositioning of existing structural elements with additions of a columellar strut capped by cartilages to provide nasal projection come close to achieving symmetry and normalcy. This procedure is usually accompanied by substantial improvement in body image (Figures 46-6 to 46-11).

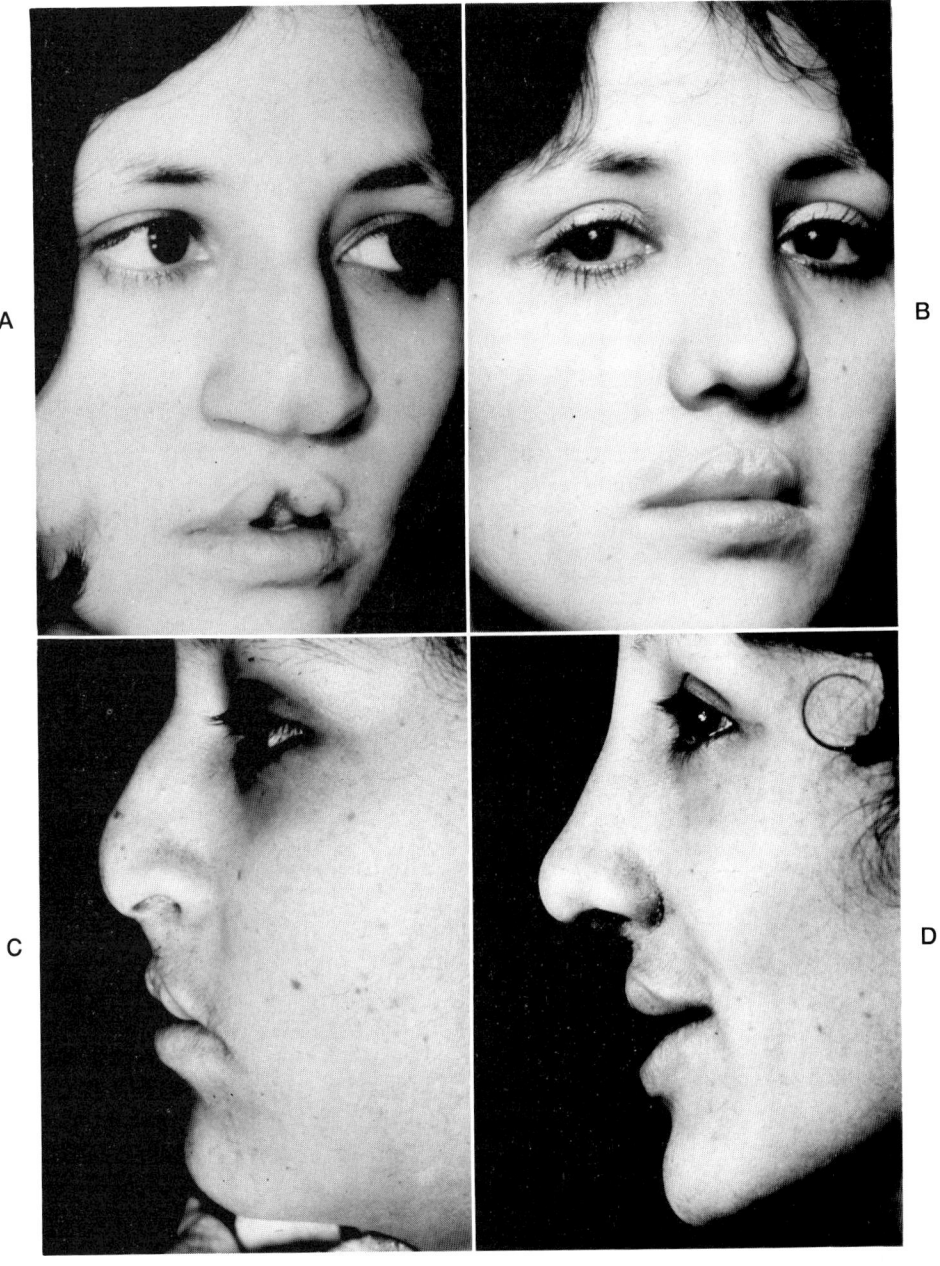

Figure 46-6. A and **B,** Preoperative and postoperative views of correction of complex nasolabial stigma with depressed bifid nose and poor lip repair. **C** and **D,** Same operation as **A** and **B.** (Courtesy of Laub, D., Chairman: Division of Plastic Surgery, Stanford University.)

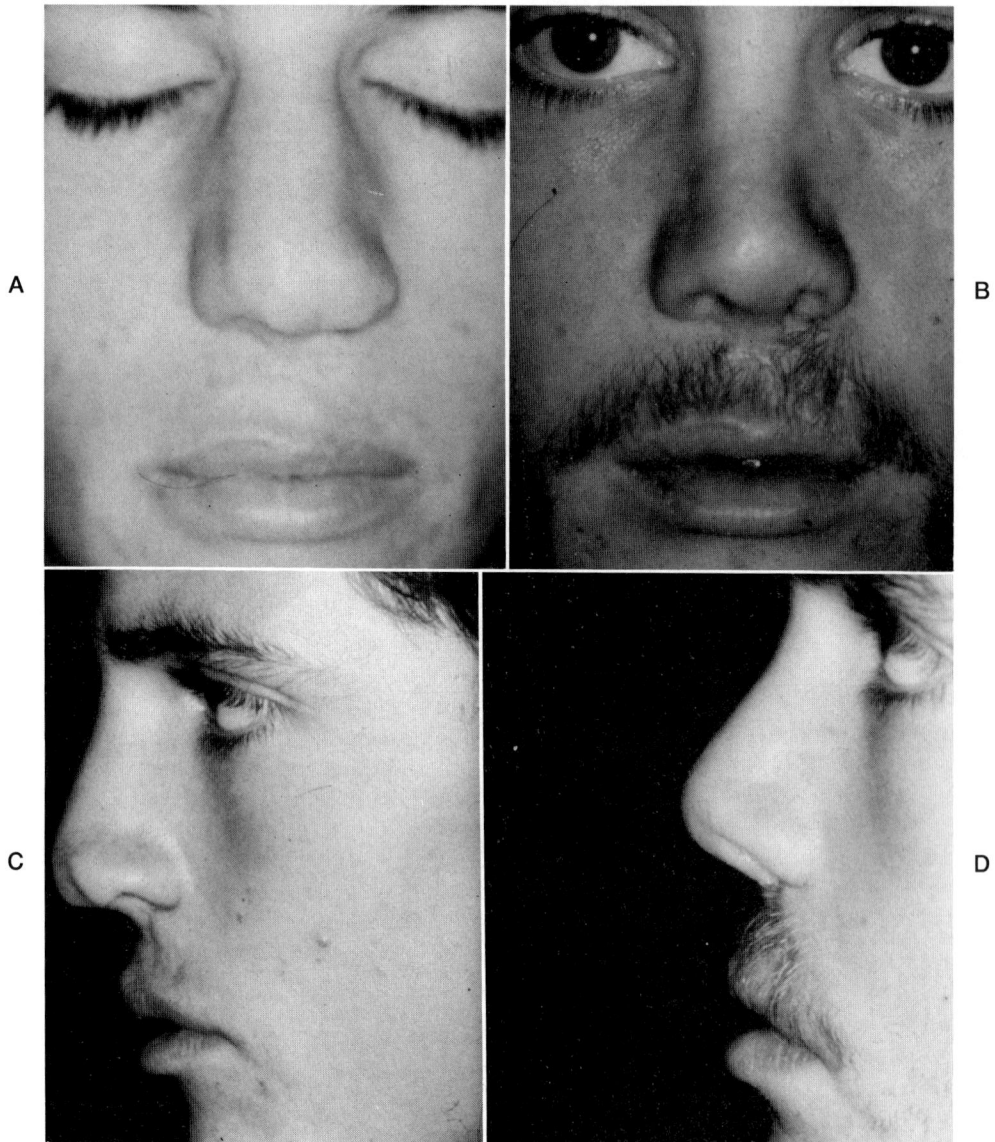

Figure 46-7. A and **B,** Correction of asymmetrical bifid nose, full face view. **C** and **D,** Full profile view.

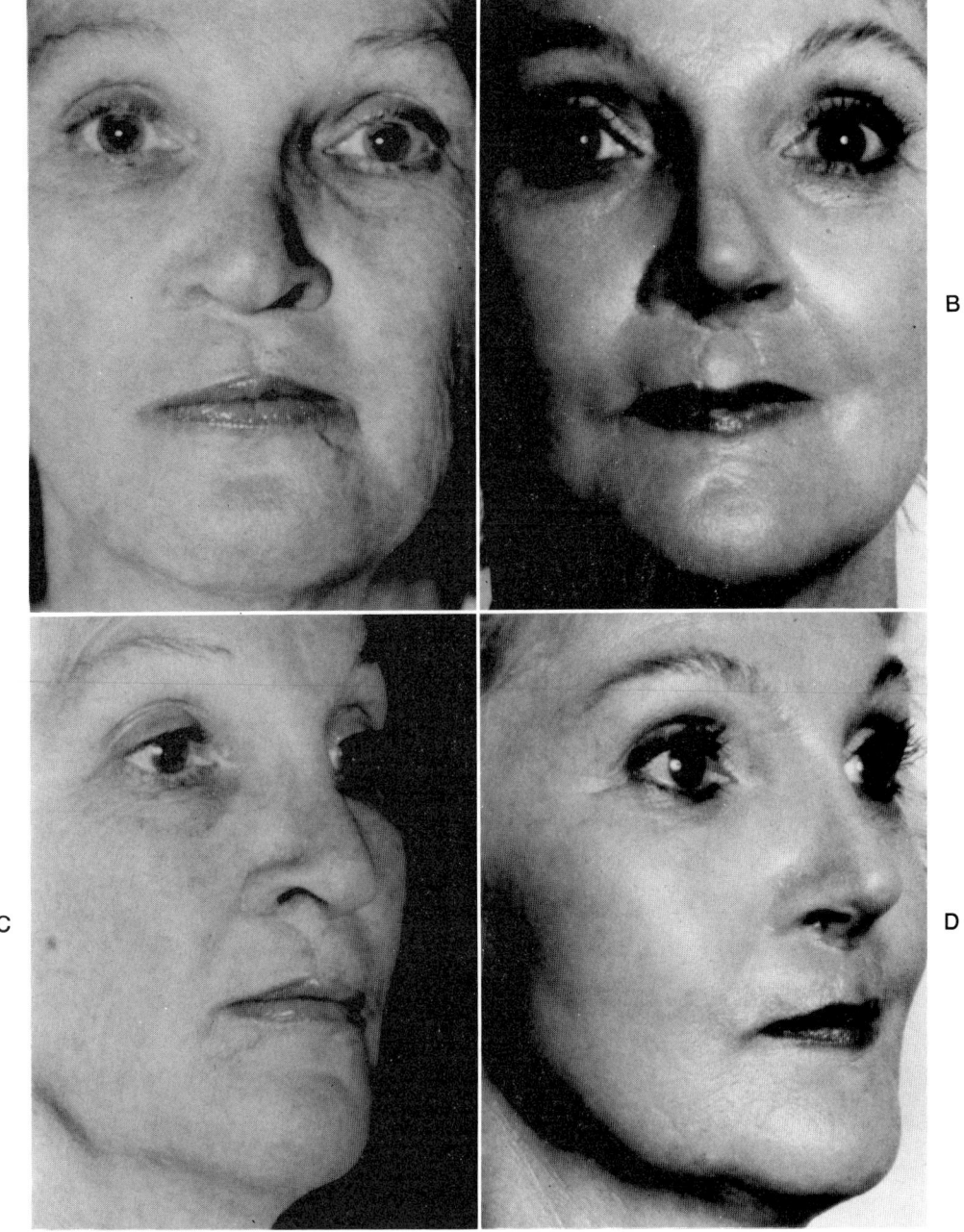

Figure 46-8. Reconstruction in a 37-year-old female through technique described in text, plus Abbe cross-lip flap. **A** and **B**, Frontal views. **C** and **D**, Semi-profile views.

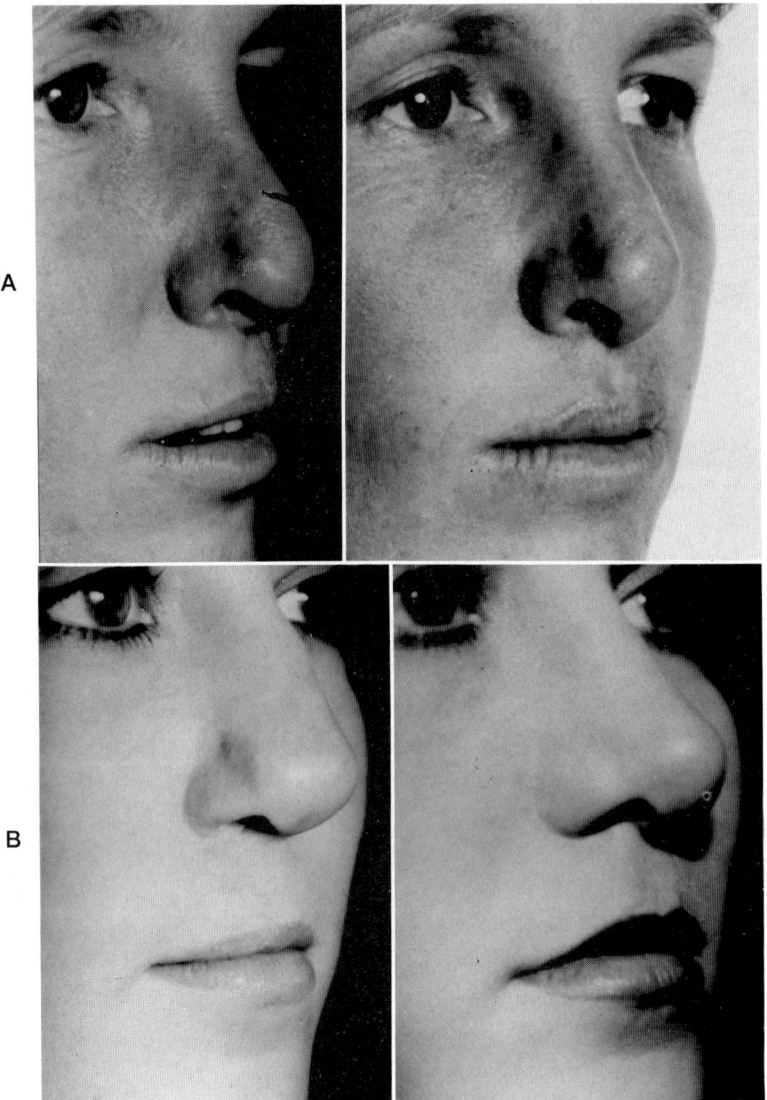

Figure 46-9. A-D, Nasal reconstruction in four different patients as described in text, plus reconstruction of philtrum with conchal graft; shown preoperatively and 5 years postoperatively.

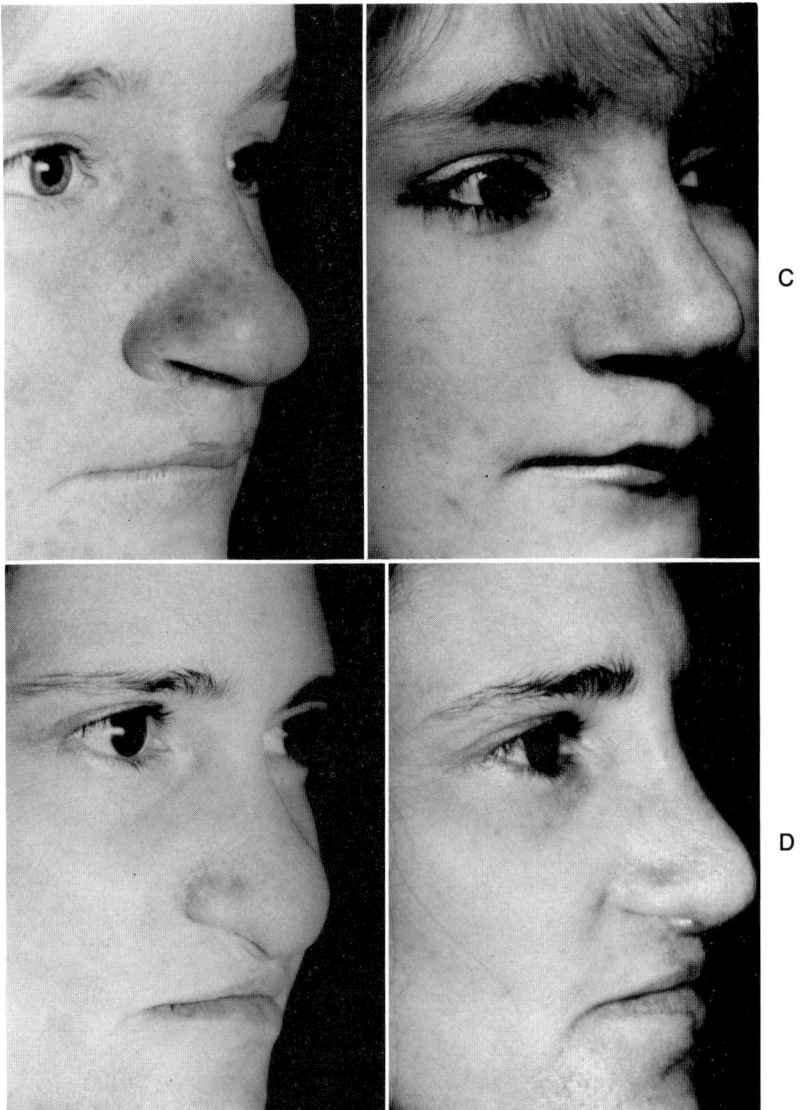

Figure 46-9, cont'd

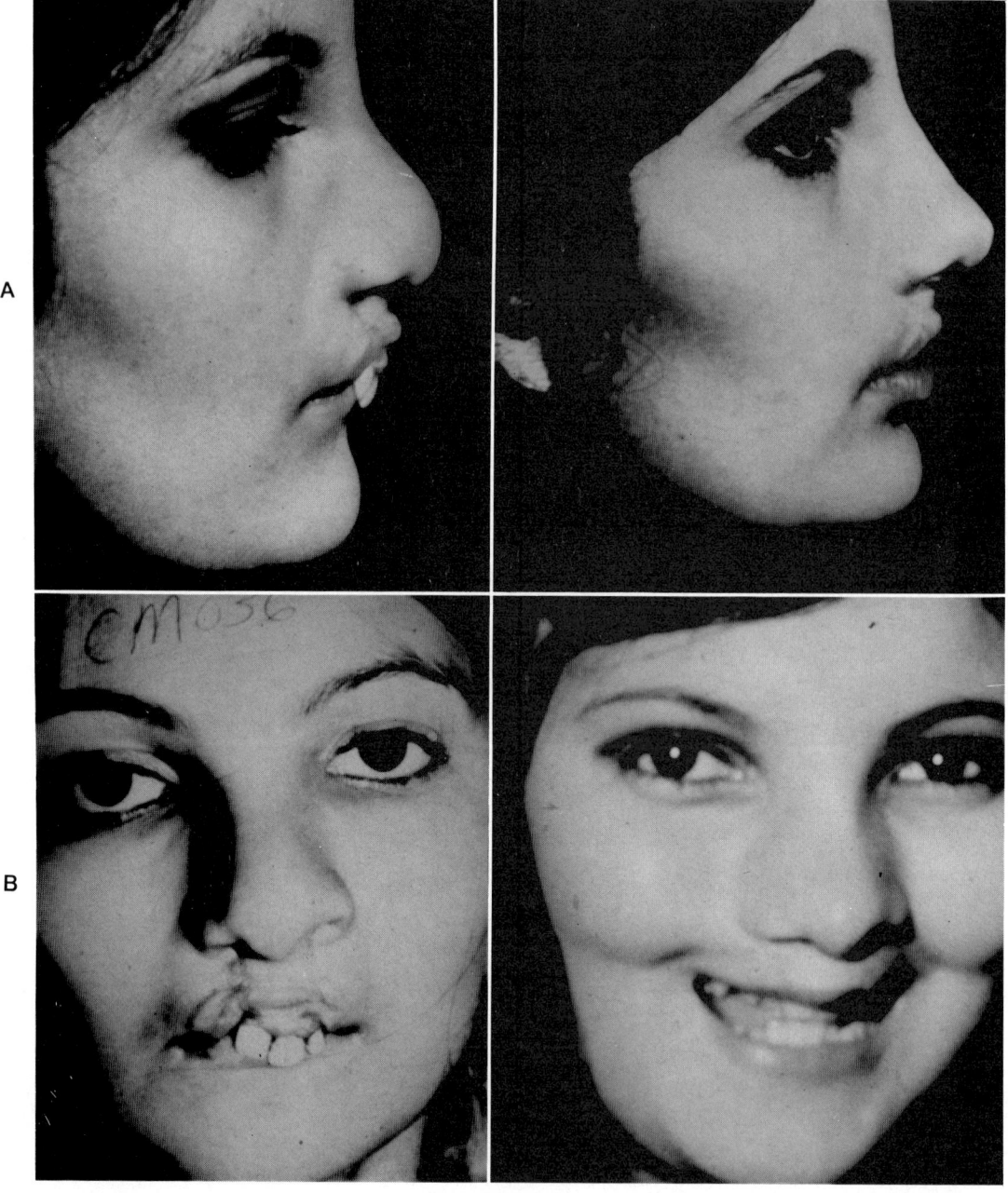

Figure 46-10. A, A 17-year-old female reconstructed by techniques discussed as well as by revision of lip and by orthognathic and prosthodontic correction; shown preoperatively and 12-years postoperatively. **B,** Same patient during arrival and departure from Stanford Plastic Surgery Service and also 6 months later, showing dramatic change in body image. (From Gorney, M.: Reconstruction of the post-cleft nasal deformity, August 1987.)

REFERENCES

1. Berkeley, W.T.: The Cleft Lip Nose, Plast. Reconstr. Surg. **23**:567, 1959.
2. Berkeley, W.T.: Correction of the unilateral cleft lip nasal deformity. In Grabb, W.C., Rosenstein, S.W., and Bzock, D.F., editors: Cleft lip and palate, Boston, 1971, Little, Brown & Co., Inc.
3. Blair, V.P.: Nasal deformities associated with congenital cleft of the lip, JAMA **84**:185, 1925.
4. Blair, V.P.: The problem of bringing forward the retracted upper lip and nose, Surg. Gynecol. Obstet. **42**:128, 1926.
5. Blair, V.P., and Brown, J.B.: Mirault operation for single hairlip, Surg. Gynecol. Obstet. **51**:81, 1930.
6. Cosman, B., and Crikelair, G.F.: Reconstruction of the unilateral cleft lip nasal deformity, Cleft Palate J. **2**:95, 1965.
7. Dibbell, D.G.: A cartilaginous columella strut in cleft lip rhinoplasties, Br. J. Plast. Surg. **29**:247, 1976.
8. Dibbell, D.G.: Personal communication, 1987.
9. Erich, J.B.: A technique for correcting flat nostril in cases of repaired hairlip, Plast. Reconstr. Surg. **12**:320, 1953.
10. Gillies, J.D., and Kilner, T.P.: Harelip operation for the correction of secondary deformities, Lancet **223**:1369, 1932.
11. Gillies, J.D., and Millard, Jr., D.R.: The principles and art of plastic surgery, Boston, 1957, Little, Brown & Co., Inc.
12. Gorney, M.: Centripetal rotation-advancement for bilateral cleft lip nasal deformities, Ann. Plast. Surg. **2**(5):374, 1979.
13. McIndoe, A.: Correction of alar deformity in cleft lip, Lancet **1**:607, 1958.
14. Millard, Jr., D.R.: The unilateral cleft nose, Plast. Reconstr. Surg. **34**:169, 1964.
15. Musgrave, R.H.: Surgery of nasal deformities associated with cleft lip, Plast. Reconstr. Surg. **28**:261, 1961.
16. Nishimura, Y.: Autogenous septal cartilage graft in the correction of cleft lip nasal deformities, Br. J. Plast. Surg. **31**:222, 1978.
17. Ortiz-Monasterio, F.: Personal communication, 1987.
18. Potter, J.: Some nasal tip deformities due to alar cartilage abnormalities, Plast. Reconstr. Surg. **13**:358, 1954.
19. Rees, T.D., Guy, C.L., and Converse, J.M.: Repair of cleft lip nose: addendum to the syncronous technique with full thickness skin grafting of nasal vestibule, Plast. Reconstr. Surg. **37**:41, 1966.
20. Reynolds, J.R., and Horton, C.F.: An alar lift procedure in cleft lip rhinoplasty, Plast. Reconstr. Surg. **35**:377, 1965.
21. Spira, M.: Repair of unilateral cleft lip nose, Cleft Palate J. **5**:356, 1968.
22. Stenstrom, S.F.: The alar cartilage and the nasal deformity in unilateral cleft lip, Plast. Reconstr. Surg. **38**:223, 1966.

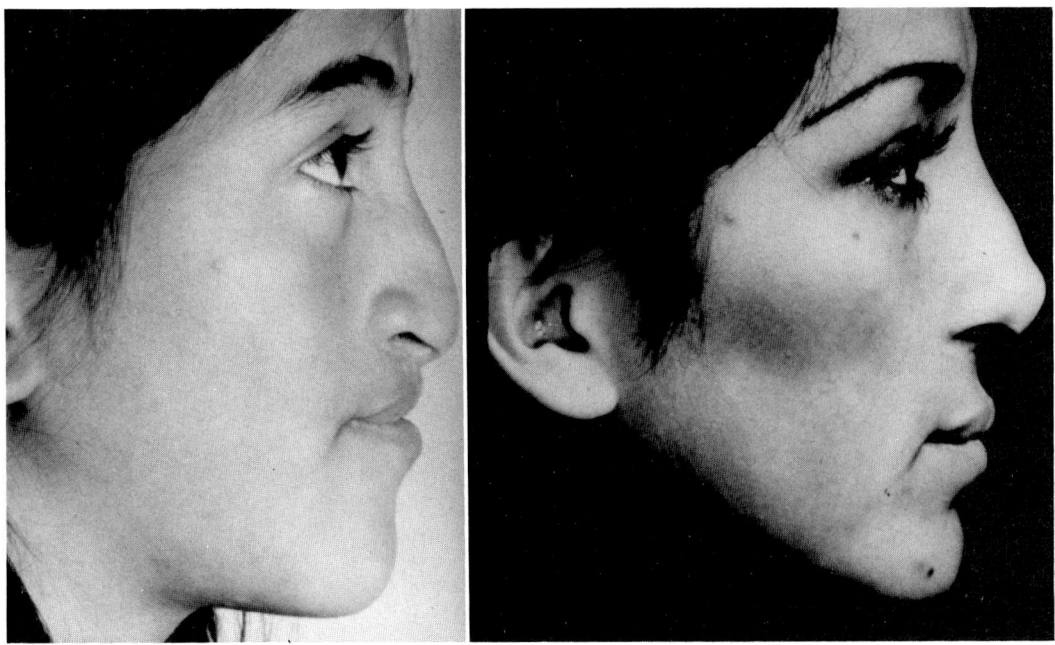

Figure 46-11. Sixteen-year-old female shown preoperatively and 14 years postoperatively. She was repaired through described technique plus crosslip Abbe flap. (From Gorney, M.: Reconstruction of the post-cleft nasal deformity, August 1987.)

Point and Counterpoint
Part XIV

Question: What is the value of x-ray interpretation in nasal fractures?

Comment (Eugene Kern): It is more important to examine the patient physically. A negative x-ray tells you that the patient does not have a severe nasal fracture. The patient can still have a severe nasal injury. The patient can also have a cartilaginous disturbance and have a negative x-ray. Obviously a positive x-ray indicates a significant fracture, and you are going to examine this patient carefully, but a negative x-ray does not mean that the patient is safe.

Comment (Claus Walter): X-rays in nasal fractures are sometimes overvalued, but they may be necessary for further or later legal actions.

Comment (Fernando Ortiz-Monasterio): X-rays, like other laboratory examinations, rarely change what we have previously diagnosed clinically. Very seldom is my treatment conditioned by the x-rays, not even in craniofacial surgery. I am more interested in the aesthetic aspect of the face. I am operating on patients, not x-rays, and the same is true for fractures.

Question: Is there a growth center in the nose, and if so, where is it?

Comment (Eugene Kern): This is really a problem for me. I have thought about it and read the literature. It was thought originally that one of the growth centers was at the junction of the perpendicular plate, the vomer, and the posterior aspect of the quadrangular cartilage in that region, but studies have found that accelerated growth occurs at the caudal end of the septum. This fits with what we see clinically. You see minor traumas to the caudal septum that cause marked deviations. This is a surprising finding.

Comment (Fernando Ortiz-Monasterio): I think we can rely on our examination and clinical research in patients over the years and conclude that there are many areas of the nose that grow. I am sure that the septum is one of them. Each one of the individual bones grows by itself, and the skin and cartilage grow by themselves. I do know that anything you take off from the nose—any interference with these areas—will affect nasal growth.

Question to Dr. Kern: There is some controversy as to whether or not cartilage and cartilaginous grafts continue growing. Do you have any beliefs about that? Particularly in reference to preservation of the perichondrium?

Comment (Eugene Kern): I think it's important to leave the perichondrium, at least in the septal space. From what we've seen in the laboratory, if you leave the perichondrium, there will be cartilaginous and bony neogenesis. I've seen this result in some of our pituitary cases (in adults) when we've gone back in a large number of cases. We have over 1,000 cases now in which we have gone back in the septal space because of a cerebrospinal fluid leak or a recurrent tumor, and there are certain areas that appear to be regrowing. The regrowth occurs because we've left the periosteum.

Comment (Fernando Ortiz-Monasterio): The donor bed area regrows cartilage; that I agree with. Now the same is true on facial cases. I operate on children under 6 months of age, and I advance the whole forehead, the orbital roof, and the lateral walls at one time. One year later, the whole bony gap is covered by new bone. But that doesn't mean a cartilage graft grows. I have never seen a graft grow myself, and I follow them for many years.

Question: A lot of experience with composite and other grafts of the nose has accumulated. Is it your impression, through long follow-up, that these grafts continue to grow, or do they just grow proportionately?

Comment (Claus Walter): I've taken these grafts with the perichondrium, and I think this is the answer to why they grow. If I had implanted mainly cartilage, then it would have been a different story.

Question: In cases of the so-called "emergency rhinoplasty" following trauma, should one wait, and how aggressive or conservative should one be?

Comment (Eugene Kern): There are times when I do an emergency rhinoplasty. To me, that term means that there is an acute nasal injury; to reconstruct this injury, I also go ahead and reconstruct the areas that are involved with previous nasal trauma or that have a congenital abnormality. I modify either the lobular cartilages or anything else that is necessary to get not only the functional, but also the aesthetic improvement. So, in those terms, I guess I do emergency rhinoplasties.

424

Question: Please explain the rationale of going in immediately after trauma and correcting the septum.

Comment (Eugene Kern): If there is septal pathology, the aim is to reconstitute normalcy; so whatever is required to do this and to replace tissues in the intraseptal space, I go ahead and do. I don't think that this action necessarily precludes a good cosmetic result. If there is a deficiency or if there are sequellae at a later date, I've already prepared the patient for a secondary procedure. I don't find a contraindication to doing the entire operation, even if there is significant septal trauma. I guess the key word is "significant."

Question to Dr. Kern: How much septal trauma are you talking about? Is it a fracture or dislocation?

Comment (Eugene Kern): If it is a fracture or dislocation with telescoping, I would do an open reduction.

Question to Dr. Kern: Would you do something to the alar cartilage as well?

Comment (Eugene Kern): If there is a lower-lateral cartilage deformity such as a broad nasal tip and there is a significant septal injury, then I would go ahead and do an open reduction on the septal injury to restore normalcy. There are times when I don't think a closed reduction can be done, so I would go ahead and do the open reduction, then modify the lobular cartilages, or do the osteotomies if and when they are necessary.

Comment (from the audience): I very respectfully disagree with Dr. Kern. To me, the rhinoplasty requires a lot of thinking and planning for each particular case. I don't know a trauma patient well enough; I haven't seen him without the edema of the trauma.

I think this surgery may be possible, but I consider it too risky for my final result. I'd much rather try to put the tissues where they belong and wait for awhile.

Comment (Eugene Kern): I certainly agree that, if the primary problem is an aesthetic problem, the time of the acute injury is not the time to correct it. But I am saying that if an osteotomy is obviously needed and if you are going to do some trimming of the upper-lateral or even the lobular cartilage, there exists no major contraindication *if swelling is minimum*. I'm thinking about a traumatic nose, not necessarily a cosmetic nose.

Comment (Claus Walter): If an acute injury to the nose has happened with an open fracture, a comminuted fracture in which you have to realign skin and torn cartilages, then you really have to go in right away. If you have a closed fracture with a lot of swelling and hematoma, you have time to wait unless you believe the hematoma in the septum may become infected. Then you have to drain it. Otherwise, you always have time—a week or two—to let this tissue settle down. Then go in, if there is a clear indication, to realign everything that has been displaced.

Question: How long do you wait after trauma before you do a rhinoplasty? What's the shortest time before you do your rhinoplasty?

Comment (Eugene Kern): No less than 3 months.

Comment (Eugene Tardy): I would take care of the acute nasal trauma immediately, and then I'd probably go back in 1 to 6 months, depending on the magnitude of the trauma.

Comment (Claus Walter): I'd say at least half a year.

Index